Brainstem Control of Wakefulness and Sleep

Brainstem Control of Wakefulness and Sleep

Mircea Steriade

Université Laval
Faculté de Médecine
Quebec, Canada

and

Robert W. McCarley

Harvard Medical School
Veterans Administration Medical Center
Brockton, Massachusetts

Plenum Press • New York and London

Library of Congress Cataloging-in-Publication Data

Steriade, Mircea.
    Brainstem control of wakefulness and sleep / Mireca Steriade and
Robert W. McCarley.
        p.   cm.
    Includes bibliographical references.
    ISBN 0-306-43342-7
    1. Sleep-wake cycle. 2. Brain stem--Physiology. 3. Sleep-
-Physiological aspects. 4. Wakefulness--Physiological aspects.
I. McCarley, Robert W., 1937-   . II. Title.
    [DNLM: 1. Brain Stem--physiology. 2. Sleep--physiology.
3. Wakefulness--physiology.   WL 310 S838b]
    QP425.S73 1990
    612.8'21--dc20
    DNLM/DLC
    for Library of Congress   89-26649
                                                               CIP

© 1990 Plenum Press, New York
A Division of Plenum Publishing Corporation
233 Spring Street, New York, N.Y. 10013

Printed in the United States of America

To Donca, Jacqueline, Claude, and Aaron,
and to Alice, Robby, and Scott

Preface

This book is part of an ongoing history of efforts to understand the nature of waking and sleeping states from a biological point of view. We believe the recent technological revolutions in anatomy and physiology make the present moment especially propitious for this effort. In planning this book we had the choices of producing an edited volume with invited chapter authors or of writing the book ourselves. Edited volumes offer the opportunity for expression of expertise in each chapter but, we felt, would not allow the development of our ideas on the potential and actual unity of the field and would not allow the expression of coherence that can be obtained only with one or two voices, but which may be quite difficult with a chorus assembled and performing together for the first time. (Unlike musical works, there is very little precedent for rehearsals and repeated performances for authors of edited volumes or even for the existence of conductors able to induce a single rhythm and vision of the composition.)

We thus decided on a monograph. The primary goal was to communicate the current realities and the future possibilities of unifying basic studies on anatomy and cellular physiology with investigations of the behavioral and physiological events of waking and sleep. In keeping with this goal we cross-reference the basic cellular physiology in the latter chapters, and, in the last chapter, we take up possible links to relevant clinical phenomenology. We are well aware of the limitations of our knowledge, and have thus chosen to write about what we know best or, in any case, what strikes us as most interesting and relevant for what we do know. We make no claim for encyclopedism in all aspects of sleep and waking and the relevant basic studies, and similarly do not apologize for including that which we do know best, namely, our own work, and for omitting some areas that have been recently reviewed elsewhere. While the reference list indicates we do not ignore the field as a whole, many of the detailed expositions are drawn from our own studies. Our wish is that the reader find the field as exciting and promising as we, and we welcome comments.

M.S.'s research benefited from the work of his many skillful and creative pre-Ph.D. and postdoctoral students and foreign research investigators over the past 20 years since he established the Laboratory of Neurophysiology at Laval University. Among these research fellows, M.S. is especially grateful to his current student and co-worker, Denis Paré, who made important contributions to the development of his laboratory. M.S. also expresses his thanks to M. Deschênes, a former student and more recently a colleague, for his participation in projects on the electrophysiology of thalamic cells; to A. Parent, for his collaboration to morphological studies on brainstem–thalamic connectivity; and to G. Oakson, for his continuous efforts in improving the statistical processing of data. M.S.'s work is supported by the Medical Research Council of Canada and by the Research Fund of Laval University. The memory of M.S.'s late teachers and friends Frédéric Bremer and Giuseppe Moruzzi has been an inspiration throughout this work.

R. W. M. thanks his colleagues and members of his Laboratory of Neuroscience in the Harvard Medical School Department of Psychiatry and the Brockton-West Roxbury VA Medical Center. These include: for the *in vivo* physiological and anatomical studies, K. Ito, A. Mitani, and S. Higo; for the *in vitro* studies, R. Greene, U. Gerber, and D. Stevens; and for the mathematical modeling, S. Massequoi. Special thanks are due to H. Haas for his role in these studies and to M. Chase and R. Fuchs for comments on Chapter 10. R.W.M. expresses his thanks to his former co-workers in the Laboratory of Neurophysiology at Harvard and Massachusetts Mental Health Center, and especially to A. Hobson, the laboratory director and a co-worker for many years. R. W. M.'s work has been made possible by grant support and a Medical Investigator award from the Medical Research Service of the Department of Veterans Affairs and by grant support from the National Institute of Mental Health.

Mircea Steriade
Robert W. McCarley

Quebec and Brockton

Contents

Chapter 4

Efferent Connections of Brainstem Neurons

Chapter 5

**Intrinsic Electrophysiological Properties of Brainstem Neurons and
Their Relationship to Behavioral Control**

Chapter 6

Neurotransmitter-Modulated Ionic Currents of Brainstem Neurons and Some of Their Targets

Chapter 7

Synchronized Brain Oscillations and Their Disruption by Ascending Brainstem Reticular Influxes

Chapter 8

Brainstem Ascending Systems Controlling Synaptic Transmission of Afferent Signals

Chapter 9

Brainstem Genesis and Thalamic Transfer of Pontogeniculooccipital Waves

Chapter 10

Motor Systems: The Brainstem Oculomotor System and Mechanisms of Motor Atonia in REM Sleep

Chapter 11

Neuronal Control of the Sleep–Wake States

Chapter 12

REM Sleep as a Biological Rhythm: The Phenomenology and a Structural and Mathematical Model

Chapter 13

Brainstem Mechanisms of Dreaming and of Disorders of Sleep in Man

Changing Concepts of Mechanisms of Waking and Sleep States

The last comprehensive reviews on the historical development of ideas on waking and sleep states were written by Moruzzi (1964, 1972) and Jouvet (1967) and dealt with experiments using electrical stimulation and electrolytic lesion techniques. Although newer, more powerful tools have been introduced in recent years for activating and destroying cellular aggregates, the concepts of the location of various brain "centers" involved in the genesis of waking and sleep states have not significantly changed since the late 1960s. What has changed is the view of neuronal mechanisms and interactions between different parts of the brain, mostly as a result of the introduction of new techniques allowing the recording of single cells in the behaving animal and, since 1980, the analysis of ionic conductances underlying intrinsic electroresponsive properties of neurons. We shall, of course, refer to earlier concepts, and we shall try to resurrect some of them from unjustified oblivion, especially when they have withstood experimental testing. But our main goal in this historical perspective and throughout this book is to examine critically the conclusions of older studies, couched in terms of large black boxes, with the more precise data gained by looking inside single cells and neuronal networks and by defining connectivities and transmitters. Our basic tenet is that the cellular approach furnishes the ultimate criterion to test hypotheses from studies conducted at more global levels.

1.1. Pioneering Steps

We begin by pointing out three major discoveries that belong to Frédéric Bremer, Giuseppe Moruzzi, and Michel Jouvet and that set the scene for more recent developments.

Since his stay at the Salpétrière in Paris during the late 1910s, Bremer was involved in clinical–pathological sleep studies related to the lethargic encephalitis (Trétiakoff and Bremer, 1920). He discovered the quite different electrographic and ocular syndromes of the *encéphale isolé* and *cerveau isolé* preparations during the 1930s (Bremer, 1935, 1937, 1938). Bremer found that a high spinal transection at C1 that disconnected the whole encephalon from the spinal cord is compatible with fluctuations between EEG patterns of waking and sleep states. In contrast, a mesencephalic transection caudal to the third nerves was associated with extremely fissurated pupils, as in normal sleep, and uninterrupted sequences of waxing and waning EEG spindle waves, much the same as during barbiturate narcosis. Bremer modified the ordinary decerebrate preparation by leaving the forebrain *in situ* after midbrain transection instead of destroying it, with the hope of demonstrating "the existence of a continuous facilitation of functional innervation of the forebrain resulting from the steady flow of ascending inputs from the spinal neuraxis and the brainstem" (Bremer, 1975, pp. 267–268).

The idea that, indeed, the structures located between the bulbospinal transection and the rostral midbrain are crucially involved in the maintenance of waking and that a sudden fall in the cerebral "tone" follows the withdrawal of the steady flow of impulses impinging on the cerebrum was extended in the studies of Bremer's disciple, Moruzzi.

Moruzzi was a visiting fellow in Bremer's laboratory during the late 1930s, thereafter worked with Adrian, and eventually went to collaborate with Magoun. Initially, Moruzzi intended to continue his analysis of paleocerebellar inhibition on the hyperexcitable state of motor cortex. To this end, Moruzzi and Magoun placed stimulating electrodes in the cerebellum and the bulbar reticular formation, which was thought to relay cerebellar impulses in their route to the cerebral cortex. To their surprise, the electrical stimulation of the brainstem reticular formation suppressed the high-amplitude slow EEG waves displayed by their *encéphale isolé* and/or chloralose-anesthetized preparations (Moruzzi and Magoun, 1949). The suppressing effect of brainstem stimulation on synchronized EEG waves resembled the α-wave blockage during attention or visual stimulation, known from Berger's (1930) and Adrian's (1936) studies. Although the chloralose-anesthetized animal was obviously not the best experimental preparation for studying arousal and activation processes, Moruzzi and Magoun decided to go far beyond observed facts and used the term "activation." This was in spite of the fact that only spontaneous EEG waves were recorded, and no sign of real cerebral activation was documented* (suppression of high-amplitude slow EEG waves may be seen in a variety of conditions that do not necessarily imply a heightened cerebral excitability). The actual demonstration of cortical facilitation during brainstem reticular stimulation came a decade later, in independent studies of thalamocortical evoked potentials conducted during the late 1950s in Bremer's and Dell's laboratories (see Chapter 8).

The discovery by Moruzzi and Magoun (1949) of an ascending brainstem reticular system with energizing actions on the forebrain was an important step forward in the physiology of states of vigilance. The progress related to the

---

*In fact, during their initial experiments, Moruzzi and Magoun were surprised by the flat aspect of the EEG during reticular stimulation and believed that "the experiments had stumbled upon some perplexing type of ascending inhibition. . . Only after some delay, and quite by chance, was the gain finally turned up, and it was then possible to see the large waves give way during reticular stimulation to the low voltage, fast activity of EEG" (Magoun, 1975, p. 524). The choice of the term *activation* in Moruzzi and Magoun's 1949 paper was better than Berger's (1933) choice to explain the blockage of α waves as a secondary diffuse *inhibition* of the cortex from a highly localized and hardly detectable enhancement of cortical activity produced by a sensory arousing stimulus. Berger's interpretation was under the influence of Pavlov's notion of negative induction.

localization of an executive system for cortical activation. On the conceptual side, the notion of nonspecificity in the activating process was introduced. Since this study was the first that attempted to localize the brainstem substrate of cortical activation, we discuss below some of the data and speculations in the 1949 paper, and we relate them to the modern findings and concepts.

Although EEG desynchronizing responses were elicited from a variety of loci in the whole brainstem tegmentum, Moruzzi and Magoun depicted the most effective area in the midbrain (see Fig. 3 in their paper). With minimal stimulation intensity, the EEG response could be localized in the sensory–motor cortex of the ipsilateral hemisphere. The cortical effect was thought to be "mediated, in part at least, by the diffuse thalamic projection system" (Moruzzi and Magoun, 1949, p. 468). All these findings have been confirmed and expanded in more recent cellular studies. Indeed, neurons recorded from the midbrain reticular formation increase their firing rates during transition from sleep to arousal, reliably preceding EEG desynchronization, and they directly excite thalamic neurons with widespread projections toward the cerebral cortex but prevalently to the sensory–motor areas (Steriade and Glenn, 1982; Steriade *et al.*, 1982a). These data are analyzed in Chapters 4 and 11. The elicitation of EEG desynchronization by stimulating a series of foci from the medulla to the midbrain occurs through lower brainstem projections to the most effective sites in the upper brainstem core (see Chapter 3).

Conceptually, the notion of a role played by *specific* sensory impulses (relayed in the spinal cord or brainstem and hypothesized by Bremer to maintain the tone of the cerebrum) was replaced after Moruzzi and Magoun's experiments by the idea of an ascending *reticular system*. By definition the reticular system was thought of as *nonspecific*, as a site of collateralization of heterogeneous sensory impulses, in a vein similar to the concept of *sensorium commune* that was localized by Jiri Prohaska, around 1750, in a region between the medulla and the diencephalon (cf. Soury, 1899). The nonspecific nature of the activating structure was supported by lesion experiments showing that the interruption of lemniscal (specific sensory) pathways did not produce the sleep or comatose syndrome of the *cerveau isolé* preparation, whereas lesions of the medial brainstem reticular formation sparing lemniscal projections produced such a syndrome (Lindsley *et al.*, 1949, 1950).* Some experimental evidence suggests that local activating processes in various thalamocortical systems can be efficiently generated by specific sensory channels, with the consequence of ultimately driving the reticular system through corticofugal projections and thus generating generalized activation processes (see Section 1.3.1).

The notion of nonspecificity and the schemes with heavy arrows depicting pathways of unknown origins acting diffusely by means of unknown transmitters on unknown targets betrayed the state of a primitive knowledge of the reticular core that persisted for three decades since the late 1940s. Spectacular advances have been achieved in this direction since 1980, and they are mainly the result of

---

*The results of more localized lesions than those reported in the late 1940s support the concept of brainstem reticular activation and the idea that EEG desynchronized patterns reliably betray the state of brain activation. Unilateral lesions confined to the midbrain reticular formation in primates induce EEG synchronization in the ipsilateral hemisphere associated with a contralateral trimodal sensory neglect (Watson *et al.*, 1974). The recovery from the unilateral neglect syndrome is concomitant with the disappearance of the EEG asymmetry (Wright and Craggs, 1978).

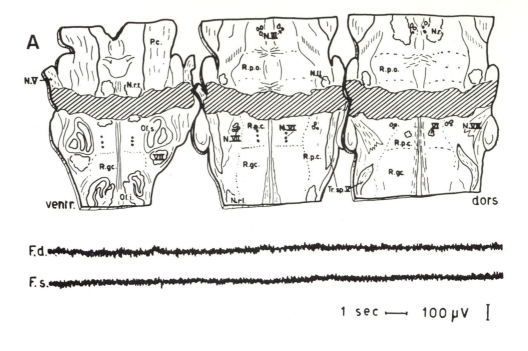

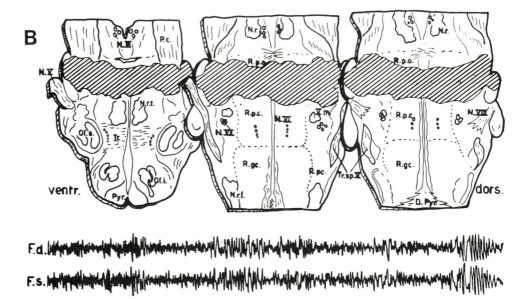

Figure 1. Electroencephalographic patterns following midpontine and rostropontine transections. Drawings of horizontal sections of the cat's brainstem. Cross-hatched areas indicate level and extent of brainstem lesions in the midpontine pretrigeminal (A) and rostropontine (B) preparations. EEG patterns typical for each preparation, as recorded from right (F.d.) and left (F.s.) frontal areas, are reproduced below each set of anatomic drawings. It can be noted that both types of transection result in the complete interruption of ascending trigeminal influences. Abbreviations: D.Pyr., decussatio pyramidum; N.l.l., nucleus lemnisci lateralis; N.r., nucleus ruber; N.r.l., nucleus reticularis lateralis; N.r.t., nucleus reticularis tegmenti pontis; N.III, V, VI, VII, VIII, root fibers of cranial nerves; Ol.i., nucleus olivaris inferior; Ol.s., nucleus olivaris superior; P.C., pes pedunculi cerebri; Pyr., pyramis;

modern tracing techniques combined with immunohistochemistry that helped to define the transmitter agents used by brainstem intrinsic, ascending, and descending projections. During the 1950s, Golgi studies and experiments with axonal degeneration following massive electrolytic lesions in the brainstem tegmentum showed axons of reticular origin that projected almost everywhere in the thalamus, without obvious differentiation among various brainstem sites of axonal origin. The same reticular neuron seemed to send bifurcating axonal branches to the spinal cord and the cerebral cortex (Scheibel and Scheibel, 1958). More recent retrograde tracing studies with double-labeling techniques and experiments with antidromic identification of brainstem reticular neurons from multiple stimulated sites have altered this viewpoint. Such pontifical reticular neurons, with ascending and descending projections controlling both cortical and spinal cord operations, are the exception rather than the rule (see Chapters 2 and 4).

Absence of data supporting the idea of such hypothetically ubiquitous projections as well as the uncertain transmitters and actions of brainstem reticular neurons caused a temporary desuetude of the ascending reticular concept. Confronted with morphological and physiological studies employing lesion and stimulation techniques that could not dissociate cell bodies from passing fibers, the reaction of some anatomists was even to deny, until quite recently, the existence of brainstem reticular projections to major thalamic nuclei (cf. Jones, 1985). The accumulating evidence of the past few years on the existence of these projections and their chemical codes are discussed in Chapter 4.

The notion of a monolithic reticular core with global and undifferentiated energizing actions on the forebrain was challenged by Moruzzi himself after crucial experiments with his team in Pisa during the late 1950s (cf. Moruzzi, 1972). The *midpontine pretrigeminal* brainstem transection is only a few millimeters behind the low collicular transection that induces the comatose syndrome of the *cerveau isolé* preparation. However, the midpontine trigeminal animal exhibits persistent EEG and ocular signs of alertness, and its eye movements follow the objects passing across the visual field (Fig. 1). In the acute conditions of these two close transections (*cerveau isolé* and midpontine pretrigeminal), "only the neurons lying between the two sections are the likely candidates for explaining the critical differences in both the EEG and ocular behavior" (Moruzzi, 1972, p. 31). We discuss in Section 1.3.1 the experimental evidence that, in chronic conditions, structures lying in the isolated cerebrum, above the mesencephalon, may be effective in maintaining wakefulness. But the demonstration of the dramatic differences displayed by the *cerveau isolé* preparation and the animal with a midpontine transection was prescient in anticipating recent findings on the brainstem substrate of ascending activation. Data presented in Chapters 4 and 10 show that brainstem cholinergic neurons with thalamic and basal forebrain projections and activating properties are concentrated in two cellular aggregates at the midbrain–pontine junction. This is precisely the region predicted by the experiments of Moruzzi and his pupils.

R.gc., nucleus reticularis gigantocellularis; R.pc., nucleus reticularis parvocellularis; R.p.c., nucleus reticularis pontis caudalis; R.p.o., nucleus reticularis pontis oralis; Tr., corpus trapezoideum; Tr.sp. V, tractus spinalis nervi trigemini; Vm, VI, VII, motor nuclei of cranial nerves. From Batini *et al.* (1959).

The enduring alert state of the midpontine pretrigeminal preparation was ascribed to the removal of inhibitory influences arising in the lower brainstem. These more disputable data, related to the concept of active inhibitory influences promoting sleep, are discussed in Section 1.3.2 together with other hypotheses of hypnogenic structures.

Finally, Jouvet (1962) discovered that the oscillator for the state of sleep with rapid eye movements (REM sleep) is located in the pontobulbar brainstem. This followed the description, during the 1950s, of periodic REM sleep episodes with low-voltage, fast EEG patterns (Aserinski and Kleitman, 1953; Dement and Kleitman, 1957; Dement, 1958). Such sleep epochs with limb and vibrissae twitches or "convulsions" have been described since antique times and were termed *sonno profondo* (deep sleep) by Fontana around 1765; they were again described as *tiefen Schlaf* with low-voltage and fast EEG waves by Klaue in the late 1930s (cf. Moruzzi, 1963; Jouvet, 1967). The notion of "deep sleep" did not imply a qualitative difference between the REM-sleep state and that of sleep with EEG synchronization. The dual nature of sleep, consisting of a quiet sleep state characterized by EEG synchronization associated with decreased transfer function of incoming messages and a brain-active sleep state characterized by EEG desynchronization and enhanced excitability of central networks, is emphasized by recent investigations at the cellular level (see Section 1.2 and Chapters 8, 11, and 12).*

Jouvet and his colleagues discovered the presence of muscular atonia and spiky pontine waves, thus establishing the signs that differentiate REM sleep from the other states of the sleep–waking cycle (Jouvet and Michel, 1959; Jouvet *et al.,* 1959). In more recent years, mechanisms of muscular atonia were first described by Pompeiano and his colleagues, who showed that both tonic and phasic inhibition of spinal reflexes occur during REM sleep in unrestrained cats (cf. Pompeiano, 1967a,b). Later on, this disclosure was substantiated by intracellular recordings of spinal motoneurons in naturally sleeping cats (Morales and Chase, 1978; Chase and Morales, 1983; Glenn and Dement, 1981; see further details in Chapter 10). As to the spiky waves recorded in the pons, lateral geniculate, and occipital cortex (therefore termed PGO waves), their neuronal progenitors have been discovered in a region at the midbrain–pontine junction (McCarley *et al.,* 1978; Sakai and Jouvet, 1980), and the thalamic projections of some PGO-on neurons have been identified by antidromic invasion (Sakai, 1985a). These data, the cellular evidence of the involvement in PGO-wave genesis of several cell classes in the pedunculopontine cholinergic nucleus (Steriade *et al.,* 1989a) and pontine reticular formation (McCarley and Ito, 1983), and the

---

*The dual nature of sleep is a recent concept, as seen from the general discussion at Lyon's 1965 symposium where some participants thought of sleep as a unitary phenomenon, emphasizing the similarities rather than the differences between EEG-synchronized sleep and REM sleep. At that symposium, which took place after the description by Dement and Jouvet of major dissimilarities between the two states of sleep, Dement commented that EEG-synchronized sleep and REM or paradoxical sleep "are as far as night and day. It is difficult to point to a single attribute that is commonly shared. . . . In terms of definition, it would seem more appropriate to regard slow-wave sleep and paradoxical sleep as entirely different states with their own specific mechanism or mechanisms. I would even go so far as to suggest that there may be some validity in questioning whether they should be subsumed under the general heading of sleep" (Jouvet, 1965b, pp. 628–629).

cellular mechanisms of thalamic PGO waves (Deschênes and Steriade, 1988; Hu et al., 1989c; Steriade et al., 1989b) are discussed in Chapter 9.

Probably the most important discovery by Jouvet came from his now classical experiments (1962, 1965a) using rostropontine transections in acute and chronic cats. These studies led to the current hypotheses of REM sleep genesis by showing that periodic episodes of muscular atonia (especially antigravity muscles), saccadic eye movements, the pontine component of PGO waves, and phasic muscle twitches occur in the prepontine preparation with a rhythmicity that is similar to that of REM sleep in the intact animal. The discovery of a brainstem sleep oscillator that operates in the absence of the forebrain has generated a series of models of REM-sleep genesis based on the interaction of different cell groups located between the midbrain–pontine junction and the bulbar reticular formation (McCarley and Hobson, 1975b; Pompeiano and Valentinuzzi, 1976). The models of oscillatory sleep–waking states and the supportive experimental data are discussed in Chapter 12.

In the next sections, we describe the physiological correlates of various behavioral states of vigilance; we define the notions of activation, deactivation, and active inhibitory influences exerted by presumed hypnogenic structures as they have appeared in the history of research on states of vigilance; we analyze the validity of data supporting the concepts of passive and active sleep; we survey the ideas on waking and sleep centers as opposed to the more encompassing (but much less testable) concept of distributed systems; and we discuss the general methodology and the criteria of cellular activities that should be applied toward the understanding of waking and sleep mechanisms.

1.2. Definition of States of Vigilance and Activation

State refers to the values assumed by the (potentially infinite) set of variables describing a system or organism (Rosen, 1970). This definition is easily understood by a computer analogy wherein the "machine state" at any point in time is completely defined by the presence of ones or zeros in the binary logic elements (see, for example, the discussion in Bartee et al., 1962, especially their Chapters 7 and 11). Appealing as this logical simplicity is, it suffers the practical complexity of requiring a specification of all the current values of the very large number of elements in the biological organism. Even the computer software engineer finds little use in the precise definition of machine state as used by his counterparts in machine design. Although complete machine state is theoretically and operationally specifiable, this description is much too detailed and complex. Instead, the software engineer abstracts certain features and uses these more global definitions of state; his "machine state" refers to global characteristics of the machine such as whether it is operating in "foreground" or "background" mode or whether it is servicing an interrupt request.

The definition of behavioral state that follows is offered as one that is in this practical spirit and one that is in accord with general usage. We first briefly discuss the terms of the definition and the rationale for including them. We use the term *indicator variable* to mean a variable that, when in a particular range of values, indicates with a high probability that *other* variables will have a particular range of values. Use of indicator variables reduces the dimensionality (number of variables) necessary to specify state. We further objectively define state as a particular *range of values of the indicator variables*. Our definition of behavioral state also includes the criteria of recurrence and temporal persistence of the state; a one-time, 1-msec condition is not a useful object for scientific study, nor is it in accord with everyday usage of state.

The definition thus becomes: *A state is a recurring, temporally enduring constellation of values of a set of indicator variables of the organism.*

The use of the term "indicator variable" makes explicit that the variables used in state definition are not themselves the state but rather are used because they efficiently imply the presence of other measures.

The three main states of vigilance (waking, quiet sleep with EEG synchronization, and REM sleep with EEG desynchronization) can be objectified by a set of three physiological signs that include EEG rhythms, muscular tone, and eye movements associated with sharp waves in brainstem–thalamocortical systems. (1) The tonic EEG desynchronization in waking is undistinguishable from that in REM sleep. This led Jouvet and his colleagues (1959) to coin the term *paradoxical* sleep for a state with the highest threshold for motoric arousal but an EEG pattern that suggested a highly active brain state. The EEG-synchronized rhythms (consisting of high-amplitude spindle oscillations at 7–14 Hz and slow waves at 0.5–4 Hz) distinguish the state of quiet or EEG-synchronized sleep from both waking and REM sleep. (2) The other tonic aspect, muscular atonia, specifically distinguishes REM sleep from the other two states. (3) Phasic eye movements are voluntary during waking and occur as involuntary saccades without relation to the visual field in REM sleep. The eye movements are accompanied by spiky PGO potentials, which originate in the pons; the neurons of the final common path for transmitting PGO waves to various thalamocortical systems are located at the midbrain–pontine junction (see Chapter 9). The PGO waves herald REM sleep and continue throughout this state. During waking, eye movement potentials (EMPs) are similar to, but much less ample than, PGO waves during REM sleep.

Note that the above three cardinal signs can be used as an easy way for objective identification of behavioral states with various degrees of vigilance. These electrographic events, however, merely represent the physiological correlates of behavioral states, and they say nothing about the psychology of the three states of vigilance. Since this monograph is mainly concerned with the brain structural and physiological bases of waking and sleep states, we in general refer to psychic activities only in passing. However, a section of Chapter 13 explicitly, although briefly, discusses mentation in sleep.

The above electrographic characterization applies only to steady, fully developed states of vigilance. More subtle features have to be used for the transitional epochs between waking and quiet sleep or vice versa and between quiet sleep and REM sleep, when most dramatic neuronal changes are expected to occur. Such neuronal activities may shed light on the mechanisms of various physiological aspects of awakening, falling asleep, and entering REM sleep. The electrographic criteria of these transitional epochs between the main states of the waking–sleep cycle are briefly presented below, and cellular investigations related to mechanisms of arousal, sleep onset, and REM-sleep genesis are treated in detail in Chapters 7 through 12. Since the data discussed in all subsequent chapters mostly derive from animal studies, we shall also mention the similarities and some differences between the main electrical signs of waking and sleep states in humans and cats, the species of choice for the study of sleep mechanisms.

The transition from EEG-synchronized sleep to arousal is usually short in duration. It may last for a few seconds and consists of decreased amplitude and increased frequency of EEG waves that precede the abruptly increased muscular tone and eye movements that occur with arousal. By contrast, the reverse transition, from waking to EEG-synchronized sleep, does not display a clear-cut picture of uninterrupted EEG synchronization but, in the cat, is marked by episodic appearance of spindle waves. Spindle waves are defined as high-amplitude waxing and waning waves at 7–14 Hz; they are grouped in sequences that last for 1.5–2 sec and recur periodically every 5–10 sec. They characteristically appear in the thalamus and cerebral cortex during the period of drowsiness and precede overt postural signs of sleep (Fig. 2C). Only at later stages do slow waves appear, usually one or several minutes after the occurrence of spindles. This occurs when quiet sleep is completely installed and when transient EEG-desynchronizing reactions no longer appear. Slow waves have a frequency of 0.5–4 Hz and are indented by the faster spindle oscillations. There is no need to discuss whether or not drowsiness has to be included within the final stage of relaxed wakefulness, as favored by some authors,* or within the initial stage of sleep. The spindle oscillations associated with repeated episodes of closing and reopening the eyes are the stigmatic event of this period of falling asleep, which should be treated as a transitional period between two main states. In man, however, the term EEG-synchronized sleep does not apply to stage I of sleep, which has a low-voltage EEG; spindles appear only later, in stage II.

The transition from EEG-synchronized to REM sleep is marked by a short period (1–2 min) during which the EEG is still synchronized, there is yet no sign of muscular atonia, but high-amplitude, single, sharp PGO waves can be recorded in the brainstem, thalamus, and cortical areas (Fig. 3). Later on, when REM sleep is fully developed, PGO waves appear as either single potentials or clusters of smaller-amplitude potentials with a frequency of about 6/sec. This phasic activity announcing REM sleep has been described in a number of mammals, but the bulk of data on cellular mechanisms of PGO waves derive from experiments on cats.

Since PGO waves related to saccadic eye movements are thought to repre-

---

*Moruzzi depicts drowsiness in the lower part of wakefulness, before sleep (see Fig. 39 in his 1972 review) and hypothesizes that "an animal's behavior during drowsiness corresponds to the appetitive phase, while sleep itself should be regarded as the consummatory action of a special instinctive behavior" (1972, p. 134). In another review article, Moruzzi (1969) analyzes the typical manifestations of the appetitive behavior and points to the period immediately preceding sleep as a stage when the animals strive for a situation, a "home" for sleep, that will facilitate sleep onset. These ethological observations and hypotheses leave little doubt that, in the natural conditions of an animal's life, sleep is preceded by a set of stereotyped or less stereotyped movements toward the search of a place to sleep. However, in the conditions of cellular investigations in an experimental animal that is sure of our good intentions and does not have to look at safer places to sleep, the period of drowsiness that precedes sleep (with transient closing and reopening the eyes) is typically associated with EEG spindle oscillations, and in the absence of unwonted stimuli, this period inevitably leads to genuine manifestations of sleep.

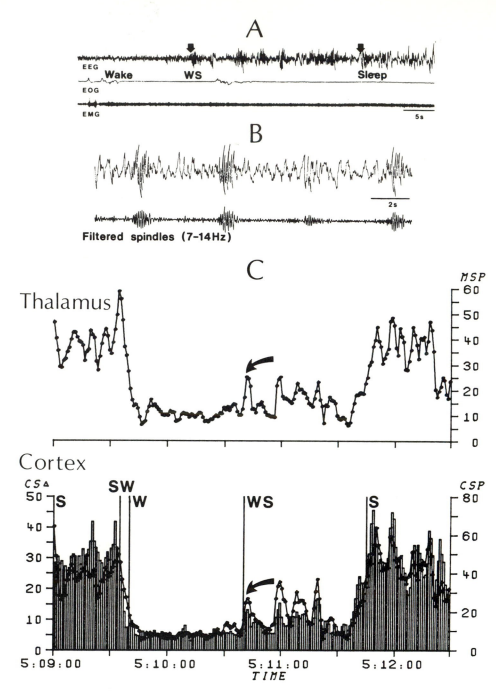

Figure 2. Electrographic criteria of wake and EEG-synchronized sleep states and characteristics of spindle rhythmicity. A: Behaving cat with chronically implanted electrodes. Electroencephalogram (EEG) from the motor (precruciate) cortex, electrooculogram (EOG), and electromyogram (EMG) of neck muscles. Spindle oscillations appear during the transitional period between waking and sleep (WS). B: Thalamic spindles in a cat with a high brainstem transection. Top trace shows the field electrical activity recorded by a microelectrode in rostral intralaminar thalamic nuclei; bottom trace shows the same period, with spindle waves filtered from 7 to 14 Hz. Note that spindle sequences recur periodically. C: Normalized amplitudes (ordinates) of simultaneously recorded focal spindle

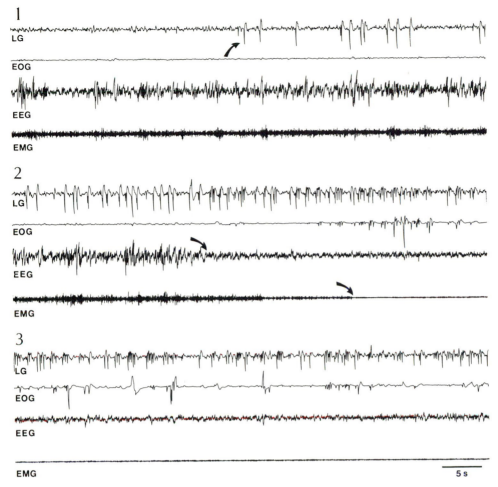

Figure 3. Electrographic criteria of transition between EEG-synchronized and EEG-desynchronized (REM) sleep states. Chronically implanted behaving cat. The four traces in 1 [LG, field potentials in the lateral geniculate (LG) thalamic nucleus; EOG; EEG recorded from the anterior suprasylvian gyrus; and EMG] are repeated in 2 and 3. Parts 1–3 are in continuation. Parts 1 and 2 represent the transition from EEG-synchronized sleep to REM sleep (in 1, oblique arrow indicates the occurrence of PGO waves; in 2, first oblique arrow points to EEG desynchronization, and second arrow points to complete muscular atonia). Part 3 depicts fully installed REM sleep. Note single PGO waves with high amplitudes during the transitional period 1 and clusters of PGO waves (at about 6 Hz) with smaller amplitudes during a later stage of REM sleep (in 3). Modified from Steriade *et al.* (1989d).

waves in the thalamus (top MSP trace) and in the cortex (bottom CSP line–circle trace depicts spindles; and bottom CSΔ bar-graph trace depicts slow waves) in a behaving cat. Spindles filtered between 7 and 14 Hz; slow waves filtered between 0.5 and 4 Hz. Abscissae indicate real time (hr, min, sec). S, EEG-synchronized sleep; W, waking; SW and WS, transitional periods from S to W and from W to S, respectively. Note EEG desynchronization with decreased wave amplitudes on awakening (SW and W); rhythmic sequences of spindles, recurring with a period of 8–10 sec in both thalamic and cortical recordings, beginning with drowsiness (WS, oblique arrows); and increased amplitudes of both spindles and slow waves beginning with S. A and C modified from Steriade *et al.* (1986);B modified from Paré *et al.* (1987).

sent a substrate of oneiric behavior during REM sleep, the question is usually raised about the similarities between REM sleep in humans and cats as well as whether animals have dreams.

The low-voltage fast EEG rhythms during the REM sleep of the adult cat are strikingly similar to the EEG rhythms directly recorded from the cerebral cortex in humans (W. Dement, unpublished findings; cf. general discussion in Jouvet, 1965b, Table I). In scalp recordings from humans, 6–8/sec rhythms appear in occipital areas. The origin of these waves in the higher range of the θ band is unknown, especially since the θ rhythm is not evident in primates and humans.

As to dreaming in animals, the usual remark is made that, since dreams are verbal reports of subjective experiences, the question must remain unanswered. However, some of the REM dream features may apply to subhuman mammals, since dreaming is a perceptual experience that does not necessarily depends on abstract thought and language. As discussed in Chapters 10 and 13, the overt behavior during REM sleep in cats with lesions in the dorsolateral part of the pontine tegmentum that suppress muscular atonia strikingly suggest oneiric behavior. The cat seems to fight with imaginary enemies or to play with an absent mouse and exhibits fear reactions associated with autonomous phenomena, episodes during which the pupils are extremely miotic and nictitating membranes are relaxed (Jouvet and Delorme, 1965). This pattern resembles that of hallucinatory oneiriclike behavior that can be elicited during the waking state by chemical stimulation of the same region at the midbrain–pontine junction (Kitsikis and Steriade, 1981), where internal signals for brain activation are generated during both REM sleep and arousal (see Chapter 9).

Under most conditions the states of waking, slow-wave sleep, and REM sleep can be specified using only three indicator variables: the voltage amplitude of the cortical EEG, the frequency of rapid eye movements, and the EMG record of antigravity muscle activity. Figure 4 illustrates this point and the use of these three indicator variables. These three are the most important and frequently used indicator variables, with animal studies utilizing PGO waves as the next most important indicator variable. The presence of hippocampal θ rhythm is often used as an important REM indicator in recordings in rodents, which have much less visual system activity than primates. Finally, we point out that the frequently used modifier "behavioral" indicates that the state is related to the external comportment of the organism and also implies an internal pervasiveness, since it usually refers to global states such as sleep and waking.

The use of indicator variables to define state as schematized in Fig. 4 (McCarley, 1980) has been concretized and implemented as a method for display of actual data and of state diagnosis by Friedman and Jones (1984). Ursin and Sterman (1981) have provided a manual of criteria for sleep-state definition in the adult cat.

In general, accurate and reliable use of waking, EEG-synchronized sleep, and REM sleep state definitions is straightforward in studies of normal, sufficiently mature, nondiseased, and nonlesioned animals. One simply looks for the presence of the three major indicator variables, and, when they are jointly present, the organism is deemed to be in the behavioral state of REM sleep. Problems arise when the central nervous system (CNS) is not intact or when a pharmacological agent is used to alter state; it is then that the presence or absence of REM sleep becomes a matter of definition of whether sufficient indicator variables are present and have the proper range of values. For our part we see little point in hermeneutics of state diagnosis. We take the viewpoint that REM sleep involves many component systems and that lesions and pharmacological agents may selectively and/or partially suppress or activate various of these systems. Following experimental procedures, the question often arises as to the definition of the ensuing state, as, for example, whether it is REM sleep or not.

We think the obvious procedure to follow with such altered states is that the set of indicator variables useful in normals must be enlarged so that the "organism state" can be specified with more precision; ideally one would measure the activity (EEG and cellular) in each component system of REM sleep. If this is not done, and it is often technically impossible to do so completely, then some uncertainty must remain about how close the match is to normal REM, with the degree of uncertainty inversely correlated with the thoroughness of the match. The reason for going into this apparently simple, straightforward line of argument in detail will become clear as lesion and REM induction studies are presented. We suggest that many disagreements arise from whether the investigator thinks the criteria for "true REM" have been satisfied and from the fact that, not surprisingly, individual definitions of "true REM" vary widely. Our reason for using "indicator variables" is to move the argument away from the hermeneutics of "true REM" and employ the descriptive, operational notation of the values of certain indicator variables after an experimental manipulation. These objectively

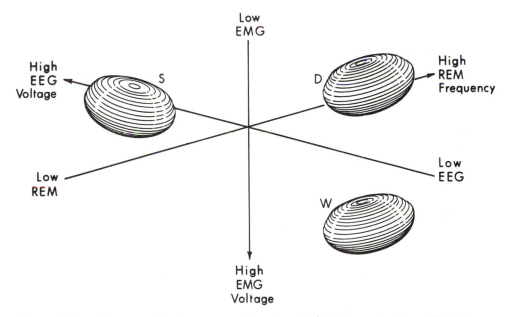

Figure 4. Three-dimensional indicator space illustrating the definition of waking (W), EEG-synchronized sleep (S), and REM sleep (labeled D, for the synonym EEG-desynchronized sleep), with the use of three indicator variables. The range of values taken on each state is indicated by an ellipsoid. This includes variability between occurrence of the state and within-state moment-to-moment variability. Modified from McCarley (1980).

describe the closeness of the match and suggest what other variables should be recorded.

The paradox that REM sleep, a state with a motoric arousal threshold higher than in EEG-synchronized sleep,* is a time when the electrical activity suggests that the cerebrum is in a highly excitable state leads us to define *activation* and *vigilance*.

Activation has to be used at the physiological, not behavioral, level. Moruzzi and Magoun (1949) referred to the activation of the EEG, but they did not equate this EEG response with arousal or waking. Activation was defined as a tonic readiness in cerebral networks that brings neuronal circuits closer to threshold, thus insuring secure synaptic transmission and quick cellular responses, a response readiness either to messages from the outside world (as during the waking state) or to internally generated drives (as during REM sleep), whether or not a motor reaction is generated (Steriade, 1984). This definition is based on data showing similar enhanced excitability of thalamic and cortical neurons to monosynaptic and antidromic volleys during both EEG-desynchronized states of waking and REM sleep (see Chapter 8). The definition does not refer, however, to inhibitory processes that insure a behavioral state with adequate, selective responsiveness. Although inhibitory processes have not been yet investigated in detail during REM sleep, the bizarre imagery during REM sleep would indicate that many sensory channels are simultaneously activated, and, correlatively, fine sculpturing inhibitory processes would probably be much less effective during this sleep state as compared to waking (see Chapter 8). The inclusion of inhibitory processes in the activating process leads to the notion of vigilance.†

Vigilance was defined by Head (1923) as a state with an increased reaction but with highly adapted responses, similarly to Dell's (1958) notion of a readiness to receive only some stimuli to the exclusion of others in order to perform efficiently. Both of these definitions implicate the presence of inhibitory processes during the active and adaptive behavioral state of wakefulness. Considering the requirement of a differential organization of cerebral networks for conscious integrative functions, Jasper (1958) concluded that, for such high processes, ascending activation should include inhibition and that "some activated cells may have an inhibitory function" (p. 341). Although cellular studies in the two decades that followed Jasper's prediction (1960s–1970s) rather claimed that a global blockage of inhibitory circuits occurs on arousal, current concepts fully agree with Jasper's assumption that some inhibitory neurons that underlie discriminatory functions are activated on natural arousal, brainstem reticular stimulation, or iontophoretic application of brainstem reticular transmitter agents. These data are fully discussed in Chapters 6 and 8.

---

*It seems that all reports agree that REM sleep is associated with the highest threshold of arousal in both cat and man. Only one study that distinguished REM sleep from various stages of non-REM (EEG-synchronized) sleep in the human found that the arousal threshold to auditory stimulation is higher in stage 4 of non-REM sleep than in REM sleep (cf. Dement, in Jouvet, 1965b).

†The term deactivation implies removal of activating influences. It is generally used by those who favor the notion of passive sleep because the idea of active inhibitory hypnogenic influences has not yet received sound experimental support at the cellular level (see Section 1.3.2).

1.3. Concepts of Passive and Active Mechanisms Promoting Sleep

Theories of passive sleep view sleep as a cessation of wakefulness. This results from forebrain deafferentation by decreased or interrupted activity either in sensory channels or in the nonspecific activating system of brainstem reticular formation. These theories have been present since antique times, appearing in Lucretius' *De Rerum Natura* (cf. Moruzzi, 1964), and were elaborated in this century by Kleitman (1929, 1963), Bremer (1935, 1938), and Moruzzi and Magoun (1949). Theories of active sleep view sleep as promoted by increased activity in systems with presumed inhibitory actions on cerebral structures maintaining the state of wakefulness. They were postulated more recently and are mainly based on two lines of evidence: the transection experiments by Moruzzi's group during the 1950s (cf. Moruzzi, 1972) and the results of lesions and pharmacological manipulations leading to the serotonergic hypothesis of sleep (Jouvet, 1972). In this section we review the roots and the current state of the passive and active hypotheses of sleep.

1.3.1. Theories of Passive Sleep

The idea that falling asleep is the simple result of negation of the active waking state is based on experiments with stimulation inducing arousal and EEG desynchronization and on clinical and animal studies with lesions followed by lethargy or coma.

The experiments with brainstem reticular stimulation by Moruzzi and Magoun (1949; see Section 1.1) led to the precise formulation of their theoretical concept of active waking and passive sleep: "The presence of a steady background of . . . activity within this cephalically directed brainstem system, contributed to either by liminal inflows from peripheral receptors or preserved intrinsically, may be an important factor to the maintenance of the waking state, and absence of such activity may predispose to sleep" (p. 470). This statement indicates that Moruzzi and Magoun did not express a clear choice between the two parts of the proposed alternative: (1) an intrinsic property of the brainstem core maintains the waking state; or (2) wakefulness requires the contribution of sensory pathways that collateralize in the reticular formation.

In fact, there is no incompatibility between the idea of a cerebral tone maintained by activities in sensory pathways and the brainstem reticular activating concept, and both factors should be considered as acting in concert. Experiments conducted in Speranski's laboratory (cf. Pavlov, 1928) have shown that the interruption of olfactory, visual, and auditory pathways at the peripheral level is followed in dog by a prolonged state of lethargy. This led Pavlov (1928) to emphasize the role of sensory impulses in the activated state of the cerebrum. Bremer's (1935, 1938) claim of a role played by sensory projections in maintaining the cerebral tone was undoubtedly strengthened by the experiments performed in his laboratory by Claes (1939), who showed a synchronizing (spindling) effect exerted on the visual cortex of cat following a bilateral section of optic nerves. The locally desynchronized electrical activity in various cortical areas, by setting into motion specific sensory projections (cf. Bremer, 1975), may become a generalized EEG activation by the action of corticofugal pathways impinging on the brainstem reticular formation. These pathways, which use excitatory amino acids as transmitter agents, are discussed in Chapter 3. Suffice it to mention the role of the corticoreticular feedback for the maintenance of the alert condition (Bremer and Terzuolo, 1954) and the depression of cell responsiveness in the upper brainstem reticular formation after a reversible cryogenic blockade of cortical sensory–motor areas (Buser *et al.*, 1969).

The emphasis on the role of brainstem structures in the diffuse cerebral activation of the waking state was the result of acute experiments. Subsequent studies on chronic *cerveau isolé* preparations (Batsel, 1960; Villablanca, 1965) have shown that, after a period of 7–10 days, the animals recover from the comatose state that appears immediately after a precollicular transection. Such chronic preparations display oscillations between EEG patterns and ocular behavior of wakefulness and sleep, with the conclusion that "a genuine state of wakefulness may be maintained in the isolated cerebrum" (Moruzzi, 1972, p. 21). The recovery of wakefulness in chronic *cerveau isolé* preparations deserves some comments concerning the activating role of supramesencephalic structures, namely, the thalamus, the posterior hypothalamus, and the basal forebrain.

A bilateral symmetrical vascular lesion that mainly affected some medial and especially the intralaminar thalamic nuclei, produced by a thrombosis at the bifurcation of the basilar artery, was followed by a state of lethargy lasting for more than 2 years (Facon *et al.*, 1958). Similar clinicoanatomic findings have been reported by Castaigne *et al.* (1962). In those studies, the thalamic lesions were associated with small vascular lesions in the midbrain periaqueductal gray. Generally, pure thalamic lesions are possible only experimentally. Villablanca (1974) performed total bilateral thalamic destruction with a midline approach that minimized cortical damage. During the first 10 postoperative days in such athalamic preparations, "although the cat behaviorally awoke . . . the EEG remained synchronized" (p. 72), and 3 months after thalamectomy, there was a delay of 10–20 sec between behavioral arousal and EEG desynchronization (see Fig. 4.16 in Villablanca, 1974). Thus, although an enduring lethargic syndrome may occur after medial intralaminar thalamic lesions combined with smaller midbrain tegmental lesions, behavioral arousal is not severely impaired after pure total thalamic lesions. However, the EEG desynchronation ordinarily accompanying arousal is absent or greatly delayed even at late postoperative stages.

Clinicoanatomic observations point to the posterior hypothalamus as a cerebral site where lesions are followed by somnolence or coma (Economo, 1929). More localized lesions than those resulting from the natural experiments created by the encephalitis lethargica became possible with the introduction of the Horsley–Clarke stereotaxic instrument and its use by Ranson through the 1930s. In experiments on macaque monkeys, Ranson (1939) observed that bilateral lesions of the lateral parts of the posterior hypothalamus that did not significantly encroach on the thalamus and the midbrain produce a state of continuous lethargy followed in later stages by a prevailing state of drowsiness and lack of motor initiative.* Ranson did not decide whether the lethargic syndrome, presumably produced by elimination of excitatory activity arising in the hypothalamus, was mediated by downward projections to the brainstem and spinal cord or by upward projections toward the cerebral cortex. The results of Ranson's experiments and the idea of a waking "center" located in the posterior hypothalamus have been revived during recent years by studies performed in Jouvet's laboratory and postulating the maintenance of the waking state by histaminergic cortically projecting neurons in the ventrolateral part of the posterior hypothalamus (Vanni-Mercier *et al.*, 1984; Lin *et al.*, 1986).

The history of cortical activating processes induced by basal forebrain structures is more recent, and it is related to the longstanding concept that ascending activation processes are largely cholinergic in nature. This concept was based on data showing that midbrain reticular stimulation or EEG-desynchronized behavioral states of waking and REM sleep are associated with a large increase in cortical release of acetylcholine (ACh) as compared with EEG-synchronized states (Szerb, 1967; Jasper and Tessier, 1971). As described a long time ago by Meynert (1872), the nucleus basalis and the adjacent basal forebrain structures of the same family were implicated in cortical cholinergic activation only recently when immunohistochemical studies showed that thalamocortical neurons, the final link in the ascending brainstem reticular system, do not use ACh as a transmitter agent. In some early kainate-induced lesion studies of the basal forebrain, there was a loss of cortical EEG desynchronization, but those results are not interpretable because there was also extensive damage to the thalamus. More precise chemical lesions of basal forebrain cell bodies in the rat, with consequent reduction in acetylcholinesterase (AChE) staining in the ipsilateral cortex, produced a large increase in slow (1–4 Hz) EEG waves during all behaviors (Buzsaki *et al.*, 1988). Similarly, EEG alterations with an increased tendency toward slow waves are seen in Alzheimer's patients (Coben *et al.*, 1983; see Fig. 8 of Chapter 13 and text discussion). These data, which are reminiscent of results obtained by means of cholinergic blockers such as atropine (Wikler, 1952), substantiate a direct cholinergic effect exerted by cortically projecting basal forebrain neurons in inducing cortical low-voltage fast activity. An indirect desynchronizing effect is mediated by basal forebrain projections to the reticular thalamic nucleus (Steriade *et al.*, 1987b) that effectively block synchronous spindle oscillations at their very site of genesis (see Chapter 7).

The point should be emphasized that the most powerful drive of all activating supramesencephalic structures arises in the upper brainstem reticular core.

---

*The syndrome of akinetic mutism was first described by Cairns *et al.* (1941) in a patient with an epidermoid cyst of the third ventricle. It can be described as a vigil coma, since the patients can be easily roused, but they lie inert and make no sound. Their eyes may follow moving objects or regard the observer steadily. Similar clinical cases have been subsequently described following hypothalamic and brainstem tegmental lesions (cf. Klee, 1961; Steriade *et al.*, 1961; Lhermitte *et al.*, 1963). The point was stressed (Steriade *et al.*, 1961) that this nosological entity should be confined to cases where there is a pathological interruption of *ascending* activating systems, excluding those cases where the lesion is diffuse and interrupts the *effector* pathways. In conditions without interruption of corticospinal or corticobrainstem pathways (as ascertained by precise motoric answers to the examiner's questions, by moving one or two fingers according to given codes and verbal instructions), the akinesia and mutism were interpreted (Steriade *et al.*, 1961) as an *Antriebsmangel*, an abolishment of incitation to action, caused by the interruption of ascending activating impulses.

This is true for ventromedial and intralaminar thalamic nuclei with diffuse cortical projections, the posterior and lateral hypothalamic areas, and the basal forebrain cell aggregates. In the intact animal, these diencephalic and forebrain neurons integrate ascending reticular impulses on their route to the cerebral cortex. The question arises as to the source of excitatory input to supramesencephalic structures in the chronic precollicular-transected preparation. This preparation displays EEG and ocular signs indicating a waking condition in the isolated cerebrum. It is known that the basal forebrain nuclei, for example, receive a projection from the amygdala (Price and Amaral, 1981), and stimulation of amygdalar nuclei induces EEG desynchronization even after complete disconnection from the midbrain reticular formation (Kreindler and Steriade, 1964). We suggest that, in a precollicular preparation, intrinsic or sensory (olfactory and visual)-induced activities of thalamic, posterior hypothalamic, and basal forebrain nuclei are effective in providing excitatory inputs for activation processes. It is also possible that denervation supersensitivity occurs in supramesencephalic structures after precollicular transection. Studies of cellular activity in supramesencephalic areas, hypothetically endowed with activating properties in the chronic stages of a *cerveau isolé* preparation, are still lacking. Such studies would provide information on the activity of neuronal networks in the isolated cerebrum.

The main difficulty facing passive theories of sleep is that sleep can be induced by stimulation of sensory receptors or central structures. Some of these experiments are discussed below.

1.3.2. Theories of Active Sleep

We shall not review data with EEG synchronization and/or sleep promoted by low-frequency (6–14/sec) peripheral or central stimulation (cf. Moruzzi, 1972) because such frequency parameters induce synchronized waves over the cortex even when applied to structures known to have activating properties. The variety of sites implicated in "sleep" simply because their stimulation led to EEG synchrony extends from the neo- and allocortex down to the medulla. Thus, if we accept this criterion, we would be forced to conclude, as remarked by Jouvet (1967), that "the whole encephalon has hypnogenic properties" (p. 135). Moreover, although rhythmic waves within the low-frequency range may outlast the stimulation period, they are probably caused by resonant activities in reciprocal thalamocortical loops (see Chapter 7) and are not necessarily related to the state of falling asleep.

We shall therefore discuss only the evidence for and against the two major cerebral sites currently postulated as active hypnogenic structures: the region of the solitary tract nucleus in the medulla and the preoptic area of basal forebrain. We consider that lesion studies inducing insomnia are more convincing for hypotheses of active hypnogenic structures than stimulation data. Although electrical stimulation should be used for the analytical purposes of identifying the input–output organization of a neuron or for studying state-dependent excitatory–inhibitory events in a cell, such synchronous stimuli are nonsensical for normal brain activity since they disturb natural patterns of neuronal discharges and thus can hardly be used to mimic natural states of sleep.

The active inhibitory role of the lower brainstem reticular formation on the rostral reticular core was hypothesized by Moruzzi and his group after the results of the midpontine pretrigeminal transection. Those experiments showed that the midpontine-transected animal displays a state of enduring alertness, about 70–90% of the total time of recording, a true experimental insomnia (Batini *et al.*, 1958; see Fig. 1). Among the numerous arguments brought by the Pisa group in favor of the synchronizing or possibly sleep-inducing influence of the lower brainstem reticular core, we mention the EEG state of desynchronization following inactivation of the lower brainstem core by intravertebral injections of barbiturates (Magni *et al.*, 1959) or by cooling the medullary floor of the fourth ventricle (Berlucchi *et al.*, 1964). At the cellular level, however, the projections from the lower to the upper brainstem reticular formation are usually described in excitatory terms, with both extra- and intracellular recordings in unanesthetized preparations (see Chapters 3 and 4). Moreover, recordings of bulbar reticular units during the waking–sleep cycle have revealed neurons with physiologically identified projections to the midbrain and/or thalamus that displayed an increased activity related to EEG desynchronization in both wakefulness and REM sleep (see Chapter 11), but no evidence was found for neurons with increased activity during drowsiness or EEG-synchronized sleep.

Electrical stimulation of the lateral preoptic region and diagonal band nuclei led to EEG synchronization and behavioral sleep in the behaving cat, even when high-frequency (150/sec) stimuli were used (Sterman and Clemente, 1962). The usual criticism of these experiments is that the latency of the hypnogenic effect was quite long (average time about 30 sec) and might well have represented "spontaneous" drowsy periods of the cat, a naturally very good sleeper. The other criticism is that with electrical stimuli, one cannot distinguish between activation of cell bodies and terminal or passing fibers. In this respect, Jouvet (1972) claimed that fibers from the serotonergic raphe nuclei terminating in the basal forebrain were implicated in the sleep syndrome produced by stimulating the basal forebrain areas. In fact, pretreatment with *p*-chlorophenylalanine (PCPA), a depleter of serotonergic terminals, suppresses the sleep effect of basal forebrain stimulation (Wada and Terao, 1970), although the nonspecificity of PCPA effects renders the significance of this result uncertain.

The hypothesis implicating the hypnogenic nature of the preoptic basal forebrain area can be traced back to Nauta's (1946) experiments showing that insomnia follows lesions of that area. Nauta's results have been confirmed by experiments with basal forebrain lesions leading to insomnia, appearing after a quite long delay (McGinty and Sterman, 1968). The long-latency appearance of insomnia and the fact that alterations of temperature regulation could appear after basal forebrain lesions led Jouvet (1972) to cast doubt on this phenomenon and to term it a "secondary insomnia" (p. 265) resulting from unknown factors but not directly induced by suppressing a sleep-promoting structure. Recently, however, a long-lasting insomnia, mostly affecting the deep stage of EEG-synchronized sleep and REM sleep, was induced in experiments performed by Jouvet's group by ibotenic lesions of perikarya in the lateral part of the preoptic area, without secondary signs of temperature disturbances (Sallanon *et al.*, 1989). Thus, the question of the possible hypnogenic role of this region was again raised. However, recordings of basal forebrain neurons show that more than 70% are waking-active or state-indifferent and that only a relatively small proportion exhibit higher discharge rates during EEG-synchronized sleep than in waking or REM sleep (Szymusiak and McGinty, 1986). Other studies have demonstrated that a more clear-cut relationship exists between the increased firing rates of basal forebrain neurons and EEG-desynchronized behavioral states (Detari *et al.*, 1987; Buzsaki *et al.*, 1988).

The active theory of sleep was also tested with the method of 2-deoxyglucose autoradiography, which was used to investigate more than a dozen brain structures postulated as "hypnogenic," including the preoptic area of the basal forebrain. No region was found to increase its metabolic rate during quiet sleep (Kennedy, 1983). It is notable that with the same method, a significant increase in metabolic activity was found in the intralaminar thalamic nuclei after stimulation of the midbrain reticular formation (Gonzalez-Lima and Scheich, 1985).

We conclude that the idea of an active hypnogenic focus still awaits consistent data at the cellular level. The neurons hypothetically endowed with such sleep-promoting functions should be physiologically identified as projecting toward, and exerting inhibitory actions on, the most likely candidates of activation processes, such as the cholinergic and noradrenergic neurons in the upper brainstem core. Although the concept of a hypnogenic focus in the basal forebrain is highly disputable in the light of the evidence discussed above, it is our

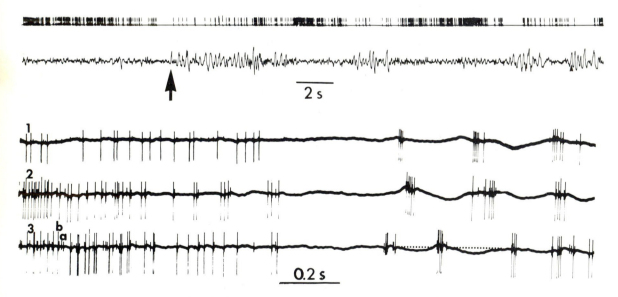

Figure 5. Changes in neuronal firing of corticofugal neurons with transition from waking (W) to sleep (S) in behaving cats. The top part (ink-written record) depicts a cortical neuron from parietal association area 5, antidromically identified from the lateral posterior thalamic nucleus. Note diminished firing rate of the neuron (first trace) prior to and during a focal spindle sequence recorded by the same microelectrode (second trace; arrow marks the onset of the first focal spindles). The bottom part depicts the original spikes of two neurons (a and b in 3) recorded from cortical area 5; both were antidromically identified from the centromedian thalamic nucleus. Traces 1–3 represent three W-to-S transitions during three successive wake–sleep cycles; increased amplitudes of both a and b discharges from periods 1 to 3, separated by about 70 min. Note that the appearance of focal spindles (dotted line in 3 tentatively indicates the baseline) is preceded by silent firing, thereafter followed by rhythmic burst discharges. Modified from Steriade (1978).

opinion that, if it exists somewhere, it is in the basal forebrain that actively hypnogenic neurons should be sought. The reasons are that descending pathways from the basal forebrain to the pedunculopontine nucleus have now been demonstrated (Swanson *et al.,* 1987) and that basal forebrain neurons are cholinergic (Mesulam *et al.,* 1983, 1984) as well as GABAergic (Nagai *et al.,* 1983; Brashear *et al.,* 1986). The presumed inhibition of waking-active brainstem neurons would be ascribable not only to GABA but also to ACh, since this exerts hyperpolarizing actions on brainstem parabrachial (Egan and North, 1986a) and pedunculopontine cholinergic (Leonard and Llinás, 1988) neurons. The latter elements are known to project widely to the thalamus (see Chapter 4).

Finally, we note that passive and active theories of sleep need not be mutually exclusive but may regarded as complementary mechanisms. Thus, the high-frequency spike bursts of thalamic and cortical neurons that result from deafferentation during drowsiness may be effective in triggering structures hypothesized to have active hypnogenic properties. Indeed, the production of high-frequency bursts in thalamocortical axons can be partly ascribed to disfacilitatory processes in brainstem–thalamic excitatory pathways, as indicated by a period of neuronal silence preceding the appearance of spike bursts (Steriade *et al.,* 1971). Similarly, at sleep onset, a period of neuronal silence lasting about 0.5–1 sec reliably precedes the spike bursts of antidromically identified corticospinal and corticobrainstem neurons associated with rhythmic focal oscillations within the spindle frequency (Fig. 5). The spike bursts in the axons of pyramidal tract or other types of corticofugal neurons are coincident, during sleep induction by vagoaortic stimulation, with phasically increased neuronal activity in the area surrounding the nucleus of the solitary tract (Puizillout and Ternaux, 1974), one of the structures postulated to cause active induction of EEG synchronization and sleep. Similar sequences may exist in other connected brain structures that initially undergo passive deafferentation effects, display postinhibitory rebound excitation, and eventually trigger active hypnogenic areas.

1.4.   Centers and Distributed Systems

Centers may be defined in a number of different ways, and anatomic, physiological, and pharmacological criteria may be used, or some combination of these. We begin by suggesting a narrow definition of a center using each of these criteria. With this concept, it will be seen that no sleep or wake state *in toto* can be said to have a center and even that few, if any, components of waking–sleep states have "a center."

Functionally, a neural center may be thought of as subserving one function and not any other. A behavioral state center would imply a group of neurons, homogeneous in their input–output organization and chemical code(s), and having the required pathways to project the generated activity to the final effectors of the events involved in that state. Furthermore, additional criteria in our restrictive definition include the following: (1) stimulation of perikarya in the center induces increased incidence of a given behavioral state or, at least, some of the crucial electrographic correlates of that state; (2) destruction of the center is necessarily followed by suppression of the implicated state; (3) the center, when deafferented from its major inputs, should continue to generate the state or to exhibit some of the defining electrographic signs of the state; and (4) neurons recorded in the center must display changes in activity in advance of the overt electrographic and behavioral aspects of the given state of vigilance. As we shall see, such rigid criteria are difficult for sleep-wake states to fulfill. They even have difficulty meeting a weaker definition of a center that uses the functional–anatomic criterion that a "center is an anatomically defined and localized set of neurons serving one function and no other."

To begin with, homogeneous cell groups are difficult to find in the mammalian brain. A few happy examples are the reticular (RE) thalamic nucleus, which consists of a single type of GABAergic cell, or the locus coeruleus of rat, which is a homogeneous collection of noradrenergic neurons; however, the same does not apply to cat, a species in which locus coeruleus contains a certain proportion of cholinergic cells. On the other hand, the heterogeneity of the so-called giant field of the pontine reticular formation, a structure strongly implicated in the genesis of REM sleep, is manifold. Conventional stainings showed that pontine giant cells are intermingled with even more numerous medium-sized and small neurons (Steriade, 1981); and intracellular staining with horseradish peroxidase (HRP) has revealed the existence of at least two cell populations with descending projections (Mitani *et al.*, 1988b), not to mention pontine reticular neurons with ascending projections that, as yet, have not been morphologically identified (see details in Chapter 4). The transmitter agent(s) used by pontine reticular neurons have not yet been defined. Other brain structures implicated in tonic and/or phasic events of EEG-desynchronized states were initially considered as purely cholinergic centers. However, it is now known, for example, that the pedunculopontine nucleus also contains catecholaminergic neurons and that nucleus basalis has a significant proportion of GABAergic neurons (see Chapter 4).

It is then difficult to conceive that such "centers" would exert functions that are sometimes depicted simply as pluses or minuses in model diagrams when the different transmitters of their neurons may exert various (even opposite) effects. The situation is made more complicated by the fact that two or more transmitters are colocalized in the same brainstem neuron (Vincent *et al.*, 1986). The nature of this coexistence (synergism or competition) is not generally understood at the present time (cf. Hökfelt, 1987).

Until now, very few cerebral structures have been found that fulfill the above criteria defining a center, and this is true for any function or state, not only states of vigilance. In a much looser sense, the pons may be thought to be the center of REM sleep since the prepontine cat displays major aspects of this state, whereas the animal with a caudopontine transection does not (see Section 1.1). In addition, studies employing all (stimulation, lesioning, and cellular recording) techniques have consistently revealed that the major events of REM sleep originate within or close to this brainstem sector (see Chapters 11 and 12). But the heterogeneity of the pontine tegmentum defies the notion of a center in a restrictive sense. It is, in fact, this heterogeneity, with interacting cell groups having different input–output organizations and using different transmitters, that probably underlies the genesis of REM sleep. The interaction of heterogeneous elements must be understood by an intensive analysis at the cellular level, taking into account the connectivity, the intrinsic neuronal properties, and the neurotransmitters, an approach we seek to further in this book.

It is similarly difficult to establish a "center" for EEG desynchronization since, as yet, no lesion in any structure has been found to abolish it for a long time during waking or, even more problematically, during REM sleep.

Confronted with the difficulties in fulfilling the rigid criteria of centers for states of vigilance or their peculiar physiological correlates, some investigators have begun to use the notion of distributed systems. This has the danger that the flexibility of this notion means a retreat into vagueness so that hypotheses concerning the role of multiple interrelated structures in the genesis of a given behavioral state cannot be proved wrong.

The RE thalamic nucleus does appear to meet the abovementioned criteria of stimulation, lesion, isolation, and cellular recording for a center (or pacemaker) of spindle oscillations, a defining electrographic feature of sleep onset. Indeed, spindles are abolished in thalamocortical systems after disconnection from RE, the deafferented RE neurons continue to oscillate *in vivo* within spindle frequencies, intracellular recordings *in vivo* demonstrate inverse images in GABAergic RE cells and their inhibited targets (the thalamocortical neurons), and stimulation of RE nucleus (with the same frequencies as those of RE spike barrages during sleep spindles) induces oscillations within spindle frequencies in thalamocortical neurons *in vitro* (see details in Chapter 7). Further light on the complex pacemaking properties of RE thalamic neurons, intrathalamic spread of spindle oscillations, and brainstem–thalamic mechanisms of spindle disruption will obviously be possible by using the isolated whole-brain preparation in which spindle sequences have been recorded (Serafin and Muhlethaler, 1988), resembling very much those observed in the intact animal. Similarly, the knowledge of REM-sleep mechanisms will be greatly advanced by using the technique of the *in vitro* perfused brainstem, whose viability was assessed by comparing the electrophysiological properties of inferior olive and pontine neurons, among others, to those observed *in vivo* (Llinás and Muhlethaler, 1988).

These new techniques provide the possibility of studying both the intrinsic properties of neurons (which are commonly investigated in brain slices) and the interactions between the cell and the entire sets of neuronal circuits that are preserved in the isolated whole-brain or brainstem preparation. One can predict that the next decade will see a true renaissance of brain studies based on the combination of the isolated whole brain in parallel with *in situ* investigations. Indeed, although the properties of neuronal networks are engraved to some extent in the intrinsic properties of their constituent single neurons, the full understanding of network characteristics depends on the knowledge of driving forces and connections between the elements of neuronal ensembles, so that different networks would generate dissimilar functional states despite the fact that their individual components have similar or identical intrinsic properties (Steriade and Llinás, 1988).

Finally, an important consideration for behavioral state control is that activated states, such as REM sleep, may result from modulation of excitability in sets of neurons subserving its many component functions such as the phenomena of saccades, muscle atonia, EEG desynchronization, and PGO waves that define this state (McCarley and Ito, 1985). Thus, behavioral state physiology may, to a large part, rest on increased knowledge of the effect of changing excitatory and inhibitory bias on defined neuronal networks, a physiology readily amenable to, and even demanding, quantitative modeling.

2

Methodological Advances in Knowledge of Morphological Substrates Underlying States of Vigilance

2.1. Early Tools and Results and Some Recent Developments

Until the 1970s, the Nissl, Golgi, and degeneration techniques were the most important tools for the knowledge of brainstem morphology and hodology.

The differentiation of the brainstem reticular core into nuclei was based on Nissl-stained sections in human (Olszewski and Baxter, 1954), cat (Brodal, 1957; Taber, 1961; Berman, 1968), and rat (Petrovicky, 1980; Newman, 1985a,b). The classical study by Olszewski and Baxter (1954) was the most important of the early signs reflecting the interest aroused among the anatomists by the discovery of Moruzzi and Magoun (1949). Olszewski and Baxter (1954) believed in a "difference in functional organization . . . [that] justifies the delineation and classification of such regions as nuclei" (p. 13). They considered, however, that the anatomic designation of reticular formation might be abandoned altogether (possibly because of the "reticularistic" flavor of the term, implying continuity between neurons) and, instead, proposed the use of the term "nuclei of unknown connections" for the newly described regions belonging to the reticular formation (see details in Section 4.1).

In those early times and even more recently, many physiologists felt that there was no need for so many reticular nuclei, differentiated on the basis of cytological differences. Ironically, when Nissl and Golgi techniques were more recently used to define the neuronal morphology in regions where retrograde labeling was observed after HRP injections into the spinal cord, at least 13 brainstem nuclei were found just in the pons and mesencephalon, and these were limited to cell groups giving rise to reticulospinal projections (Newman, 1985b).

At variance with the tendency toward an analytic dissection of brainstem nuclei by means of Nissl staining, Golgi studies emphasized the uniform morphology of reticular neurons and suggested a cellular archetype based on dendroarchitectonics. The brainstem reticular neuron was defined by its radiate, relatively long, and rectilinear dendrites that transcend the limits of the nucleus in which the soma lies and that overlap with dendrites of other reticular cells (Scheibel and Scheibel, 1958; Leontovich and Zhukova, 1963; Ramon-Moliner and Nauta, 1966). The term *isodendritic* was introduced (Ramon-Moliner and Nauta, 1966) for its topognostic value, the dendritic configuration allowing not only the identification of Golgi-stained cells as belonging to the brainstem reticular formation but also permitting the recognition of similar neurons in distant (thalamic, subthalamic, and hypothalamic) territories that are connectionally and functionally related to the brainstem core (Ramon-Moliner, 1975; Fig. 1). Obviously, the considerable degree of dendritic overlap in the brainstem core suggests that reticular neurons are not likely to receive specialized inputs

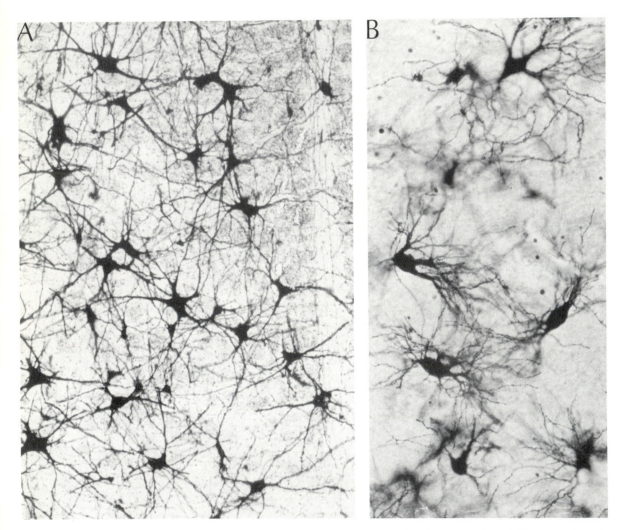

Figure 1. Different dendritic patterns of brainstem reticular neurons and thalamic relay neurons in Golgi impregnations. A: Gigantocellular field of pontine reticular formation in kitten. ×180; reproduced at 68%. B: Lateral geniculate thalamic nucleus in kitten. ×240; reproduced at 68%. Courtesy of Dr. E. Ramon-Moliner.

and that they offer a substrate for integration of afferents from heterogeneous sources.

The typical radiating dendritic pattern of brainstem reticular cells was first seen in newborn animals. In some brainstem nuclei of the medullary reticular formation, this pattern is rearranged during maturation, eventually forming complexes of dendritic bundles that surround running fascicles of myelinated fibers (Fig. 2; Scheibel and Scheibel, 1975). The protospines of dendrites increase in number during the course of early development and peak near 11 days of age, but later on they decline, and eventually many are resorbed onto the dendritic surface (Melker and Purpura, 1972; Hammer *et al.,* 1981; see Chapter 4).

In the Scheibels' study (1958), the Golgi method also helped to rule out the earlier hypothesis that the brainstem reticular core essentially consists of chains of short-axoned cells. Their stainings revealed, on the contrary, that "no short-axoned Golgi type II cells exist in the brainstem core" (p. 37) and that "bulbar magnocellular elements usually emit axons which course dorsomedially toward the region of the MLF (medial longitudinal bundle) . . . , and bifurcate into caudad- and rostrad-running fibers, which may reach the spinal cord and the mesencephalon or diencephalon, respectively" (pp. 38–39). As yet, there are no

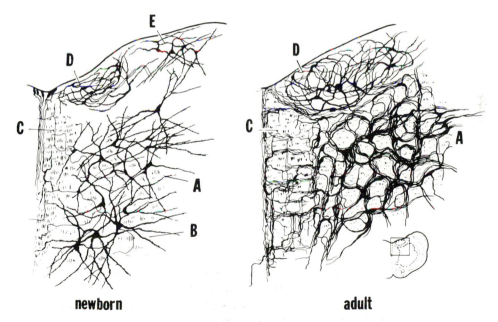

newborn   adult

Figure 2. Cross sections through the dorsal half of the lower medulla oblongata in newborn and adult cats to show the difference in dendrite patterns of reticular neurons. Neurons of the rostral part of the nucleus reticularis parvocellularis (A) and of the nucleus reticularis magnocellularis (B) show familiar radiating dendrites bearing many excrescences in the newborn. In the adult, the dendrites have been "resculpted" to form characteristic bundles that surround the rostrocaudal running fascicles of myelinated fibers. Other abbreviations include: C, medial longitudinal fasciculus; D, nucleus prepositus hypoglossi; E, medial vestibular nucleus. Drawn from cat brainstem material stained by variants of the rapid Golgi method. From Scheibel and Scheibel (1975).

data from studies with more powerful tools (such as intracellular HRP staining) indicating the presence of short-axoned neurons in the brainstem core. As to the second statement concerning the long conductors branching both rostrally and caudally, this feature may characterize the brainstem reticular projections in the newborn (up to 7–10 days old) animals from which the Scheibels' material derived, but it is certainly not valid in adult animals in which neurons with ascending or descending projections are rather segregated (see Chapter 4). Nonetheless, the Scheibels' studies were the first to emphasize the projections of single brainstem reticular neurons to distant sites and, thus, to provide data on the substratum of brainstem core control on spinal cord and diencephalic operations.

The capriciousness of the Golgi method and the lack of quantitative data in earlier studies were compensated by attempts at determining the real shape and the actual dimension of the neuronal soma and dendrites of Golgi-stained elements by photogrammetric representations using different stages of illumination in serial sections (Mannen, 1975) and by tridimensional reconstruction using computer analyses (Glaser and van der Loos, 1965; Llinás and Hillman, 1975; Cowan *et al.*, 1975). Such studies have been performed on various cellular types in the cerebellum, hippocampus, and neocortex, but detailed analyses of the brainstem core have not so far been undertaken.

That Golgi technique can be combined with many other, more recent methods, including electron microscopy (EM), retrograde transport of HRP, and immunocytochemistry, was demonstrated in a series of elegant studies by Somogyi and his colleagues performed on visual cortex and striatonigral neurons (Somogyi, 1978; Somogyi *et al.*, 1979, 1983). A neuronal circuit was identified by Golgi staining and anterograde degeneration under EM analysis as involving three successive links from geniculostriate degenerated axons to two Golgi-stained cortical targets in layer IV (a small pyramidal cell and a spiny stellate); in turn, some of the axonal arborizations of these two types of Golgi-stained neurons were found to establish asymmetric contacts on large nonspiny stellate cells (Szomogyi, 1978).

There are limitations of the above method of tracing neuronal chains since the Golgi technique does not usually stain myelinated axons and little information is obtained about the local-circuit or long-axoned character of the third neuron in the circuit. This led to staining with the Golgi method of neurons that had been retrogradely labeled by HRP transport; then EM was used to identify the type of synapses on the efferent neuron. Thus, Golgi staining is used to identify the soma shape and dendritic patterns of a neuron (say *X*) whose projections were identified by means of retrograde HRP transport from a distant site, and the input to cell *X* is studied by EM-identified synapses of degenerating boutons after a lesion in a given structure (Somogyi *et al.*, 1979). The immunohistochemical localization of glutamate decarboxylase (GAD) in neurons that have also been processed with the Golgi procedures and the EM identification of synaptic contacts made by GAD-positive boutons on Golgi-impregnated neurons have also been used. This approach has demonstrated that GABAergic short-axoned cortical neurons receive powerful excitatory inputs and that some of them are contacted by other GABAergic neurons, a presumed basis for disinhibition in target pyramidal cells (Szomogyi *et al.*, 1983). These methods of tracing neuronal networks should now be applied to brainstem circuits between cholinergic and monoaminergic neurons with identified (ascending and descending) projections that have been hypothesized to play a role in the genesis of behavioral states of vigilance and in the regulation of state-dependent neuronal activities in the cerebral cortex, thalamus, and spinal cord.

During the past decade, the more powerful tool of intracellular or intraaxonal staining technique was added to the Golgi method for the characterization of soma shape, dendritic domains, and axonal collateralization. In addition to details gained for the knowledge of cellular morphology, this method allows knowledge of neuronal structure to be obtained in physiologically identified elements. First employed in the visual cortex of cat by Kelly and Van Essen (1974), who used the fluorescent dye procion yellow as the marker, the method was greatly developed with the use of intracellular HRP injection in a great variety of central structures from the cerebral cortex to the spinal cord. After electrophysiological characterization of the neuron through a glass micropipette filled with HRP, the marker is injected by using direct current for several minutes while continuously monitoring cell's responses to assure that the pipette remains intracellular. Within the brainstem, the intracellular HRP staining helped to demonstrate autapses (i.e., a synapse between a neuron and a collateral of its own axon; cf. van der Loos and Glaser, 1972) in thalamically projecting neurons in substantia nigra pars reticulata (Karabelas and Purpura, 1980), the soma–dendritic profile, axonal trajectory, and branching of tectobulbospinal neurons (Grantyn and Grantyn, 1982), and the soma size, orientation of dendrites, and axonal collateralization in two distinct classes of pontine and bulbar reticulospinal neurons (Mitani *et al.*, 1988b,c).

Finally, the anterograde degeneration technique was used by Nauta and Kuypers (1958) to demonstrate ascending projections from the brainstem reticular core to intralaminar thalamic nuclei, subthalamic fields, and hypothalamic areas. Since the electrolytic lesions giving rise to axonal degeneration involve not only cell bodies but also passing fibers, this method was abandoned in favor of more advanced tracing methods, which are described in the next section.

2.2. Anterograde and Retrograde Tracing Techniques

The autoradiographic tracing technique, introduced around 1970 (Lasek *et al.*, 1968; Cowan *et al.*, 1972), is based on the anterograde axonal transport of macromolecules that have incorporated radiolabeled amino acids injected in the vicinity of projection neurons. The radioactive label is transported up to the axonal terminals (see Rogers, 1979, for technical procedures). This method has been widely used to reveal descending and ascending projections of brainstem reticular neurons. The anterograde transport technique is still the only tracing technique that unequivocally avoids the fiber-of-passage problem. Thus, the exact termination in the spinal gray matter of axons originating in various nuclei of the brainstem (including direct projections to the motoneuronal cell groups) was determined by means of radioactive amino acid tracers, which avoided the possible uptake of the retrograde HRP tracer by damaged axonal terminals (see

below) and proved to be much more sensitive than the anterograde degeneration technique (Holstege and Kuypers, 1987).

However, when the ascending brainstem reticular projections were studied,
the anterograde autoradiographic technique proved to be less powerful than the
retrograde transport techniques. Indeed, autoradiographic experiments revealed that midbrain and pontine reticular neurons project to medial, intralaminar, and reticular thalamic nuclei, but major sensory and motor relay
thalamic nuclear groups remained unlabeled, such as the medial and lateral
geniculate, ventrobasal, and ventrolateral nuclei (Edwards and DeOlmos, 1976;
Graybiel, 1977a; Robertson and Feiner, 1982; Jones and Yang, 1985). Clear
signs of facilitated synaptic transmission were seen in these relay thalamic nuclei
following stimulation of the upper brainstem reticular formation, but the pathways underlying the potentiating effect remained to be elucidated. The disclosure of brainstem reticular projections to virtually all relay and associational
thalamic nuclei was made possible by using injections of retrograde tracers strictly confined within the limits of those thalamic nuclei (see Fig. 4 and Chapter 4).

Since 1984, the *Phaseolus vulgaris* leukoagglutinin (PHA-L) has been employed as an anterograde axonal tracer to reveal the axonal trajectory and terminals and has sometimes been combined with the EM analysis of synaptic profiles
(Gerfen and Sawchenko, 1984; Wouterlood and Groenewegen, 1984). The
PHA-L method was used to trace efferent projections from the upper brainstem
cholinergic nuclei (Satoh and Fibiger, 1986; Mitani *et al.*, 1988d), and it can be
combined with immunohistochemical labels on the same brain section (Woolf *et
al.*, 1986).

The retrograde tracers consist of the enzyme HRP, a series of fluorescent
dyes, and labeled transmitter-related compunds. These three categories of retrograde markers are briefly presented below.

The demonstration of retrograde transport of intramuscularly injected
HRP to spinal cord motoneurons was accomplished by Kristensson and Olsson
(1971), and the retrograde transport in the centrifugal control pathway from the
isthmooptic nucleus to the chick's retina was shown by LaVail and LaVail (1972).
Since then, the sensitivity of this method has been greatly improved with the
introduction of tetramethylbenzidine (TMB) as the chromogen; this proved to
be superior to all other methods in tracing projections at the light-microscopic
level (Mesulam, 1978; Mesulam and Rosene, 1979). The conjugation of HRP
with the lectin wheat germ agglutinin (WGA) has the advantage of a much more
potent tracing for neuronal connections, especially when minute amounts of
tracer have to be injected (cf. Mesulam, 1982).

The problems involved in studies with HRP injections mainly concern the
uptake by passing fibers and the precise delineation of the injected territory.
Although there is virtually no uptake or transport by intact axons coursing
through the injection site, entry of HRP does occur into severed axons (axons e
and f, respectively, in Fig. 3; Mesulam, 1982). The absence of uptake by intact
axons was documented in a study that showed lack of retrogradely labeled cells
in habenular nuclei in spite of the fact that the HRP injection into the center
median-parafascicular thalamic complex also covered the passing retroflex bundle (Paré *et al.*, 1988). A precaution to avoid HRP entry into severed axons is a
delayed injection through a previously implanted cannula, allowing about 24–36

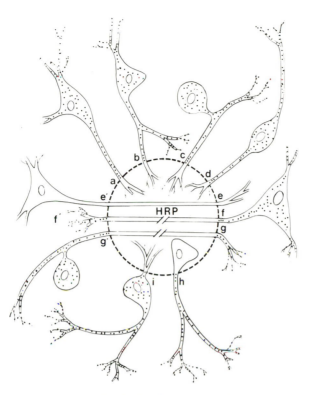

Figure 3. Types of HRP transport. The broken line contains the injection site. a: Uptake into intact terminals results in retrograde transport to the perikaryon and dendrites. b: The same type of uptake also results in labeling of axonal collaterals. c: Uptake into intact peripheral sensory terminals results in labeling of the ganglion cell as well as in transganglionic labeling of central sensory terminals. d: A similar complex transport occurs along bipolar neurons. e and e′: There is virtually no uptake or transport by intact axons passing through the injection site. f and f′: There is entry of HRP into severed axons; entry into the proximal stump results in retrograde labeling; the labeling is granular and occurs within membrane-delimitated organelles if the perikaryon is at a distance from the point of injury or if the survival time is sufficiently long; labeling of the distal axonal stump is mostly by cytoplasmic diffusion. g and g : Entry into an injured peripheral sensory axon results in retrograde, anterograde, and transganglionic labeling; the resulting transganglionic labeling almost always occurs as a consequence of active vesicular transport. h: Uptake into an intact perikaryon results in anterograde transport into terminal fields. i: Uptake into intact dendrites may result in labeling of the perikaryon and its axonal branches. From Mesulam (1982).

hr for axonal cicatrization or degeneration, to preclude the HRP transport. As to the site of the HRP injections, its size is greater (and probably overestimated) when the TMB procedure is used as compared to the diaminobenzidine (DAB) procedure. It is generally believed that only the center of the injection corresponds to the region of effective uptake.

One of the most difficult assessments as to the critical localization of HRP injections concerns the various thalamic nuclear groups (Fig. 4A,B), which are quite closely located on the thalamic map, each being interposed within distinct sensory and motor modalities or systems with general regulatory functions. In those cases, in addition to the histological examination of HRP injection sites on counterstained sections to facilitate the recognition of nuclear boundaries, the evidence that the injection was strictly localized within a given nucleus comes from the differential patterns of retrograde and anterograde labeling in various cortical areas known to have reciprocal connections with the injected thalamic nucleus (Fig. 4C,D). Thus, for example, after an injection in anterior nuclei, massive retrograde cell labeling occurs in the retrosplenial gyrus but not in the pericruciate cortex, indicating that the injection did not encroach on the adjacent centrolateral and ventromedial thalamic nuclei. The localization of HRP injections within the limits of various sensory thalamic nuclei was necessary because very great percentages (70–90%) of retrogradely labeled brainstem reticular cholinergic neurons are uniformly distributed in a circumscribed region at the midbrain–pontine junction regardless of the thalamic location of HRP injection (Steriade *et al.*, 1988).

In addition to the retrograde tracing, HRP is comparable to the amino acid autoradiographic technique for anterograde tracing (Mesulam and Mufson, 1980). The validity of HRP histochemistry for both retrograde and anterograde tracing is especially fruitful for the disclosure of reciprocal connections between two structures. For example, when WGA–HRP is injected in a thalamic relay or associational nucleus, retrograde labeling is found in neurons of cortical layer VI, whereas the fine-grained extraperikaryal product reflecting the anterograde HRP transport is mainly seen in middle layer IV and supervening part of layer

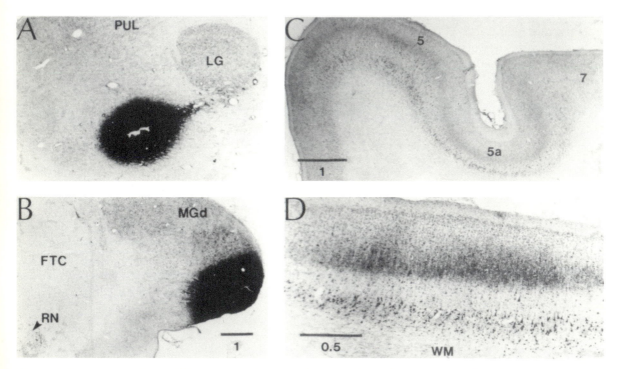

Figure 4. Localization of WGA–HRP injections in various thalamic relay nuclei of cat. A and B: Oblique injections in the ventroposterior and medial geniculate nuclei, respectively. C and D: Anterograde and retrograde labeling in suprasylvian gyrus (C) and coronal gyrus (D) after WGA–HRP injections in the lateral posterior and ventroposterior thalamic nuclei, respectively. Horizontal bars indicate millimeters. Modified from Steriade *et al.* (1988).

III (see Fig. 4C,D). The anterograde transport of HRP was also used to reveal a superficial diffuse cortical projection of the ventromedial thalamic nucleus to the outer third of layer I (Glenn *et al.*, 1982), in line with data obtained by means of the autoradiographic experiments of Herkenham (1979). In some cases, the HRP method proved to be more sensitive than the autoradiographic one. With injections of [³H]proline into the intralaminar centrolateral nucleus, Cunningham and LeVay (1986) found anterograde labeling in layers V and VI of visual cortical areas 17 and 18 in the cat (Fig. 5A,B), whereas the use of the anterograde transport of WGA–HRP led, in addition, to a distinct band of terminal labeling in layer I as well as, occasionally, the labeling of a thalamocortical axon traversing the cortical layers vertically (Fig. 5C).

The fluorescent dyes were introduced by Kuypers and his colleagues and are especially suited for the demonstration of axonal collateralization to different structures by means of multiple-labeling methods (Kuypers *et al.*, 1980; Van der Kooy *et al.*, 1978). The most employed compounds are fast blue and nuclear yellow, which are useful for retrograde transport in long pathways. This method was applied to test the hypothesis of ascending and descending projections of the same brainstem reticular neuron. One fluorescent dye was injected in the spinal cord and another dye in the cerebellum or in the diencephalon; the results showed that very few reticulospinal cells of the pontine gigantocellular field also provide collaterals to the cerebellum or to the diencephalon (Waltzer and Martin, 1984). The same method was recently used to demonstrate that a significant number of monkey's basal forebrain neurons send axon collaterals to both the reticular thalamic nucleus and the cholinergic peribrachial area in the upper brainstem core; however, no basal forebrain neurons were found to send branching axons to the brainstem core and the cerebral cortex (Parent *et al.*, 1988).

Lastly, retrograde tracing can be obtained by using some transmitters or related molecules that, after having been selectively taken up by the axon terminals, migrate toward the perykaryon where they are accumulated. By contrast with HRP or other retrograde tracers that label nonselectively all neurons with terminals within the injected area, only neurons with an affinity uptake mechanism for a given transmitter or precursor will be retrogradely labeled after the injection of the tritiated transmitter marker into the projection area. The first experiments with this method have been performed on the pigeon optic tectum by Hunt and his colleagues in Cuénod's laboratory (Hunt *et al.*, 1976). Since then, a series of studies succeeded in demonstrating the retrograde transport of tritiated serotonin* in the pathways between the nucleus raphe dorsalis and substantia nigra or caudoputamen (Streit, 1980), glutamate/aspartate in corticothalamic pathway (Baughman and Gilbert, 1980, 1981; Rustioni *et al.*, 1983), and choline in the pigeon's thalamo-Wulst projection (Bagnoli *et al.*, 1981) and in the pathway between the brainstem core and the basal forebrain (Jones and Beaudet, 1987b). The results of other studies on the retrograde transport of transmitter-related compounds are reported in Chapter 4.

---

*The problems with retrograde labeling of serotonin involve the crossed specificity of serotonin and catecholamine uptake mechanisms and, above a certain serotonin concentration, the quite unspecific labeling of all inputs to the injected area, much the same as with HRP (Cuénod *et al.*, 1982).

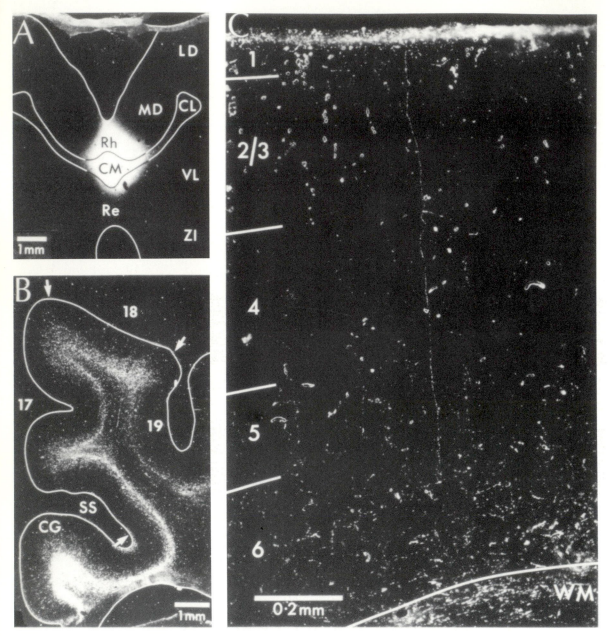

Figure 5. Projections of intralaminar thalamic nuclei centralis lateralis (CL) and centralis medialis (CM) to primary visual cortex in the cat studied by means of anterograde labeling after [³H]proline injection (A and B) or WGA–HRP injection (C) in the CL or CM nuclei. A: Site of [³H]proline injection in the CM nucleus; there is some spread into the adjacent rhomboidal (Rh) nucleus. Darkfield. LD, LP, MD, Re, Rt, VL, VPL, ZI: laterodorsal, lateral posterior, mediodorsal, reuniens, reticular, ventrolateral, ventral posterolateral, and zona incerta thalamic nuclei. B: Low-power darkfield micrograph of autoradiograph labeling pattern in visual cortex and cingulate gyrus (CG). Coronal section of right hemisphere at about stereotaxic plane A3. The midline is at the left of the figure.

The arrows mark the boundaries of areas 17 and 18. Note the heavy labeling of fibers in the white matter underlying the cingulate gyrus (cingulum bundle) and the fibers looping around the fundus of the splenial sulcus (SS) to approach the visual areas. Terminal labeling is restricted to the deep layers of the cortex except for some labeling of layer I at the fundus of the SS just outside the ventral boundary of area 17. C: Labeling pattern in area 17 after WGA-HRP injection of CL nucleus. Darkfield. Sparse terminal labeling is seen in layers 6 and 5 and the upper part of layer 1. A labeled fiber ascends through the cortical layers in the center of the field. The other structures in layers 2–3 and 4 are artifactually labeled blood vessels. WM, white matter. Modified from Cunningham and LeVay (1986).

2.3. Immunohistochemical Identification of Various Cell Groups and Disclosure of Their Projections by Combined Retrograde Tracing and Immunohistochemistry

The history of research on the chemical code of neurons in various groups of the brainstem core began in the 1960s with the use of formaldehyde histo-fluorescence method (Dahlström and Fuxe, 1964) and continued with the introduction of the glyoxylic acid fluorescence method (Lindvall and Björklund, 1974; Lindvall *et al.*, 1974). Both of these methods were successful in identifying monoamine-containing neurons and their projections. However, the catecholaminergic system was better visualized than the serotonin-containing system, and among catecholaminergic systems, the noradrenergic component could not be clearly distinguished from the dopaminergic one.

More recently, immunohistochemical methods were introduced by using antisera raised against synthesizing enzymes of catecholamines (Hökfelt *et al.*, 1984) and, finally, directly against each of monoamine transmitters: serotonin (5-HT) (Steinbusch, 1981), norepinephrine (NE) (Geffard *et al.*, 1986), and dopamine (DA) (Onteniente *et al.*, 1984).

In the past few years, chemically identified projections of monoaminergic systems have been studied by combining the retrograde transport of HRP with immunohistochemical methods using, for example, the synthesizing enzyme of catecholamines, tyrosine hydroxylase (TH). These data are reported in Chapter 4.

The cholinergic systems could be formally identified only during the 1980s with the production of monoclonal antibodies reactive to choline acetyltransferase, the synthetic enzyme of acetylcholine (ACh), a highly specific marker for cholinergic neurons and fibers.

The ascending projections of the brainstem reticular formation have long been hypothesized to be cholinergic on the basis of Shute and Lewis' (1967a,b) studies of the trajectories of fibers containing acetylcholnesterase (AChE), the degradative enzyme of acetylcholine. Since the documentation of AChE-stained projections was usually based on diagrams or on coronal sections that preclude a satisfactory evaluation of ascending brainstem pathways, a new perspective was recently provided by employing a three-dimensional photographic characterization of the dorsal tegmental pathway, which originates in the midbrain and pontine reticular core (Wilson, 1985).

There is a specificity problem related to the use of AChE histochemistry as a marker of cholinergic elements. For example, the ventral tegmental component of the ascending brainstem pathway, originally described as cholinergic, is now known to arise mainly from dopaminergic neurons (Butcher *et al.*, 1975; Moore and Bloom, 1978).

Nonetheless, studies in different brain regions emphasize the similarities between the results obtained by means of AChE histochemistry and those employing monoclonal antibodies to ChAT. Thus, studies comparing AChE histochemistry with ChAT immunohistochemistry revealed that intense AChE staining of neurons in some cerebral structures, such as the neostriatum and the basal forebrain, can be reliably used for identifying cholinergic elements (Levey *et al.*, 1983b). Also, the pattern of AChE staining in the thalamus (Olivier *et al.*, 1970; Jones, 1985; Steriade *et al.*, 1988; Fig. 6) is generally similar to the distribution of ChAT-immunoreactive fibers (Levey *et al.*, 1987a). Despite these similarities, it is accepted that the correspondence between the two methods is not complete.

CAT

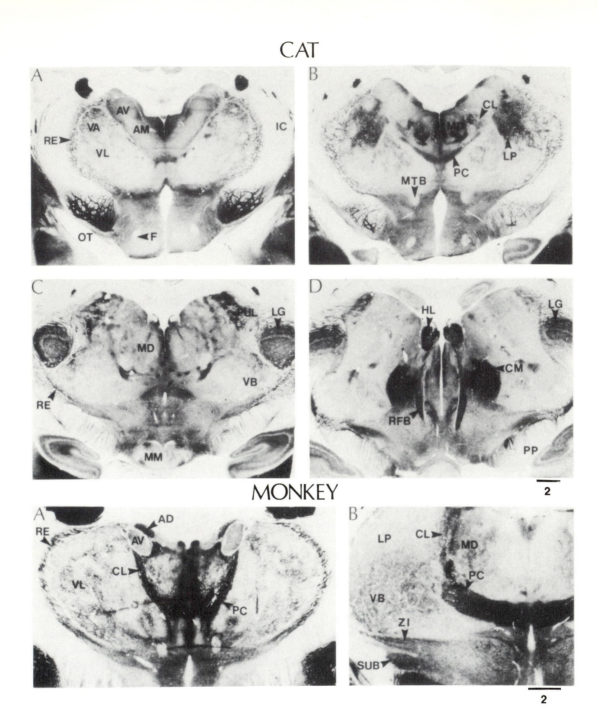

MONKEY

Figure 6. Distribution of acetylcholinestarase (AChE) activity in thalamic nuclei in the cat and macaque monkey. Staining according to Gomori's technique. Four levels rostral to caudal (A–D) in cat and two levels (A and B) in monkey. Horizontal bar indicates millimeters. AD, AM, AV, anterodorsal, anteromedial, and anteroventral thalamic nuclei; CL and CM, central lateral and centrum medianum thalamic nuclei; IC, internal capsule; F, fornix; HL, LG, LP, lateral habenula, lateral geniculate, lateral posterior thalamic nuclei; MM, medial mammillary nucleus; MTB, mammillothalamic bundle; OT, optic tract; PC, paracentral thalamic nucleus; PP, pes pedunculi; RE, reticular thalamic nucleus; RFB, retroflex bundle; SUB, subthalamic nucleus; VA, VB, VL, ZI, ventroanterior, ventrobasal, ventrolateral, zona incerta thalamic nuclei. From Steriade *et al.* (1988).

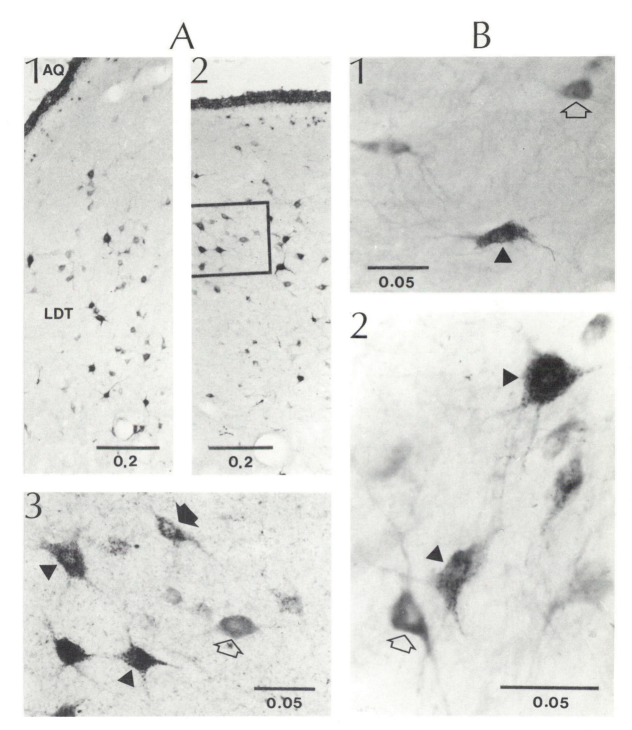

Figure 7. Microphotographs showing examples of the three types of cells analyzed in cat material processed according to TMB procedure combined with ChAT immunohistochemistry: HRP-positive cells (black arrows); ChAT-positive neurons (open arrows); and double-labeled neurons (triangles). A1 and A2 are low-power photographs depicting retro-gradely labeled cells in brainstem LDT nucleus after a WGA–HRP injection in the MD thalamic nucleus; the area marked by rectangle in A2 is enlarged in A3. B1 and B2 depict double-labeled and simple cholinergic cells in the brainstem PB area after an injection in the VM thalamic nucleus. From Steriade *et al.* (1988).

The most reliable results concerning the identification of basal forebrain and brainstem cholinergic cell groups have been obtained with ChAT immunohistochemistry. The first description (Kimura *et al.*, 1981) used an antiserum raised in rabbit against human ChAT. Since then, monoclonal antibodies to ChAT have been introduced (Eckenstein *et al.*, 1981; Levey *et al.*, 1983a) and used to map brain cholinergic neurons in rat (Armstrong *et al.*, 1983), cat (Vincent and Reiner, 1987), and macaque monkey (Mesulam *et al.*, 1984).

In recent years, the various brainstem reticular cholinergic cell groups and their efferent connections to the thalamus and the basal forebrain have been investigated by combining the retrograde transport of HRP or fluorescent tracers with ChAT immunohistochemistry. The combined ChAT plus HRP technique reveals three types of elements: simple HRP-positive cells with small blue HRP granules in both perikarya and dendrites; simple ChAT-positive cells displaying a diffuse light brown immunostaining throughout the cell body and its processes; and double-labeled neurons containing both retrogradely transported HRP and ChAT (Fig. 7). The first study used large injections of HRP in the thalamus of rat (Sofroniew *et al.*, 1985). Two subsequent studies on rat used more localized injections of fluorescent (Woolf and Butcher, 1986) or HRP (Hallanger *et al.*, 1987) tracers into various thalamic nuclei. Finally, ChAT immunoreactivity combined with WGA–HRP retrograde transport has been used to demonstrate that brainstem cholinergic neurons project to virtually all sensory and motor, associational (Steriade *et al.*, 1988), intralaminar, and reticular (Paré *et al.*, 1988) thalamic nuclei of cat and to major associational thalamic nuclei of macaque monkey (Steriade *et al.*, 1988) as well as to the pontine reticular formation (Mitani *et al.*, 1988d). Two studies have been focused on the visual thalamus of cat, one of them dealing with all (lateral geniculate, lateral posterior, and perigeniculate) sectors (Smith *et al.*, 1988), the other one providing the first detailed comparative analysis of brainstem cholinergic and monoaminergic projections to the lateral geniculate nucleus (DeLima and Singer, 1987). The results of all these studies are reported in Chapter 4.

Immunoreactivity for somatostatin, substance P, cholecystokinin, and other peptides was demonstrated in a series of brain structures from the spinal cord up to the cerebral cortex (cf. Bjorklund and Hökfelt, 1985). In the brainstem, the presence of substance P and other peptides was described in cholinergic reticular neurons with ascending projections (Vincent *et al.*, 1983, 1986). In the thalamus, the somatostatinlike immunoreactivity was first shown in reticular neurons (Graybiel and Elde, 1983), colocalized with GAD immunoreactivity in the same elements (Oertel *et al.*, 1983). And immunoreactivity for all abovementioned peptides was recently demonstrated especially in the intralaminar and reticular thalamic nuclei (Molinari *et al.*, 1987). The colocalization of peptides in brainstem and thalamic neurons using more conventional transmitters is further discussed in Chapter 4.

3

The Origin of Afferents to the Brainstem Core

We now discuss the inputs to brainstem core neurons as revealed by morphological and electrophysiological studies. Since neurons in the classical brainstem reticular fields (either identified immunohistochemically as cholinergic or using transmitters as yet unidentified) have morphological and functional characteristics that are dissimilar to monoaminergic neurons, these two groups of elements are dealt with separately. Although cholinergic nuclei of various species also contain a minority of monoaminergic cells, and some monoaminergic nuclei possess a certain number of cholinergic cells (see Chapter 4), the presence of ACh or of one of the three monoamine transmitters defines one or the other of these two nuclear categories. The parabrachial nucleus, i.e., the caudal part of the neuronal group that surrounds the brachium conjunctivum and contains both cholinergic and aminergic neurons, is conventionally included among brainstem reticular nuclei. An initial section (3.1) discusses extrabrainstem sources of reticular afferents, and a subsequent section (3.2) examines brainstem sources of reticular afferents, including intrinsic reticuloreticular connectivity. Details of brainstem oculomotor system anatomy, which critically involves the reticular formation, are reviewed in Chapter 10 in conjunction with discussion of the physiology of the saccade-generating system. The final section (3.3) of this chapter discusses the afferents of monoaminergic nuclei.

3.1. Afferents from Extrabrainstem Sources to Brainstem Reticular Neurons

The order used in this section is simply anatomic and does not reflect the power of different types of inputs onto brainstem reticular neurons. Input strength is considered in Section 3.2 in discussion of pontine reticular afferents and reticuloreticular connectivity.

3.1.1. Afferents from Spinal Cord and Sensory Cranial Nerves

Since the first decade of our century there has been evidence, based on axonal degeneration and Golgi impregnation, that fibers originating in the spinal cord end exclusively in the brainstem reticular formation or collateralize within it while the parent axon ascends further to the thalamus. These afferents are probably involved in alerting responses to noxious stimuli. The early literature on this topic was comprehensively reviewed by Pompeiano (1973). We shall discuss only data accumulated during the past decade.

There are interspecies differences as to the origin of spinoreticular pathways. Electrophysiological studies show that, in cat, the spinoreticular tract is mostly crossed and originates in laminae VII and VIII, i.e., in the *ventral* part of the spinal cord (Albe-Fessard *et al.*, 1974; Maunz *et al.*, 1978). Most of these data resulted from antidromic activation of cat spinal neurons by stimulating the bulbar gigantocellular field and the nucleus reticularis pontis caudalis. The median of axonal conduction velocities is around 45 m/sec. Stringent limitations on stimulus intensity and failure to activate spinal neurons from more rostral (mesodiencephalic) sites indicated that the axons of those neurons probably end in the lower brainstem reticular formation and do not ascend to more rostral levels (Maunz *et al.*, 1978).

At variance with cat, the spinoreticular axons of rat originate in two neuronal groups in the *dorsal* half of the cord: the dorsolateral funiculus nucleus (DLF) and the dorsal horn, within or around the nucleus proprius and within lamina I (Menetrey *et al.*, 1980). Those neurons were antidromically activated mostly from both nuclei reticularis pontis caudalis and oralis and from the rostral (peribrachial) and caudal (parabrachial) regions around the brachium conjunctivum in the midbrain reticular formation and at the midbrain–pontine junction (Fig. 1). These projection sites were corroborated by the same authors using retrograde tracing experiments following localized HRP injections. The rat spinoreticular neurons are heterogeneous. The DLF cells project to the midbrain or the midbrain–pontine junction with slow conduction velocities (mean around 3.5 m/sec) and are driven by stimulation of subcutaneous or deep structures. The dorsal horn cells project to both pontine and midbrain levels with higher conduction velocities (mean around 13 m/sec), are driven by both innocuous and noxious stimulation, and are subject to descending inhibitory influences from the bulbar reticular formation and the nucleus raphe magnus (Menetrey *et al.*, 1980).

Figure 1. Spinoreticular neurons in rat. A: Locations of the active brainstem reticular sites for antidromic activation of spinal neurons. Each dot corresponds to an activated unit. Contralateral (filled circles) and ipsilateral (open circles) activations have been separated. The stereotaxic levels of various coronal sections are indicated by figures. From rostral to caudal, abbreviations correspond to colliculus superior (CS), colliculus inferior (CIF), cuneiformis area (CU), subcuneiformis area (CUS), subnucleus dissipatus (DI), nucleus reticularis pontis oralis (RPO), nucleus reticularis pontis caudalis (RPC), nucleus parabrachialis (PB), nucleus reticularis gigantocellularis (RG), nucleus raphe magnus (RM), and nucleus paragigantocellularis (RPG). B: Criteria for demonstrating antidromic activation (1), antidromic latencies (2), and location of spinoreticular neurons (3). The demonstration of antidromic activation is shown in 1. This cell responded to a single reticular shock with a constant latency (upper line, ten superimposed responses) and followed two pulses (600 Hz) without any change in latency (third line, ten superimposed sweeps). Antidromic spikes were occluded by the presence of orthodromic spikes in the critical period (equal to twice the antidromic latency plus one refractory period). Occlusion indicated by arrowheads on second and fourth lines. In 2, top histograms corresponds to dorsal horn neurons, bottom histogram to the dorsolateral funiculus cells. In 3, locations of 55 spinoreticular cells. Modified from Menetrey *et al.* (1980).

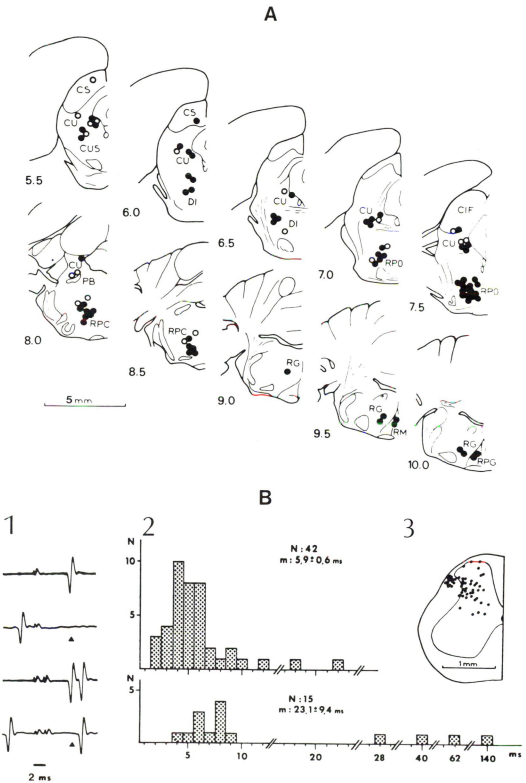

The monkey spinoreticular projections are more similar to those of rat than to those of cat. This similarity also concerns the collateral projections of spinothalamic axons to the brainstem reticular core. Indeed, both electrophysiological and HRP tracing experiments show that the lumbar spinothalamic tract of rat and monkey originates in the dorsal horn (Albe-Fessard *et al.*, 1974; Giesler *et al.*, 1979), whereas the source of the same tract of cat is mainly found in neurons of the ventral horn, with only some additional cells in lamina I (Albe-Fessard *et al.*, 1974; Carstens and Trevino, 1978). In monkey, the collateralization of spinothalamic axons toward the brainstem core was estimated by multiple stimulation sites and differences in antidromic response latencies, and it seems to take place in the medullary reticular formation where the branch crosses the midline and terminates in the reticular core ipsilateral to the soma (Giesler *et al.*, 1981).

The response decrement in brainstem reticular neurons to body surface stimuli at frequencies higher than 0.25–0.5 Hz indicates the inability of these neurons to relay efficiently rapidly recurring peripheral volleys and was interpreted as a sign of behavioral habituation (Peterson *et al.*, 1976).

In addition to transmitting impulses from noxious and some nonnoxious receptors to brainstem reticular neurons with ascending projections and alerting functions, spinal afferents arising in lamina I innervate the brainstem parabrachial nucleus and thus contribute to a series of vegetative processes mediated by this nucleus in response to nociceptive stimuli. The role of parabrachial nucleus in cardiovascular and respiratory reactions has been revealed in both rat and cat (cf. Fulwiler and Saper, 1984). Anterograde and retrograde HRP tracing showed that neurons of spinal cord lamina I project to a series of parabrachial subnuclei (Cechetto *et al.*, 1985). So far it is not precisely determined whether lamina I cells that give rise to the spinothalamic tract (Willis *et al.*, 1979) collateralize to the brainstem parabrachial nucleus or if there are two distinct populations of lamina I neurons with thalamic or brainstem projections, as double-labeling experiments with fluorescent dyes on cat suggest (Panneton and Burton, 1985). In either case, many spinoparabrachial neurons that receive afferent terminals immunoreactive to substance P (cf. Cechetto *et al.*, 1985) are probably the afferent source of cardiovascular and pulmonary reactions mediated by the parabrachial nucleus in response to nociceptive stimuli.

The termination of spinal afferents at the level of the medullary and pon-

Figure 2. Electrophysiological identification, somadendritic profile, and axonal trajectory of tectobulbospinal neurons (TBSNs) in the cat. A: Schematic diagram of experimental arrangement for antidromic activation of TBSNs. B to D: specimen recordings of antidromic spikes to show identification of axonal projection into the contralateral predorsal bundle (Fpd_c), anterior funiculus (FA_c), and collaterals to perioculomotor zone of the central gray (SGC_c). E: Soma, dendrites, and axon (a) of a representative TBSN. Complete reconstruction from serial sections after intrasomatic HRP injection. F: Axonal pattern of TBSN labeled by HRP injection into the main axon near the dorsal tegmental decussation. Schematic drawing in parasagittal plane. INJ: injection site. Solid lines: part of axonal tree reconstructed on the basis of HRP staining. Dotted line: extension of the main axon into the medulla as demonstrated by antidromic response to contralateral predorsal bundle stimulation at point 5 (record 5). Presence of collaterals in the bulbar tegmentum proved by antidromic response to stimulation at point 3 located 1.7 mm from midline (record 3. threshold 50 μA). 1,3,4: First-order collaterals of the main axon within the mesencephalic reticular formation. 2: The main ascending branch. Modified from Grantyn and Grantyn (1982).

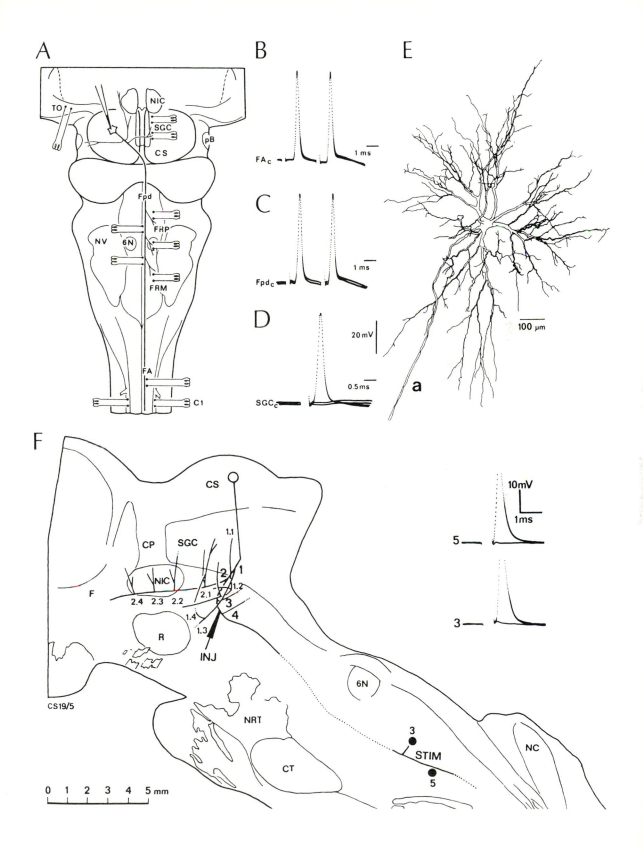

tine reticular neurons of gigantocellular fields was studied at the electron microscopic level (Bowsher and Westman, 1970; Westman and Bowsher, 1971). Degenerating presynaptic terminals are in contact with both soma and dendrites. Some calculations estimated that only one in 1000 presynaptic endings on polydendritic reticular neurons are of spinal origin.

Brainstem reticular neurons are also the targets of collaterals of axons of sensory cranial (mainly trigeminal, vestibular, acoustic, and optic) nerves (cf. Brodal, 1957).

One of the interposed relay stations through which the optic afferents reach the brainstem reticular neurons is the superior colliculus (SC), from which tectoreticular projections originate (Edwards, 1980). Grantyn and Grantyn (1982) made intracellular HRP injections in neurons located in the intermediate and deep SC layers with antidromically identified projections to the rhombencephalon and the spinal cord (tectobulbospinal neurons, TBSNs) (Fig. 2). Superior colliculus projections to brainstem reticular formation are also discussed in conjunction with the oculomotor system in Chapter 10. These studies revealed that TBSNs send axonal collaterals to the midbrain reticular territory and an ascending branch that could be traced up to the caudal diencephalon in the field of Forel.

Another structure that relays visual and auditory impulses in their collateralization to the brainstem reticular core is the cerebellum. The observations by Snider and his colleagues, during the early 1940s, that impulses of retinal and acoustic origin reach certain cerebellar areas challenged the Sherringtonian concept that the cerebellum is solely the headganglion of the proprioceptive system. The distribution of teleceptive responses in the cerebellar vermis and the hodology of cerebellopetal impulses of visual and auditory origin were reviewed in detail by Fadiga and Pupilli (1964). The cerebellofugal projections from vermal areas that receive auditory afferents (lobules VI and VII) do not reach the secondary areas of the cat auditory cortex through the medial geniculate thalamic nucleus but through a relay in the upper brainstem reticular formation (Steriade and Stoupel, 1960) that probably transmits further the information through the intralaminar thalamic nuclei. In those early studies, the projections from the vermal cerebellar surface to the upper brainstem reticular formation were studied by the evoked potential method, and the intermediate relay in deep cerebellar nuclei was not investigated. There is now morphological evidence that the fastigial nuclei, which are the obvious candidates for relaying impulses from the auditory–visual vermal areas, project to the midbrain reticular formation (Kievit and Kuypers, 1972). In addition, deep cerebellar nuclei modulate the activity of the deep layers of the superior colliculus through topographically organized projections (Roldan and Reinoso-Suarez, 1981).

3.1.2. Afferents from Diencephalon and Telencephalon

The following sources of descending inputs to the more rostral brainstem reticular core will be considered, as they may be involved in behavioral state control: thalamic nuclei, posterior and anterior hypothalamic areas, basal forebrain and related structures, and cerebral cortex.

3.1.2.1. Thalamic Nuclei

The thalamic projections to the midbrain reticular formation essentially originate in the intralaminar, reticular thalamic, and zona incerta nuclei. These descending projections have been revealed by both morphological and antidromic invasion techniques.

Horseradish peroxidase or WGA–HRP injections in the rostral midbrain reticular core or within the limits of the cholinergic peribrachial nucleus led to retrograde labeling of neurons in the centromedian–parafascicular (CM-PF) and centrolateral–paracentral (CL-PC) intralaminar nuclei (Parent and Steriade, 1981; Steriade *et al.*, 1982b). Neurons in those caudal and rostral components of the thalamic intralaminar complex can be antidromically activated from the midbrain reticular formation, with response latencies usually ranging between 1 and 3 msec (Fig. 3), suggesting axonal conduction velocities around 3–4 m/sec. Such conduction velocities are similar to those found in the reciprocal pathway from the midbrain core to intralaminar thalamic nuclei (Ropert and Steriade, 1981). These thalamobrainstem pathways may account for the monosynaptic responses elicited in midbrain reticular neurons by stimulation of intralaminar or other thalamic territories, responses that can faithfully follow 100/sec volleys (Steriade *et al.*, 1980). Another possibility is that such responses merely represent axon-reflex activation of spinothalamic projections or superior colliculus projections to intralaminar thalamic nuclei. These axons may branch and collateralize into the midbrain reticular core. Longer-latency (>10 msec) synaptic responses to brainstem reticular neurons to thalamic stimulation may be ascribed to circuitous pathways, including thalamocortical and corticoreticular projections.

Until recently, the projection from the reticular thalamic nucleus (RE) to the upper brainstem core was a matter of controversy. In cat and squirrel monkey, this projection was described by means of the retrograde transport of HRP and fluorescent tracers and was further substantiated in the same study with antidromic responses of RE cells to midbrain reticular stimulation (Parent and Steriade, 1984; Fig. 4). The very long latencies of antidromic responses (median around 12 msec) suggest that the conduction velocities of RE axons to the midbrain core are about 1 m/sec. In rat, however, this descending projection was ruled out on the basis of negative results of retrograde labeling after HRP injections in the midbrain reticular formation, with the conclusion that interspecies differences mark the organization of RE projections to the brainstem core (Berry *et al.*, 1986). The same study in the rat also reported that ascending brainstem reticular projections to the RE nucleus are extremely sparse or even absent (Berry *et al.*, 1986). It is now demonstrated that, in both cat (Paré *et al.*, 1988) and rat (Hallanger *et al.*, 1987), cholinergic and noncholinergic brainstem reticular projections innervate the RE nucleus (see Chapter 4).

A major diencephalic input originates in zona incerta (ZI), a lens-shaped nuclear field that continues laterally with the RE thalamic nucleus, with which it shares a common origin from the ventral thalamus (cf. Jones, 1985). The input–output relationships of the ZI place it as an integrator of very heterogeneous messages transmitted by spinothalamic, deep cerebellar, brainstem reticular, hypothalamic, and corticofugal projections. Retrograde transport experiments showed that ZI projects to the superior colliculus and periaqueductal gray (Grofova *et al.*, 1978) and to the central tegmental field of the midbrain reticular core (Steriade *et al.*, 1982b). The projections from ZI to the midbrain reticular formation exceed those from the RE thalamic nucleus. The morphological demonstration of ZI projections to the midbrain reticular formation was corroborated by the antidromic invasion of ZI cells, the axonal conduction velocities being around 11 m/sec (Steriade *et al.*, 1982b), twice as high as the values found

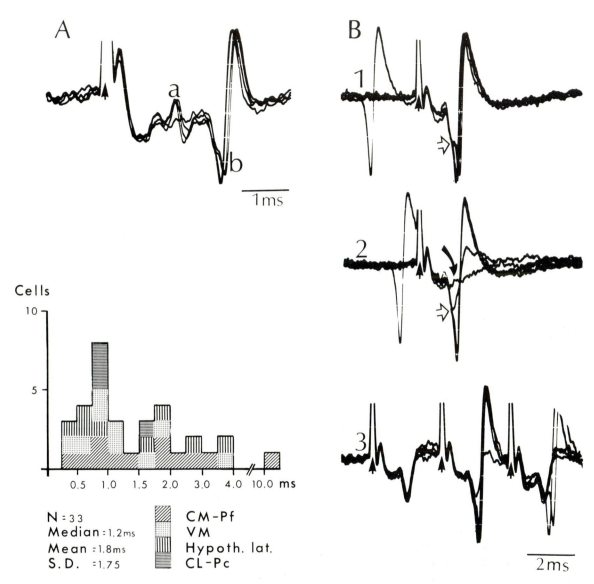

Figure 3. Antidromic identification of neurons in the lateral area of the posterior hypothalamus, centromedian parafascicular (CM-Pf), centrolateral paracentral (CL-Pc), and ventromedial (VM) thalamic neurons projecting to the midbrain central tegmental field (FTC). Stimulation was applied to the peribrachial (PB) and more rostral areas in FTC ipsilateral to the recorded diencephalic neurons. Specimen recordings of antidromic responses shown in A (neurons a and b recorded from CM-Pf) and B (neuron recorded from posterior hypothalamus). Stimulus artifacts indicated by arrows. Histogram of response latencies for antidromic responses to various sites of stimulation, as indicated by symbols. Open arrows in B point to break between initial segment (IS) and somadendritic (SD) spikes of antidromic responses. Oblique arrow in B2 shows collision of antidromic response with a preceding spontaneous discharge. Modified from Paré *et al.*, (1989b).

in the reciprocal pathway from the midbrain core to the ZI (Ropert and Steriade, 1981).

The caudally directed ZI axons may eventually synapse with colliculopontine neurons (Edwards, 1975) involved in eye movement commands, with brainstem reticular neurons projecting to the anterior or lateral funiculi of the spinal cord (Tohyama *et al.,* 1979a,b) that are involved in phasic and/or postural events of axial and limb musculature, and also with brainstem reticular neurons with ascending axons and arousing properties. The probable involvement of these projections in motor operations was shown by significantly increased firing rates of antidromically identified ZI–brainstem neurons during epochs with waking movements, as compared with periods without movements (Steriade *et al.,* 1982b). And a large proportion of ZI neurons of monkey were found to be activated when the animal reached for objects of interest (Crutcher *et al.,* 1980). The speculation may then be advanced that the reciprocal pathway between ZI and the upper brainstem reticular core is one of the elements that contribute to the attendance to relevant stimuli and thus prepare the motor commands.

3.1.2.2. Hypothalamic Areas

Massive retrograde labeling is observed in the ventromedial and ventrolateral parts of the posterior hypothalamus of the cat after HRP injections in the rostral midbrain reticular formation or, more caudally, in the peribrachial area at the midbrain–pontine junction (Steriade *et al.,* 1982b; Paré *et al.,* 1989b; Fig. 5). The paraventricular hypothalamic nucleus has even more widely distributed projections, extending to a series of brainstem core nuclei as well as to the spinal cord (Holstege, 1987). The descending projections from the paraventricular and lateral hypothalamic nuclei were also traced to the rat parabrachial nucleus and related to the presence of substance-P-like immunoreactivity in axon terminals that form asymmetric synapses with dendrites of parabrachial neurons (Milner and Pickel, 1986). The projections from the posterior hypothalamus, an area that has been strongly implicated in alertness (see Section 1.3.1), may be related to defense–aggression instinctive behavior elicited from the hypothalamus (Chi and Flynn, 1971) and are a possible source of tonic impingement on midbrain reticular neurons involved in the maintenance of thalamocortical activation processes (see Chapter 11).

The projections from the anterior hypothalamus to the midbrain reticular core arise in the medial and lateral parts of the preoptic area (Mizuno *et al.,* 1969; Morrell *et al.,* 1981; Swanson *et al.,* 1987). During the early 1960s the preoptic area was hypothesized to be an active sleep-promoting structure and to exert this role by an inhibitory influence on the rostral brainstem reticular neurons (see Section 1.3.2). However, recordings of midbrain neuronal responses to preoptic stimuli in the nonanesthetized animal showed direct excitatory actions (Ropert and Steriade, 1981), much the same as with the other inputs onto brainstem reticular cells.* Other afferents originate in the suprachiasmatic nuclei

---

*The only inhibitory inputs from extrabrainstem structures to brainstem reticular neurons are plausibly those from the GABAergic reticular thalamic neurons (see Fig. 4) and those from the basal forebrain neurons (see Fig. 6). The latter elements use as synaptic transmitter(s) GABA and/or ACh, which presumably exert hyperpolarizing actions on brainstem neurons surrounding the brachium conjunctivum (see Section 3.1.2.3). Both reticular thalamic and basal forebrain neurons may represent dampening factors in preventing the overexcitation of rostral brainstem reticular neurons on arousal.

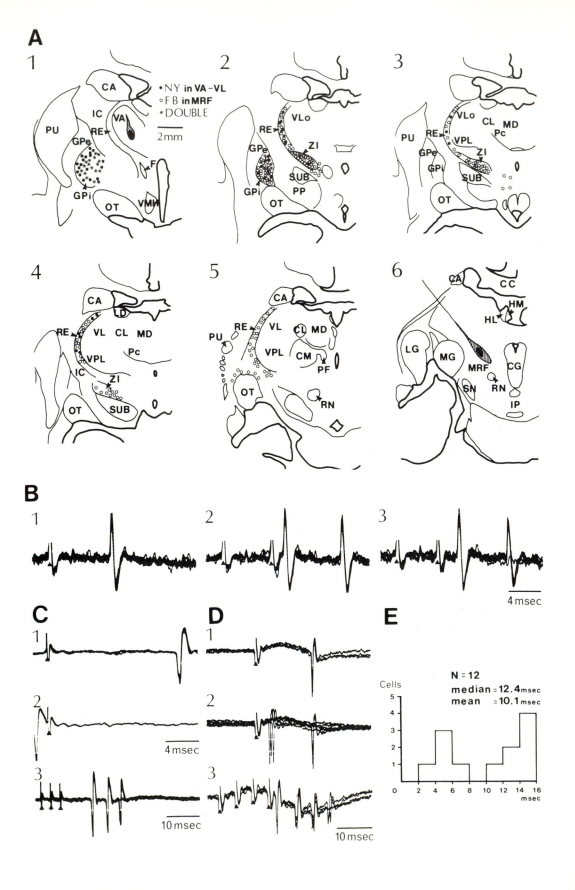

(Kucera and Favrod, 1979; Stephan *et al.*, 1981). Suprachiasmatic nuclei display circadian periodicity in action potential generation (Inouye and Kawamura, 1979), and lesions of these hypothalamic nuclei are followed by a disruption of normally occurring oscillation between non-REM sleep and REM sleep states (Ibuka *et al.*, 1977; Yamoaka, 1978). The link between suprachiasmatic nuclei and the brainstem oscillator of sleep states has not yet been elucidated.

3.1.2.3. Basal Forebrain and Related Systems

The basal forebrain consists of a series of structures, such as substantia innominata whose magnocellular elements constitute the nucleus basalis (NB) of Meynert, the vertical and horizontal branch of diagonal band nuclei (DBv and DBh, respectively), and the medial septum. These nuclei contain cholinergic and noncholinergic (among them GABAergic) neurons (see Section 1.3.2). Recent morphological and electrophysiological studies have disclosed reciprocal projections between the basal forebrain and the rostral brainstem reticular formation as well as monoaminergic nuclei. We discuss here the basal forebrain inputs to the upper reticular core. As the amygdaloid complex receives projections from cholinergic (Kitt *et al.*, 1987) and GABAergic (Zaborski *et al.*, 1986) basal forebrain neurons and, in turn, send axons back to this input source (Russchen *et al.*, 1985), we also mention the projections from the amygdala to the rostral reticular core, because such connections may be involved in the organization of some phasic events that are characteristic of REM sleep state.

The projection from the basal forebrain to the brainstem reticular core was disclosed by means of retrograde HRP tracing in rat and squirrel monkey (Divac, 1975). This projection was confirmed in rat with the method of anterogradely transported PHA-L and was found to terminate in and around the peribrachial (PB) area of the pedunculopontine nucleus (Swanson *et al.*, 1984) and in the laterodorsal tegmental (LDT) nucleus (Satoh and Fibiger, 1986). The PB and LDT nuclei mainly consist of cholinergic neurons and are termed Ch5 and Ch6 groups in the nomenclature introduced by Mesulam *et al.* (1983).

Recently, experiments were undertaken in cat and monkey by combining ChAT immunohistochemistry with the retrograde transport of WHA–HRP to determine the amount of cholinergic basal forebrain neurons with brainstem projections, and with retrograde double labeling by means of fluorescent tracers to determine the degree of collateralization of basal forebrain axons directed to the brainstem, thalamus, and cerebral cortex (Parent *et al.*, 1988).

Figure 4. Midbrain projections of thalamic reticular (RE) neurons in monkey and cat. A: Schematic drawings illustrating retrograde labeling after injections of fluorescent tracers in squirrel monkey. Nuclear yellow (NY) was injected in ventroanterior–ventrolateral (VA–VL) thalamic complex (panel 1), and fast blue (FB) was injected in the peribrachial (PB) area of the midbrain reticular formation (MRF; panel 6). Various symbols are indicated in 1. Retrograde labeling of RE neurons projecting to MRF is shown in panels 2 to 5. Note lack of double-labeled neurons in RE nucleus as compared to a large number of double-labeled neurons in internal part of globus pallidus (GPi; panels 1 and 2). B to D: Antidromic identification of three different RE thalamic neurons projecting to MRF in the cat. Note fixed latencies, collision with spontaneously occurring (C2) or orthodromically evoked (D2) discharges, and faithful following of fast stimuli (B2, C3, and D3). Median and mean of antidromic response latencies in a sample of 12 RE neurons are shown in E. Latencies were measures from the middle of the initial phase of stimulus artifact (arrowheads) and initiation of discharge. Modified from Parent and Steriade (1984).

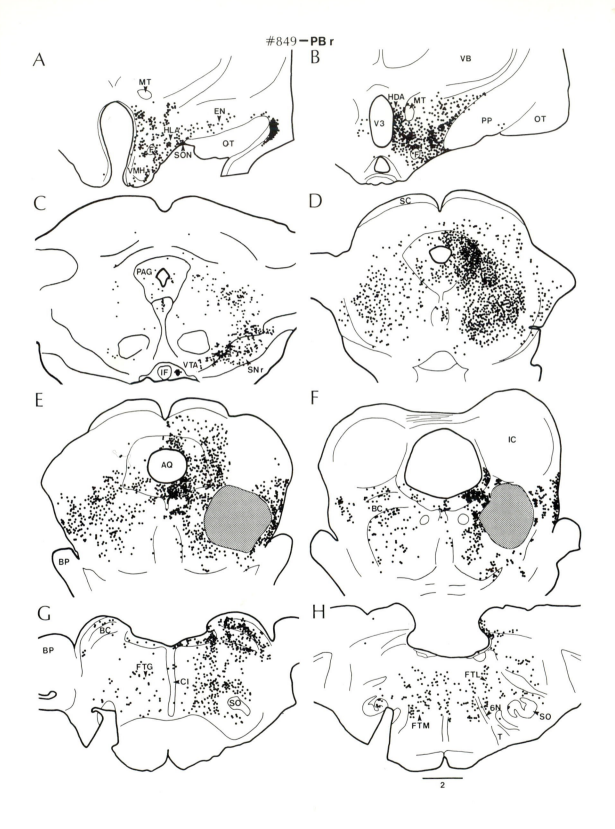

After WGA–HRP injections in the brainstem PB area, numerous retrogradely labeled cells were found in the preoptic area, a moderate number in
substantia innominata, and a small number in the ventrolateral part of the DBh,
but only 10% of HRP-positive cells in NB of substantia innominata were identified as cholinergic. The candidate transmitter of the remaining, large majority
of basal forebrain neurons with brainstem projections is probably GABA, since
numerous GABAergic elements are found intermingled with cholinergic cells in
DB nuclei and in substantia innominata of rat and squirrel monkey (Nagai *et al.*,
1983; Brashear *et al.*, 1986; Smith *et al.*, 1987). Electrophysiological studies show
that both excitatory and inhibitory responses are recorded in pedunculopontine
(or PB) neurons after stimulation of the substantia innominata (Swanson *et al.*,
1984). The probable transmitter for inhibition is GABA, but excitatory responses are not necessarily evoked by ACh since *in vitro* studies revealed that
ACh exerts hyperpolarizing actions on neurons surrounding the brachium conjunctivum in the rat (Egan and North, 1986a; Leonard and Llinás, 1989).

After simultaneous injections of the fluorescent dyes fast blue (FB) in the
brainstem PB area and nuclear yellow (NY) in the rostrolateral part of the RE
thalamic nucleus, about 10% of all retrogradely labeled neurons in the substantia
innominata and adjacent structures of the same family contained both FB and
NY tracers (Fig. 6). Double labeling was not obtained, however, when FB was
injected in the PB area and NY was injected either in other thalamic territories
or in the cerebral cortex.

Reciprocal connections also exist between the upper brainstem reticular
areas (such as the peribrachial, parabrachial, and LDT nuclei) and amygdala
nuclei (Hopkins and Holstege, 1978; Takeuchi *et al.*, 1982). The bulk of amygdaloid projections to those areas at the midbrain–pontine junction arise in the
central nuclei of the amygdala (CNA). During REM sleep of cat, CNA stimulation significantly increases the number of PGO waves and their cluster density
(Calvo *et al.*, 1987). It is known that the final common path for transmission of
PGO waves to the thalamus originates in and around the peribrachial area (see
Section 1.1 and Chapter 9). The amygdala-induced facilitation of this phasic
component of REM sleep in cat may be related to the elicitation of dreaming
sensations by electrical stimulation of amygdala and other limbic structures in
man (Halgren *et al.*, 1978).

3.1.2.4. Neocortical Areas

Golgi studies, anterograde degeneration, and retrograde tracing techniques
showed that the projections of neocortical neurons to the brainstem core mainly

Figure 5. Posterior hypothalamic and brainstem core afferents to the peribrachial (PB) area in the
cat. A to H: Eight frontal sections, rostral to caudal. The site of WGA–HRP injection shown in panels
E and F. Each dot represents one retrogradely labeled neuron. Note, in A and B, retrograde labeling
in dorsomedial, ventromedial and lateral areas of the posterior hypothalamus (HDA, VMH, HLA,
respectively). Retrograde labeling in substantia nigra pars reticulata (SNr) shown in C. Note massive
retrograde labeling in deep layers of the superior colliculus (SC) and the midbrain central gray and
central tegmental field, both ipsilaterally and contralaterally to the injection site (D and E). Retrograde labeling also seen in the caudal pontine gigantocellular tegmental field (FTG), magnocellular
field (FTM), and lateral tegmental field (FTL), ipsilaterally and contralaterally (G and H). Horizontal
bar indicates millimeters. Modified from Paré *et al.*, (1989b).

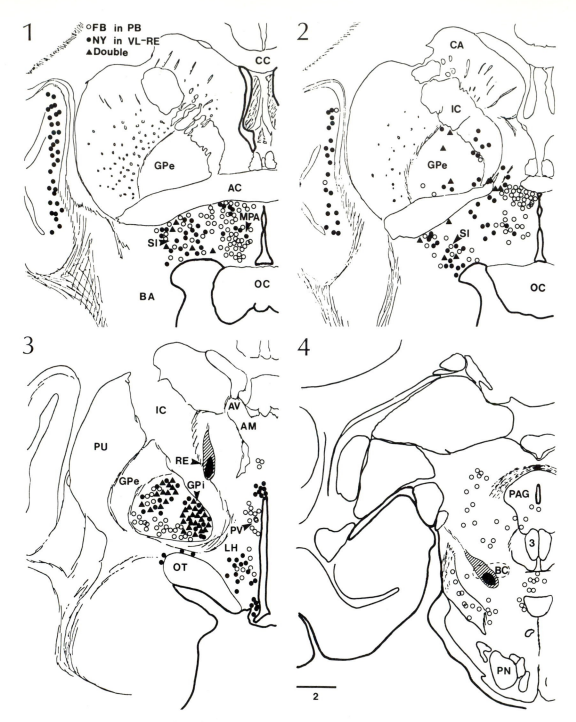

Figure 6. Basal forebrain neurons with branching axons to the RE thalamic nucleus and brainstem PB area in the squirrel monkey. Drawings of four transverse sections through the basal forebrain (1–3) and upper brainstem (4) showing the injection sites and the distribution of retrogradely labeled cells after injection of the fluorescent tracers fast blue (FB) in the PB area and nuclear yellow (NY) in the rostrolateral sector of the RE thalamic nucleus. The symbols are explained in the upper left portion of the figure, and the injection sites are illustrated by dark and hatched areas. From Parent *et al.* (1988).

arise in motor–sensory areas and terminate in the midbrain reticular formation and in pontomedullary reticular fields (Rossi and Brodal, 1956; Kuypers, 1958; Valverde, 1962; Catsman-Berrevoets and Kuypers, 1975, 1981). This projection is excitatory, as all of the 20% of midbrain reticular formation neurons that responded to cortical stimulation (51 out of 243 tested neurons) were directly excited, the great majority being activated at latencies shorter than 5 msec (Ropert and Steriade, 1981). The corticoreticular feedback projections have been implicated in the maintenance of the alert condition (see Section 1.3.1).

3.1.2.5. Convergent Inputs onto Single Brainstem Reticular Neurons

The convergence of various types of inputs from sensory pathways and central structures onto lower brainstem reticular neurons has been demonstrated by the Scheibels in Moruzzi's laboratory (Scheibel *et al.,* 1955). Those rhombencephalic reticular cells may periodically function as part of one network and then of another network, as they display cyclic variations in responsiveness to multiple volleys of somatic and visceral origin (Scheibel and Scheibel, 1965). The midbrain reticular neurons are the site of convergences between inputs arising in the cerebral cortex, preoptic area, some thalamic nuclei, and bulbar reticular formation (Steriade, 1981). Figure 7 shows that the responses of midbrain reticular neurons display very slight latency dispersion and may follow high-rate volleys. More importantly, the common feature of midbrain reticular neurons receiving multiple converging inputs is the dissimilar discharge patterns and temporal evolution of the excitatory–inhibitory sequence evoked in the same neuron by several testing stimuli (Fig. 7A). This suggests that each of those inputs reaches different parts of the somadendritic membrane and differentially sets into motion various sources of inhibition acting on midbrain neurons. Synaptic convergences from multiple sites were more often seen in midbrain reticular neurons that remained unidentified by antidromic invasion than in midbrain reticular neurons with antidromically identified projections to distant sites (Fig. 7B,C).

3.2. Afferents from Intrabrainstem Sources to the Reticular Formation

3.2.1. Afferents to the Pontine Reticular Formation

3.2.1.1. Anatomic Studies

In examining the afferents to the pontine reticular formation (PRF), it is helpful to provide an overview by describing a recent HRP/WGA–HRP study that systematically tabulated the relative percentage of retrogradely labeled neurons in the different regions sending projections to PRF in the rat (Shammah-Lagnado *et al.,* 1987). In looking at these data it must be kept in mind that the "relative percentage of projecting neurons," although an essential measure, is only one way of measuring importance of connections to PRF. Other chapters in this monograph make clear the importance of neuronal groups with particular

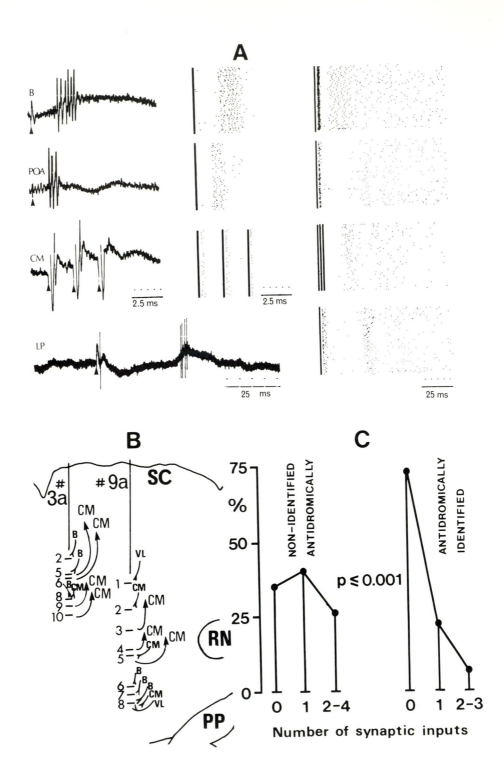

chemical codings that may powerfully modulate excitability and be of consequent importance for behavioral state changes, although the number of projecting neurons is relatively few; the cholinergic neurons discussed in Chapter 4 are excellent examples. Shammah-Lagnado *et al.* (1987) studied retrogradely labeled neurons from what they termed "the medial magnocellular pontine reticular formation," which included a rostral non-giant-cell portion (FTP in the nomenclature of Berman, 1968), which they termed nucleus reticularis pontis oralis (RPO), and a giant cell portion, the caudal nucleus reticularis pontis caudalis (RPC), corresponding to the giant-cell field (FTG) of Berman. In our illustration of the results we will follow their use of RPO and RPC.

The major finding was that almost one half of the labeled neurons come from regions within the brainstem reticular core, including the midbrain, intrapontine connections, and bulbar reticular formation. These data provide a strong anatomic basis for the recent physiological data (discussed below) indicating dense reticuloreticular connections and point to dense reticuloreticular connectivity as a major feature of reticular formation. Crossed, contralateral, and homotopic reticuloreticular input is important for both caudal and rostral PRF; this input constitutes 7–13% of the labeled neurons. There is also a dense interconnectivity between rostral and caudal PRF (8–14% of labeled neurons). Midbrain input is predominantly ipsilateral and from the area designated by Berman as FTC, with some input from nucleus cuneiformis. Bulbar input is predominantly from the giant cell field (BFTG), with some input from ventralis, parvocellularis, paragigantocellularis, and magnocellularis areas.

With respect to nonbrainstem input, the diencephalic zona incerta and field of Forel provide the most important rostral input (14%) to RPO and 4% to RPC. This diencephalic zone may be regarded as a rostral extension of the brainstem reticular core.

Cerebral corticoreticular connections, primarily from frontal lobe, account for 5% of the labeled neurons. The superior colliculus is the source of 15% of neurons with input to both rostral (ipsilateral predominance) and caudal portions of PRF (contralateral predominance). The central gray of midbrain, predominantly periaqueductal gray (including what was termed the midbrain extrapyramidal area by Rye and colleagues, 1988), contains 10% of neurons with projections to RPO and 4% of neurons with projections to RPC. Cerebellum contributes 2%. The spinal cord is the source of 13% of neurons with input to RPC but of very few projecting to RPO.

Figure 7. Convergent synaptic excitation of midbrain reticular neurons in cat. A: A neuron in central tegmental field was excited synaptically following stimulation of the bulbar reticular formation (B), preoptic area (POA), center median (CM) and lateral posterior (LP) thalamic nuclei. Original spikes (left) and 50-sweep dotgrams at fast (middle) and slow speed (right) to show dissimilar latencies, discharge patterns, and suppressed firing–rebound sequences following stimulation of different sites; three-shock train to the CM. B: Two descents (3a and 9a) drawn from sagittal sections (lateral plane 3). Target structures (oblique arrows) were identified by antidromic invasion, and excitatory inputs (forked symbols) were recognized from synaptically elicited discharges at short latencies. PP, pes pedunculi; RN, red nucleus; SC, superior colliculus; VL, ventrolateral thalamic nucleus. The graph in C depicts the percentage (ordinate) of cells with various degrees of synaptic convergence in two neuronal populations (which could not be or have been antidromically identified from structures outside the midbrain reticular formation). 0 indicates neurons that have not been synaptically excited, and 1–4 indicate the number of stimulated sites that induced synaptic excitation. Modified from Steriade *et al.* (1980) and Ropert and Steriade (1981).

With respect to projections from nuclei suspected of roles in modulating reticular excitability, retrogradely labeled neurons were found in dorsal raphe, raphe magnus, locus coeruleus, laterodorsal tegmental nucleus, and parabrachial complex.

The main findings were essentially paralleled in a study in the cat (Leichnetz *et al.*, 1987), which used a transcannular method of depositing WGA–HRP (in an attempt to avoid labeling of fibers of passage) in the medial pontine reticular formation.

3.2.1.2. Electrophysiology of Inputs from Other Brainstem Reticular Formation Areas to the Pontine Gigantocellular Tegmental Field

A series of studies has also been done by Ito and McCarley (1987) and McCarley *et al.* (1987) surveying the physiological nature of input to pontine FTG by means of intracellular recording in PFTG in the unanesthetized, undrugged animal and with microstimulation of other brainstem reticular areas. The initial, monosynaptic responses of medial pontine reticular neurons to microstimulation of bulbar (Ito and McCarley, 1987), contralateral pontine, and midbrain (McCarley *et al.*, 1987) reticular formation are initially depolarizing excitatory postsynaptic potentials (EPSPs) in proportions from 75% to 90%. The initial PSPs that were IPSPs evoked by midbrain or contralateral pontine stimulation represented only about 4% of responses, statistically significantly less than the IPSPs in response to stimulation of the bulbar gigantocellular or magno-

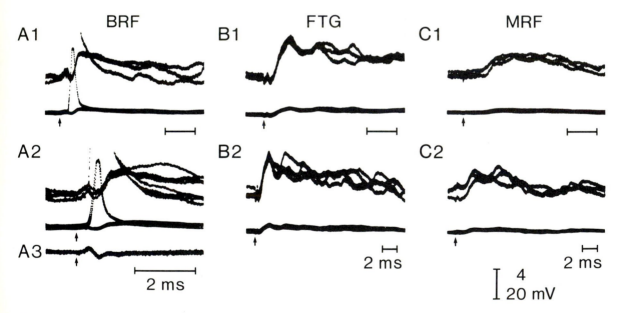

Figure 8. Typical responses of an intracellularly recorded medial pontine reticular formation neuron to microstimulation of bulbar reticular formation (BRF, column A), contralateral pontine giant cell field (cFTG, column B), and mesencephalic reticular formation (MRF, column C). Part A3 shows the extracellular field response following BRF stimulation (4 mV calibration); note, in particular, the presence of an antidromic field potential temporally coincident with the antidromic responses shown in A1 and A2 (A2 has same time base as A3). Antidromic field potentials are also seen in the intracellular potential records with cFTG stimulation (column B) but not with MRF stimulation (column C). Note the presence of short-latency EPSPs in all records; stimulation of BRF and cFTG produces EPSPs with a faster rise time than with stimulation of MRF. Adapted from McCarley *et al.* (1987).

cellular tegmental fields (about 12%). The shape of the EPSPs varied as a function of the stimulated sites: the EPSPs from the contralateral pontine and the bulbar reticular fields had a rapid rise time and a relatively constant latency, whereas those evoked by midbrain reticular stimulation had a less rapid rise time and a longer plateau (Fig. 8). These results were collected from pontine neurons that, in a subsample with intracellular HRP labeling, proved to have in their great majority (80%) a soma diameter greater than 40 μm (McCarley et al., 1987).

At variance with data on midbrain reticular neurons that suggested a relative segregation between receivers of multiple inputs and projection neurons (Ropert and Steriade, 1981; see Fig. 7), the intracellular studies of pontine reticular neurons suggest an identity of input and output pontine reticular neurons with respect to synaptic response properties (Ito and McCarley, 1987; McCarley et al., 1987). The type and latency of initial PSPs in pontine reticular neurons are diagramatically indicated in Fig. 3.9.

3.2.1.3. Electrophysiology of Intrinsic Pontobulbar Reticular Formation Connections in Morphologically Characterized Neurons

The anatomic data described above indicate the presence of dense and reciprocal pontobulbar interconnections but do not, of course, indicate whether these are excitatory or inhibitory or whether there is any input differentiation for neurons with different projection pathways, such as those with and without axons in medial longitudinal fasciculus (MLF) and ventral funiculus (VF), the

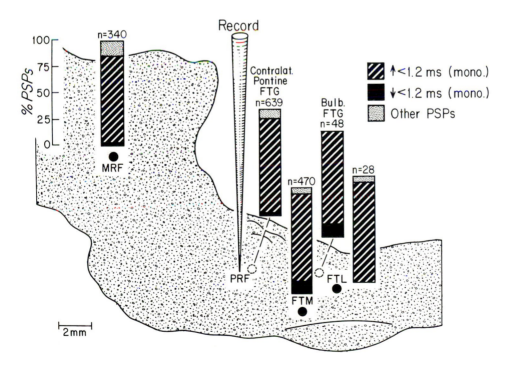

Figure 9. Summary of type and latency of initial PSPs produced in mPRF neurons by stimulation of various reticular regions. Note (1) the presence of dense monosynaptic excitatory input from almost all reticular regions and (2) that the maximum percentages of monosynaptic inhibitory PSPs occur with stimulation of bulbar FTM and FTG. Adapted from McCarley et al. (1987).

medial reticulospinal projection pathway. Electrophysiological studies performed by Mitani, McCarley, and co-workers on the same neurons, morphologically characterized with intracellular HRP injections, have answered these questions.

Pontine FTG neurons uniformly respond to stimulation of the bulbar FTG with an initial short-latency excitatory postsynaptic potential (EPSP) response that has the short latency, rapid rise time, and faithful following indicative of monosynaptic connections. This is true of PFTG neurons identified by intracellular HRP injection as sending axons in MLF (Fig. 10) and also of those sending axons into bulbar reticular formation when no antidromic response was present (Fig. 11).

Similarly, bulbar FTG neurons respond to microstimulation of the ipsilateral pontine FTG with initial EPSPs that also have the characteristics of

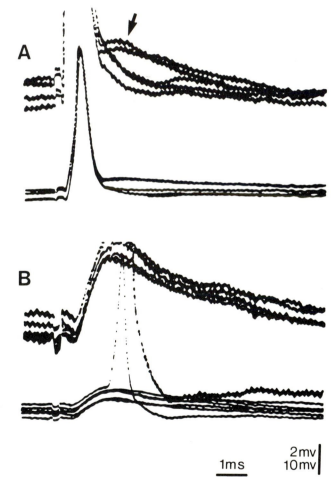

2mv
1ms   10mv

Figure 10. Intracellular recording of a pontine gigantocellular field neuron with axon descending in MLF (intracellular HRP labeling). A: Antidromic spike potentials with a latency of 0.3 msec were elicited by MLF stimulation; EPSPs (solid arrow) were also produced. B: EPSPs with a monosynaptic latency of 0.7 msec were evoked by microstimulation of bulbar FTG. AC-coupled recordings in upper traces in A and B (calibration bar = 2 mV) and DC-coupled recordings in lower traces (calibration bar = 10 mV). Resting membrane potential was −58 mV. Adapted from Mitani *et al.* (1988b).

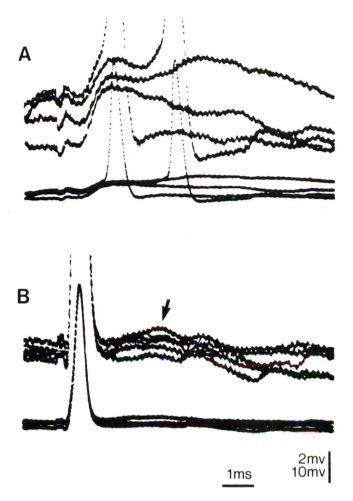

Figure 11. Intracellular recording of a pontine gigantocellular field neuron with axon descending in BRF (intracellular HRP labeling). A; EPSPs with a latency of 0.8 msec were evoked by MLF stimulation; antidromic spike potentials were not present. B: Antidromic spike potentials with a latency of 0.35 msec were evoked by stimulation of bulbar FTG; EPSPs (solid arrow) were also produced. Calibration and AC and DC coupling as in Fig. 10. Adapted from Mitani *et al.* (1988b).

monosynaptic responses. This initial monosynaptic EPSP response to PFTG microstimulation is seen in all types of BFTG neurons identified by intracellular HRP injection, including those sending axons to MLF and those with axons descending in the bulbar reticular formation (Fig. 12). Longer-latency hyperpolarizing responses frequently followed these initial EPSPs in both bulbar and pontine neurons.*

*From the data of these and other connectivity studies using electrical stimulation (e.g., Eccles *et al.*, 1976), one cannot alone determine whether the recorded PSP is from stimulation of neuronal somata or fibers of passage, even at low current levels and with minimal current spread. The percentage of initial excitatory PSPs, however, is so high for reticular stimulation and recording sites within reticular formation that regardless of any fibers of passage the presence of excitatory reticuloreticular synapses is suggested, especially since input from other reticular zones is known to predominate in reticular formation (see Section 3.2.1.1).

3.2.2. Afferents to the Midbrain and Bulbar Reticular Formation

CHAPTER 3

3.2.2.1. Reticuloreticular Connections

After the demonstration, based on Golgi staining, of long-axoned neurons coursing from the lower to the upper brainstem reticular core (Scheibel and Scheibel, 1958), autoradiographic studies have shown projections from rhombencephalic reticular nuclei to the upper brainstem core (Graybiel, 1977a) and from the midbrain reticular formation to the rostral pons and, less substantially, to the bulbar reticular formation (Edwards, 1975). An autoradiographic and retrograde transport study that focused on the bulbopontine reticular projections of the rat indicated that the bulbar magnocellular tegmental field projects ipsilaterally to the ventromedial part of the pontine reticular formation (FTG zone) with a decreasing density of projections toward more rostral pontine sites, whereas the rostral portions of the bulbar gigantocellular field send bilateral projections throughout the pons and, further, to the forebrain (Zemlan *et al.,* 1984). Reticuloreticular projections from pontine sites to bulbar FTG have recently been quantified (Mitani *et al.,* 1988a) and found to be most dense from

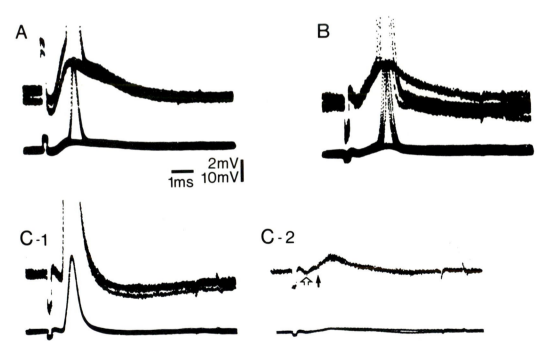

Figure 12. Intracellular recordings of bulbar gigantocellular reticular formation neurons labeled by intracellular HRP injections. Part A is from a neuron sending its axon in contralateral MLF (cMFL neuron); part B from a neuron with axon coursing in ipsilateral MLF (iMLF neuron); and part C from a neuron with an axon coursing in ipsilateral bulbar reticular formation (iBRF neuron) and with a bifurcating axonal branch to ipsilateral pontine gigantocellular reticular formation (PFTG). In A and B, EPSPs with laten- cies of 0.5 msec (A) and 0.6 msec (B) were evoked by PFTG stimulation. C-1: In this iBRF neuron PFTG stimulation (0.10 mA) elicited antidromic spike potentials with a latency of 0.6 msec. C-2: At a lower stimulus amplitude (0.04 mA) EPSPs were elicited (solid arrow, 1.1 msec latency); open arrow shows the antidromic field component. Calibration and AC and DC coupling as in Fig. 10. Adapted from Mitani *et al.* (1988c).

pontine FTG, which accounts for 70% of the retrogradely labeled neurons, with approximately equal ipsi- and contralateral distribution. Projections from FTP, primarily contralateral, accounted for 24%, and predominantly ipsilateral projections from FTL and the parabrachial regions accounted for about 2% each.

Antidromic identification studies on bulbar reticular neurons of cat revealed that the afferents to midbrain reticular projections mainly arise in magnocellular field, whereas both magno- and gigantocellular bulbar neurons project to medial and intralaminar thalamic nuclei (Steriade *et al.,* 1984b).

Massive retrograde labeling occurs in rostral midbrain, paramedian pontine reticular formation, and gigantocellular as well as magnocellular bulbar reticular fields after WGA–HRP injections localized within the limits of the cholinergic PB area at the midbrain–pontine junction (Paré *et al.,* 1989b; see Fig. 5 in Section 3.1.2.2).

In earlier electrophysiological studies, some controversial data resulted from attempts at characterizing the nature of these reticuloreticular projections. The IPSPs described in lower brainstem reticular neurons as responses to midbrain stimulation (Ito *et al.,* 1970) were contrary to the midbrain-evoked short-latency (1–3 msec) depolarizing potentials in bulbar reticular neurons (Mancia *et al.,* 1974). The IPSPs could well be caused by collaterals in the ascending pathway (toward unidentified inhibitory sources) since the antidromic invasion of medullary neurons from the midbrain occurred before the IPSP (Ito *et al.,* 1970). On the other hand, the IPSPs produced in midbrain reticular cells by bulbar stimulation (Mancia *et al.,* 1974) and interpreted in the light of the hypothesized inhibitory linkage from the lower to the upper brainstem reticular core (see Section 1.3.2) may be ascribed to costimulation of medullary monoaminergic neurons. Indeed, immunohistochemically identified adrenergic neurons project to rostral sites at the midbrain–pontine junction (Guyenet and Young, 1987; see also Section 3.3.1).

Studies conducted in chronically implanted behaving cats reported monosynaptic excitatory responses of midbrain reticular neurons to pontine or bulbar reticular stimulation (Ropert and Steriade, 1981).

3.2.2.2. Reciprocal Connections between Reticular Nuclei and Substantia Nigra

The connections between substantia nigra (especially its pars reticulata, SNr) and brainstem reticular nuclei, in particular the peribrachial (PB) area of the pedunculopontine nucleus, are direct or through an intermediate relay in the superior colliculus (SC). These connections play a key role in some physiological correlates of behavioral states of vigilance.

The reciprocal connections between SNr and PB were established by means of anterograde and retrograde tracing techniques (Jackson and Crossman, 1981; Beckstead and Frankfurter, 1982; Saper and Loewy, 1982; Beckstead, 1983; Moon-Edley and Graybiel, 1983; Sugimoto and Hattori, 1984) as well as by intracellular analysis (Noda and Oka, 1984). Small HRP injections localized in the lateral and dorsal parts of the PB nucleus led to retrograde labeling mostly in SNr, with only occasional cells lying in the pars compacta of SN (Moon-Edley and Graybiel, 1983). The reciprocal connections are reflected electrophysiologically by antidromic activation of midbrain–pontine neurons surrounding the brachium conjunctivum (PB cells) after SN stimulation, suppression of PB-cell discharge by SN stimulation (SNr cells are GABAergic), and prevalently excitatory effects in SN neurons by PB stimulation (Scarnati *et al.,* 1987). The latter study was conducted in chronically decorticated rats to preclude axon-reflex activation of descending corticofugal fibers giving off collaterals to both SN and PB.

The indirect connections between SNr and PB are mediated by a relay of SNr axons in the SC. The nigrotectal pathway was studied by retrograde tracing methods (Rinvik *et al.,* 1976; Graybiel, 1978a,b; May and Hall, 1986). A comparative analysis showed that, in the rat, the SNr–SC projection arises in a ventral stratum of SNr and is almost exclusively ipsilateral, whereas crossed SNr–SC projections are visible in the cat and even more substantially in the monkey (Beckstead *et al.,* 1981). The GABAergic nature of SNr–tectal pathway was revealed by combined retrograde tracing and histochemical techniques (Childs and Gale, 1983; Araki *et al.,* 1984), and the inhibitory effects on SC neurons were assessed by SNr stimulation and GABA iontophoresis (Chevalier *et al.,* 1981a,b). In turn, the cells in intermediate and deep SC layers send axons caudally that give off collaterals to the PB area (Grantyn and Grantyn, 1982; see Fig. 2).

The SNr–SC connection is involved in orienting reactions. Novel sensory stimuli are accompanied by a decrease in the firing rates of SNr cells, which releases from inhibition the target SC neurons and eventually leads (through SC projections to premotor pontine reticular neurons) to eye movements toward the signal (Hikosaka and Wurtz, 1983a,b). On the other hand, the inhibitory projections from SNr neurons to PB neurons may be one of the decisive factors for hyperpolarizing some PB elements during REM sleep. The consequence would be postinhibitory rebound bursts that are indeed the characteristic discharge patterns of a few PB elements, known as PGO-on burst neurons (see Chapter 9).

3.3. Afferents to Brainstem Monoaminergic Nuclei

3.3.1. Locus Coeruleus

Until 3 years ago, the locus coeruleus (LC) was described as a site of convergence from a great variety of pathways. The retrograde HRP transport experiments by Cederbaum and Aghajanian (1978) were performed in rat, a species in which LC is well defined and is homogeneously composed of NEergic elements. A series of manipulations were undertaken to ascertain the accurate placement of the HRP deposit, such as recording of single cells with discharges (fairly regular, with a rate of 0.5–5 Hz) known to characterize LC neurons and control injections in adjacent structures, including the parabrachial nucleus. That study reported that afferents to LC arise in the marginal zones of the dorsal horn of the spinal cord, fastigial nuclei of the cerebellum, various brainstem nuclei (the solitary tract nuclei, medullary areas that correspond to A1–A2 catecholamine groups, several cell groups located dorsal and lateral to the superior olive, the dorsal raphe nucleus, and parts of classical reticular fields), paraventricular and lateral hypothalamic areas, medial and lateral preoptic areas, the central nucleus of amygdala, and a highly restricted band of cerebral cortex containing areas 13 and 14 around and dorsal to the rhinal sulcus.

In cat, similar afferents from medullary (presumed catecholaminergic) cell groups and hypothalamus reach the ventrolateral part of the LC, whereas the dorsomedial or principal part of the LC receives afferents from the contralateral LC, fastigial nuclei, dorsal raphe nucleus, and mesencephalic central gray but not from the bulbar reticular formation or the pontine gigantocellular field (Sakai *et al.*, 1977b), although more sensitive WGA–HRP methods indicate projections from these reticular zones (A. Mitani and R. McCarley, unpublished data). The projection from the midbrain reticular formation to the LC of cat was also documented with the anterograde labeling method (Edwards, 1975).

The projection from the dorsal raphe is probably one of the sources of immunocytochemically identified serotonergic fibers that surround the perikarya and dendrites of NEergic LC neurons (Pickel *et al.*, 1977). The sources of other inputs, among them those originating in various hypothalamic areas and/or the brainstem medullary core, are neurons containing enkephalin and substance P (Pickel *et al.*, 1979), β-endorphin (Bloom *et al.*, 1978), or neurophysin (Swanson, 1977).

After these reports of afferents to LC from so many sources, from the spinal cord up to the cerebral cortex, it was recently reported that the rat LC has a restricted afferent control, mainly consisting of two medullary nuclei, paragigantocellularis and prepositus hypoglossi, the connection being predominantly ipsilateral (Aston-Jones *et al.*, 1986). The nucleus paragigantocellularis (termed PGCL by Andrezik *et al.*, 1981a,b) is located in the ventrolateral part of the medulla, is involved in processes of autonomic integration, and contains the somata of bulbospinal neurons that provide the excitatory drive to the vasoconstrictor preganglionic neurons (Guyenet and Brown, 1986). The NRPG is a pleomorphic nucleus and has neurons that contain serotonin, norepinephrine/-epinephrine, enkephalin, as well as more typically reticular neurons; a major input is the pontine and bulbar FTG, and there is also strong connectivity with regions associated with the autonomic nervous system and nociception (see Andrezik *et al.*, 1981a,b; Satoh *et al.*, 1980; Khachaturian *et al.*, 1983; Ross *et al.*, 1985; Gray and Dostrovsky, 1985; Ruggiero *et al.*, 1985). As to the nucleus prepositus hypoglossi (PH), it is involved in oculomotor system control (see Chapter 10) and is a site of afferents from quite diverse sources. Recent data suggest the PH zone may also be heterogeneous, with neurons at the rostral pole being important for LC projections (G. Aston-Jones, personal communication).

In addition to massive retrograde labeling in PGCL and PH nuclei after WGA–HRP injections in the LC, much weaker retrograde labeling was found in the paraventricular hypothalamic nucleus and intermediate gray of the spinal cord. These somewhat controversial results (Aston-Jones *et al.*, 1986) were attributed to a more precise localization of the tracer injection into the LC, whereas the previous results were ascribed to diffusion of the tracer outside the LC limits, particularly in the parabrachial nucleus. Some comments can be made with regard to these recent data: (1) the criteria used for retrograde labeling ("at least ten TMB reaction granules," p. 234) may dismiss elements with axonal collaterals, which usually display very few reaction granules (the so-called diluting collateral effect); (2) the parabrachial nucleus was injected in a control experiment by Cederbaum and Aghajanian (1978), and although retrograde labeling was found in preoptic area, ventromedial–dorsomedial hypothalamic areas, and dorsal raphe nucleus after LC injections, the same areas remain unlabeled after parabrachial injections (see Table 2 in that paper); (3) this restrictive view of LC input has also been criticized on the grounds that input to the large LC dendritic extensions outside the compact nuclear zone of the somata was neglected and that the extracellular techniques used to cross-validate input physiologically were insensitive compared with intracellular recordings, which detect PSPs as well as action potentials.

The short-latency robust excitatory responses of LC neurons (73%) to PGCL stimulation (see Fig. 4 in Aston-Jones *et al.*, 1986) have recently been characterized as subject to blocking by the excitatory amino acid (EAA) antagonists kynurenic acid and γ-D-glutamylglycine but not the more specific NMDA EAA antagonist 1-amino-7-phosphonoheptanoic acid (AP7) and the preferential quisqualate receptor antagonist glutamate diethyl ester (GDEE) (Ennis and Aston-Jones, 1988).

The nonexcitatory, suppressive responses to PGCL stimulation may result from a PGCL–LC projection originating from phenylethanolamine-N-methyltransferase-immunoreactive cells (C1 adrenergic cluster); data by Guyenet and Young (1987) and Williams *et al.* (1985; see Chapter 6) show that the effect of NE on LC cells is a powerful hyperpolarization mediated by α_2 receptors (Cederbaum and Aghajanian, 1976; Williams *et al.*, 1985). In fact, the effects exerted by PGCL on LC neurons are not simply inhibitory or excitatory because of the complexity of transmitters used by the heterogeneous PGCL neurons. After the pharmacological blockade of PGCL-evoked excitation, LC neurons display purely inhibitory responses to PGCL stimulation (Ennis and Aston-Jones, 1988) that may also be attributable to the adrenergic hyperpolarization of LC cells.

3.3.2. Raphe Nuclei

The serotonergic raphe nuclei that are mainly involved in the control of the sleep–waking cycle are raphe dorsalis, other midbrain raphe nuclei, and raphe medianus. Their major afferents seem to arise in the rostral part of the nucleus of the solitary tract, LC, substantia nigra, lateral part of posterior hypothalamus and preoptic area, lateral habenula, hippocampus, and prefrontal cortex (Nauta, 1958; Aghajanian and Wang, 1977; Sakai *et al.*, 1977a). The pathway from the lateral habenula to the dorsal raphe is inhibitory, probably GABAergic, as the effect induced by electrical stimulation of the habenula can be blocked by picrotoxin (Wang and Aghajanian, 1977).

As to the transmitter-specified afferents to the nucleus raphe dorsalis, disclosed by means of immunocytochemistry, the serotonin-immunoreactive fibers (Steinbush, 1981) originate partly in the dorsal raphe itself (Mosko *et al.*, 1977) and in other raphe nuclei. The noradrenergic fibers that make synaptic contacts with dorsal raphe neurons (Baraban and Aghajanian, 1981) probably originate in the LC.

3.3.3. Ventral Tegmental Area

Dopamine (DA)-containing neurons with connections to widespread areas of the cerebral cortex are located in the ventral tegmental area (VTA), and DA-containing neurons projecting to the striatum are located in substantia nigra pars compacta (SNc). Since we shall deal in other chapters with the dopaminergic modulation of the cerebral cortex, we refer here to the afferent connections of VTA.

In rat, they originate in LC, parabrachial nucleus, various raphe nuclei (mainly dorsalis and magnus), posterodorsal hypothalamus and preoptic area, substantia innominata and diagonal band nuclei, amygdala, nucleus accumbens, and various cortical areas, especially the dorsal bank of the rhinal sulcus and the prefrontal cortex (Phillipson, 1979). Antidromic invasion studies in rat indicate that in addition to innervating the VTA, prefrontal cortical neurons send axon collaterals to the mediodorsal thalamus, SN, and central gray (Thierry *et al.*, 1983).

In cat, VTA afferents arise in the spinal cord, deep cerebellar nuclei, several raphe nuclei, LC, mammillary nuclei, basal forebrain structures, and some cortical areas such as the medial sigmoid gyrus (Tork *et al.*, 1984).

These sources of inputs point to the VTA as a site of convergences from a variety of brain structures. In addition to the more conventional projections and transmitters, there are probably seven amines and at least ten peptides that modulate VTA neurons (cf. Oades and Halliday, 1987).

4

Efferent Connections of Brainstem Neurons

In this chapter we describe both immunohistochemically identified and nonidentified brainstem neuronal aggregates and their projections within and outside the brainstem core. We dissociate cholinergic from monoaminergic systems not only because of their chemical distinctness but also because of their dissimilar projection patterns to rostral brain structures. Whereas the ascending projections arising in brainstem cholinergic neurons are overwhelmingly relayed in the thalamus, monoaminergic neurons project much less densely to thalamic nuclei but have direct access to cortical neurons.

We first analyze the brainstem reticular nuclei, which consist of quite circumscribed populations of cholinergic neurons at the midbrain–pontine junction and a series of nuclei whose chemical transmitter(s) remain(s) largely unidentified (Section 4.1). The projections of cholinergic as well as noncholinergic brainstem reticular neurons to rostral sites (thalamus and basal forebrain) are thereafter discussed on the basis of modern tracing techniques combined with choline acetyltransferase (ChAT) immunoreactivity (Section 4.2). Brainstem and spinal cord efferents of the cholinergic mesopontine and noncholinergic pontobulbar reticular formation are discussed in Section 4.3. The intrinsic morphology of pontobulbar reticular formation neurons and the correlations with anatomic projections are discussed in Section 4.4. In the final sections (4.5 to 4.7) we discuss the nuclear arrangements of norepinephrine (NE)-containing, dopamine (DA)-containing, and serotonin (5-HT)-containing neurons and their projections to extrabrainstem (rostral and caudal) structures.

The actions of various transmitters of brainstem neurons on thalamic, cortical, and spinal cord neurons and the synaptic influences exerted on those distant targets by stimulating brainstem projection pathways are examined together with the intrabrainstem transmitter actions in Chapter 6. The hypothesized interactions between brainstem cholinergic and monoaminergic neurons that may underly oscillations in states of vigilance are discussed in Chapter 12.

4.1. Systematization of Cholinergic and Noncholinergic Brainstem Reticular and Basal Forebrain Nuclei

We first analyze the recently identified cholinergic cell groups in the brainstem reticular formation and the related basal forebrain family. The nuclear groups of neurons in the brainstem and in the basal forebrain are reciprocally connected. These morphological relationships as well as the common innervation of some thalamic nuclei by brainstem and basal forebrain cholinergic neurons play a crucial role in the cholinergic activation of thalamic and cortical processes (see Chapters 7 and 8).

The brainstem and basal forebrain nuclear systematization and cytoarchitecture described below derive from studies in rat (Mesulam *et al.*, 1983), cat (Vincent and Reiner, 1987), and macaque monkey (Mesulam *et al.*, 1984). Other studies have been focussed on distinct cholinergic nuclei in the mesopontine tegmentum and have studied the interdigitation of cholinergic with catecholamine neurons in the cat (Jones and Beaudet, 1987a) and rat (Rye *et al.*, 1987).

The nomenclature (Ch1 to Ch6) proposed by Mesulam *et al.* (1983), with subsequent additions made by the same group (Mufson *et al.*, 1986), is adopted here to designate various basal forebrain and brainstem core cholinergic nuclei. We describe in more detail cholinergic groups whose neurons are implicated in the genesis of wake–sleep states and in the regulation of state-dependent processes of sensorimotor integration. The ChAT-positive neurons of oculomotor nuclei and of other brainstem nuclei are described elsewhere (see Vincent and Reiner, 1987).

4.1.1. Basal Forebrain Cholinergic Nuclei

The cholinergic nuclei of the basal forebrain are designated Ch1 to Ch4.

The Ch1 sector consists of small-sized ChAT-positive neurons grouped in the medial septum. In both rat and monkey, the medial septum also contains a sizable proportion of noncholinergic neurons, at least half of the total neuronal population (Mesulam *et al.*, 1983). The noncholinergic cells are probably GABAergic elements (Onteniente *et al.*, 1987). Scattered single ChAT-positive neurons are also found in the lateral septum of cat (Vincent and Reiner, 1987).

The Ch2 and Ch3 sectors consists of ChAT-positive cells within, respectively, the vertical and horizontal branches of the diagonal band nuclei (DBv and DBh). These neurons are multipolar and of larger size than Ch1 neurons. Here also, cholinergic neurons are intermingled, at least in rat, with GABAergic elements (Brashear *et al.*, 1986). There are no definite boundaries between Ch2 and Ch1 or between Ch3 and the following basal forebrain sector, Ch4.

The Ch4 group mostly corresponds to nucleus basalis (NB) of Meynert, but cholinergic cells are also found in the larger region known as substantia innominata (SI) that forms a neuronal band located ventrally to the anterior commissure with extensions that surround the internal part of the globus pallidus (termed entopeduncular nucleus in cat). The Ch4 neurons are larger and hyperchromic as compared to Ch1 to Ch3 neurons, and 90% of NB cells are cholinergic in rat and monkey (Mesulam *et al.*, 1983). Caudally, SI neurons extend into the anterior part of the preoptic area and the amygdaloid complex, with few cholinergic cells within the central nucleus of amygdala in cat (Vincent and Reiner, 1987).

4.1.2. Brainstem Reticular Cholinergic Nuclei

The two brainstem cholinergic cell groups, Ch5 and Ch6, extend from the caudal part of the midbrain to the rostral pons.

The Ch5 group is located within the central tegmental field (FTC) of the caudal midbrain. In rat, many authors include it within, or simply term it, pedunculopontine tegmental nucleus (PPT). The PPT was first described in human material and thereafter in other primates. It consists of medium- to large-sized darkly stained neurons that appear from the decussation of brachii conjunctivi rostrally to the level of locus coeruleus and subcoeruleus caudally. The PPT is not a cytoarchitecturally distinct cell group in the cat (Moon-Edley and Graybiel, 1983), and its close association with the brachium conjunctivum should be emphasized. We use interchangeably the term PPT or the descriptive term of peribrachial (PB) area, part of the PPT nucleus, for the cat Ch5 group. The PB area should not be confused with the *parabrachial* nucleus, which is an elongated nuclear mass located more caudally in the brainstem and characteristically aligned lateral to the caudal portion of brachium conjunctivum. These distinctions should be kept in mind in our discussion of the cytoarchitecture and cytochemistry of PPT. Whereas the PPT is one of the major sources of generalized projections to virtually all (specific relay, associational, intralaminar, and reticular) thalamic nuclei (see Section 4.2) and to pontine and bulbar reticular formation, the parabrachial nucleus is mainly specialized in relaying taste and visceral information to the forebrain.

In cat, PPT neurons are medium-sized (soma surface 400–600 μm^2) and fusiform or polygonal in shape. A detailed analysis in rat (Rye *et al.*, 1987) showed that in Nissl-stained sections, the rostral third of the PPT nucleus consists of medium- to large-sized neurons (mean perikaryal longest axis of 20 μm), the middle third consists of smaller neurons (16 μm) with rounder shape, and the caudal third has a dense cell group (around 19 μm) that corresponds to the PPT pars compacta described in several investigations on rat. The comparative analysis of Nissl-stained and ChAT-positive neurons reached the conclusion that the large multipolar neurons in the rat PPT nucleus, as they appear on Nissl-stained sections, are entirely cholinergic neurons (Rye *et al.*, 1987). In addition to the population of medium- to large-sized cholinergic neurons, the rat PPT contains smaller noncholinergic perikarya intermingled with the cholinergic ones. The ChAT-positive neurons have angular to pyramidal somata, three to five primary radiating dendrites that divide into two or three secondary dendrites with irregularly spaced swellings resembling varicosities. The axon usually originates from a proximal dendrite.

The admixture of cholinergic and catecholaminergic neurons in the PPT area was investigated in cat (Jones and Beaudet, 1987a) and rat (Rye *et al.*, 1987) with ChAT and tyrosine hydroxylase (TH) immunohistochemical techniques on the same or adjacent sections. In cat, ChAT-positive and TH-positive cells in the

PPT area are morphologically similar, and both are medium in size. At rostral PPT levels (frontal planes anterior 2 to 0), there are very few TH-positive neurons. Significant percentages of TH-positive neurons appear at more caudal levels of the PPT (Fig. 1; Jones and Beaudet, 1987a). Within the *parabrachial* nucleus, TH-positive neurons are as numerous as ChAT-positive neurons. In rat, the rostral pole of the PPT cell group is distinct from the TH-positive cells belonging to the substantia nigra (SN) and retrorubral field (respectively A9 and A8 groups of monoamine-containing neurons), but the dendritic arbors of PPT neurons overlap with those of the most caudal SN cells. In the middle part of the PPT, its medial aspect is traversed by TH-positive ascending axons. And in the caudal third of the PPT, ChAT-positive neurons are admixed with TH-positive perikarya extending from the rostral pole of the locus coeruleus (Rye *et al.*, 1987). Thus, it seems that both in cat and rat a significant population of TH-positive neurons only appears within the caudal third of PPT.

In both cat and rat, the caudal part of the PPT merges dorsomedially into the Ch6 group (laterodorsal tegmental nucleus, LDT), embedded in the periaqueductal–periventricular gray (Fig. 2). In cat, the cholinergic LDT neurons are similar in size to PPT neurons but more roundish in shape. As in the rostral part of the PPT area, the number of ChAT-positive neurons by far exceeds that of TH-positive neurons in the LDT nucleus (Jones and Beaudet, 1987a).

Approximately 15% to 30% of rat PPT and LDT cholinergic neurons also display substance P, corticotropin-releasing factor (CRF), bombesin/gastrin-releasing peptide, and atriopeptinlike immunoreactivity (Vincent *et al.*, 1983, 1986; Saper *et al.*, 1985; Standaert *et al.*, 1986). Many PPT and LDT cholinergic cells also display intense nicotinamide adenine dinucleotide phosphate (NADPH)–diaphorase activity in double-staining experiments (Vincent *et al.*, 1986). The functional significance of ChAT and neuropeptide colocalization is still obscure. Because cholinergic neurons in Ch5–Ch6 cell groups are strongly implicated in processes of thalamocortical activation (see Section 4.2 and Chapter 11), it may be of interest to mention that bombesin and CRF can produce EEG and/or behavioral signs of arousal (Sutton *et al.*, 1982; Ehlers *et al.*, 1983; Rasler, 1984).

In addition to Ch5–Ch6 groups, virtually all neurons in the parabigeminal (PBG) nucleus, located at the extreme lateral part of the midbrain tegmentum, are cholinergic. The PBG nucleus was designated as Ch8 by Mufson *et al.* (1986) in their experiments on mouse and was also identified as a cholinergic nucleus in the cat (Vincent and Reiner, 1987; Smith *et al.*, 1988). The PBG projects to the superior colliculus (Graybiel, 1978b) and to lamina C of the lateral geniculate thalamic nucleus (Hughes and Mullikin, 1984). WGA–HRP retrograde tracing combined with ChAT immunoreactivity revealed that cholinergic neurons are the sources of the PBG–tectal (Mufson *et al.*, 1986) and PBG–geniculate (Smith *et al.*, 1988) projections.

The complex arrangements of neurons and fibers in the mesopontine re-

Figure 1. Distribution of ChAT-positive (filled circles) and TH-positive (open circles) neurons through the upper and middle brainstem of cat, represented on schematic drawings of sections at approximate 1-mm intervals. The respective stereotaxic levels and most neuroanatomical labels conform to those of the cat brainstem atlas of Berman (1968). Modified after Jones and Beaudet (1987a).

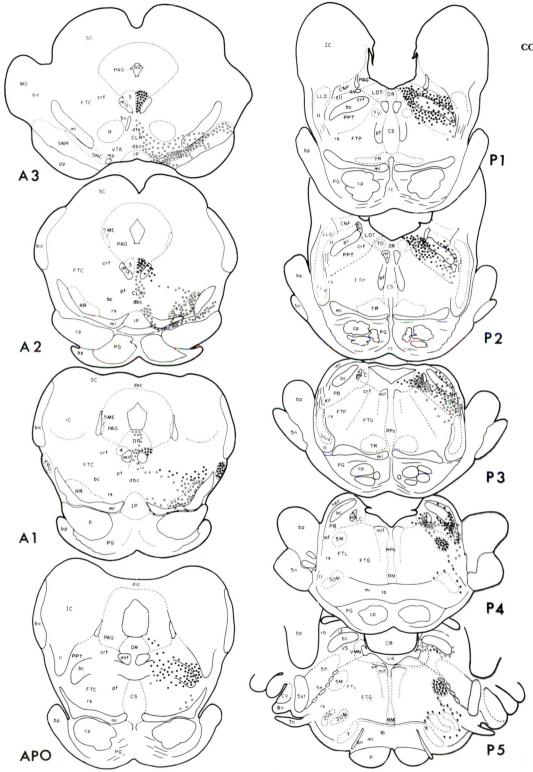

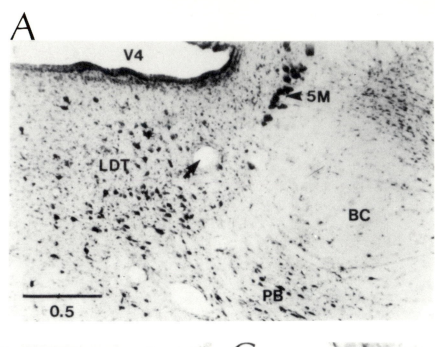

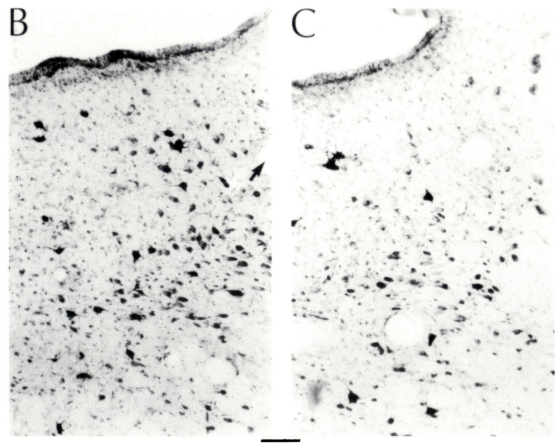

ticular core challenge prior views that assumed that the effects induced on thalamocortical systems are simply cholinergic in nature (see Section 1.3.1). First, in most electrophysiological experiments conducted during the 1960s and the 1970s, stimulation was applied in the rostral midbrain core where there are virtually no cholinergic perikarya. In those cases, stimulation was applied, at best, to the axons arising in cholinergic neurons located more caudally, at the midbrain–pontine junction. Although substance-P-containing and histaminergic neurons have been identified in some territories of the rostral mesencephalon (see Section 4.1.3), the transmitter(s) of most upper midbrain reticular neurons remain(s) largely unknown. Second, even when stimuli have been applied in more recent studies within the PB (or PPT) area, it must be acknowledged that this cholinergic territory also contains a certain number of TH-positive neurons and that it is traversed by catecholaminergic axons issuing from locus coeruleus. As discussed in Chapter 6, ACh and NE similarly exert depolarizing actions on some thalamic neurons studied *in vitro*. Muscarinic and nicotinic blockers can ascertain the cholinergic nature of the phenomena, but, with some exceptions (see Chapters 7, 8), the synaptic effects elicited by rostral brainstem reticular stimulation *in vivo* are rarely entirely blocked by one or the other cholinergic blocker. In those cases, the colocalization of peptides in cholinergic neurons may be the factor that accounts for the observed failure of blockage. The physiological actions of various peptides whose colocalization was described in immunohistochemical studies of brainstem cholinergic neurons are almost completely unknown. Lastly, in any study conducted on the deep layer C of the cat's lateral geniculate neurons, the cholinergic effects elicited by PPT stimulation may be caused by costimulation of fibers arising in the PBG (Ch8) nucleus.

4.1.3. Brainstem Reticular Nuclei with Unidentified Transmitters

The principal nuclei of the midbrain, pontine, and bulbar reticular formation, other than the recently identified cholinergic groups at the midbrain–pontine junction, have been described since the 1950s on the basis of Nissl-stained preparations (see Chapter 2). Some terminological differences arose from various authors' preferences to use nuclear designations according to neuronal size (parvo-, magno-, and gigantocellular) or to their position on the brainstem map (dorsal, ventral, rostral, caudal).

4.1.3.1. Midbrain

At rostral (perirubral) levels, the midbrain reticular core is termed the central tegmental field (FTC; Berman, 1968). The FTC is a large territory extending between the substantia nigra (SN) and the deep layers of the superior colliculus (SC). Many authors consider the large neurons of the deep SC layers as

Figure 2. Features of retrograde cell labeling in brainstem peribrachial (PB) area and laterodorsal tegmental (LDT) nucleus after a WGA–HRP injection into the mediodorsal (MD) thalamic nucleus in the cat. Arrow in A points to the same blood vessel as indicated in the enlarged photograph in B. C is an adjacent more posterior section. Abbreviations: BC, brachium conjunctivum; 5M, mesencephalic nucleus of the fifth nerve; V4, fourth ventricle. From Steriade *et al.* (1988).

more closely related to the reticular formation than to the SC because of their isodendritic patterns and heterogeneity of sensory inputs (Grofova *et al.*, 1978; Edwards, 1980).

The FTC cells of the cat are prevalently small-sized (soma surface 200–400 μm^2). This fits in with their slow axonal conduction velocities as determined by antidromic invasion of FTC neurons from intralaminar thalamic nuclei and zona incerta (Steriade, 1981). Caudally to the red nucleus, the ventral border of FTC is contiguous with the retrorubral field (RRF), occupied in part by the catecholamine group A8. It should be emphasized that, at least in the cat, the FTC territory, located dorsally to the RRF, does not contain catecholaminergic neurons (Parent, 1984). The distinction between FTC and RRF also results from their different connections. The rostral part of the FTC essentially projects to the thalamus (mediodorsal, intralaminar, and zona incerta nuclei), whereas RRF projections are directed to the head of the caudate nucleus (Paré *et al.*, 1988). More caudally, at the level of the trochlear nucleus, the cholinergic PB (PPT) nucleus appears in the lateral part of the FTC, around the brachium conjunctivum. The cuneiform nucleus can be regarded as a dorsal extension of the FTC. It appears at the caudal pole of the trochlear nucleus, and its relations are the inferior colliculus dorsally, the nucleus sagulum and dorsal nucleus of the lateral lemniscus laterally, and the PPT area ventrally.

The transmitters of FTC neurons are largely unknown. Some studies report a number of substance-P-containing neurons in nucleus cuneiformis (Ljungdahl *et al.*, 1978) and histaminergic neurons located more ventrally in the midbrain reticular formation (Brownstein, 1975; Schwartz *et al.*, 1980). The elucidation of transmitter(s) used by the great number of neurons in the huge territory of the rostral mesencephalic reticular formation is a matter of future investigations. It may be predicted that the major transmitter of thalamically projecting rostral midbrain reticular neurons will be found to be an excitatory substance since, as discussed in Section 4.3, the effect of stimulating that midbrain region (after chronic degeneration of passing fibers) is a monosynaptic excitation of thalamocortical neurons.

4.1.3.2. Pons

The continuation of the midbrain FTC in the pontine tegmentum was termed paralemniscal tegmental field (FTP) by Berman (1968) in his atlas on cat brainstem. The FTP might be differentiated from the parvocellular FTC by the presence of scattered medium-sized and very few large-sized neurons. The FTP occupies the largest part of the rostral pontine tegmentum, and it is replaced more caudally (posterior planes 3–4) by a lateral tegmental field (FTL) and a paramedian gigantocellular tegmental field (FTG). The FTL contains cells of all sizes, well below those of FTG neurons. But FTG is also heterogeneous, with giant neurons (soma large diameter around 60 μm) interspersed with medium-sized neurons (30–40 μm) and small neurons (around 20 μm). Intracellular HRP staining revealed that giant cells of the paramedian pons prevalently project to the spinal cord, whereas medium-sized and smaller neurons are reticuloreticular elements (Mitani *et al.*, 1988a,b). Although not yet formally identified, evidence based on antidromic invasion suggests that the smaller pontine neurons are those with ascending projections to the thalamus (Fuller, 1975).

The heterogeneity of pontine reticular neurons is the reason why some prefer to use the topographical terms reticularis pontis oralis (RPO) and reticularis pontis caudalis (RPC) to designate the nuclei of the pontine core. The RPO extends from the caudal pole of the inferior colliculus to the trigeminal motor nucleus. A Golgi analysis of rat RPO (Newman, 1985b) distinguished a medial and a lateral part of this nucleus: (1) the medial part contains neurons with triangular or polygonal somata usually ranging between 30 μm and 50 μm in length and with medially directed dendrites that occasionally enter the nucleus raphe centralis superior; (2) the lateral part contains neurons with somata between 20 μm and 80 μm and dendrites coursing laterally and frequently intersecting with the axons of the lateral lemniscus. The RPC extends caudally to the rostral pole of facial nucleus, where it merges with the bulbar reticular core.

4.1.3.3. Medulla

The bulbar reticular formation consists of three main territories: the gigantocellular (Gc) nucleus in the dorsal paramedian region, the magnocellular (Mc) nucleus in the ventral paramedian zone, and the parvocellular (Pc) nucleus in the dorsolateral area. These nuclei are synonymous with FTG, FTM, and FTL fields described by Berman (1968). The sizes of neurons in various bulbar reticular regions fit in with their axonal conduction velocities, the antidromically identified Gc neurons having significantly higher conduction velocities than Mc neurons (Steriade *et al.*, 1984b).

4.2. Rostral Projections of Brainstem Reticular Cholinergic and Noncholinergic Nuclei

The projections of brainstem reticular neurons are described as a function of rostral (diencephalic and telencephalic) targets. In many instances, the same target area is afferented from both cholinergic and noncholinergic, upper and lower, brainstem reticular neurons.

As originally described by fiber degeneration techniques (Nauta and Kuypers, 1958) and Golgi studies (Scheibel and Scheibel, 1958) and subsequently elaborated and confirmed by autoradiography (Jones and Yang, 1985), long ascending projections from the giant-cell fields of the bulb and pons as well as from FTP and FTC ascend as Forel's tegmental fascicles into the diencephalon where this diffuse band of fibers splits into a dorsal and a ventral leaf. The dorsal system supplies the intralaminar and midline nuclei of the thalamus, whereas the ventral division distributes fibers to subthalamus (especially nucleus of the field of Forel) and (especially lateral) hypothalamus and beyond to basal forebrain.

4.2.1. Are There Direct Cortical Projections?

The ascending axons of cholinergic neurons at the midbrain–pontine junction (Ch5–Ch6 groups) and noncholinergic reticular neurons of midbrain, pontine, and medullary fields are overwhelmingly relayed in the thalamus. This stands in contrast to the direct cortical projections of monoaminergic brainstem nuclei (see Sections 4.5 to 4.7). The absence of direct cortical projections of nonmonoaminergic brainstem neurons (using ACh or other, as yet nonidentified, transmitters) was especially reported in studies conducted in cat, but the scarcity of such projections is also reported in studies in rat and squirrel monkey. The only species that seems to have a significant brainstem reticular projection to the visual cortex is the chimpanzee. This should be emphasized because reports continue to accumulate in the literature referring to direct reticulocortical projections without qualifications about their importance and their widespread or localized character and without dissociating the classical reticular (cholinergic and noncholinergic) fields from the monoaminergic systems.

After large injections of retrograde tracers in cat visual cortex, no nonmonoaminergic neurons were labeled in the brainstem reticular formation, but a significant number of 5-HT-positive or TH-positive neurons were also HRP-positive in the dorsal raphe or locus coeruleus (Sakai, 1985a). The absence of retrogradely labeled brainstem reticular neurons was also reported in other experiments using retrograde tracer injections in cat visual cortex (Tigges and Tigges, 1985) as well as large HRP injections in motor (pericruciate) and parietal associational (suprasylvian) neocortical areas and posteroventral hippocampus of cat (Steriade *et al.*, 1988).

In rat, after [³H]proline injections in the upper brainstem reticular formation, the projections to the cerebral cortex were sparse and difficult to visualize (Jones and Yang, 1985). Only isolated fibers were anterogradely labeled in the cortex, and confined to the infralimbic area, after WGA–HRP and PHA-L injections in the cholinergic LDT nucleus (Satoh and Fibiger, 1986). Recently, a study dealt in detail with rat "reticulocortical" systems as disclosed by retrograde transport of fluorescent tracers or WGA–HRP (Newman and Liu, 1987), but the notion of reticular formation was extended to include monoaminergic nuclei. Table 2 in that study shows that: (1) no cell or one occasional neuron was labeled in midbrain and pontine reticular cholinergic or noncholinergic nuclei (PPT pars compacta or Ch5 and both RPO and RPC nuclei; LDT or CH6 group was not mentioned) after retrograde tracer injections in somatosensory or visual cortices, which was in sharp contrast with about 50 to 100 labeled cells in various raphe and locus coeruleus nuclei; (2) after tracer injections in motor, premotor, or cingulate cortices, the approximate ratios between labeled cells in the cholinergic or noncholinergic mesopontine reticular nuclei and those found in monoaminergic nuclei were 1/10 to 1/30; and (3) only after prefrontal injections, significant numbers of labeled cells were found in Ch5 group (about one to five with respect to those found in monoaminergic nuclei).

In squirrel monkey, brainstem core neurons were labeled after HRP injections into different visual cortical areas, but they were found in "the medial portion of the formatio reticularis pontis oralis (RF) which adjoins the nucleus raphe centralis superior. . . This region of the RF corresponds to that described as containing the serotonergic cell group S9 . . ." (Tigges *et al.*, 1982, p. 31). In the chimpanzee, a similar arrangement of retrogradely labeled neurons was found in the pontine tegmentum after HRP injections in the occipital lobe (namely, coextensive with labeled neurons in the nucleus raphe centralis superior), but, in addition, HRP-positive cells were described within the ventral mid-

4.2.2. Thalamic Projections

There is a general consensus that the great majority of ascending brainstem reticular axons are synaptically relayed in the thalamus. The other, less massive contingent is directed to the basal forebrain nuclei (see Section 4.2.3). The thalamic projections have been investigated by using anterograde and retrograde tracing techniques, corroborated by antidromic identification experiments that provided information about axonal conduction velocities, and the cholinergic sources of these projections have been recently disclosed by retrograde transport techniques combined with ChAT immunoreactivity of brainstem reticular neurons.

Generally, the rostral targets of brainstem reticular neurons were thought in earlier studies to be limited to some medial, intralaminar, reticular, and zona incerta thalamic nuclei, whereas major sensory and motor relay thalamic nuclei remained unlabeled in autoradiographic experiments on the pontine and mesencephalic reticular formation (Edwards and DeOlmos, 1976; Graybiel, 1977a,b; Robertson and Feiner, 1982). And, despite some indications that the brainstem peribrachial (PB) area of the PPT nucleus projects to dorsal lateral geniculate (LG) and lateral posterior (LP) nuclei of the cat visual thalamus (Graybiel, 1977a; Moon-Edley and Graybiel, 1983), the same thalamic nuclei remain unlabeled after similar midbrain injections with tritiated amino acids in the rat (Jones and Yang, 1985). Since until quite recently (1987–1988) there was no certain morphological evidence for brainstem reticular projections to thalamic relay nuclei (cf. Jones, 1985), the facilitatory and presumed cholinergic effects induced by stimulating the midbrain reticular formation on neurons recorded from the LG, LP, ventroposterior (VP), ventrolateral (VL), and other thalamic relay and associational nuclei remained something of a mystery and awaited the clarification of the underlying pathways as well as their chemical signature.

We now know that: (1) cholinergic nuclei at the midbrain–pontine junction (Ch5–Ch6 groups) project to virtually *all* thalamic nuclei; (2) in addition to Ch5–Ch6 projections, some associational and especially intralaminar nuclei receive a massive projection from the noncholinergic neurons located in the rostral midbrain FTC territory and in the rostral pontine reticular formation; and (3) medullary reticular neurons also project to some medial and intralaminar thalamic nuclei.

4.2.2.1. Specific Relay and Associational Nuclei

Here, we analyze in some detail the brainstem reticular projections to the sensory and motor relay nuclei—medial geniculate (MG), dorsal part of the LG, VP, ventromedial (VM) and ventroanterior–ventrolateral (VA–VL)—and to the associational pulvinar–lateroposterior (PUL–LP) and mediodorsal (MD) thalamic nuclei. The analysis of brainstem projections to some or all of these nuclei was performed in studies on rat (Hallanger *et al.*, 1987), cat, and macaque monkey (Steriade *et al.*, 1988). Other studies focused on the visual thalamic nuclei of cat (Smith *et al.*, 1988), with comparisons between cholinergic and monoaminergic projections to the LG nucleus (DeLima and Singer, 1987).

Specific relay sensory and motor (MG, LG, VP, VA–VL, VM) nuclei receive less than 10% of their brainstem reticular afferents from noncholinergic neurons located at rostral midbrain (perirubral) levels (frontal levels A4–A3 in the cat). Instead, they receive 85–95% of their brainstem afferents from a region concentrated around 3 mm between A1 and P1, where cholinergic PPT and LDT (Ch5–Ch6) nuclei are maximally developed (Fig. 3; see the localization of WGA–HRP injections strictly confined within the limits of relay thalamic nuclei in Fig. 4 of Chapter 2). The only exception to this peaked localization between A1 and P1 is the VM nucleus, which receives approximately 40% of its brainstem innervation from posterior levels P3–P4. Double staining (ChAT plus HRP) in cat material revealed that the percentages of retrogradely labeled cholinergic brainstem neurons from the total number of simply HRP-positive elements were between 73% and 87% in the case of sensory (MG, LG, VP) nuclei and around 60% after injections in VA–VL and VM motor nuclei. The ratios between the number of double-labeled neurons in PPT (Ch5) and those in LDT (Ch6) were much higher for sensory thalamic nuclei (LG, 40; MG, 15; VP, 8) than in motor VA–VL (2) and VM (4) nuclei. And, although the afferent projections arise predominantly from the ipsilateral brainstem reticular nuclei, the contralateral projections are surprisingly high, from 20% to 40% of the ipsilateral projection (Steriade *et al.*, 1988).

Antidromic identification studies by careful threshold mapping at closely spaced foci in the LG laminae also indicated that brainstem neurons with LG projections are located around the brachium conjunctivum in the region of Ch5 group, and the conduction velocities from the stimulated sites of the parent axons to the PPT cell bodies were estimated to be around 1–3 m/sec (Ahlsén, 1984).

The elegant study by DeLima and Singer (1987) used the retrograde transport of rhodamine-labeled latex spheres injected in the LG thalamic nucleus combined with immunohistochemistry techniques for ChAT, 5-HT, and TH. These data thus provide quantitative data not only for projections arising in cholinergic nuclei but also for projections of monoaminergic systems to the LG nucleus of cat, thus allowing a comparison between the power of these distinct brainstem systems impinging on the principal thalamic visual relay station. Compared to the total number of retrogradely labeled ChAT-positive cells found between stereotaxic planes A3 and P5, 5-HT-positive neurons in the dorsal raphe represent only about 10%, and TH-positive neurons in the locus coeruleus cells about 20% (Fig. 4). Probably there are species differences concern-

Figure 3. Brainstem reticular projections to relay and associational thalamic nuclei in the cat. The parasagittal section shows some of the thalamic nuclei where WGA–HRP was injected and the main brainstem reticular territories where retrogradely labeled neurons were found (FTC, PB, and LDT nuclei). Frontal stereotaxic planes are indicated (A4–P4). The three computer-generated graphs show the percentage (ordinate) of HRP-positive cells at various rostrocaudal levels (abscissa) from the total number of labeled neurons in the upper brainstem reticular core. For abbreviations of thalamic nuclei, see text. Other abbreviations: AC, anterior commissure; IC, inferior colliculus; MM, medial mammillary nucleus; OC, optic chiasm; PAG, periaqueductal gray; RFB, retroflex bundle; RN, red nucleus; SC, superior colliculus. From Steriade *et al.* (1988).

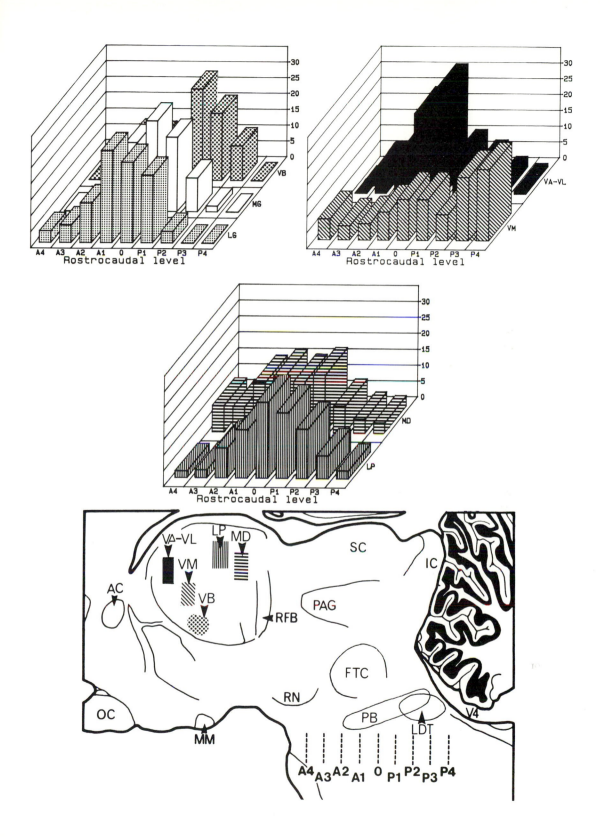

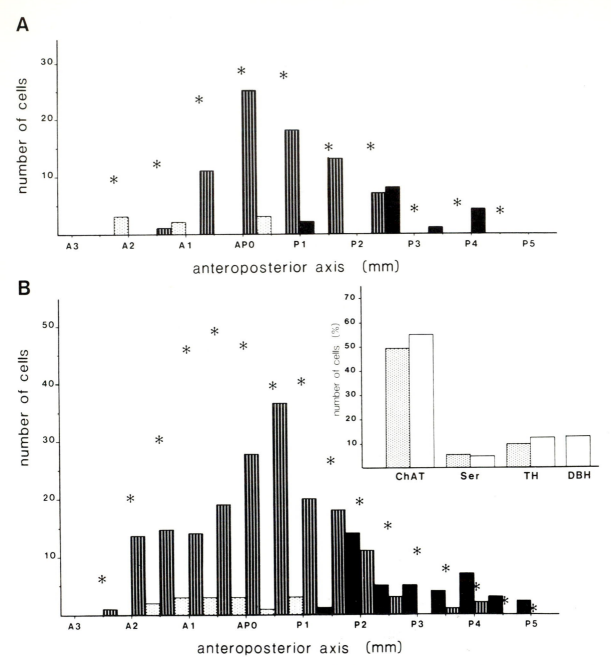

Figure 4. Brainstem cholinergic and monoaminergic projections to the lateral geniculate (LG) thalamic nucleus in the cat. A: Histogram quantitatively representing the distribution of all double-labeled cells in the anteroposterior axis. Each bar corresponds to the number of cells in one section. Punctate bars correspond to serotonergic double-labeled cells; black bars correspond to noradrenergic (TH⁺) cells; and black-and-white bars correspond to cholinergic (ChAT⁺) cells. The crosses indicate the mean of the total retrogradely labeled cells in the immunostained adjacent sections. B: Histograms indicating the proportion of double-labeled cells in each series of immunostained sections relative to the total retrogradely labeled cells in the respective series. Punctate and white bars represent the results of two experiments. ChAT, choline acetyltransferase; Ser, serotonin; TH, tyrosine hydroxylase; DBH, dopamine-β-hydroxylase; TH and DBH probably labeled the same population of cells. See also text. Modified from DeLima and Singer (1987).

ing these relative proportions of cholinergic and monoaminergic brainstem neurons projecting to the LG, since in rat the number of dorsal raphe neurons is at least 40% of those found in Ch5–Ch6 groups (see Table 1 in Hallanger *et al.*, 1987). At any rate, these data indicate that the thalamic projections of cholinergic nuclei by far exceed those of monoaminergic nuclei.

The ChAT-positive fibers form dense networks within the main LG laminae (Stichel and Singer, 1985). Since the basal forebrain does not participate in the cholinergic innervation of the LG nucleus, these cholinergic fibers probably arise in the brainstem Ch5 group (see above). In lamina A, ChAT-positive terminals participate in synaptic contacts with the dendrites of LG relay cells in the extraglomerular neuropil and also in the complex synaptic arrangements of glomeruli, where they have access to presynaptic dendrites of local-circuit LG cells (DeLima *et al.*, 1985).

The brainstem reticular projections to thalamic associational nuclei are more massive than those to the specific relay nuclei. WGA–HRP injections in the PUL–LP or MD nuclei of cat led to three to eight times more retrograde cell labeling in the brainstem core than did injections into the relay nuclei (Fig. 5). By contrast to the LG projection, which arises almost exclusively in the Ch5 group, the LP nucleus receives an important projection from both Ch5 and Ch6 groups (Smith *et al.*, 1988; Fig. 5A). The ratio between retrogradely labeled cells in the Ch5 and Ch6 groups was 40 in the case of LG, whereas it was 2 in the case of the LP injection. In monkey too, the projection to the PUL–LP thalamic complex arises in cholinergic neurons of the medial part of Ch5 and the adjacent Ch6 group (Steriade *et al.*, 1988). The massive brainstem–MD projection is not accounted for by a greater contribution from PPT and LDT cholinergic nuclei but by the massive labeling in noncholinergic parts of the midbrain and rostral pontine reticular formation (Fig. 5B). Moreover, numerous cells in the periaqueductal gray project to MD in both cat and monkey. Note that the rich innervation of MD with ChAT-positive fibers (Levey *et al.*, 1987a) does not exclusively originate in the brainstem, since MD as well as a limited number of other thalamic nuclei receive a cholinergic innervation from the basal forebrain (Steriade *et al.*, 1987b; Parent *et al.*, 1988; see Section 4.2.2.3).

4.2.2.2. Intralaminar, Reticular, Zona Incerta, Ventral Lateral Geniculate and Limbic Thalamic Nuclei

Whereas brainstem reticular projections to relay thalamic nuclei modulate the synaptic transmission of impulses from various sensory and motor modalities, the projections to intralaminar and reticular thalamic nuclei are involved in generalized processes of activation and oscillation in thalamocortical systems. The caudal intralaminar (centromedian–parafascicular, CM-PF) nuclei are essentially related to the striatum. In addition to their efferent connections to the caudate nucleus, the rostral intralaminar (centrolateral–paracentral, CL-PC) neurons project over widespread cortical territories, where they exert depolarizing actions and thus represent an important link in the activating circuit from the brainstem reticular formation to the cerebral cortex. The reticular thalamic nucleus (RE) is a pacemaker of spindle oscillations and the main source of long-range inhibition of thalamocortical neurons during EEG-synchronized sleep (see Chapter 7). The brainstem cholinergic projections to the RE nucleus are an

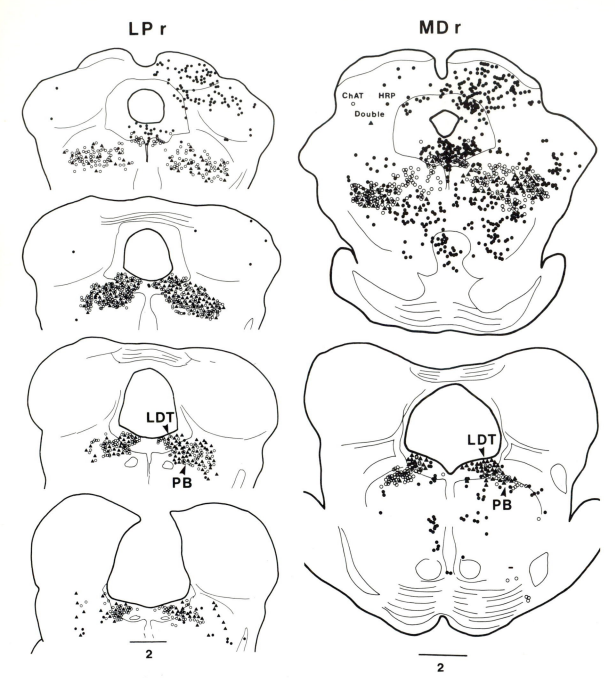

Figure 5. Cholinergic and noncholinergic brainstem reticular projections to the right lateroposterior (LP) and mediodorsal (MD) nuclei in the cat. In the LP case, four levels at stereotaxic planes A1, P0.5, P1, and P2.5. Three types of neurons are represented (ChAT⁺, HRP⁺, and double-labeled; see symbols in top section of the MD case), as found on one section after combining the TMB procedure for retrogradely labeled WGA–HRP with ChAT immunohistochemistry. In the MD case, same type of graph as for LP nucleus, but each of the two drawings represents labeled cells found on two sections. Camera lucida localization. LP modified from Smith *et al.* (1988). MD modified from Steriade *et al.* (1988).

important factor in the disruption of synchronized spindle oscillations upon arousal. The zona incerta (ZI) nucleus, which is sometime included in the subthalamic region, has the same developmental history as the RE nucleus, both originating from the ventral thalamus. The anterior (anterodorsal–anteroventral–anteromedial, AD–AV–AM) nuclei project over the whole limbic cortex (anterior and posterior cingulate gyri, retrosplenial gyrus, pre- and parasubiculum) and are part of a basically different network than most dorsal thalamic nuclei, as they are interposed in the circuit between the hippocampus, mammillary nuclei, and the cingulate cortex.

All brainstem reticular fields, from the medulla to the rostral midbrain, send projections to the CM-PF and CL-PC intralaminar nuclei. This is quite different from the brainstem reticular innervation of most specific relay nuclei, which receive afferents almost exclusively from the circumscribed brainstem region of Ch5–Ch6 groups (see Fig. 3). The contribution of the whole brainstem reticular formation to the afferentation of intralaminar thalamic nuclei, already indicated in axonal degeneration studies and in early autoradiographic experiments (see Chapter 2), has been repeatedly confirmed.

Thus, in anterograde and retrograde transport experiments, the source of CM-PF and CL-PC afferents was found not only in the upper brainstem reticular core but also in rostral and caudal pontine reticular nuclei and in medullary reticular gigantocellular (Gc) and magnocellular (Mc) fields; by contrast, few of the projections from the medullary parvocellular (Pc) nucleus ascend beyond the midpons (Zemlan *et al.*, 1984; Jones and Yang, 1985; Vertes *et al.*, 1986). Antidromic identification experiments revealed that: (1) the midbrain-to-intralaminar axons conduct between 3.5 and 4.6 m/sec (Ropert and Steriade, 1981), in keeping with the small-sized neurons in the mesencephalic FTC; (2) the larger pontine reticular neurons project to intralaminar nuclei with conduction velocities around 7 m/sec (Fuller, 1975); and (3) Gc and Mc bulbar reticular neurons project to intralaminar nuclei with conduction velocities of 20 m/sec and 7–14 m/sec, respectively, also as a function of the larger size of Gc, compared to Mc, neurons (Steriade *et al.*, 1984b).

In more recent years, the cholinergic nature of brainstem reticular projections from the PPT and LDT nuclei to intralaminar nuclei was revealed by a series of methods. Transmitter specific labeling was used to investigate the retrograde transport of [³H]choline from CM-PF nuclei mainly to PPT and LDT nuclei of rat (Wiklund and Cuénod, 1984). In the opposite sense, the anterograde labeling of LDT projections to PF and more rostral (CL-PC) intralaminar nuclei was shown after injections of WGA–HRP and PHA-L (Satoh and Fibiger, 1986). The demonstration of brainstem cholinergic projections to both (caudal and rostral) components of the intralaminar nuclei was eventually achieved by combining the retrograde transport of HRP or fluorescent tracers with ChAT immunohistochemistry in rat (Woolf and Butcher, 1986; Hallanger *et al.*, 1987), cat (Paré *et al.*, 1988), and dog (Isaacson and Tanaka, 1986).

The considerably more numerous brainstem reticular neurons labeled after WGA–HRP injections into the cat CM-PF nuclei or CL-PC nuclei, as compared to the number of brainstem reticular cells labeled after injections in relay sensory and motor thalamic nuclei, result from a dissimilar distribution of retrogradely labeled neurons. In addition to massive projections from the Ch5–Ch6 groups, the intralaminar nuclei receive a substantial proportion of afferents from noncholinergic neurons in the rostral midbrain (planes A4–A3) and in the paramedian rostral pontine reticular formation (Paré *et al.*, 1988; Figs. 6 and 7). In rat too, there were two or three times more numerous cells labeled in midbrain FTC and pontine reticular formation than in Ch5–Ch6 groups after WGA–HRP injections in CM or CL thalamic nuclei (see Table 1 in Hallanger *et al.*, 1987). The noncholinergic neurons labeled in the periaqueductal gray after the CM injection (Fig. 7) may use aspartate as synaptic transmitter, since injections of [^{3}H]aspartate into the CM-PF nuclear complex leads to retrograde labeling in the small-sized cells of the midbrain periaqueductal gray (Wiklund and Cuénod, 1984). The axons of Ch5 cells form asymmetric synaptic contacts with dendrites of CM-PF and CL neurons (Sugimoto and Hattori, 1984).

The distribution and number of retrogradely labeled brainstem reticular neurons after WGA–HRP injections in the rostral pole or rostrolateral districts of cat RE thalamic nucleus are similar to those found after tracer injections in relay nuclei (Fig. 6). Of all retrogradely labeled neurons in the brainstem reticular core, 50% were also ChAT-positive. The demonstration of a substantial brainstem cholinergic and noncholinergic projection to the rostral RE nucleus in both rat (Woolf and Butcher, 1986; Hallanger *et al.*, 1987) and cat (Paré *et al.*, 1988) settles the controversial issue of interspecies differences between rat and cat related to the RE thalamic nucleus (see Section 3.1.2.1).

In addition, WGA–HRP injections confined within the limits of the perigeniculate (PG) part of the RE nucleus result in retrograde labeling in PPT and LDT nuclei, with 73% of PPT neurons also being ChAT-positive (Smith *et al.*, 1988; Fig. 8). Ahlsén's (1984) antidromic identification study revealed that of three PPT cell types encountered, one sends axons exclusively to the LG nucleus, another to the PG nucleus (and/or to the overlying RE sector subserving the PUL–LP thalamic nuclei), and a third group projects to both LG and PG nuclei, probably being involved in the control of intrinsic LG inhibitory processes as well as the control of the recurrent inhibitory loop between PG and LG (Fig. 9).

The upper brainstem core projections to ZI have been shown with anterograde (Edwards and DeOlmos, 1976) and retrograde (Shammah-Lagnado *et al.*, 1985) transport techniques and in electrophysiological experiments (Steriade *et al.*, 1982b). The territory of origin for brainstem–ZI axons extends down to the pontine reticular formation, but this projection exclusively arises from small- and medium-sized pontine reticular cells; no giant cell was found retrogradely labeled after tracer injections in ZI, much the same as after injections in intralaminar thalamic nuclei (Paré *et al.*, 1988).

The ventral lateral geniculate nucleus* (VLG) has been recently shown to receive a dense input from PPT in a study using both anterograde (WGA–HRP) and double-labeling retrograde ChAT techniques (Higo *et al.*, 1989a,b). PPT is the site of neurons that transfer PGO-wave-related activity from brainstem to thalamus (see Chapter 9), and although there yet has been no physiological study

---

*The VLG connectivity is quite different from the dorsal LG. The VLG receives input from the retina but does not project to cortex; instead the VLG sends axons to a number of subcortical structures, including ventral thalamus and oculomotor/visual system-related areas (Nakamura and Kawamura, 1988). The VLG provides input to both rostral and caudal intralaminar nuclei (CL, PC, CM) and to the pulvinar and LP; its caudal projections include the ZI, the pretectal area, and superior colliculus.

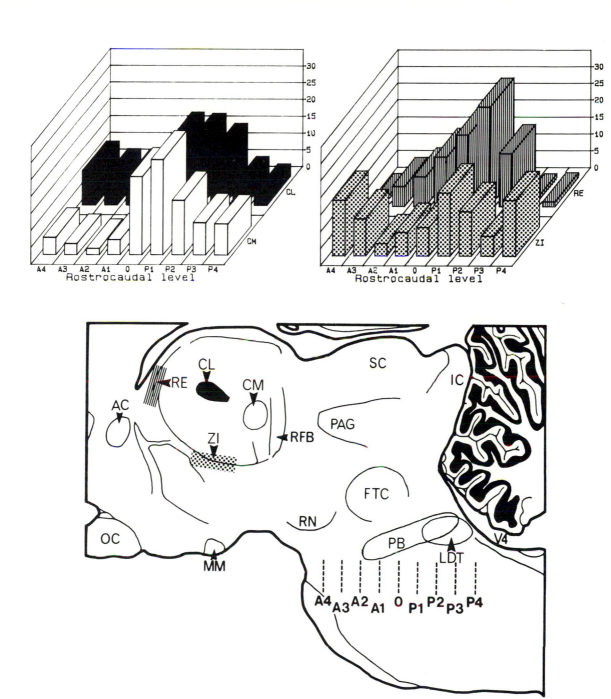

Figure 6. Brainstem reticular projections to intralaminar, RE, and ZI thalamic nuclei of cat. The parasagittal section shows the thalamic nuclei where WGA–HRP was injected (CM-PF, CL-PC, rostral pole of RE, and ZI) and the main brainstem territories where retrogradely labeled neurons were found (FTC, PB, and LDT). Frontal stereotaxic planes are indicated (A4–P4). The two computer-generated graphs at top show the percentage (ordinate) of HRP+ cells at vari- ous rostrocaudal levels (abscissa) from the total number of retrogradely labeled elements in the brainstem core. Note that the peak of retrogradely neurons is at A0–P2 for the CM-PF and RE injections, that a significant proportion of cells was found at most rostral level (A4) of the midbrain in the case of the CL-PC injection, and that three peaks were found after the ZI injection (at A4–A3, P1–P2, and P4). For abbreviations, see legend of Fig. 3. From Paré *et al.* (1988).

819—CM

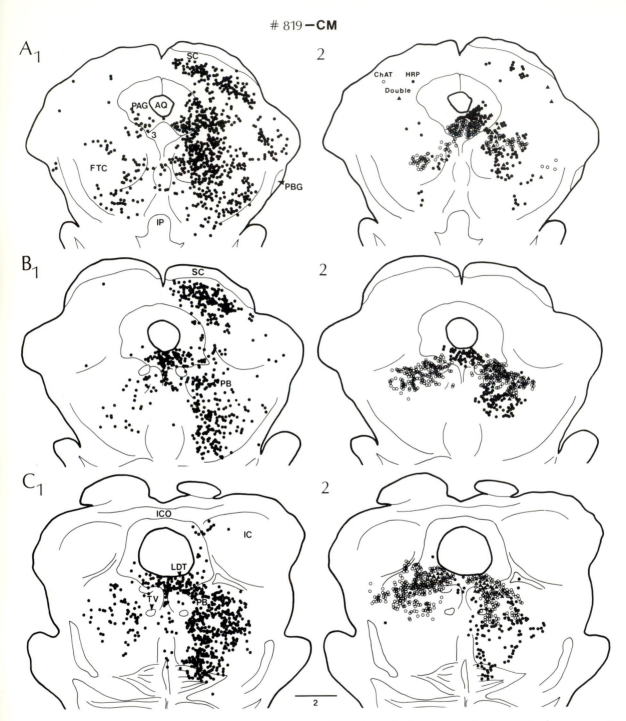

Figure 7. Cholinergic and noncholinergic brainstem core neuron projections to the right CM-PF thalamic nuclei of cat. A, B, and C: Three levels, from rostral to caudal. At each level, left column depicts the total number of retrogradely labeled neurons as found in five successive sections after TMB procedure counterstained with neutral red. Right column depicts the same levels, with the three types of cells (ChAT+, HRP+, and double-labeled; see symbols in A2), as found in two sections after TMB procedure combined with ChAT immunohistochemistry. Right part in brainstem drawings ipsilateral to thalamic injection. From Paré *et al.* (1988).

of VLG neurons in sleep, the PPT–VLG projections provide an anatomical substrate for transfer of PGO-wave-related activation to VLG and thence to VLG projection targets. The PPT-VLG projections have an ipsilateral dominance and are topographically organized with rostral PPT projecting to medial VLG and caudal PPT to lateral VLG. Reciprocal VLG–PPT projections provide an ana-

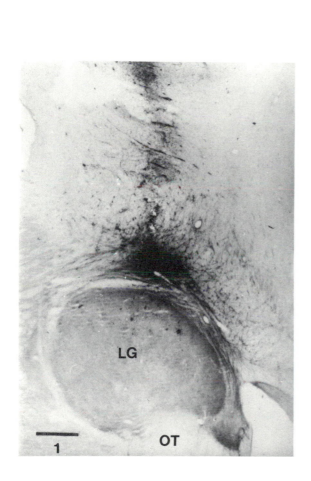

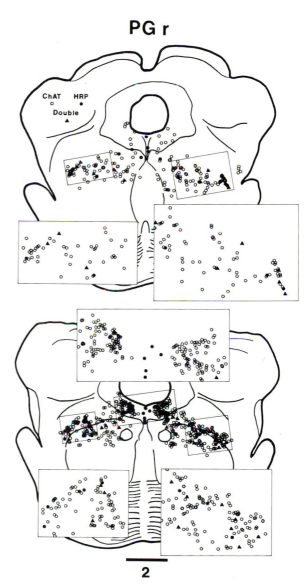

Figure 8. Cholinergic and noncholinergic brainstem reticular cells projecting to the right perigeniculate (PG) sector of the RE nuclear complex of cat. Localization of WGA–HRP injection in PG is depicted in the left microphotograph. Bar indicates millimeters. LG, lateral geniculate nucleus; OT, optic tract. Right column depicts two levels (A1 and P0.5) with the three cell types (CHAT⁺, HRP⁺, and double-labeled; symbols in top drawing) as found on one section (WGA–HRP procedure combined with ChAT immunohistochemistry). Localization of cells by means of a computer-assisted microscope. The areas delimitated by rectangles are shown at higher magnification. Modified from Smith *et al.* (1988).

a

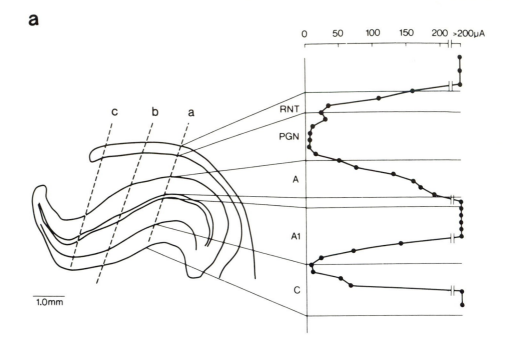

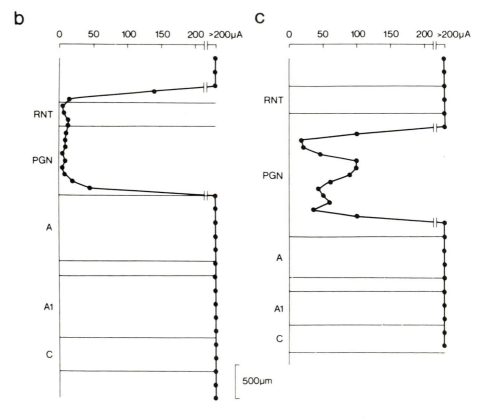

b

c

tomical substrate for the physiological observation of monosynaptic activation of PGO burst neurons in PPT by stimulation in the area of the lateral geniculate nuclear complex (see, for example, Nelson *et al.*, 1983).

The AD–AV–AM nuclear group receives projections from cholinergic and noncholinergic neurons of the upper brainstem reticular core. The anterior thalamic complex in cat is heavily afferented from the Ch6 group (Steriade *et al.*, 1988). Indeed, the ratio between Ch5- and Ch6-labeled neurons after a WGA–HRP injection into AV–AM nuclei is 1, whereas for all other thalamic nuclei such ratios range from 2 to 40 (see Section 4.2.2.1). Moreover, in rat the labeled Ch6 cells outnumber those in the Ch5 group (Woolf and Butcher, 1986; Hallanger *et al.*, 1987).

4.2.2.3. Thalamic Nuclei Receiving Cholinergic and Noncholinergic Projections from Both Brainstem and Basal Forebrain

It was recently demonstrated that basal forebrain nuclei contribute to the cholinergic innervation of a limited number of nuclei in the medial and rostral thalamus. Although the rostral pole of RE nucleus, MD, and AM nuclei of cat and macaque monkey receive projections from cholinergic and noncholinergic neurons of different basal forebrain cell groups (Steriade *et al.*, 1987b; Parent *et al.*, 1988), only the RE nucleus is afferented from the basal forebrain in the rat (Levey *et al.*, 1987b). Recently, Asanuma (1989) demonstrated that basal forebrain neurons project to RE nucleus by using PHA-L anterograde labeling of single axons from basal forebrain neurons and intracellular staining of RE thalamic cells. The basal forebrain projection to the RE thalamic nucleus is crucial in EEG desynchronization processes since, in addition to the brainstem–RE projection, it is a source for disruption of synchronized spindle oscillations at their very site of genesis, the RE nucleus (see Chapter 7). As to the basal forebrain projection to the MD nucleus, it can be involved in the modulation of memory and learning processes.

After WGA–HRP injections in the rostral pole of cat RE nucleus, retrograde labeling mostly occurred in the horizontal branch of diagonal nuclei (DBh) and in substantia innominata (SI), where 16–18% of HRP-positive cells were also ChAT-positive (Fig. 10; Steriade *et al.*, 1987b).

A similar distribution of labeled basal forebrain neurons was found after MD injections in cat. After the MD injection in the macaque monkey (Fig. 11), the vast majority of HRP-positive cells occurred medially in the vertical branch of the diagonal band nuclei (DBv), ventrally in DBh, and dorsolaterally in the SI, with double-labeled (HRP plus ChAT) cells ranging from 11% to 23% (Parent *et al.*, 1988). The projection from basal forebrain to MD thalamic nucleus was also observed with the anterograde transport of tritiated amino acids in monkey (Hreib *et al.*, 1985) and with PHA-L transport in rat (Ray and Price, 1987).

Figure 9. Antidromic identification of a brainstem peribrachial neuron with projections to the laminae A1 and C of the cat lateral geniculate nucleus, the perigeniculate nucleus (PGN), and the sector of the reticular thalamic nucleus (RNT) located dorsally to the PGN. Threshold mapping; stimulus intensities indicated at top, in each of the three microelectrode penetrations (a, b, and c). Note different types of axonal termination in three microelectrode tracks: in RNT, PGN, and A1/C interlaminar plexus (a); in RNT and PGN (b); and only in PGN (c). From Ahlsén (1984).

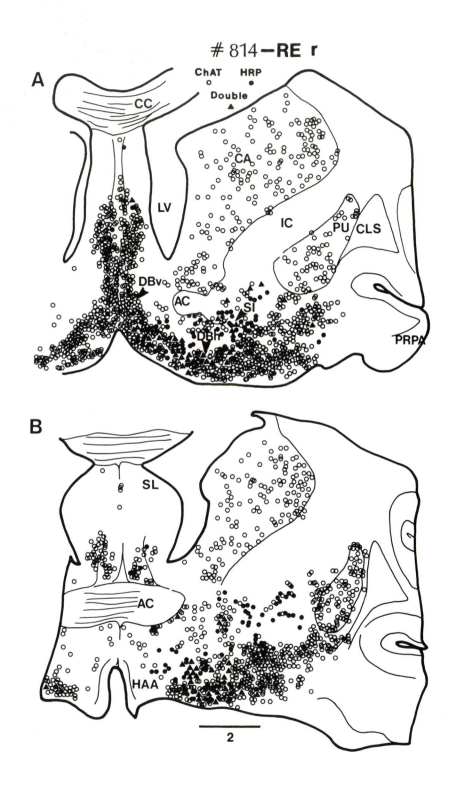

The salient finding after AV–AM injections was that the number of labeled cells was much higher in DBv (compared to those found after RE or MD injections), where neurons also displaying ChAT immunoreactivity reached 27% of the total number of retrogradely labeled elements (Parent *et al.*, 1988). Finally, after VM injections, HRP-positive cells were observed in SI and lateral part of the preoptic area, but no double-labeled (HRP plus ChAT) cell was detected. As discussed in Section 3.1.2.3, the great majority of noncholinergic basal forebrain neurons with thalamic projections are probably GABAergic.

4.2.2.4. The Final Corticopetal Link of Brainstem–Thalamic Projections

As yet, there is no formal morphological evidence that axons originating in the brainstem cholinergic or noncholinergic reticular nuclei contact thalamocortical neurons. Such successive links can be established by combining various methods such as anterograde degeneration, retrograde transport, and immunohistochemistry under electron-microscopic analysis (see Somogyi's studies in Section 2.1). Nonetheless, the two (brainstem–thalamic and thalamocortical) links of the circuit have been identified electrophysiologically by inducing monosynaptic excitation of intralaminar CL or PC thalamic neurons from the rostral midbrain FTC or the PPT area at the midbrain–pontine junction and by identifying antidromically the CL or PC neurons from motor or parietal association cortical areas. This has been achieved in unanesthetized animals in which the pontine tegmentum was chronically lesioned to allow degeneration of passing fibers through the stimulated PPT region (Fig. 12; Steriade and Glenn, 1982).

Such circuits probably exist for all cortically projecting neurons in the dorsal thalamus, since there are brainstem reticular projections from Ch5–Ch6 groups to virtually all thalamic nuclei, and, for many nuclei, additional projections arise from the noncholinergic FTC, rostral pontine, and medullary Gc and Mc fields. These ascending fibers must have access to cortically projecting thalamic neurons because they represent at least 70% of thalamic neurons in cat and reach much higher proportions in the rat.

Whereas specific relay thalamic nuclei project over relatively *circumscribed* cortical territories, especially to midlayers IV–III or with a trilaminar pattern (including minor projections to layer VI or I), two groups of nuclei project *diffusely* over the neocortex: the intralaminar CL-PC over layer I and VI and the VM nucleus to the outer third of layer I (Herkenham, 1979; Glenn *et al.*, 1982; Jones, 1985; Cunningham and LeVay, 1986; see Fig. 5 of Chapter 2).

The cortical projections of CL-PC and VM nuclei represent the required substratum for the generalized activation of cortical processes by stimulating the rostral reticular core (Steriade, 1984), since both rostral intralaminar and VM thalamocortical nuclei receive massive projections from the brainstem reticular

Figure 10. Distribution of cholinergic and noncholinergic basal forebrain neurons projecting to the rostral pole of the right RE thalamic nucleus in the cat. Symbols of the three types of cells (Chat+, HRP+, and double-labeled) indicated in A. Two basal forebrain levels (A16 in A, and A14.5 in B). Abbreviations of DBh, DBv and SI, explained in text. Other abbreviations: AC, anterior commissure; CA, caudate nucleus; CC, corpus callosum; CLS, claustrum; HAA, anterior hypothalamic area; IC, internal capsule; LV, lateral ventricle; PRPA, anterior prepyriform area; PU, putamen. Bar indicates millimeters. From Steriade *et al.* (1987b).

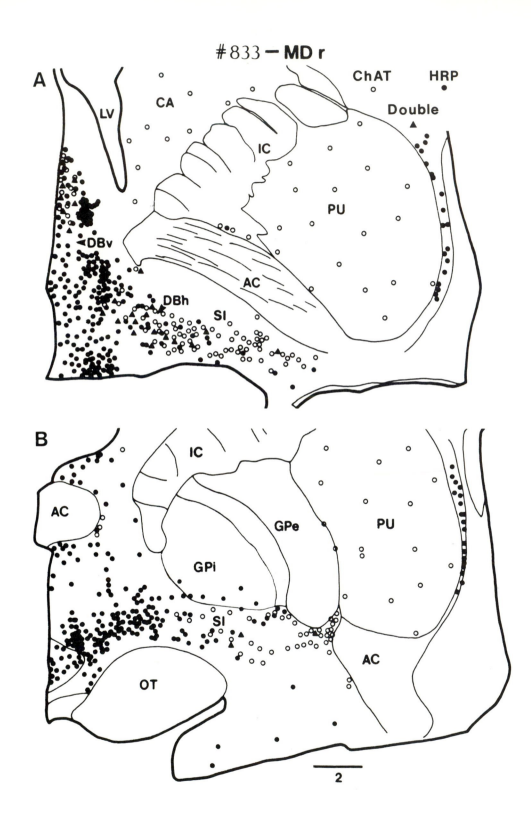

#833 — MD r

core, and their neurons make asymmetric synaptic contacts with dendritic shafts and spines of cortical neurons (Donoghue and Ebner, 1981; Cunningham and LeVay, 1986) and exert depolarizing actions on their targets (Endo *et al.*, 1977). The excitatory nature of thalamocortical neurons is also ascertained by retrograde labeling with transmitter-related compounds, indicating that they use aspartate as synaptic transmitter (Streit, 1980; Ottersen *et al.*, 1983).

The diffuseness of the intralaminar–cortical projection concerns the rostral intralaminar CL-PC nuclei as a whole. By contrast, double-labeling experiments (Bentivoglio *et al.*, 1981; Macchi *et al.*, 1984) and antidromic identification studies (Steriade and Glenn, 1982) indicate that a very small proportion of individual CL or PC neurons project to more than one cortical region or to both the caudate and the cerebral cortex. About 20% of single VM neurons that project to the insular (anterior sylvian) cortex send axon collaterals to the precruciate (motor) fields, but very few branched cells were found in other combinations of cortical areas examined (Minciacchi *et al.*, 1986).

4.2.3. Basal Forebrain Projections

The demonstration of linkages between the rostral brainstem reticular core and various groups of basal forebrain cholinergic systems with widespread cortical projections is important for the notion of the brainstem-induced cholinergic activation of the cerebral cortex, since, as mentioned above, thalamocortical neurons use aspartate as transmitter agent but not ACh.

Autoradiographic experiments in squirrel and rhesus monkeys showed projections from the peripeduncular nucleus (compared to the nucleus of brachium of the inferior colliculus in other species) to nucleus basalis (NB) of Meynert (Jones *et al.*, 1976). In that study, the brainstem source of projection to the basal forbrain was regarded as part of the central auditory pathway.

More recently, evidence has been accumulated that cholinergic and noncholinergic neurons in PPT–LDT nuclei and adjacent brainstem reticular fields project to the basal forebrain. The AChE-containing fibers of the rat dorsal tegmental pathway, which originates in Ch5–Ch6 groups, end in substantia innominata (SI) and related areas (Wilson, 1985). Also in rat, retrograde labeling of caudal midbrain and oral pontine tegmental neurons, especially in PPT and LDT (Ch5 and Ch6) nuclei, occurs after injections of [³H]choline covering the whole basal forebrain (Jones and Beaudet, 1987b). A study using more localized infusions of fluorescent tracers combined with ChAT immunohistochemistry showed that ChAT-positive cells in LDT nucleus and very few such cells in the PPT nucleus project to the medial septum (Ch1 group), DBv (Ch2 group), and the magnocellular preoptic area (Woolf and Butcher, 1986). That the projection from the brainstem to the basal forebrain is predominantly noncholinergic, even when retrogradely labeled neurons in LDT and PPT nuclei are considered, is a common conclusion from recent studies. After injections of a fluorescent tracer

Figure 11. Distribution of cholinergic and noncholinergic basal forebrain neurons projecting to the right mediodorsal (MD) thalamic nucleus of the *Macaca sylvana* monkey. Two frontal sections (A more anterior than B). Symbols of the three types of cells (ChAT⁺, HRP⁺, and double-labeled) indicated in A. GPe and GPi, external and internal segments of globus pallidus. For other abbreviations, see legends of previous figures. From Parent *et al.* (1988).

in SI and ventral pallidum, about 20% of neurons in PPT pars compacta (Ch5) were ChAT-positive, whereas less than 10% of retrogradely labeled cells in the LDT where ChAT-positive (Martin *et al.,* 1987). Similarly, the retrograde transport of WGA–HRP injected in cat DBh (Ch3) labeled many midbrain FTC, PPT, LDT, parabrachial, pontine oralis neurons, and especially dorsal raphe and centralis superior raphe neurons (Fig. 13), but very few neurons in PPT or LDT

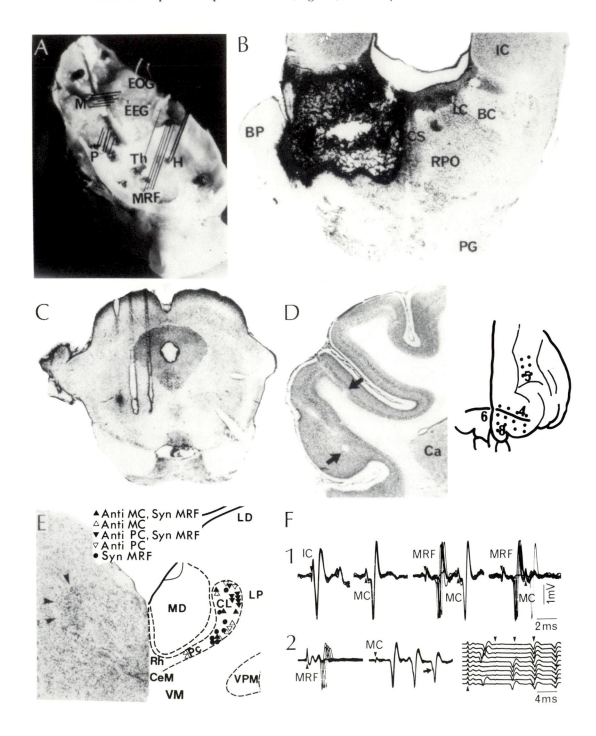

nuclei were ChAT-positive (D. Paré, Y. Smith, A. Parent, and M. Steriade, unpublished data).

The widespread cortical projections of cholinergic and noncholinergic basal forebrain neurons are well known (e.g., Rye *et al.*, 1984). In rat and monkey, individual basal forebrain neurons do not collateralize to different cortical areas and have quite circumscribed (less than 2 mm) territories of projection (Price and Stern, 1983; Saper, 1984; Walker *et al.*, 1985). It seems that, in cat, large polymorphic cells in nucleus basalis have more extensive axonal fields, innervating the precruciate, postcruciate, and/or cingulate gyri (Boylan *et al.*, 1986). It is not known whether the noncollateral versus collateralized projection represents an interspecies difference between rat and cat or if it results from a different methodological approach, namely, more extensive tracer injections used in the study on cat. Branching of basal forebrain neurons to multiple cortical areas was regarded (Boylan *et al.*, 1986) as the substratum of the low incidence of antidromic invasion of basal forebrain neurons to cortical stimulation (Aston-Jones *et al.*, 1984), since action potentials can be blocked at axonal branching points.

Ultrastructural studies indicate that cholinergic fibers to the cerebral cortex that probably originate in nucleus basalis and related areas have pleomorphic synaptic vesicles at symmetrical junctions (Houser *et al.*, 1985).

4.3. Brainstem and Spinal Cord Projections of the Cholinergic Mesopontine and Noncholinergic Pontobulbar Reticular Formation

4.3.1. Cholinergic Projections to Pontine FTG

The natural source of cholinergic input to pontine reticular formation is of interest for the physiology of rapid eye movement (REM) sleep because microin

Figure 12. Neocortical projections of intralaminar thalamic neurons and their monosynaptic excitation from upper brainstem reticular core in cat. A: Calvarium with last recording thalamic microelectrode (Th) and chronically implanted stimulating electrodes in pericruciate motor cortex (M), parietal association cortex (P), and midbrain reticular formation (MRF). EOG and EEG, silver balls for recording eye movements and EEG rhythms; H, electrodes for recording hippocampal rhythms. B: Lesion of the ipsilateral pontine tegmentum for chronic degeneration of ascending systems coursing through MRF. Abbreviations: BC, brachium conjunctivum; BP, brachium pontis; CS, nucleus raphe centralis superior; IC, inferior colliculus; LC, locus coeruleus; PG, pontine gray; RPO, nucleus reticularis pontis oralis. C: Array of stimulating electrodes in the caudal part of the MRF, within the peribrachial area of the pedunculopontine nucleus; the most lateral electrode track was found in an anterior section. D: Location of precruciate stimulating electrodes within deep layers of medial parts of areas 8 and 6. In the diagram, black dots indicate the whole territory of pericruciate and anterior suprasylvian gyri (various cytoarchitectonic areas are indicated). E: Location of a sample of CL-PC thalamic neurons. Anti and Syn, antidromic and synaptic responses to stimulation of motor cortex, parietal cortex, and MRF. Abbreviations: CeM, Rh, VM, and VPM, central medial, rhomboidal, ventromedial, and ventoposteromedial thalamic nuclei. F: Electrophysiological identification of CL-PC thalamic cells. 1 and 2, two different neurons antidromically activated form the internal capsule (IC) or motor cortex (MC) and synaptically driven from MRF. Stimulus artifacts marked by arrowheads. In 2, only first stimulus of MC three-shock train at 250/sec is marked; arrow indicates fractionation of antidromically elicited discharges to last stimulus in MC train. Collision between cortically elicited antidromic spikes and MRF-evoked synaptic discharges shown in right superimposition (1) and in ten-sweep sequence (in 2). Modified from Steriade and Glenn (1982) and Glenn and Steriade (1982).

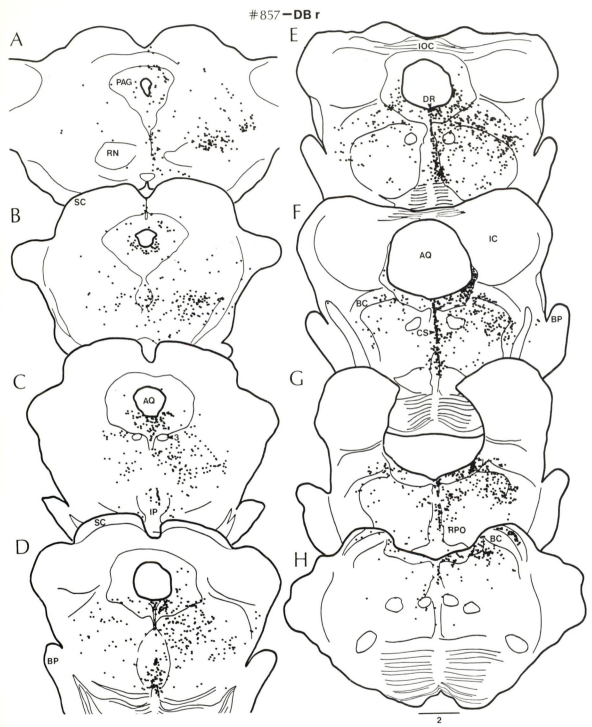

Figure 13. Projections of brainstem neurons to the diagonal band (DB) nuclei of cat. Injection of WGA-HRP in the medial part of the horizontal branch of DB, at right. TMB procedure. Eight brainstem levels (A to H, rostral to caudal) are depicted. Note massive projections from the rostral midbrain reticular formation (A), peribrachial area of the central tegmental field (B–D), and raphe nuclei at the midbrain–pontine junction (E to G). Abbreviations: CS, centralis superior raphe nucleus; DR, dorsal raphe nucleus. For other abbreviations, see preceding figures in this chapter. Unpublished data by D. Paré, Y. Smith, A. Parent and M. Steriade.

jection of cholinergic drugs into the pontine reticular formation of the cat activates a state that has, depending on the injection site, either all or some of the components of natural REM sleep, which include rapid eye movements, pontogeniculooccipital (PGO) waves, and a suppression of postural muscle tone with superimposed distal muscle twitches (see Chapters 9, 10, and 11).

A recent study by Mitani, McCarley, and co-workers (1988d) has demonstrated that the laterodorsal tegmental nucleus (LDT) and pedunculopontine tegmental nucleus (PPT) both provide cholinergic projections to the cat pontine reticular formation gigantocellular tegmental field (PFTG). Neurons of the LDT and PPT were double labeled utilizing choline acetyltransferase (ChAT) immunohistochemistry combined with retrograde transport of horseradish peroxidase conjugated with wheat germ agglutinin (WGA–HRP; Fig. 14). In LDT the percentage of cholinergic neurons retrogradely labeled from PFTG was 10.2% ipsilaterally and 3.7% contralaterally, whereas in PPT the percentages were 5.2% ipsilaterally and 1.3% contralaterally (Fig. 15). Double-labeled neurons were observed throughout the rostral–caudal extent of the LDT and PPT, and no apparent preferential topographic localization was observed in those nuclei. These projections and their relative density have recently been confirmed in a double-labeling study by Shiromani and co-workers (1988a).

The Mitani *et al.* study also used *Phaseolus vulgaris* leukoagglutinin (PHA-L) anterograde transport technique to show that PHA-L-positive fibers projecting from LDT into the PFTG spread ventrally from the injection site and enter the ipsilateral PFTG, although some crossed the midline and entered the contralateral PFTG (Fig. 16, part 1). PHA-L-positive fibers and varicosities were also observed in the raphe nucleus and contralateral LDT. The PHA-L-positive fibers from PPT injections course ventromedially from the injection site and enter the ipsilateral PFTG, although some cross the midline and enter the contralateral PFTG (Fig. 16, part 2). On both sides of the PFTG, the PHA-L-positive fibers from both LDT and PPT give rise to boutonlike varicosities (Fig. 14F) suggestive of termination within the PFTG.

As measured by the percentage of double-labeled cholinergic neurons, the density of cholinergic LDT-to-PFTG projections observed appears to approximate that of cholinergic LDT-to-thalamus projections in rat (Hallanger *et al.*, 1987), where, ipsilaterally, a mean of 10% of ChAT-positive LDT neurons were double labeled after WGA–HRP injections of comparably small size in thalamus, as compared with the ipsilateral percentage of about 10% in the Mitani *et al.* LDT–PFTG study. Cholinergic PPT-to-PFTG projections appear to be somewhat less dense than described for PPT to thalamus in rat, where ipsilateral double labeling averaged 22% of PPT neurons (range 3–47%, Hallanger *et al.*, 1987). Although the basic techniques of injection, processing, and counting were similar in Hallanger's and Mitani's studies, the percentages should, of course, be taken only as approximate comparisons of projection strengths, since the species were different and the size of WGA–HRP injections in the zones of interest varied.

These cholinergic inputs to PFTG likely form the basis of induction of REM sleep by PFTG neostigmine injections (Baghdoyan *et al.*, 1985), which presumably act on the acetylcholine released by these inputs. Pathology of these projections may be responsible for the abnormalities of muscarinic receptor binding in PFTG observed in canine narcolepsy (Boehme *et al.*, 1984; see Chapter 13). Finally, as will be discussed later, these LDT/PPT projections may be important

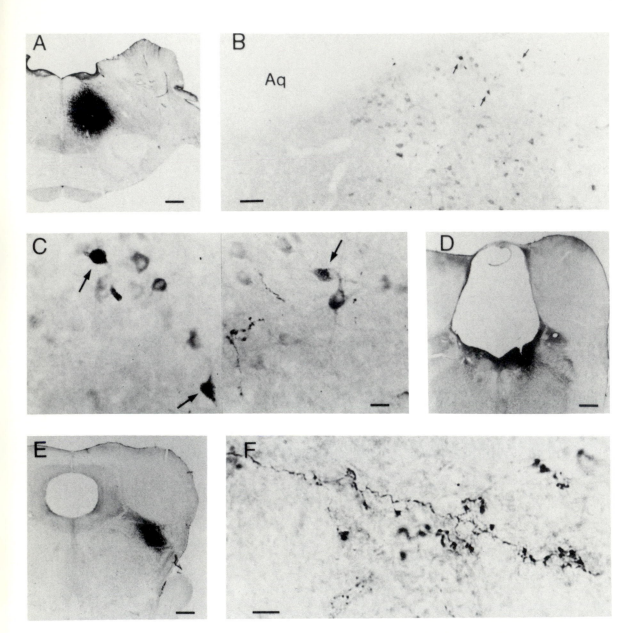

Figure 14. A: Site of WGA–HRP injection in the pontine gigantocellular tegmental field (PFTG) of the cat. B: Double-labeled neurons (solid arrows) with both ChAT immunoreactivity and retrogradely transported WGA–HRP were found in the LDT together with neurons stained only for ChAT (level corresponds to C in Fig. 15). C: A higher magnification of three double-labeled neurons shown in upper part of B. Note the black granular HRP reaction product in the double-labeled ChAT-positive neurons (solid arrows) but not in the single-labeled ChAT-positive neurons near them. D: Photograph of PHA-L injection site in the laterodorsal tegmental nucleus. E: PHA-L injection site in the pedunculopontine nucleus (pars compacta). F: Labeled fine axons and boutonlike varicosities in the ipsilateral PFTG after PHA-L injection into the laterodorsal tegmental field (level corresponds to Fig. 16, part 1B) Calibration bars: A,D,E, 1 mm; B, 100 μm; C, 20μm; F, 10 μm. Abbreviation: Aq, cerebral aqueduct. From Mitani *et al.* (1988d).

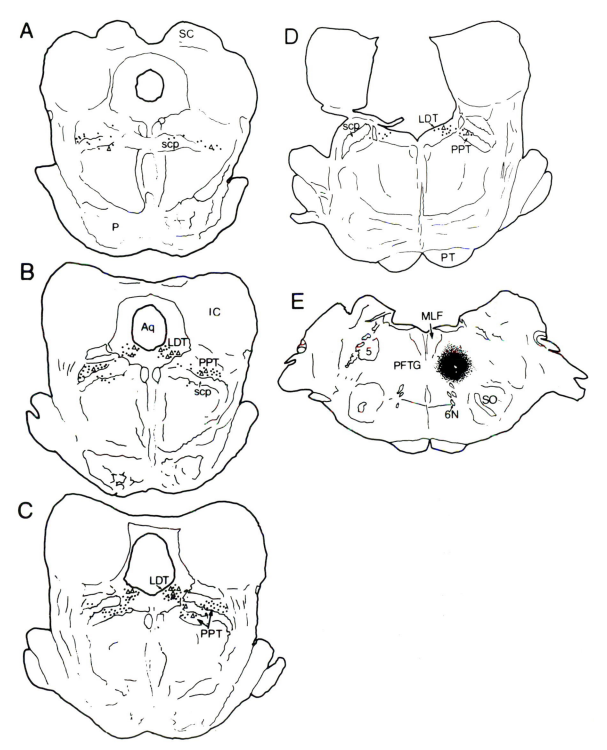

Figure 15. A–D: The distribution of LDT and PPT neurons double labeled with both retrogradely transported WGA–HRP and ChAT immunocytochemistry (open triangles), and single labeled with ChAT immunocytochemistry (black dots). E: representation of the PFTG injection site of WGA–HRP. Abbreviations: IC, inferior colliculus; LDT, laterodor-sal tegmental nucleus; MLF, medial longitudinal fasciculus; P, pontine nuclei; PFTG, pontine gigantocellular tegmental field; PPT, pedunculopontine tegmental nucleus; PT, pyra-midal tract; SC, superior colliculus; scp, superior cerebellar peduncle; SO, superior olive; 5, trigeminal nucleus; 6N, ab-ducens nerve. From Mitani *et al.* (1988d).

in the induction and maintenance of various components of normal REM sleep and of other behavioral states. The presence of LDT/PPT projections to other pontine reticular nuclei remains to be determined.

4.3.2. Bulbar and Spinal Cord Cholinergic Projections

Utilizing autoradiographic anterograde tracing and retrograde HRP/-WGA–HRP techniques in conjunction with ChAT immunohistochemistry, a

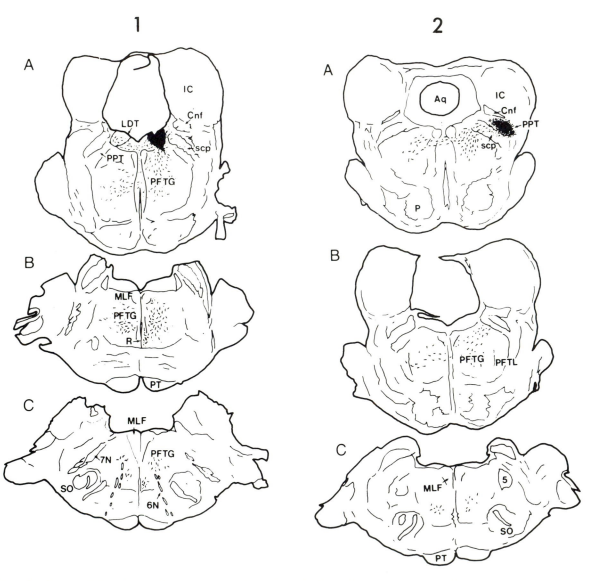

Figure 16. Part 1 (left column): Distribution of labeled fibers and terminals (broken lines) after an iontophoretic injection of PHA-L into the laterodorsal tegmental nucleus in the cat. Injection site is represented in A. Abbreviations: Cnf, cuneiform nucleus; R, raphe nucleus; 7N, facial nerve. Part 2 (right column): Distribution of labeled fibers and ter- minals (broken lines) after an iontophoretic injection of PHA-L into the pars compacta of the pedunculopontine teg- mental nucleus. Injection site is represented in A. Abbrevia- tion: PFTL, pontine lateral tegmental field. From Mitani *et al.* (1988d).

recent study in the rat has characterized the bulbar and spinal efferents from the mesopontine junctional region that includes the cholinergic PPT nucleus and the noncholinergic mesopontine tegmentum (Rye *et al.*, 1988). Figure 17 summarizes the anatomy of this region and the major descending pathway. Rye *et al.* (1988) label the major descending pathway as Probst's tract, and we follow this terminology. Probst's tract descends in the dorsolateral reticular formation in close apposition to the nucleus of the solitary tract (Fig. 17) and has several branches. (1) A *ventrolateral* branch of Probst's tract courses alongside the spinal trigeminal nucleus and is the primary projection pathway of the parabrachial nucleus, particularly the Kolliker–Fuse nucleus. (2) A *ventromedial* branch of Probst's tract contains fibers from PPT, the subcoeruleus region, as well as an adjacent portion of FTC that has reciprocal connections with entopeduncular nucleus and substantia nigra and afferents from globus pallidus, which was termed the midbrain extrapyramidal area by Rye and colleagues (1987). The ventromedial branch courses through the pons to bulb, where its fibers distribute to the ipsilateral bulbar gigantocellular field. This ventromedial branch closely corresponds to the "lateral tegmentoreticular tract" described by Russell (1955) and Sakai *et al.* (1979) as descending from the subcoerulear region and is physiologically important because of its role in the postural atonia in sleep.

Both Sakai's and Rye's papers indicate the presence of a projection of the ventromedial branch to the reticular zone just dorsal to the caudal two-thirds of the inferior olive, termed the "magnocellular tegmental field" by Sakai and his colleagues. However, Rye and co-workers suggest that the designation of this area as "magnocellular tegmental field" is not in accord with Berman (1968) and Kalia and Fuxe (1985), who indicate that this is a ventral portion of the gigantocellular tegmental field. While this may seem a trivial point, it is in fact not, since the pathway and its projection zone are important for muscle inhibition in sleep. For example, Chase *et al.* (1986) characterize a portion of BFTG as involved in muscle atonia during REM sleep, and this description is often thought to be in conflict with Sakai's description of the area, but, in fact, the apparent conflict is simply one of terminology and not physiology. Rye's paper indicates further that this subcoerulear projection is noncholinergic.

Rye and co-workers (1988) did note a ventromedial pathway that crosses the midline shortly after origin and descends in a ventral paramedian position through the contralateral bulbar magnocellular field, but this crossing cholinergic pathway is apparently not critical for REM atonia. Most of the spinal projections of this mesopontine zone arise from the noncholinergic midbrain extrapyramidal area, but no cholinergic neurons project to spinal cord. Retrograde HRP studies suggest that the spinal fibers arising from this zone course in the lateral funiculus (Tohyama *et al.*, 1979b; Mitani *et al.*, 1988a).

Rye and colleagues (1988) found the PPT cholinergic projection to bulbar reticular formation to be dense, with 18% of the cholinergic PPT neurons double labeled after a BFTG injection of WGA–HRP, with an ipsilateral : contralateral ratio of about 2 : 1. Rye *et al.* do not describe LDT as a significant source of projections to bulbar reticular formation; however, their Fig. 12 indicates that at least 12 LTD neurons were double labeled after an injection centered in BFTG, approximately 10% of the PPT double labeling on the same sections. The crossed cholinergic PPT projection to the magnocellular bublar nucleus was about one-fourth as dense as that of the ipsilateral PPT-to-BFTG

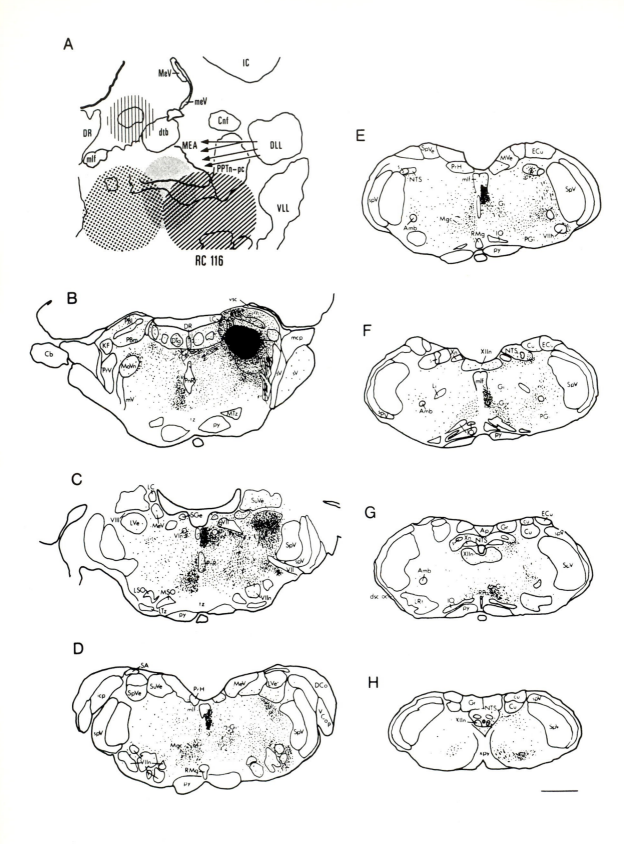

projection. This study did not evaluate the density of cholinergic projections to other bulbar reticular nuclei.

103

EFFERENT
CONNECTIONS

projection. This study did not evaluate the density of cholinergic projections to other bulbar reticular nuclei.

4.3.3. Brainstem and Spinal Cord Projections of the Noncholinergic Pontobulbar Reticular Formation

Recent anatomic advances have more clearly characterized the descending pathways from the giant-cell-field portion of the pons (PFTG) and bulb (BFTG) and have made it apparent that particular pathways arise preferentially from reticular elements of different size. It is consequently useful to follow this division in discussion of the pathways, for which we will present only the major projections, which are epitomized in Fig. 18.

Before going into a more detailed description, we believe it is useful to provide the following overview. Large and giant neurons form the predominant source of the descending projections in the medial longitudinal fasiculus (MLF) in both the pontine and the bulbar reticular formation, and these projections descend in the spinal cord in the ventral funiculus (VF). In contrast, neurons of medium and small size in PFTG project primarily and densely to ipsi- and contralateral bulbar reticular formation, especially the BFTG. Neurons of small and medium size in BFTG send descending axons in the lateral funiculus (LF).

Because of the possibility of terminological confusion, it is also useful at this point to review the terminology associated with the midline fiber tracts of the pons and bulb, the trajectory taken by many reticulospinal fibers. The dorsalmost portion is consistently termed the medial longitudinal fasciculus (MLF) and is comprised of caudally and rostrally coursing fibers associated with the oculomotor and vestibular systems (see Chapter 10). Traveling more ventrally in the same central white matter area are fiber bundles that have been termed the tectospinal tract and the medial reticulospinal tract, after their presumed sites of origin and termination, a terminology based on earlier studies and followed by classic anatomic texts (e.g., Ranson and Clark, 1953, Fig. 153; Crosby *et al.*, 1962, Figs. 140, 145; Elliott, 1969, Plates XXI–XXIII). However, more recent ante-

Figure 17. Five major descending pathways of the dorsolateral tegmentum in the rat. Part A shows anatomy of tritiated AA injection site of RC116 as indicated by heavy oblique lines—other shadings in inset correspond to other injection sites. Note the position of the pedunculopontine tegmental nucleus pars compacta (PPTn-pc) and midbrain extrapyramidal area (MEA); arrows indicate fascicles of the commissure of the lateral lemniscus (DLL). Parts B–H show the five major descending pathways: (1) Probst's tract descending in the dorsolateral reticular formation in close relation to the nucleus of the solitary tract (NTS, D–G). (2) A ventrolateral branch of Probst's tract that extends ventrolaterally alongside the spinal trigeminal nucleus (SpV, C–G). (3) A ventromedial branch of Probst's tract that extends ventromedially throughout the gigantocellular field of the medulla (Gi, C–G). This ventromedial branch is often termed the "lateral tegmentoreticular tract" and contains fibers thought to be important in the muscle atonia of REM sleep (see Chapter 10). (4) The medial reticulospinal tract, which descends in parallel with the medial longitudinal fasciculus (mlf, C–E) and turns ventrolaterally along the dorsal surface of the inferior olive (F–G) to enter the ventrolateral funiculus of the spinal cord. (This pathway arises primarily from pontine tegmental fields, including the gigantocellular field). (5) A crossed ventromedial pathway that descends in a ventral paramedian position through the magnocellular field of the medulla (Mgc, B–E). All except the crossed ventromedial pathway were labeled bilaterally with a strong ipsilateral predominance. Calibration bar, 0.5 mm for A and 1 mm for B–H. Modified from Rye *et al.* (1988).

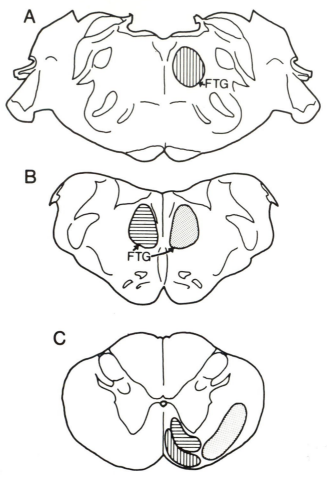

Figure 18. Summary diagram of the course of the major reticulospinal pathways from the pontine FTG (A) and bulbar FTG (B). C: Approximate location of the reticulospinal pathways in C1. Pontine reticulospinal fibers (vertical lines) descend in the ipsilateral ventromedial part of the ventral funiculus. Crossed bulbar reticulospinal fibers (horizontal lines) descend in the contralateral dorsolateral part of the ventral funiculus. Uncrossed bulbar reticulospinal fibers (stipples) descend in the ventral part of the ipsilateral lateral funiculus. See text for description of the sizes of the cells of origin of each pathway. From Mitani *et al.* (1988a).

rograde tracing studies (Figs. 19 and 20) and intracellular HRP injections (also illustrated below) have refined our conception of the course taken by pontine and bulbar reticulospinal fibers. This book, in agreement with the terminological convention of Holstege and Kuypers (1982), has taken the course of using the MLF as a convenient terminological reference point for the pontine and bulbar central white matter while letting the data speak for themselves about the exact reticulospinal fiber course within this midline substantia alba.

4.3.3.1. Reticulospinal Pathways from Pontine FTG Coursing in the Ipsilateral MLF-VF

In the pons, ipsilateral VF pathways have been indicated by autoradiographic studies in the cat (Holstege and Kuypers, 1982), opossum (Martin *et al.*,

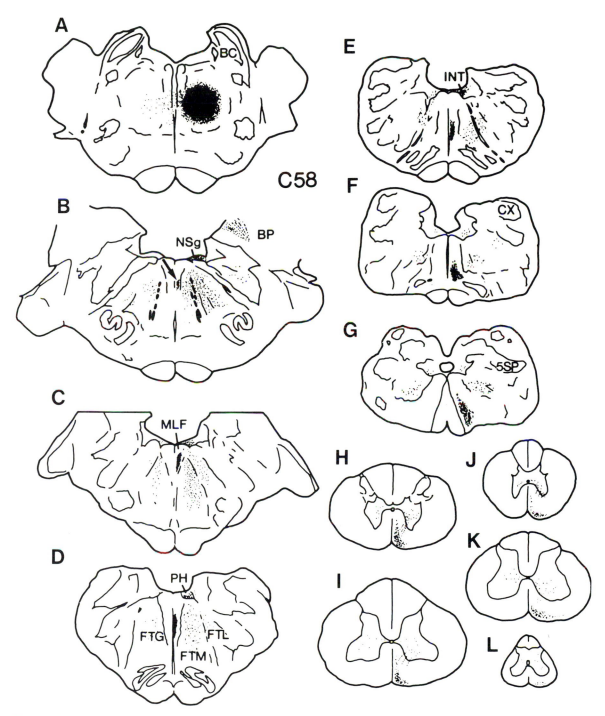

Figure 19. Anterogradely labeled descending fiber course for pontine FTG WGA–HRP injection, case C58. Sections H–L are at spinal cord C1, C7, T5, L4, and S3, respectively. Note fibers descending ipsilaterally in the medial longitudinal fasciculus (MLF)–ventral funiculus and bilaterally to the bulbar reticular formation. 5SP, spinal trigeminal nucleus; 7G, genu of the facial nerve; BC, brachium conjunctivum; BP, brachium pontis; CX, external cuneate nucleus; INT, nucleus intercalatus; NSg, n. supragenualis; PH, n. prepositus hypoglossi. From Mitani *et al.* (1988a).

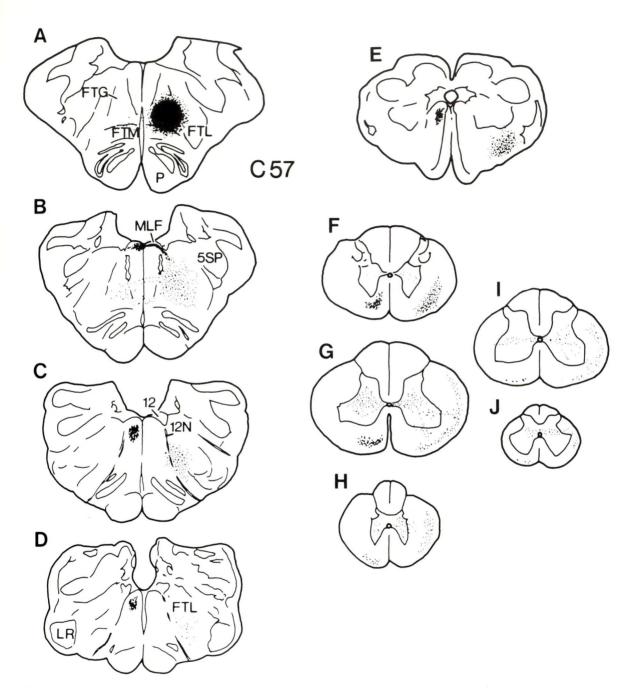

Figure 20. Anterogradely labeled descending fiber course for injection in bulbar FTG, case C57. Sections F–J are at C1, C7, T5, L4, and S2, respectively. Note fibers descending both in the contralateral medial longitudinal fasciculus–ven-tral funiculus and the ipsilateral bulbar reticular formation–lateral funiculus. 12, hypoglossal nucleus; 12N, hypoglossal nerve; LR, lateral reticular nucleus. From Mitani *et al.* (1988a).

1979), and rat (Jones and Yang, 1985) and a retrograde HRP study in the cat (Tohyama *et al.*, 1979a). Recent anterograde WGA–HRP and intracellular HRP injection studies in the cat (Mitani *et al.*, 1988a) have provided a more detailed description of the fiber trajectory: PFTG reticulospinal fibers enter the ipsilateral MLF, descend through the ventral part of the MLF in the bulb and the ventromedial part of the VF in the upper cervical cord, and continue in the VF to all spinal levels. All studies suggest distribution to laminae V–X with a main distribution to laminae VII and VIII. Jones and Yang (1985) noted in their study on rat that reticulospinal fibers from the PFTG descend not only into the ipsilateral VF but also into the contralateral VF; the contralateral descending fibers cross over dorsally to enter the contralateral MLF after leaving the injection site. However, in the anterograde WGA–HRP study of Mitani *et al.* (1988a), reticulospinal fibers descending into the contralateral MLF–VF from the PFTG in the cat were only observed when the WGA–HRP deposit extended into levels caudal to the abducens nerve (as described below for bulbar FTG), and Figure 5 of the Jones and Yang (1985) paper suggests that this may also be true in the rat.

4.3.3.2. Reticulospinal Pathways of Bulbar FTG in the Contralateral and Ipsilateral MLF–VF

The initial autoradiographic study in the cat of Basbaum *et al.* (1978), as well as subsequent autoradiographic studies in the cat (Holstege and Kuypers, 1982) and rat (Zemlan *et al.*, 1984; Jones and Yang, 1985), indicate bulbar reticulospinal neurons send axons bilaterally in MLF–VF with a contralateral predominance. The course of BFTG reticulospinal fibers in the contralateral MLF–VF has been detailed with anterograde WHA–HRP and intracellular HRP studies (Mitani *et al.*, 1988a,c) and is congruent with the findings of the previous studies: fibers course dorsomedially to the floor of the fourth ventricle, cross the midline, turn caudally, descend in the dorsal part of the contralateral MLF, and then continue in the contralateral VF. Reticulospinal fibers in the contralateral MLF–VF descend to all spinal levels, although they are diminished in number at lumbosacral levels (Basbaum *et al.*, 1978). Distribution is principally to laminae VII–VIII.

4.3.3.3. Pontine and Bulbar FTG Descending Pathways Not in Ventral Funiculus

In contrast to the predominantly large and giant neurons sending axons in MLF–VF, the dense PFTG-to-BFTG projections arose from small and medium neurons (Mitani *et al.*, 1988a,b). The density of this projection has also been seen in autoradiographic studies in the cat (Jones and Yang, 1985). The HRP studies indicate that there is a slight contralateral preference and that density of pontine reticular formation retrograde labeling after HRP injections into the BFTG is approximately threefold greater in PFTG compared with other pontine reticular nuclei (FTP > FTL) and with the midbrain FTC (Mitani *et al.*, 1988a).

A non-VF descending fiber system has been described in the cat (Basbaum *et al.*, 1978; Holstege and Kuypers, 1982) and rat (Zemlan *et al.*, 1984; Jones and Yang, 1985) and consists of fibers descending in the ipsilateral lateral funiculus (LF) of the spinal cord. Basbaum *et al.* (1978) suggested there was an initial course of fibers in MLF, and Mitani *et al.* (1988a) observed that the relatively small-diameter fibers directly descended in BRF, whereas those descending in the ipsilateral MLF were mainly of relatively large diameter, findings directly confirmed with intracellular HRP injections (Mitani *et al.,* 1988c).

The relative preponderance of reticulospinal projections onto motoneurons as opposed to other spinal cord neurons is unknown. However, a recent auto-radiographic–EM study in rat with injection zones including bulbar FTG and magnocellularis (as well as other ventral reticular structures) reported evidence that more than 50% of medial reticular formation synaptic terminals studied in lumbar spinal cord contact motoneurons, and preferentially their proximal dendrites; the motoneurons had been retrogradely labeled by HRP injected in the muscle (Holstege and Kuypers, 1987). Electrophysiological mapping of reticular projections to spinal motoneurons has shown the presence of several different projection zones within the pontobulbar reticular formation (Peterson, 1977).

4.4. Intrinsic Morphology of Pontobulbar Reticular Formation Neurons and Correlations with Anatomic Projections

The neuronal morphology of reticular neurons in the cat has been examined by the Golgi method (Scheibel and Scheibel, 1958; Valverde, 1961; Ramon-Moliner and Nauta, 1966). Scheibel and Scheibel (1958), using the Golgi method in young mammals, described neurons in the pontobulbar FTG region with axons that bifurcated into ascending and descending branches and also gave off richly branching collaterals to the cranial nerve nuclei and reticular formation. For many years their camera lucida drawing (Fig. 21) was often used to represent "the canonical reticular formation neuron" until studies in adult animals found less of the exuberant axonal branching and a relative paucity of neurons with both ascending and descending branching. The Scheibels further suggested that the dendritic fields of PFTG neurons had a characteristic flattening in the anterior–posterior direction, which was described as a "poker chip" configuration.

Morphology is of special interest in FTG both from the standpoint of intrinsic interest—the giant cells are among the largest in the brain—and also from the standpoint of whether any functional or projection specialization might be indicated by size. As an example, after the discovery of REM-sleep-related activity in this region, an initial speculation was that the "giant cells" served to convey this excitation to many regions, presupposing that it was the giant cells of the FTG that had the effulgent branching represented by the Scheibels' "canonical reticular neuron." Recent evaluations by McCarley and co-workers of pontobulbar reticular neurons in the giant-cell field using electrophysiological recording and stimulation techniques combined with intracellular HRP injection to reveal the morphology have begun to allow more definitive answers about FTG morphology and its functional linkage, and we here sketch this information. The data from the intracellular HRP labeling studies were always in agreement with the extracellular antero- and retrograde tracing studies described previously (unless otherwise stated these data are from Mitani *et al.,* 1988a–c).

4.4.1. Cell Size Distribution within the Pontine and Bulbar FTG

The discussions in this chapter make it clear that the large and giant neurons in PFTG and BFTG apparently tend to have different functional connections (to MLF–VF) and an absence of collaterals. In this regard and for future studies it is important to have quantitative data on the cell sizes in the pontobulbar FTG, and the cytoarchitectural observations of a recent study are of interest (Mitani *et al.*, 1988a). On Nissl-stained sections from two cats, 1-mm square areas of FTG were randomly selected at every 1-mm distance from posterior 2.0 mm to posterior 11.0 mm, and the diameters of all FTG neuronal cell bodies with a nucleolus were measured. The FTG neuronal cell bodies were classified as (1) *small,* average diameters (AD) < 20 μm; (2) *medium,* AD < 40 μm; (3) *large,* AD < 60 μm; and (4) *giant,* AD > 60 μm. The percentage of each size was then calculated in each of the ten 1-mm square areas of each brainstem. The average percentages were: small (57%), medium (35%), large (6%), and giant (2%). Thus, in general, the giant-cell field has a few large and giant neurons that are scattered among many small and medium neurons (see also Section 1.4). Although the absolute values of the soma sizes will vary somewhat (perhaps 10–20%) with differences in anatomic and measurement technique, and hence the boundary values listed here should not be taken as rigid absolutes, it is likely true that the relative proportions of neurons of different sizes are accurate and

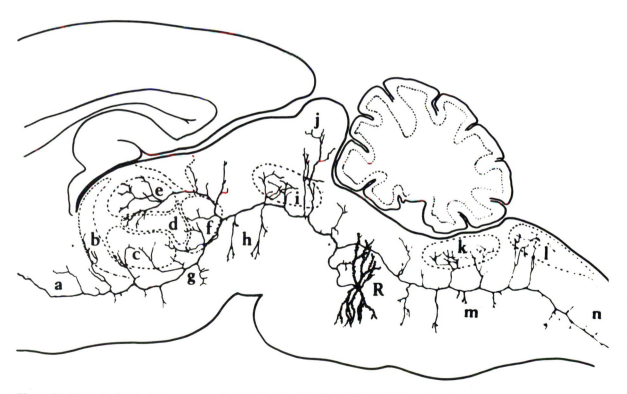

Figure 21. Extend of reticular neuron as depicted by the Scheibels (1958). Golgi preparation.

should be taken into account in modeling function and interpreting results. For example, because of the sampling bias of microelectrodes for medium to large neurons, we know much more about the physiology of medium to giant neurons than of the numerous small neurons in FTG.

4.4.2. Morphology of Pontine FTG Neurons

The morphology of reticuloreticular pontine neurons (antidromically identified from the bulbar reticular formation) and of reticulospinal pontine neurons was recently studied by means of intracellular HRP injections (Mitani *et al.*, 1988a). The pontine reticular neurons projecting to bulbar reticular fields have soma diameters (mean 40 μm) smaller than pontine neurons projecting in MLF (around 60 μm), thinner axons, and smaller, slightly oblate dendritic fields. Quantitative data indicated that, by contrast to previous Golgi studies on young mammals by the Scheibels (1958) and Valverde (1961), who assumed that the reticular dendritic field is flattened in the anteroposterior plane, the mean anteroposterior extent of the dendritic field of intracellularly stained pontine reticular cells in the adult cat is at least 16% less than the dorsoventral and mediolateral extents. Although no pontine neurons projecting in MLF were observed to have axon collaterals, 36% of pontobulbar reticular neurons have axon collaterals projecting to the ipsilateral abducens nucleus or the adjacent pontine gigantocellular field. The collaterals to the abducens nucleus may be involved in the generation of horizontal saccades (Igusa *et al.*, 1980; Sasaki and Shimazu, 1981), whereas the collaterals to the adjacent pontine reticular fields and the bulbar reticular formation may subserve the spread and maintenance of membrane depolarization in the reticular population during the REM sleep state (Ito and McCarley, 1984).

4.4.2.1. Pontine FTG Neurons Sending Axons in the Ipsilateral MLF (PFTG-to-iMLF Neurons)

Figure 22 is a composite photomicrograph of an intracellularly HRP-labeled giant cell neuron in PFTG. The ellipsoid–polygonal soma measures 100 × 50 μm (long × short axis) with an average soma diameter of 75 μm; even in the photograph, dendritic field diameter is seen to extend some 2 mm in the dorsoventral and mediolateral directions. Such HRP-stained neurons are clearly visible in sections viewed without the aid of a microscope. Figure 23 shows a camera lucida reproduction of another giant cell with soma measurements of 103 × 41 (mean = 72) μm and a dendritic field diameter of about 2 mm with the axonal course in ipsilateral MLF labeled in part B. Both of these neurons were antidromically activated from stimulating electrodes placed in ipsilateral bulbar MLF. Most PFTG neurons sending axons in iMLF have large ellipsoid–polygonal somata (mean 60 μm) and thick axons (average diameter 3 μm). Slightly oblate large dendritic fields are also typical, with mean anteroposterior extent of 1500 μm, a mean mediolateral extent of 1800 μm and a mean dorsoventral extent of 1600 μm. No neurons sending axons in MLF were observed to have axon collaterals.

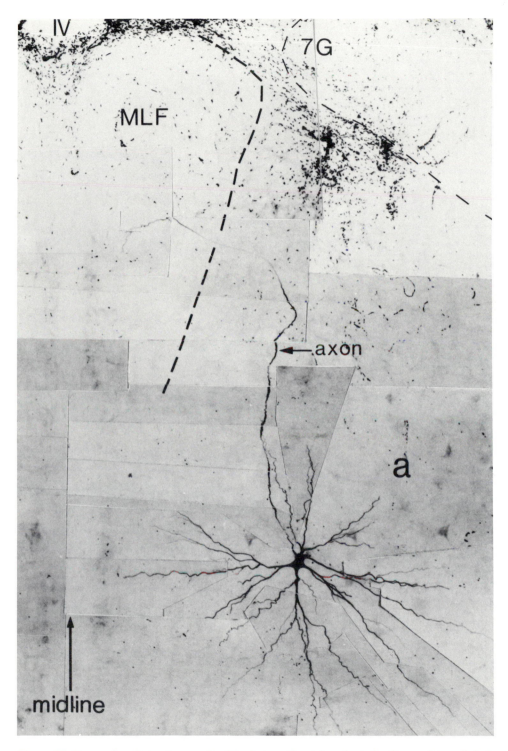

Figure 22. Composite photomicrograph of brainstem (frontal section) showing an intracellularly stained large PFTG neuron (a) with axon entering MLF. Note the axon courses caudodorsomedially in the PFTG and enters the ipsilateral MLF at a level near the genu of the facial nerve (7G). Note the large extent of the dendritic field, over 2 mm. IV, fourth ventricle. From Mitani *et al.* (1988b).

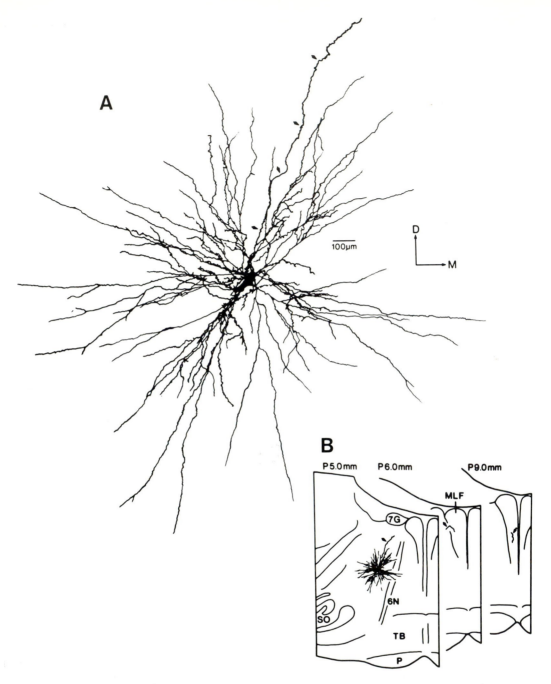

Figure 23. Camera lucida drawing of pontine FTG neuron sending its axon in ipsilateral MLF (frontal sections); the cell body, dendrites, and proximal axon are shown in (A) and neuronal location and axon course in (B). Note the large ellipsoid–polygonal cell body (major axis 103 μm and minor axis 41 μm with average diameter 72 μm) with the major axis slanted from dorsomedial to ventrolateral. The dendrites were nonspiny and had extensive branching. The dendritic field was large, extending 2100 μm in the M–L direction and 2030 μm in the D–V direction; the axis of the dendritic field was tilted from dorsomedial to ventrolateral. The axon (solid arrows in A and B) originated from the cell body, ran dorsomedially, then turned caudally into the ipsilateral MLF and descended toward the spinal cord (B). No axon collaterals were observed. The average axon diameter was 3.3 μm. Abbreviations: P(posterior) 5.0 mm, 6.0 mm, and 9.0 mm are frontal coordinates of labeled neuron and axons in Berman Atlas (the plane of this section ran 40° caudal to the Berman perpendicular plane). SO, superior olivary nucleus. From Mitani *et al.* (1988b).

Figure 24 is a camera lucida drawing of horizontal section with a PFTG neuron whose axon projects directly to BRF and does not collateralize. The neuron was of medium size (mean soma diameter 38 μm), with an axon diameter of 1.6 μm. The dendritic field, although large, is only 10% reduced in the anteroposterior direction (1400 μm) as compared with the mediolateral direction (1500 μm) and hence does not resemble a "poker chip." Figure 25 shows another PFTG neuron whose axon courses directly into BRF; this axon, like that of 36% of the BRF-projecting neurons, was collateralized, in this case with projections to abducens nucleus. Overall, PFTG neurons whose axons projected directly to BRF had, in comparison to those with axons in MLF, smaller ellipsoid–polygonal somata (mean, 40 μm), thinner axons (average diameter 2.3 μm), and slightly smaller dendritic fields with a mean anteroposterior extent of 1300 μm, a mean mediolateral extent of 1500 μm, and a mean dorsoventral extent of 1200 μm. All of these neurons were antidromically activated from BFTG but not from MLF.

The trajectories of axon collaterals of the PFTG-to-BRF neurons that projected to the ipsilateral abducens nucleus resembled those of HRP-stained reticular neurons in the cat (Grantyn *et al.*, 1980), HRP-intraxonally-stained reticular neurons in the monkey (Strassman *et al.*, 1986), and Golgi-impregnated neurons in young mice (see Fig. 11, neuron b, in Scheibel and Scheibel, 1958). However, intracellularly labeled PFTG neurons with projections to both the abducens nucleus and the spinal cord, as reported by Grantyn *et al.* (1980, 1988), were not observed. As described in Chapter 9, the Grantyn *et al.* data were from a physiologically selected and specialized population. Since the anterograde WGA–HRP study (Mitani *et al.*, 1988a) also found that fibers of PFTG neurons descending in the BRF could not be traced as far as the spinal cord, it is likely that the neurons described by Grantyn *et al.* may be from a relatively small subpopulation.

A specific orientation preference of the major soma axis was present only in PFTG-to-iMLF neurons (Mitani *et al.*, 1988b). The major axis of these neurons was angled from dorsal/dorsomedial to ventral/ventrolateral in frontal sections (67%), from dorsocaudal to ventrorostral in parasagittal sections (76%), and from medial to lateral in horizontal sections (91%). The finding in frontal sections agrees with previous work by Newman (1985b), but preferences in parasagittal and horizontal sections had not previously been studied.

4.4.2.3. Dendrites

The findings that PFTG dendrites repeatedly gave off two or three branches and extended for long distances are in agreement with data from Golgi studies (Scheibel and Scheibel, 1958; Valverde, 1961; Newman, 1985b). The "dendritic index" is defined by dividing the total number of terminal branches by the total number of trunks (Edwards *et al.*, 1987) and, when high, indicates a high degree of branching. The dendritic indices were high for both PFTG-to-iMLF neurons (mean = 16) and for PFTG-to-BRF neurons (mean = 14) and did not significantly differ but were higher than for some bulbar reticular neurons (see below).

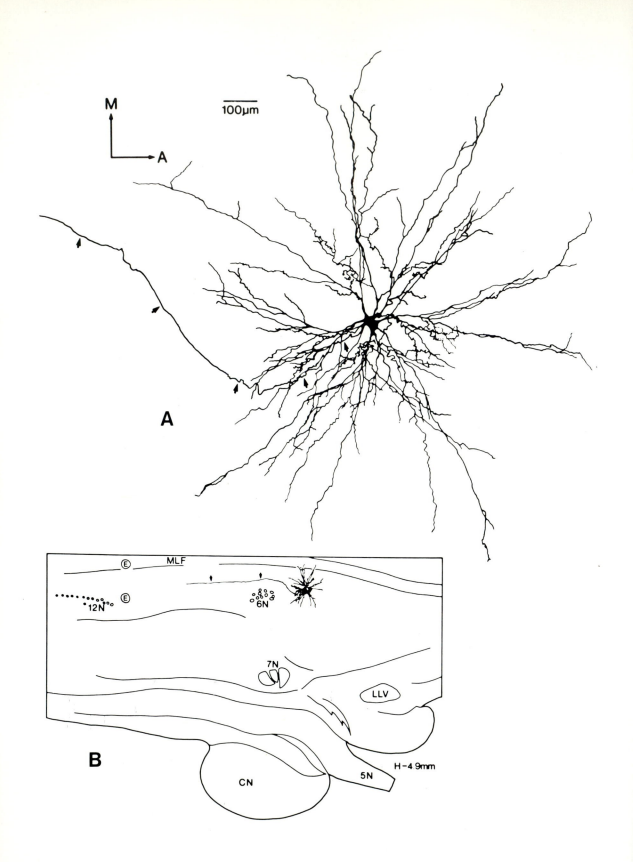

M

A

100μm

A

MLF

Ⓔ

Ⓔ

12N

6N

7N

LLV

CN

5N

H-4.9mm

B

4.4.3. Morphology of Bulbar FTG Neurons

4.4.3.1. Bulbar FTG Neurons Sending Axons in the Ipsilateral MLF (BFTG-to-iMLF) Neurons or Contralateral MLF (BFTG-to-cMLF) Neurons

As was true for PFTG neurons, Mitani *et al.* (1988c) found that BFTG neurons with axons traveling in MLF had somata that were predominantly in the large to giant size range and, also like the PFTG, had axons that did not collateralize. The BFTG-to-iMLF neurons closely resembled the PFTG-to-iMLF neurons with large ellipsoid–polygonal somata (mean 60 μm), thick axons (average diameter 3 μm), mostly nonspiny dendrites, and dendritic fields that were only slightly flattened in the anteroposterior direction. The BFTG-to-cMLF neurons were similar in soma size (mean 57 μm) and in having thick axons (average diameter 3 μm) and mostly nonspiny dendrites (Fig. 26 and 27). They were, however, different from both pontine and bulbar neurons sending axons in iMLF in that BFTG-to-cMLF neurons had dendritic fields flattened in the anteroposterior direction, where mean extent was 1100 μm compared with 1700 μm in the mediolateral direction and 1400 μm in the dorsoventral direction. The mean anteroposterior extent was thus 32% and 20% less than the mean mediolateral and dorsoventral extents, respectively.

4.4.3.2. Bulbar FTG Neurons That Send Axons Directly into the Ipsilateral Caudal Bulbar Reticular Formation (BFTG-to-iBRF Neurons)

Compared with bulbar and pontine iMLF and cMLF neurons, most BFTG-to-iBRF neurons had smaller ellipsoid–polygonal somata (mean 39 μm) and thinner axons (average diameter 1.8 μm) and dendritic fields that were flattened in the anteroposterior direction, where mean extent was 1200 μm, 35% and 30% less than the mediolateral mean extent of 1900 μm and the mean extent of 1800 μm in the dorsoventral direction, respectively.

In contrast to neurons sending axons in cMLF and iMLF, axon collaterals were present in BFTG-to-iBRF neurons and were much more frequent than in PFTG-to-BFTG neurons: 73% of BFTG-to-iBRF neurons have axon collaterals. Bifurcated axon collaterals with both anterior and posterior projections were also common in the BFTG-to-iBRF neuronal population, being present in about half of BFTG-to-iBRF neurons (Fig. 28). In these neurons antidromic spike potentials were elicited by stimulation of the ipsilateral PFTG.

The "dendritic index" (defined above) was smaller in BFTG neurons (means of cMLF, iMLF, and iBRF neurons were 8, 7, and 9, respectively) than in

---

Figure 24. Camera lucida drawing of pontine FTG neuron with axon descending in BRF but not in MLF (horizontal section). This neuron had an ellipsoid–polygonal cell body of medium size (major axis 45 μm and minor axis 31 μm with average diameter 38 μm). The dendrites were nonspiny. The dendritic field extended 1360 μm in the A–P direction and 1520 μm in the M–L direction. The axis of the longest extent was tilted from medial to lateral. The axon (solid arrows in A and B) originated from the dendritic trunk and after curving laterally for a short distance coursed caudally and entered the BRF. No axon collaterals were observed. The average axon diameter was 1.6 μm. H −4.9 mm is the horizontal coordinate of labeled neuron in Berman Atlas (this horizontal plane of section is approximately parallel to floor of fourth ventricle). From Mitani *et al.* (1988b).

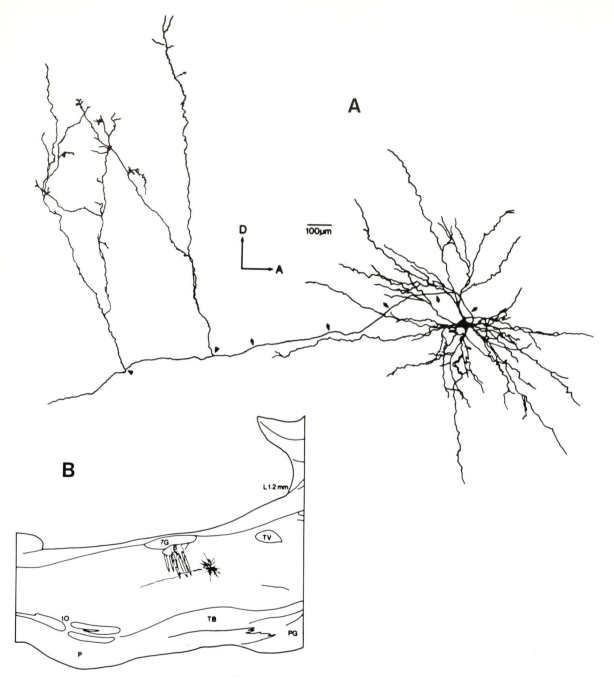

Figure 25. Camera lucida drawing of a pontine FTG neuron with axon descending in BRF but not MLF (parasagittal section). This neuron had an ellipsoid–polygonal cell body of medium size (major axis 55 μm and minor axis 39 μm with average diameter 47 μm). The dendrites were nonspiny. The dendritic field extended 1350 μm in the A–P direction and 1470 μm in the D–V direction, and the axis of the longest extent was tilted slightly from dorsocaudal to ventrorostral. The axon (solid arrows) originated from the dendritic trunk, and coursed dorsally for a short distance, then turned caudally and entered the BRF. Axon collaterals originated from the main axon (solid triangles in A) and projected into the ipsilateral abducens nucleus (B). Average main axon diameter was 1.7 μm, and average axon collateral diameter was less than 1.0 μm. L1.2 mm is parasagittal coordinate of labeled neuron (Berman Atlas coordinate). TV, ventral tegmental nucleus. From Mitani *et al.* (1988b).

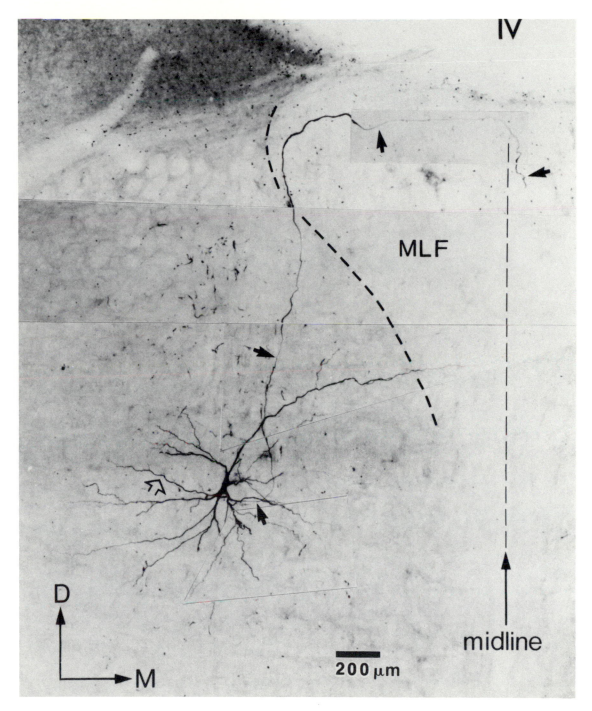

Figure 26. Composite photomicrograph showing an intracellularly stained bulbar FTG neuron with axon descending in cMLF. This frontal section shows a neuron whose axon (solid arrows) coursed dorsally and entered the ipsilateral MLF, then turned medially and crossed the midline to descend in the dorsomedial part of the contralateral MLF. IV, fourth ventricle; d, dorsal; M, medial; MLF, medial longitudinal fasciculus. From Mitani *et al.* (1988c).

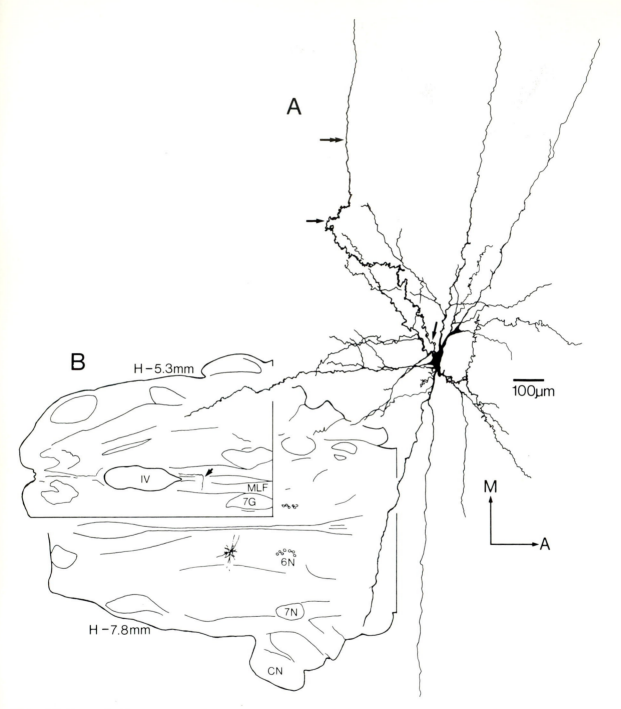

Figure 27. Camera lucida drawing of a bulbar FTG neuron with axon descending in cMLF (horizontal section). Note the ellipsoid–polygonal soma (major axis 62 μm and minor axis 38 μm with average diameter 48 μm) and slant of the major axis from medial to lateral. The dendritic field extended 1330 μm in the A–P direction and 2230 μm in the M–L direction; the longest extent of the dendritic field was mediolateral. The axon originated from the soma and coursed dorsally while curving (corresponding to the part between the two solid arrows in A), then turned medially (double-headed arrow in A), entered the ipsilateral MLF (arrow), crossed the midline (solid arrow in B), and descended in the medial part of the contralateral MLF toward the spinal cord. No axon collaterals were observed. The average axon diameter was 3.1 μm. Abbreviations: H(horizontal) −5.3 mm and −7.3 mm are horizontal coordinates of labeled neuron and axon in Berman's Atlas (horizontal plane of section approximately parallel to floor of fourth ventricle). 7N, facial nerve; CN, cochlear nerve. From Mitani *et al.* (1988c).

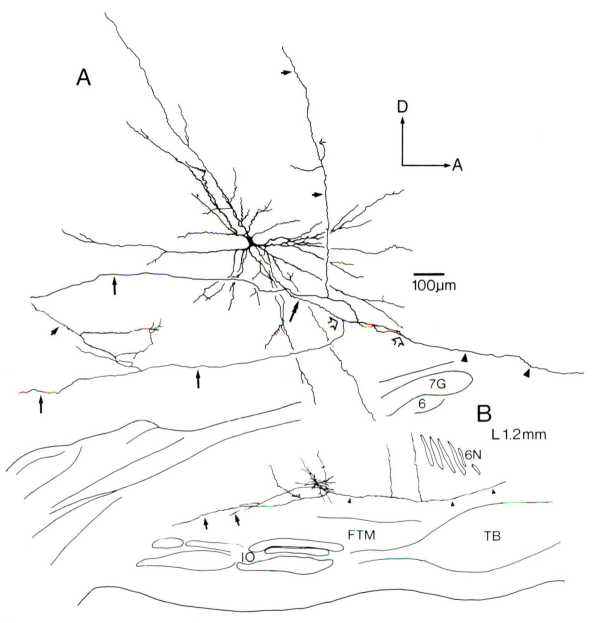

Figure 28. Camera lucida drawing of a bulbar FTG neuron with axon descending in iBRF and with extensive collaterals (parasagittal section). This neuron had an ellipsoid–polygonal soma of medium size (major axis 39 μm and minor axis 20μm with average diameter 30 μm). The dendrites were nonspiny. The dendritic field extended 1170 μm in the A–P direction and 1610 μm in the D–V direction, and the axis of the longest extent was tilted slightly from dorsocaudal to ventrorostral. The axon originated from the dendritic trunk and coursed anteriorly for a short distance (double headed arrow in A), then bifurcated (open arrows) into an ascending branch (solid triangles in A and B) and two descending branches (solid arrows in A and B); the ascending axon entered the pons, and the descending axons descended in the bulbar reticular formation. Both ascending and descending axonal branches gave off dorsally coursing axon collaterals (B) (some of them are indicated by small arrows in A). From Mitani *et al.* (1988c).

PFTG neurons (means of two types of PFTG neurons were 16 and 14). These results indicated that BFTG neurons had fewer branching dendrites and were similar to those reported for bulbar reticular neurons near the raphe magnus (Edwards *et al.*, 1987).

4.4.4. General Comments on Morphology

The large neurons with large, noncollateralized axons coursing in the MLF and the VF would seem ideally suited for rapid, secure transmission of information. The phylogenetic homology is of course with the Mauthner neurons and other giant reticulospinal neurons of fish and other lower vertebrates. In the cat, these large neurons with axons in VF may be involved in locomotion. A study of bulbar medial reticular formation neurons (most within FTG) in alert cats during treadmill walking showed that it was the neurons antidromically identified as reticulospinal by stimulation of ventral cord at L2 that showed predominance of EMG- and locomotor-related discharge; these neurons had high conduction velocities (approximately 100 m/sec), compatible with a large soma size (Drew *et al.*, 1986). In contrast, neurons of smaller and medium-sized neurons in both PFTG and BFTG appear to be the carriers of reticuloreticular information in addition to their other targets. It should be emphasized that there is some overlap of soma size of PFTG- and BFTG-to-MLF neurons with neurons sending axons in BRF; in the studies cited, this was about 10%, and thus the size distinctions are not absolute. The previously cited studies (Section 4.2.2.2) suggest that rostral PFTG and BFTG projections also arise predominantly from nongiant neurons. The bulbar projections descending in the ventrolateral funiculus may mediate the muscle atonia during REM sleep (see Chapter 10 and Pompeiano, 1976).

Scheibel and Scheibel (1958) concluded from their Golgi studies of young mammals that the reticular dendritic field was flattened in the anteroposterior plane and assumed a nearly two-dimensional configuration they described as resembling "poker chips." The Golgi study in young mammals by Valverde (1961) also described dendritic fields, especially those in the pontine and rostral bulbar reticular formations, as being more prominent in a transverse direction. However, the quantitative data of the present HRP intracellular study in adult cats modify these conclusions.

In PFTG, there is only a tendency to a "poker chip" configuration in a few neurons. The mean anteroposterior extent of the population of PFTG neurons was only 16% less than the mean dorsoventral and 3% less than the mean mediolateral extent. Furthermore, only 15% of PFTG neurons showed a flattening of the A–P dendritic fields that was between 30% and 39%, a degree of flattening much less than shown in Fig. 3 of Scheibel and Scheibel (1958). In fact, the dendritic field extent of 19% of PFTG neurons was slightly longer in the A–P direction than in the M–L or D–V direction.

However, a tendency toward anteroposterior flattenting, although not quite as strong as in the Scheibels' material (1958), was present in the BFTG-to-cMLF and BFTG-to-iBRF neuronal classes of BFTG neurons. The mean anteroposterior extent of the BFTG-to-cMLF and BFTG-to-iBRF neurons is 31% and 35% less than their respective mean mediolateral extent and 20% and 30% less than their respective mean dorsoventral extent. In contrast, dendrites of

BFTG-to-iMLF neurons showed only a small trend to anteroposterior flattening, less than 16% and thus less than half of that seen in cMLF and iBRF neurons and similar to that of PFTG neurons.

4.4.5. Speculations on Organization of Ascending and Descending (Bifurcating) Collaterals in Bulbar FTG

With respect to the extent of collateralization of FTG neurons, it is of interest that double-labeling experiments have shown that only relatively few (<4%) bulbar FTG neurons project to both spinal cord and cerebellum (Martin and Waltzer, 1984a) or to both cerebellum and diencephalon (Waltzer and Martin, 1984) or to both spinal cord and diencephalon (Martin and Waltzer, 1984b), also a finding of Jones and Yang (1985). This is also in accord with the older physiological studies of Magni and Willis (1963) and of Eccles *et al.* (1975). This paucity is, however, in marked contrast to the 55% of non-MLF-projecting BFTG axons that had bifurcating collaterals and suggests that in the adult the neurons with bifurcating collaterals have one branch that is shortened, i.e., terminates before arrival in diencephalon or spinal cord. Our supposition from the intracellular HRP data is that it is the rostral branch that ascends only a relatively short distance. Given the strong tendency of bulbar neurons to project to the spinal cord, the preliminary observation of "frequent" double labeling of BFTG neurons from midbrain and spinal cord is of interest (Jones and Yang, 1985). The actual axonal BFTG-to-PFTG tracings with boutonlike terminations, the presence of antidromic activation of BFTG neurons from PFTG, and the 100% monosynaptic excitatory responsiveness of PFTG neurons to BFTG microstimulation (Mitani *et al.*, 1988b,c) lead to the inference that pontine FTG neurons are heavily innervated by the class of BFTG neurons with ascending collaterals.

4.5. Norepinephrinergic Systems

Norepinephrinergic (NE) neurons are located in the pons and medulla, with about 60% of them in the locus coeruleus (LC)–subcoeruleus complex. In rat, the LC almost exclusively consists of NE elements, contains about 1500 neurons, and is divided into a ventral part with multipolar neurons and a dorsal part with smaller densely packed fusiform cells (Swanson, 1976; Grzanna and Molliver, 1980). Colocalization of tyrosine hydroxylase immunoreactivity with neuropeptide Y immunoreactivity was recently found in approximately 23% of rat's LC neurons (Holets *et al.*, 1988). In cat, the LC is more loosely arranged, with an LC proper (corresponding to the dorsal compact part of the rat LC and containing about 5300 NE cells on each side) and more scattered NE cells extending into the parabrachial nucleus and the subcoeruleus and Kolliker–Fuse nuclei (Wiklund *et al.*, 1981; Bjorklund and Lindvall, 1986).

The rostral projections of NEergic cells ascend mostly ipsilaterally via the dorsal tegmental bundle, with a minor projection taking a ventral course. In the midbrain, the bundle gives off collaterals to the ventral tegmental area, dorsal regions of the central tegmental field, and inferior and superior colliculi. Most of

the ascending NE fibers enter the medial forebrain bundle at the caudal diencephalic level and enter the thalamus via the retroflex bundle or the mammillothalamic tract, and other fibers ascend along the zona incerta and radiate within the internal and external medullary laminae. The NE fibers distribute to various hypothalamic areas, thalamic nuclei, septum, amygdala, hippocampus and pyriform cortex, and neocortical areas (cf. Lindvall and Bjorklund, 1974; Pickel *et al.,* 1974; Jones and Moore, 1977; Foote *et al.,* 1983).

In contrast with the congruent results on the cholinergic innervation of different thalamic nuclei in rat, cat, and monkey (see Section 4.2), the density of NE projections to the thalamus varies greatly from nucleus to nucleus and from species to species. Whereas the LG thalamic nucleus of rats is one of the most important targets of LC nucleus, the associative visual thalamic nuclei (pulvinar and lateral posterior) only receive a sparse to moderate NE input (Swanson and Hartman, 1975). A reverse picture is seen in some primates (squirrel monkey and cynomolgus monkey) that display a striking paucity of NE fibers in the LG nucleus although pulvinar and lateral posterior thalamic nuclei are densely innervated; the reticular thalamic nucleus is very densely innervated throughout its extent (Morrison and Foote, 1986).

The corticopetal NE fibers have been found to leave the main bundle at rostral hypothalamic levels, to continue their course up to the frontal lobe, and to distribute caudally for the entire length of the hemisphere (Morrison *et al.,* 1981). Earlier autoradiographic studies (Jones and Moore, 1977) and more recent antidromic identification experiments (Sakaguchi and Nakamura, 1987) indicate, however, that some fibers originating in the LC nucleus reach the occipital lobe without coursing through the frontal lobe. The interspecies differences that characterize NE projections to the thalamus are also observed in the cerebral cortex, and the degree of regional and laminar variation increases with the phylogenetic development. Thus, although the NE innervation of rat's neocortex is quite constant throughout the cortex and the axons seem to ramify in all layers (Levitt and Moore, 1978; Lindvall *et al.,* 1978), marked laminar variations are seen in striate and extrastriate cortices of primates (Morrison *et al.,* 1982). In particular, sudden changes in the density and laminar profiles of NE fibers are seen by passing from area 17 to area 18: in area 18, a distinct lamination pattern emerges, with the highest density of NE axons in layers III and V and the lowest density in layers I and IV (Morrison and Foote, 1986). Antidromic activation of rat's LC neurons can be elicited from many target cortical areas, and most LC–cortical axons conduct with wide range and very low (<0.6 m/sec) velocities (Aston-Jones *et al.,* 1980; see also Nakazato, 1987, for cat experiments), suggesting thin nonmyelinated fibers, but a significant population of monkey's LC neurons was found to exhibit conduction velocities greater than 1 m/sec (Aston-Jones *et al.,* 1985).

In earlier studies by Descarries and his colleagues (1977), a very low proportion of NE axons were seen to be engaged in genuine synaptic relations, and it was claimed that NE is released in a neurohumoral type, over great distances, as in the peripheral nervous system (Beaudet and Descarries, 1978). More recently, however, conventional synaptic profiles have been found in at least 50% of NE terminals (Olschowska *et al.,* 1981; Freund *et al.,* 1984). Probably, synaptic and nonsynaptic release coexist (for further details and methodological issues concerning junctional versus nonjunctional relations of NE terminals in the cortex, see Beaudet and Descarries, 1984).

The descending projections of LC neurons run dorsomedially in the pontine tegmentum, and varicosities are present in pontine reticular formation, including giant-cell field. A lateral group enters the cerebellum through the brachium conjunctivum, and the fibers terminate in the molecular layer as well as around the Purkinje cells (Pickel *et al.*, 1974). In the pons and medulla, the prime targets of LC axons are sensory nuclei, namely, the pontine gray nuclei, the cochlear nuclei, and the principal sensory trigeminal nucleus (Levitt and Moore, 1979). The projections to the spinal cord originate in the ventral part of the LC and in nucleus subcoeruleus, descend in the ventral and ventrolateral funiculi, and distribute bilaterally to the ventral horn, intermediate gray, and ventral part of the dorsal horn (cf. Bjorklund and Lindvall, 1986).

A significant proportion of LC cells give rise to axons that collateralize to different structures. About 10% to 30% of LC neurons are double labeled when one fluorescent tracer is injected in the spinal cord and the other one into the cerebellum (Nagai *et al.*, 1981), cortex, or thalamus (Room *et al.*, 1981).

4.6. Serotonergic Systems

The serotonergic (5-HT) neurons are located in the brainstem raphe system, which consists, at midbrain–pontine levels, of the centralis superior (or medianus), linearis, and dorsalis nuclei; at pontobulbar levels, it comprises the magnus, obscurus, and pallidus nuclei (see details on their systematization and cytoarchitectonics in Steinbusch and Nieuwenhuys, 1983).

The heterogeneity of raphe nuclei, with both 5-HT and non-5-HT neurons, was repeatedly emphasized (Aghajanian *et al.*, 1978; Belin *et al.*, 1979; Steinbusch *et al.*, 1980). Among non-5-HT raphe cells, there are GABAergic (Belin *et al.*, 1979) and dopaminergic (Descarries *et al.*, 1986) elements. The heterogeneity of the dorsal raphe nucleus is reflected in the different firing patterns, electrophysiological properties, and morphology of its constituent neurons. Aghajanian and co-workers (1978) have initially distinguished three types of dorsal raphe neurons: type 1 are medium-sized 5-HT cells (disappearing in animals treated with the selective toxin 5,7-dihydroxytryptamine, 5,7-DHT) with spontaneous firing rates of 0.5–1.5 Hz; type II cells (almost silent) and type III (rapidly firing) are still recordable in experiments after lesions produced by 5,7-DHT and are probably non-5-HT neurons. The rapidly firing neurons (100–130 Hz) have been recently recorded intracellularly, stained with HRP, and compared to slowly firing neurons (Park, 1987). The action potentials of rapidly firing cells have a repolarization that is about five times faster than that in slowly firing 5-HT cells. Intracellular labeling revealed that type III fast-discharging dorsal raphe neurons have small (10–15 μm) somata (Park, 1987), similar to GABAergic neurons of the dorsal raphe nucleus (Belin *et al.*, 1979).

The ascending projections originate in dorsal raphe (DR) and centralis superior (CS) nuclei. The major organizational features of the ascending raphe projections to the hypothalamus, diencephalic periventricular gray, striatum, globus pallidus, diagonal band nuclei, septum, hippocampus, and glomerular layer of the olfactory bulb have been revealed in the rat by light-microscope autoradiography after intraventricular administration of tritiated 5-HT (Parent *et al.*, 1981). The CS raphe projections to septum and hippocampus of rat have also been identified by antidromic invasion, and the results showed conduction velocities of 0.8 m/sec as well as branching axons to both the fornix and the medial septum (Crunelli and Segal, 1985). An autoradiographic study of efferent raphe projections in cat disclosed some differences between DR and CS nuclei, with preferential DR projections to striatum, amygdala, pyriform lobe, and olfactory bulb, whereas CS nucleus was found to project rather selectively to the mammillary body and hippocampus (Bobillier *et al.*, 1976).

The axons issuing from DR and CS nuclei ascend to the thalamus mostly along the retroflex bundle, the mammillothalamic tract, and stria terminalis. The 5-HT projections to the rat thalamus have been demonstrated by combining retrograde transport techniques with 5-HT immunohistochemistry (Consolazione *et al.*, 1984). The thalamically projecting neurons are confined within the lateral DR wing. The highest density of the 5-HT innervation is found in the ventral part of the lateral geniculate (LG) nucleus and the intrageniculate leaflet, whereas other thalamic nuclei display low to moderate density of 5-HT fibers (Cropper *et al.*, 1985). The low density of 5-HT fibers in the rat thalamus is paralleled by low levels of the two types of 5-HT receptors (Pazos and Palacyos, 1985; Pazos *et al.*, 1985). In cat, DR cells with projections to the dorsal part of LG nucleus are not restricted to a particular sector of the DR nucleus (DeLima and Singer, 1987; Smith *et al.*, 1988), and the density of 5-HT fibers is moderate to high in the ventral part of the LG and intralaminar nuclei but rather low in A and C laminae of the dorsal LG nucleus (Mize and Payne, 1987). In primates, Morrison and Foote (1986) have found a relatively uniform distribution of 5-HT fibers in various visual thalamic nuclei, which was at variance with the marked nuclear variations of NE fibers.

The 5-HT fibers that reach the cortex traverse the septum, sweep around the genu of the corpus callosum, and continue in the cingulum. In rat, the 5-HT innervation does not display regional differences or laminar preferences (Lidov *et al.*, 1980), whereas in primates 5-HT fibers are concentrated in layer IV of striate area 17 and are homogeneously distributed in area 18 (Morrison *et al.*, 1982; Morrison and Foote, 1986). In both rat and monkey, 5-HT innervation of the cerebral cortex is more dense than the NE input. At this time, the innervation of cat cerebral cortex has not been systematically studied with immunohistochemistry. Biochemical investigations indicate that the highest concentration of 5-HT is in the pyriform cortex and the lowest in the visual cortex of cat (Gaudin-Chazal *et al.*, 1979; Reader *et al.*, 1979).

The descending projections of DR and CS are mostly directed to pontine and bulbar core structures, whereas the 5-HT projections to the spinal cord derive from magnus, obscurus, and pallidus raphe nuclei (cf. Steinbusch and Nieuwenhuys, 1983).

4.7. Dopaminergic Systems

The dopamine (DA)-containing brainstem neurons are grouped in the substantia nigra pars compacta (SNc) or A9 group of Dahlstrom and Fuxe (1964), the ventral tegmental area (VTA) or A10 group, the retrorubral (RR) area corresponding to group A8, and the periaqueductal gray (PAG) thought to be a caudal extension of group A11. In addition, DA cells are found in the dorsal raphe nucleus of both cat (Wiklund *et al.*, 1981) and rat (Descarries *et al.*, 1986). Extensive interconnections are established among SNc, VTA, and RR cell groups (Deutch *et al.*, 1986) and may integrate the forebrain projections of the DA aggregates.

The use of a polyclonal antibody raised against DA-glutaraldehyde-lysyl-protein conjugate (Geffard *et al.*, 1984) helped to describe the distribution and fine morphological features of the SNc, VTA, RR, and PAG cell groups in the squirrel monkey (Arsenault *et al.*, 1988) and to study the rostral projections of immunocytochemically identified DA neurons in the rat (Voorn *et al.*, 1986; Séguéla *et al.*, 1987).

The thalamus is largely bypassed by DA axons. As classically known, axons from SNc project to the striatum. Retrograde double-labeling studies in squirrel monkeys point to a complex mosaic pattern of SNc cell clusters that project either to the caudate or to the putamen (Carter and Fibiger, 1977; Parent *et al.*, 1983). The VTA efferent connections distribute caudally to various districts of the brainstem core and to the spinal cord, whereas rostrally they are mostly directed toward the septohippocampal complex, amygdala, accumbens, bed nucleus of stria terminalis, and prefrontal (pregenual) and insular (suprarhinal) cortices (cf. Oades and Halliday, 1987). Distinctly from SNc single axons that are highly collateralized to telencephalic target structures, VTA neurons, are predominantly single labeled after injections of three retrograde tracers into the caudate–putamen, septum, and frontal cortex (Fallon, 1981). Finally, the RR group contributes to the dorsal mesostriatal pathway in rodents (cf. Bjorklund and Lindvall, 1984) and cat (Paré *et al.*, 1988).

Intrinsic Electrophysiological Properties of Brainstem Neurons and Their Relationship to Behavioral Control

The properties of neuronal circuits controlling behavior are determined not only by their anatomic connectivity but also by the intrinsic properties of the constituent neurons, including voltage- and transmitter-sensitive membrane currents. Historically there has been relatively little "cross talk" between physiologists interested in analysis of behavior from a macropotential or even cellular perspective in the behaving mammal and those physiologists exploring cellular properties in *in vitro* preparations, including slices and dissociated neuronal cultures. One of the purposes of our book is to facilitate and promote information transfer between these still largely separate domains of work by emphasizing areas of potential and demonstrated commonality of interest. We believe the future course of brainstem investigation will be toward increasing joint use of both techniques to understand mechanisms of behavior.

This chapter also presents data from thalamic and basal forebrain neurons since these are both important targets of brainstem influences and also furnish contrasts with properties of brainstem neurons. We begin with a discussion of the properties of cholinoceptive and cholinergic reticular core neurons (Sections 5.1 and 5.2), we summarize *in vitro* data on monoaminergic neurons (Section 5.3), and we compare the intrinsic properties of brainstem neurons with those of thalamic and basal forebrain cells (Sections 5.4 and 5.5).

5.1. Medial Pontine Reticular Formation Neurons

Figure 1 illustrates the plane of section of the pontine reticular formation (PRF) slice preparation, first described in Greene, Haas, and McCarley (1986) and with details of physiology described by Gerber *et al.* (1989a). Unless otherwise stated, these references apply to the data of this section. The PRF slice preparation utilized 500-μm-thick transversely cut brainstem slices from young Sprague–Dawley rats; slices were totally submerged in perfusate in a modified Haas recording chamber (Haas *et al.,* 1979). When the preparation was viewed under a binocular dissecting microscope, identifying anatomic landmarks were readily observable; these were primarily white matter tracts and include sixth nerve rootlets, the seventh nerve, and the medial longitudinal fasciculus. Use of young, 7-to 13-day-old animals facilitated tissue viability (slices remained viable throughout the 8-to 16-hr recording sessions) and was also appropriate in that the behavior of principal interest, REM sleep, is some four to five times more abundant in young than in adult animals (Jouvet *et al.,* 1968). Recordings of medial pontine reticular formation neurons described in this section were made in the giant-cell field zone (FTG).

5.1.1. Neuronal Classes of the Medial PRF: Overview

Our classification of mPRF neurons will be based on the presence of different kinds of firing pattern as influenced by the presence of different voltage-sensitive membrane currents. Two main neuronal classes have thus far been defined by the presence of two types of firing pattern in response to current injection (Fig. 2 and Table 1). We first summarize data on these main types before proceeding with more detailed descriptions. Later sections also include brief primers of terminology and technical aspects of cellular physiology for the reader not working in this field. We note in passing the presence of a third type of neuron, one with a high-threshold burst. Since this type is rare (5%), we will not discuss it here, but refer the interested reader to Gerber *et al.* (1989a).

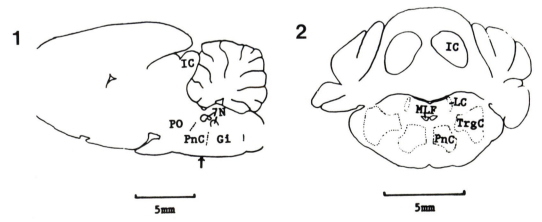

Figure 1. Schematic representation of the *in vitro* recording zone in the medial pontine reticular formation (nucleus reticularis pontis caudalis, PnC) in sagittal and coronal sections, with the latter having the same orientation as the slices used for recording. Gi, bulbar nucleus reticularis gigan-tocellularis; IC, inferior colliculus; LC, locus coeruleus; MLF, medial longitudinal fasciculus; PO, nucleus reticularis pontis oralis; TrgC, trigeminal complex; 7N, seventh nerve. From Gerber *et al.* (1989a).

These neurons generated a low-threshold burst (LTB) firing pattern that was caused by the presence of a low-threshold calcium spike (LTS). As shown in Fig. 2A, the LTS was visible as a slow potential on which rode a burst of fast (sodium-dependent) action potentials, the low-threshold burst. LTBN also produced a *nonburst* (NB) firing pattern consisting of a relatively regular series of action potentials (Fig. 2A, column 3). Production of the LTB pattern was dependent on a sufficiently hyperpolarized baseline membrane potential that deinactivated the LTS, as described in detail below.

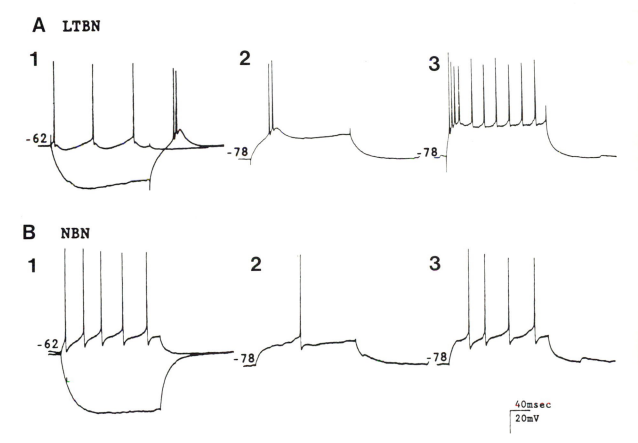

Figure 2. Two patters of repetitive firing in the two main classes of mPRF neurons recorded *in vitro*. Part A shows voltage traces from a low-threshold burst neuron (LTBN) illustrating the presence of a low-threshold burst (LTB) and nonburst (NB) patterns. A1: A depolarizing current pulse of 200 pA amplitude and 200 msec duration (same duration throughout figure) evokes a nonburst (NB) repetitive firing pattern. A hyperpolarizing current pulse of 400 pA amplitude evokes a rebound low-threshold burst (LTB). A2 and A3: With a hyperpolarized membrane potential (−78 mV), depolarizing current pulses of 300 pA and 500 pA evoke low-threshold bursts (LTB), which, with 500-pA current in- jection, are followed by a nonburst pattern (NB). Part B shows voltage traces from a nonburst neuron (NBN) evincing an NB pattern but no LTB pattern: there is no rebound LTB seen in B1 even with the same amplitude hyperpolarizing pulse as in A1, and no LTB results from depolarizing pulses in B2 and B3 of the same magnitude and from the same hyperpolarized membrane potential in A2 and A3. Note, however, the delay in depolarization evident in B2 and B3 compared with B1; evidence indicating that this delay is caused by A current is described in the text. Modified from Gerber *et al.* (1989a).

Table 1. Characteristics of Medial Pontine Reticular Formation Low-Threshold Burst Neurons (LTBN) and Nonburst Neurons (NBN)

	NBN	LTBN
Firing pattern		
Low-threshold burst	0	+
Nonburst	+	+
Calcium action potentials		
Low threshold	0	+
High threshold		
in control media	0	0
with K(Ca) antagonists	+	+
Outward potassium currents		
Early transient, A current	+	+
Delayed, calcium dependent	+	+

In addition to the LTS, LTBN also showed a *high-threshold calcium spike* (HTS); this HTS was dependent on a calcium current, but one with a higher threshold for activation than the LTS. Both the LTS and HTS were visualized in the presence of tetrodotoxin (TTX), a blocker of sodium action potentials, and the HTS also required the presence of potassium current blockers. We note that whereas the LTS is not so common in neuronal populations throughout the brain, the HTS is quite common, and the calcium current associated with it is often triggered by the depolarization associated with the sodium action potential. LTBN constituted about 45% of the recorded mPRF neurons.

5.1.1.2. Nonburst Neurons (NBNs)

These neurons showed only a nonburst (NB) firing pattern (Fig. 2B) and an HTS. They did not show an LTS or associated LTB. The action potential frequency of the NB pattern was principally controlled by a calcium-dependent potassium conductance and the latency to occurrence of the first spike by A current, an early outward (hyperpolarizing) current that opposed the depolarization leading to the initial spike. NBNs constituted about one-half of the neurons recorded.

5.1.1.3. Biophysical and Morphological Characteristics of the Two PRF Neuronal Classes

These two neuronal classes did not show statistically significant differences in input resistances or resting membrane potentials. Resting membrane potentials averaged −65 mV, and input resistances (measured by the change in membrane potential resulting from a 200-msec hyperpolarizing current pulse) were about 65 MΩ. The observed lack of correlation between input resistance and the neuronal type as identified by firing pattern suggests that the two patterns resulted from recordings in different neurons rather than from recordings obtained from different zones of the same neuron; e.g., patterns characteristic of an LTBN might be elicited from the soma and patterns characteristic of an NBN from the dendrites. There was also no association of age of preparation and the frequency of occurrence of the different classes. Use of recording site marker lesions and Nissl staining showed that the different classes were not preferentially localized to any particular portion of the pontine FTG.

Carboxyfluorescein injected intracellularly into mPRF neurons enabled computation of mean soma diameters as the average of long and short axes (cf. studies in cat described in Chapter 4). Diameters ranged from 20 to 50 μm, and there was a tendency ($P < 0.10$) for LTBNs to have larger somata (mean diameter 37 μm) than NBNs (30 μm). It was particularly notable that 80% of neurons with somata >35μm were LTBNs. For comparison of the soma sizes of the sample of intracellularly recorded neurons with all mPRF neurons, and to compare young (10-day-old) with adult animals, soma size measurements were performed on neurons on Nissl-stained sections from young and adult rats. Average soma diameters were not statistically different for young (25 μm) and adult (28 μm) rats. In terms of comparability of results to those obtained in the adult cat (Mitani *et al.*, 1988a), the soma size percentile distributions, based on three subdivisions (large, medium, and small neurons), were remarkably similar. Neurons in the upper 8% had diameters larger than 40 μm in cat and 39 μm in young rats, the next 35% had diameters of 20–40 μm in cat and 24–39 μm in rat, and the smallest 57% of the sampled neurons had diameters less than 20 μm in cat and 24 μm in rat. The majority of cat mPRF neurons with soma sizes greater than 45 μm project to the spinal cord without collaterals (Mitani *et al.*, 1988a,b); if a similar association of size and efferent projection pattern exists in the rat, then these data suggest that the LTB pattern predominates in the class of noncollateralized reticulospinal neurons.

5.1.2. Low-Threshold Burst Neurons and the Low-Threshold Calcium Spike

For those readers not familiar with calcium action potentials a brief review may be useful. Soon after the sodium action potential was described, Fatt and Ginsborg (1958) found that muscle fibers in crab legs utilized a "calcium spike," an action potential based on the inflow of calcium rather than sodium ion during the depolarization of the action potential upstroke. Llinás and colleagues have described low-threshold calcium spikes and associated low-threshold burst firing patterns in mammalian neurons (cf. Llinás, 1988, for a review). Neurophysiological studies have shown that, in general, calcium channels activate (open) with membrane depolarization and also show inactivation (i.e., closing of channels) with time courses slower than for the sodium channels involved in fast action potential production (see review in Hille, 1984). Of particular importance for low-threshold calcium spikes is the concept of *deinactivation,* a process leading to removal of inactivation so that the current may be activated under the proper conditions, such as membrane depolarization. Deinactivation or removal of inactivation may be analogized to the "cocking of a gun": the process itself does not cause a dramatic change but, with depolarization, *permits* activation of the currents causing the calcium spike or, in the analogy used, permits pressing the trigger to be effective.

In mPRF neurons (Fig. 2A) the slow potential seen as a rebound after a hyperpolarization (A1) or elicited by a depolarizing pulse from a hyperpolarized base-line potential (A2) will be shown to represent a calcium spike, and the burst of fast (sodium-dependent) action potentials riding on the calcium spike (e.g., the low-threshold burst, LTB) occur because the calcium spike depolarizes the membrane past the threshold for generation of sodium spikes. The subsequent discussion further dissects the various factors involved in production of calcium spikes. The calcium spike associated with the LTB pattern is termed a *low-threshold spike* because of the low threshold for activation of this calcium current and spike and is to be contrasted with the higher-threshold calcium spike to be described later.

It is to be noted that the LTB pattern is characterized by a sensitivity to base-line membrane potential (Fig. 2A). A depolarizing current pulse from a base-line membrane potential more negative than −75 mV activates a low-threshold slow spike (the calcium spike) with a burst of two to five fast action potentials superimposed on it. Larger-amplitude current pulses (Fig. 2A3) evoke similar bursts of action potentials, but they are followed by an NB pattern of firing. LTB patterns were not usually activated with depolarizing current injection from a base-line membrane potential more positive than −65 mV (Fig. 2A1); they instead elicited only an NB pattern. Note further (Fig. 2A1) that a rebound LTB is evoked following current pulses that hyperpolarize the membrane to potentials more negative than −75 mV (300-msec pulse durations).

The number of action potentials generated during an LTB, the intensity of a burst, was strongly controlled by the factors illustrated in Fig. 3. Increasing the amplitude of depolarizing current (amplitude of activation) (Fig. 3A) produced an LTB with more action potentials. The threshold for activation of the LTB, obtained by a visual estimation of the inflection point on the membrane-potential charging trajectory, was about −60 mV. Another important factor in the intensity of an LTB was the degree of removal of inactivation (deinactivation), dependent on the degree and duration of hyperpolarization (Fig. 3B,C) prior to a rebound LTB. Maximal LTBs averaged about five action potentials per burst.

Figure 4, columns 2 and 3, shows the calcium dependence of the LTS and associated LTB firing pattern. (Effects on the nonburst pattern illustrated in column 1 are discussed below.) Figure 5A shows the effects of addition of tetrodotoxin (TTX), a blocker of sodium-dependent action potentials; the abolition of the LTB clearly reveals the time course of the calcium spikes resulting from a rebound hyperpolarization (A1) or depolarization from a hyperpolarized membrane potential (A2), and A3 shows the abolition of the slow calcium spikes in perfusate containing no calcium. Figure 5A1 shows that the LTS amplitude increased and its latency to peak decreased in direct relationship to the magnitude of the preceding hyperpolarization. By comparison of Fig. 3 with Fig. 5A1 it can be seen that the graded increase of the LTS produced by increasing hyperpolarization of the membrane potential was similar to the graded increase in the number of action potentials observed in the rebound LTB.

5.1.2.1. Modulation of the LTS by a 4-Aminopyridine-Sensitive Current

The LTS was not "an island unto itself" but interacted with other currents to shape firing pattern; one of these currents appeared to be similar to the A current first described in gastropod mollusks (Neher, 1971; Connor and Stevens, 1971) and present in mammalian central nervous system neurons from many different regions (Gustafsson *et al.*, 1982; Williams *et al.*, 1984; Yarom *et al.*, 1985; Champagnat *et al.*, 1986). The A current is so named because of its sensitivity to blockage by 4-aminopyridine (4-AP) (Thompson, 1977) and is also known as the transient outward current. The A current is activated when a neuron is depolarized *after* a period of hyperpolarization; since it is an outward potassium current, it tends to counteract depolarizing, inward currents such as the calcium current associated with the LTS. Figure 6B shows how the threshold and size of an LTS in LTBNs was influenced by interaction with a 4-AP-sensitive conductance. Blocking the 4-AP-sensitive current by perfusion with 4-AP (500 μM) increased the peak amplitude of the LTS by at least 30% compared with no-4-AP control conditions. Further, in the presence of 4-AP and starting with a base-line membrane potential of −76 mV (A current inactivation removed), depolarizing currents elicited a more rapid LTS rise than the no-4-AP control.

Since the putative A current and the current responsible for the LTB had similar voltage sensitivities for both activation and inactivation, this interaction

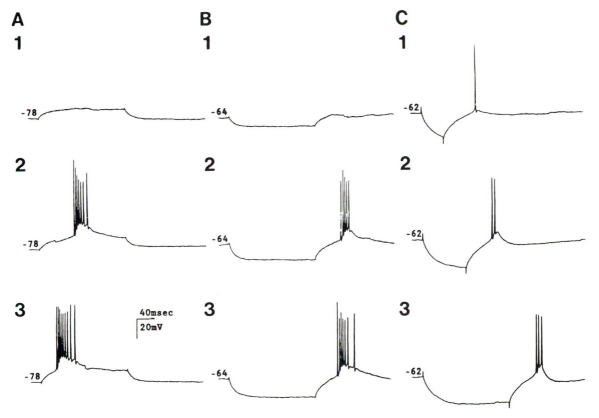

Figure 3. Activation and the removal of inactivation of the low-threshold burst response of mPRF neurons recorded *in vitro*. Column A illustrates graded activation of the LTB with voltage traces of responses to depolarizing current pulses of 200 msec duration and 200 (A1), 250 (A2), ad 300 (A3) pA amplitude, all applied from a hyperpolarized membrane potential of −78 mV. Column B illustrates the voltage sensitivity of the removal of inactivation with the responses to hyperpolarizing pulses of 200 msec duration and 300 (B1), 500 (B2), and 600 (b3) pA amplitude applied on a base-line membrane potential of −64 mV. Note the increased number of action potentials with greater hyperpolarization. Column C illustrates the time dependence of the removal of inactivation with the responses to hyperpolarizing pulses of the same amplitude (300 pA) but of increasing duration: 100 msec in C1, 200 msec in C2, and 400 msec in C3. Modified from Gerber *et al.* (1989a).

may be especially important in the control of the LTB. Depending on the relative amplitudes of these two currents, depolarization from a hyperpolarized membrane potential may produce either a state of decreased excitability when A current predominates or increased excitability with a burst response when low-threshold calcium current predominates.

5.1.2.2. The High-Threshold Calcium Spike

Not only was an LTS present in LTBNs, there was also a higher-threshold calcium spike (HTS) that was revealed with the addition to the perfusate of 5–10 mM tetraethylammonium (TEA), an antagonist of a number of outward po-

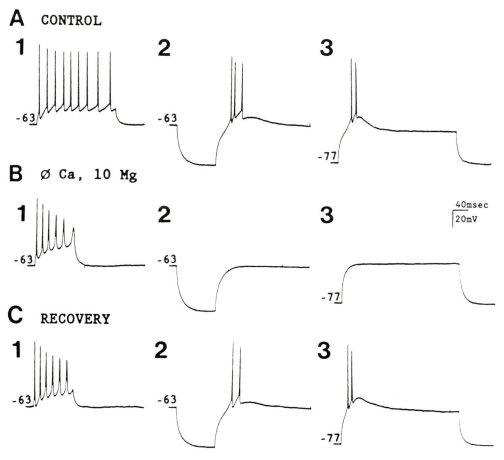

Figure 4. Calcium dependence of repetitive firing patterns of a low-threshold burst mPRF neuron recorded *in vitro*. Row A is during perfusion with control medium. In A, column 1, there is a *nonburst* response to a depolarizing current pulse of 300 pA amplitude from a base-line membrane potential of −63 mV. In A, column 2, a rebound *low-threshold burst* response follows a hyperpolarizing pulse of 500 pA amplitude. In A, column 3, there is a *low-threshold burst* response to a depolarizing pulse of 400 pA amplitude delivered from a hyperpolarized base line. Row B, during perfusion with medium containing 10 mM magnesium and no calcium, shows the absence of the low-threshold burst response in B2 and B3; the increased frequency of the nonburst pattern in B1 and other alterations are addressed in Section 5.1.3. and Fig. 12 of Gerber *et al.,* (1989a). Row C shows partial recovery 5 min after returning to perfusion with control media. Modified from Gerber *et al.* (1989a).

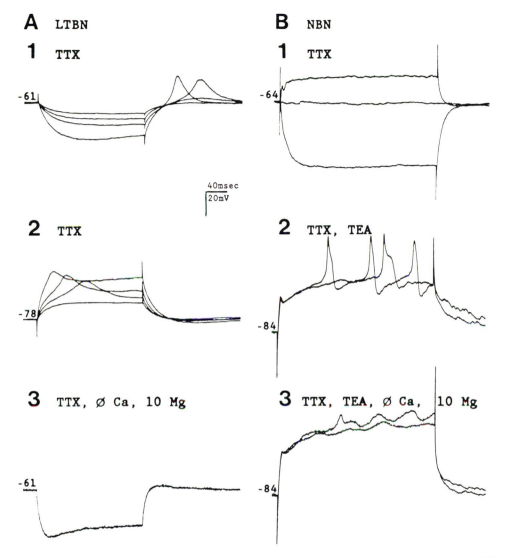

Figure 5. Tetrodotoxin-resistant, calcium-dependent action potentials (calcium spikes) of mPRF neurons recorded *in vitro*. Voltage traces from a low-threshold burst neuron (LTBN) are shown in column A and from a nonburst neuron (NBN) in column B. A1: In the presence of TTX, increasingly greater hyperpolarization of the membrane potential (current amplitudes of 100, 200, 300, and 500 pA) results in increasingly greater amplitude of rebound low-threshold calcium spikes. A2: From a base-line potential of −78 mV, increasingly greater depolarization (current pulse amplitudes of 200, 400, 600, and 800 pA amplitude) also evoked increasingly greater amplitude low-threshold calcium spikes. A3: The low-threshold calcium spike is abolished in the presence of 10 mM magnesium and no calcium. B1: In the NB neuron no calcium spikes were evoked even by large-amplitude current pulses (+600 pA and −600 pA) in the presence of TTX. B2: With the addition of TEA (10 mM), depolarizing current pulses (+1000 and 1200 pA) evoke high-threshold calcium spikes. B3: High-threshold calcium spikes are abolished when calcium is replaced by 10 mM magnesium (B3) and identical current pulses are applied. Calibration bar is 80 msec for A3. Modified from Gerber *et al.* (1989a).

tassium currents including both the calcium-dependent potassium channel (Hermann and Gorman, 1981) and the calcium-independent delayed rectifier (Stanfield, 1983). Column B of Fig. 5 shows the presence of HTS in response to depolarizing pulses in the presence of TEA (TTX was added to eliminate fast sodium action potentials); these HTSs (B2) were calcium dependent since they disappeared when calcium was replaced by 10 mM magnesium (B3). The threshold for the TTX-resistant HTS was −33 mV for LTBNs, easily distinguishable from the LTS threshold, which was approximately 30 mV more hyperpolarized (Fig. 5A). The HTS and LTS were also distinguished by the selective antagonism of the LTS by magnesium; in the presence of 10 mM magnesium and 2 mM barium (an outward potassium current antagonist), the LTS was reversibly abolished, but the HTS was still readily evoked by depolarizing current pulses. This was directly analogous to the effects of these treatments on the LTB and NB firing patterns.

The most likely explanation for the differences between the LTS and HTS is that two distinct types of calcium channels control the calcium fluxes on which

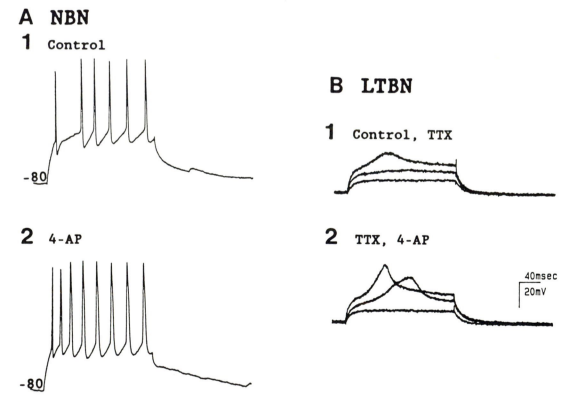

Figure 6. In mPRF neurons recorded *in vitro,* 4-AP reduces the latency to the first action potential, shortens the interspike interval between the first and second action potentials, and reduces the threshold and increases the amplitude of the low-threshold calcium spike. A: Voltage traces of responses to depolarizing pulses of 400 pA in a nonburst neuron before (A1) and during (A2) application of 4-AP (0.5 mM). B: Responses of a low-threshold burst neuron to depolarizing current pulses of 200, 400, and 600 pA amplitude applied before (B1) and during (B2) 4-AP exposure (0.5 mM) in the presence of TTX and from a base-line membrane potential of −79 mV. Note that in all cases the subthreshold responses to the current pulses were not affected by 4-AP. Calibration: 20 mV and 40 msec. Modified from Gerber *et al.* (1989a).

they depend. The voltage sensitivities of the LTS and HTS were similar to those of calcium channels described as low-voltage-activated (Carbone and Lux, 1984; Yaari *et al.*, 1987) or T type (Nowycky *et al.*, 1985) and high-voltage-activated or L type, respectively.

5.1.2.3. Effects of Antagonists of Delayed Hyperpolarizing Potassium Currents on the LTS and the HTS

The amplitude and duration of the LTS, and hence the number of action potentials in the LTB, were controlled not only by the depolarizing calcium-dependent conductance but also by an interaction with delayed hyperpolarizing (outward) potassium conductances. In the presence of TTX, application of blockers of delayed outward potassium currents, including TEA, barium, or intracellular cesium, resulted in an LTS of sufficient amplitude to surpass threshold for the HTS; in this case these TTX-resistant action potentials reached membrane potentials more positive than +5 mV, a level never reached without TEA, barium, or intracellular cesium. However, the inability to elicit the LTS from depolarized membrane potentials without a preceding hyperpolarization was not affected by these antagonists. Cesium in the presence of TTX had the additional effect of eliciting a rebound LTS followed by repetitive HTSs; these continued until hyperpolarizing current was applied.

5.1.3. Nonburst Neurons and Factors Controlling the Nonburst Firing Pattern

As noted in the previous section, both nonburst neurons (NBNs) and LTBNs generated a nonburst pattern, and the discussion here pertains to the NB pattern in both types of neuron. The nonburst pattern was characterized by a relatively constant interspike interval during depolarizing current injection (Fig. 2A1,B1,B3,C1, which are to be compared to Fig. 2A2,A3,C2,C3). With increased amplitude of current injection, some accommodation was apparent, but never to the extent of complete cessation of action potential firing, nor was there any evidence of an associated long-duration (greater than 0.5 sec) after-hyperpolarization (AHP). This was in marked contrast to the accommodation and associated long-duration AHP observed in hippocampal CA1 and CA3 neurons (Hotson and Prince, 1980; Schwartzkroin and Stafstrom, 1980; Madison and Nicoll, 1984; Lancaster and Nicoll, 1987; Storm, 1987).

As shown in Fig. 5B, NBNs had no LTS, but large-amplitude depolarizing pulses in the presence of TEA and TTX demonstrated the presence of an HTS whose threshold was similar to the HTS in LTBNs.

In contrast to the direct dependence of the LTB pattern on a calcium spike, the NB pattern was indirectly controlled by a high-threshold inward calcium conductance that, in turn, activated an inhibitory (outward) calcium-dependent potassium conductance. Thus, calcium-free media altered the nonburst pattern in both LTBNs (Fig. 4) and NBNs (see Fig. 12 in Gerber *et al.*, 1989a) in that spike frequency was increased and the AHP reduced. The calcium conductance mediating these effects was shown to be different than for the LTS conductance because neither NB firing frequency nor the AHP was altered by high magnesium in control concentrations of calcium, although this treatment antagonized the LTB/LTS (Fig. 5A). The effects of addition of 5 mM TEA (Fig. 7), an antagonist of calcium-dependent potassium currents, were similar to those following exposure to calcium-free media, suggesting that a calcium-dependent potassium current mediated both effects. The presence of a calcium-dependent outward current was also indicated by the fact that large current pulses in the presence of TTX did not depolarize the membrane potential positive to −38 mV (Fig. 5B1); the removal of calcium from the perfusate abolished this effect.

The high-threshold calcium current may indirectly control the repetitive firing of the NB pattern by the following sequence of events: under physiological conditions, the TTX-sensitive sodium currents of the fast action potential elicit sufficient membrane depolarization to exceed the threshold of the high-threshold calcium current. The influx of calcium, in turn, leads to a calcium-dependent potassium current, which then contributes to action potential repolarization and the AHP. Similar effects of calcium-dependent potassium current have been observed in the vertebrate peripheral nervous system (Adams *et al.*, 1982) and in hippocampal neurons (Lancaster and Nicoll, 1987; Storm, 1987). Other factors controlling the NB pattern, not yet directly examined in mPRF neurons, may include the calcium-independent delayed outward rectifier and the removal of sodium inactivation (Adams *et al.*, 1980).

There may be more than one calcium-dependent potassium conductance, as has been demonstrated in other neurons. In hippocampal neurons repolarization of the action potential and fast AHP (<10 msec duration) has been at-

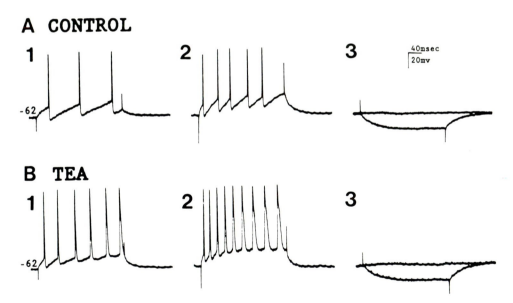

Figure 7. A TEA-sensitive outward current modulates the excitability of the nonburst firing mode of mPRF neurons recorded *in vitro*. Responses of a nonburst neuron to depolarizing current pulses of 300 pA (column 1) and 500 pA (column 2) and to a hyperpolarizing pulse of 300 pA (column 3). After the addition of TEA (10 mM in row B), the frequency and number of action potentials evoked are increased compared to control condition (row A) despite an unaltered input resistance as measured in column 3. Note also that action potential amplitude is increased and that with successive firing action potential duration is also increased. From Gerber *et al.* (1989a).

tributed to a TEA- and charybdotoxin-sensitive calcium-dependent potassium conductance (Lancaster and Nicoll, 1987; Storm, 1987), but a medium AHP (<200 msec) is calcium insensitive. In contrast, in neurons of the sensorimotor cortex (Schwindt *et al.*, 1988) and spinal cord (Barrett and Barrett, 1976; Walton and Fulton, 1986), action potential repolarization is not dependent on calcium flux across the membrane (although it is antagonized by TEA in both cases), but the medium-duration AHP is calcium dependent. In mPRF neurons, repolarization of action potential, the medium-duration AHP, and restriction of the LTS are all mediated to some extent by one or more calcium-dependent potassium conductances. However, additional investigation of the voltage and pharmacological sensitivities of these phenomena is needed before more precise statements can be made.

When NBNs were hyperpolarized to membrane potentials negative to −65 mV and then depolarized, there was a delay in reaching action potential threshold in association with a (outwardly rectifying) deviation from the membrane charging trajectory seen with current pulses applied from more depolarized base lines (compare Fig. 2B1 to B2 and B3). Since this is consistent with an activation of A current (cf. previous discussion), the effect of 4-AP, an antagonist of A current, was tested using the same experimental procedures (Fig. 6A). Compared with control conditions, exposure of NBNs to 4-AP (200–500 μm) reduced the delay to threshold of the first action potential and the first interspike interval when base-line membrane potential was maintained at levels negative to −65 mV, but when examined from a membrane potential of −60 mV, 4-AP had no effect. These effects are consistent with the known characteristics of A current: inactivation at membrane potentials of −60 mV and more positive, removal of inactivation at more hyperpolarized potentials, and activation at potentials more positive than −60 mV (Connor and Stevens, 1971; Neher, 1971). Further, the 4-AP antagonism affected only the early part (<150 msec) of the firing pattern and did not alter input resistance, again arguing for a specific blocking of A current.

5.1.4. Role of Baseline Membrane Potential in Controlling Repetitive Firing Properties of mPRF Neurons and Implications for Behavior

Identical inputs to LTBNs and NBNs can result in markedly different responses when the membrane potential is sufficiently hyperpolarized. An excitatory input can evoke an LTB response in LTBNs, and if the excitatory input continues, the LTB will be followed by an NB pattern. However, in NB neurons at the same baseline membrane potential, the same excitatory input may fail to elicit even a single action potential because of an unopposed A current; if input continues, the A current will finally inactivate, and an NB pattern will emerge. This heterogeneity and specialization of response may be important to the physiological organization of the mPRF in waking for both oculomotor and somatomotor systems. In particular, the reader's attention is directed to the examples given in Chapter 10 of quick activation of oculomotor system neurons from a base line of absence of firing and presumed membrane hyperpolarization. The presence of an LTS may be functionally advantageous in permitting a quick recruitment of action potential discharge from a hyperpolarized membrane potential level.

Furthermore, the change of baseline membrane potential during behavioral state changes may have important consequences for firing patterns in these states. In passage from waking and slow-wave sleep to EEG-desynchronized sleep, neurons of the mPRF depolarize 7 to 10 mV (Ito and McCarley, 1984). This depolarization may inactivate both the LTS and the A current. Under such conditions, LTB and NB neurons will respond similarly to excitatory input with an NB firing pattern. Overall, excitability may be increased as membrane potential depolarizes towards action potential threshold, but the specificity of response to excitatory input that distinguishes NB from LTBNs in waking may be decreased, and burst firing may be absent. Consistent with this, analysis of the firing pattern of mPRF neurons *in vivo* indicates an increased firing frequency in association with an absence of burst discharges during REM sleep (McCarley and Hobson, 1975a).

5.2. Pedunculopontine Tegmental Neurons

The location of these cholinergic neurons and their thalamic projections are discussed in Chapter 4 (see Figs. 3–8 of Chapter 4). Those data, obtained by combining retrograde tracing with ChAT immunohistochemistry (see Section 4.2.2), have been confirmed in guinea pig slices containing the pedunculopontine tegmental (PPT) nucleus (Leonard and Llinás, 1988, 1989). The PPT neurons were retrogradely labeled after injections of rhodamine-labeled microspheres prior to the preparation of the slice. Intracellular injection of Lucifer yellow in retrogradely labeled PPT cells showed that their shape and soma–dendritic size are similar to cholinergic PPT neurons described in rodents by Rye *et al.* (1987). The results of experiments performed by Leonard and Llinás (1987, 1988, 1989), dealing with the intrinsic properties of thalamically projecting PPT cells, are described below. Three major neuronal classes have been observed.

One class of PPT neurons did not spontaneously fire action potentials after impalement, but they fired a spike train under depolarizing current pulses (Fig. 8A). If the membrane was hyperpolarized sufficiently, the same depolarizing pulse elicited an LTS crowned by a burst of two to five fast action potentials (Fig. 8B). The conductance underlying this burst was TTX insensitive (Fig. 8C) but was blocked by cobalt and cadmium, thus indicating that it is calcium mediated. This neuronal type was designated as generating purely LTS responses. Similar LTS-generating neurons have been found by Wilcox *et al.* (1987) in the other brainstem cholinergic group, the lateral dorsal tegmental nucleus.

The second neuronal type described by Leonard and Llinás (1987, 1988, 1989) in the PPT nucleus also displayed an LTS but, unlike the first type, did fire spontaneously on impalement and, at resting membrane potential, did not show a rebound excitation at the break of a hyperpolarizing pulse. At rest, these cells had a transient outward A current, which delayed the return to base line of the voltage trace after the termination of a hyperpolarizing pulse (see also Section 5.1). This cellular class was then designated as "LTS+A."

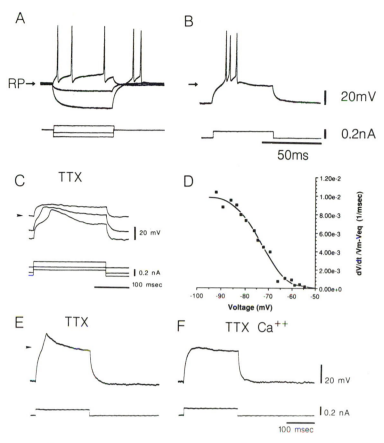

Figure 8. Low-threshold spiking (LTS) neuron recorded from the pedunculopontine tegmental (PPT) nucleus of guinea pig *in vitro*. A, top trace: Neuron fires repetitively during depolarization from resting potential. Following hyperpolarizing current pulses (bottom trace) of sufficient magnitude, the neuron demonstrates rebound bursts of action potentials. B: Hyperpolarization from resting potential elicits for subsequent depolarizing steps a burst-mode firing. C: This spike burst is mediated by an LTS, is insensitive to TTX, and is inactive at resting potential (arrow) but becomes progressively deinactivated as the membrane potential is hyperpolarized. D: Maximum rate of rise of the LTS is plotted as a function of membrane potential. The spike is half-maximally active at -75 mV membrane potential. E and F: Calcium dependency of the LTS (E) is demonstrated by its blockage with 500 mM CdCl (F). Modified from Leonard and Llinas (1989).

The third cellular type did not display LTS responses but had the outward potassium conductance termed A current. Such neurons were regarded as particularly suited to the relatively slow, tonic repetitive firing observed in some PPT neurons explored *in vivo*. On intracellular current injection, these neurons fired repetitively (Fig. 9A). Following a hyperpolarizing current pulse from resting potential, the membrane potential displayed a delay in the return to base line, typical for A current. The A conductance was inactivated at resting membrane potentials and was progressively deinactivated by brief hyperpolarizing prepulses (Fig. 9B). Single-electrode voltage-clamp records (Fig. 9C,D) showed that the outward current peaked rapidly (within 6 msec) and decayed more slowly (about 200 msec). The A conductance was normally inactivated at resting membrane potentials (Fig. 9E) and was deinactivated during the AHP of the action potential. Thus, this conductance leads to an increased duration of the AHP and consequently to a lengthening of the interspike interval.

The first two cell classes (LTS and LTS+A current) may be related to the burst firing of PPT neurons whose activity underlies the thalamic component of the phasic pontogeniculooccipital waves of REM sleep (see Chapter 9), whereas the third cellular type (A current) probably corresponds to the tonically firing neurons in PPT that may be involved in the tonic aspect of EEG desynchronization during both waking and REM sleep (see Chapter 11). As to the PGO-wave production in some brainstem PPT bursting neurons, it is of interest that octanol, a high-molecular-weight alcohol that specifically blocks the LTS of inferior olive neurons (Llinas and Yarom, 1986), was also found to block the PGO-like waves induced in the LG thalamic nucleus by brainstem peribrachial (PB) stimulation (Fig. 10; Llinas *et al.*, 1987). In these *in vivo* experiments, octanol was injected systemically, and therefore, the blockage of the all-or-none PGO-like component of the PB-LG response (appearing at a latency of about 50–80 msec after the PB stimulation) could well be caused by the blockage of brainstem or thalamic LTS. The suppressing effect of octanol on PGO waves may be related to the fact that REM sleep is partially suppressed by acute doses of alcohol and continues to be suppressed for longer periods if the dosage is increased.

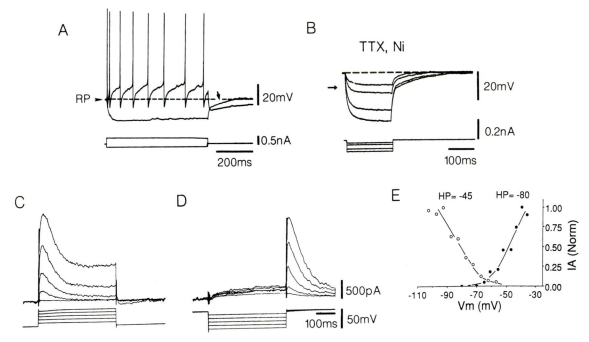

Figure 9. g_A-Type neuron in the guinea pig PPT nucleus *in vitro*. A: Repetitive firing elicited by depolarizing current pulses. The delay in the return of the membrane potential to rest following hyperpolarizing current pulses characterizes the presence of g_A. B: The g_A is not blocked by TTX and nickel, is inactive at resting potential, and increases with membrane hyperpolarization. C: Single-electrode voltage-clamp recording of A-current activation in TTX from other neuron of this class. Progressively larger depolarizing steps produce larger fast transient outward currents of increasing amplitude (−80 mV holding potential). D: Hyperpolarizing voltage steps from a holding potential of −45 mV rapidly reactivate I_A. E: Peak I_A plotted as a function of membrane potential. From a holding potential of −80 mV, this current is half-maximally activated by voltage steps to about −50 mV. From a holding potential of −45 mV, this current is half-maximally reactivated by a voltage step to about −75 mV. Modified from Leonard and Llinás (1989).

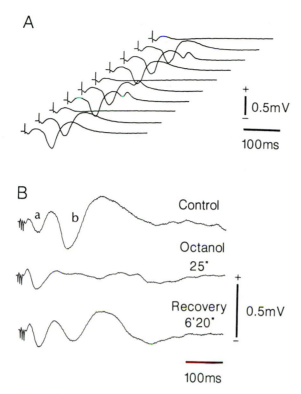

Figure 10. Octanol-induced blockage of all-or-none (PGO-like) component of field potential evoked in the lateral geniculate (LG) thalamic nucleus by stimulation of the brainstem peribrachial (PB) area in cat. A: Ten-sweep sequence showing the all-or-none character of the second component of PB-evoked LG field potential. B: Effect of octanol on second component of LG field potential evoked by midbrain reticular stimulation (three-shock train). Reserpine-treated (2 mg/kg) *encéphale isolé* preparation with deafferentation of trigeminothalamic pain pathways. Second component (b) disappeared 25 sec after octanol administration (despite no alteration in a component) and recover 6 min 20 sec later. Unpublished data by D. Paré, M. Deschênes, R. Llinás, and M. Steriade.

5.3. Neurons of the Locus Coeruleus and the Dorsal Raphe

5.3.1. Locus Coeruleus Neurons

Chapter 4 has detailed the widespread projections of the locus coeruleus (LC), and subsequent chapters will indicate the strong behavioral state dependence of its neuronal discharge: LC neurons slow and virtually arrest discharges with the approach and advent of REM sleep. A further striking characteristic of extracellular recordings *in vivo* of LC neurons is their slow, regular discharge pattern, which has suggested the possibility of pacemakerlike activity determined by intrinsic membrane properties. Thus, intracellular *in vitro* recordings are of great importance for determining the mechanisms of this pacemakerlike discharge pattern and the existence of modulatory mechanisms that would account for its dramatic alteration with change in behavioral state. This section presents data supportive of the hypothesis that LC neurons have intrinsic pacemaker activity at certain membrane potential levels and that calcium-dependent currents play a key role in this pacemaker activity. The data also are supportive of the general hypothesis that behavioral state changes may alter discharge pattern and discharge rate through the modulation of membrane potential and consequent changes in voltage-sensitive membrane currents (McCarley and Ito, 1985; McCarley and Massequoi, 1986a; Greene *et al.*, 1986). Certain potassium conductances of LC neurons are discussed in Chapter 6, together with ligand-activated potassium conductances.

The slice preparation and the data in this section, except where otherwise indicated, are described in detail by Williams *et al.* (1984). Adult rat brainstem slices were cut in the transverse (coronal) plane, and the slice with the maximum lateral extent of the LC was used for recording. The zone of the LC was identified as a translucent area using transmitted light in the slice in the recording chamber, and the identity of this area with the anatomically defined LC was confirmed both by Nissl staining and by intracellular injections of sample neurons in the presumptive LC zone with Lucifer yellow; the morphological characteristics of the injected neurons were the same as previously described for noradrenergic LC neurons.

In the *in vitro* preparation, almost all LC neurons were found to be spontaneously active, with a firing threshold of about −55 mV and membrane potentials otherwise ranging from −55 to −65 mV. As can be seen in Fig. 11, action potentials arose from a slowly declining (depolarizing) membrane potential (rate of change, 7 mV/sec). There were two components of the rising phase of the action potential (AP): an initial calcium-dependent slow depolarization (72 V/sec) followed by a rapid depolarization of the sodium-dependent action potential proper (351 V/sec); the peak height attained by the action potential averaged 82 mV. The falling phase showed an initial repolarization of membrane potential, a calcium-dependent shoulder, followed by a more rapid repolarization. Mean duration of the AP measured at threshold was 1.4 msec. The AP was followed by an AHP that carried the membrane potential 15–20 mV negative to the AP threshold. The AHP had an initial period of rapid decay (depolarization) followed by a slower depolarization phase that merged into the interspike depolarization.

Of interest with respect to the *in vivo* recording data showing virtual arrest of spontaneous LC neuronal discharges in REM sleep was the finding that, *in vitro,* hyperpolarization to about −60 mV arrested LC spontaneous firing, suggesting a strong voltage dependence of the spontaneous activity. The presence of intrinsic pacemaker activity was further suggested by the absence of any evidence for spontaneous synaptic potentials driving the depolarization and repetitive discharges. In a few neurons (<10%) small spikelike depolarizations were evident on hyperpolarization; these occasionally reached AP threshold and vanished in calcium-free, high-magnesium solutions, suggesting that they were spontaneously occurring dendritic calcium spikes. The frequency of spontaneous discharge activity did not change with the addition of TTX to the perfusate, indicating both the lack of significance of synaptic input from sodium-dependent APs for driving the depolarization/regular discharge of LC neurons and also demonstrating the importance of ion(s) other than sodium in the generation of one component of the LC action potentials. The APs after TTX were of lesser amplitude (46 mV) and had a slower maximal rate of rise (21 V/sec), and interference with calcium currents eliminated these TTX-resistant smaller, slower spikes: they were not present in perfusates either containing the calcium channel blockers cobalt or magnesium or containing no calcium (Fig. 12), data

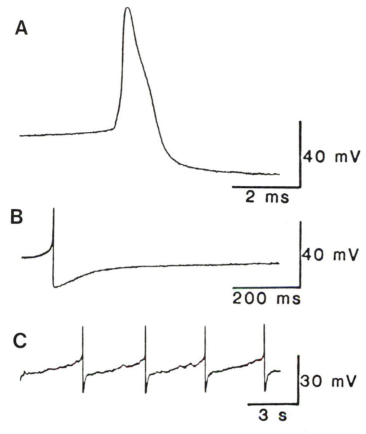

Figure 11. Spontaneous action potentials of locus coeruleus neurons recorded *in vitro*. A: In control perfusate a change in slope on the rising phase is visible (see text), as well as a shoulder on the falling phase. B: The spontaneous action potential (full height not shown) was followed by an afterhyperpolarization, which merged into the interspike depolarization, seen more clearly at the slower recording speed of C. Modified from Williams *et al.* (1984).

agreeing with the formulation that the initial component of the LC action potential was a calcium spike.

Analysis of membrane properties with single-electrode voltage-clamp (SEVC) techniques showed a steady-state slope conductance that was relatively constant at membrane potentials from −90 to −70 mV, then progressively less with depolarization, and negative at about −55 mV (Fig. 13). The negative-slope conductance* at −55 mV was analyzed further as to the nature of the current responsible for the change.

*Slope conductance is simply the slope of the line tangent to each point of the I/V curve; a positive slope means that net outward current flow is increasing for small depolarizing changes in membrane potential. For example, potassium ion (K$^+$) current flow from inside the neuron to the outside, called outward current, is, by convention, labeled positive; in general, an increase in the movement of positive ions outward via channel openings is termed outward or positive current. Similarly a negative slope means that inward current increases for small depolarizing changes; an increase in channel openings leading to positive ion flow from outside to the inside of the membrane is by convention labeled inward current and has a negative sign. It will be noted that a decrease in channel openings and a resultant decrease in positive ion flow from outside to inside may also be viewed as a decrease in inward current. In Fig. 14 the early portion of the curve shows a decrease in inward current, with an increase occurring at about −55 mV.

As shown in Fig. 14, blockade of inward calcium currents by cobalt abolished the negative-slope conductance. The negative-slope conductance at about −55 mV was also abolished by calcium-free high-magnesium solutions. Other data indicated that a later outward current (associated with the AHP) was a calcium-dependent potassium current.

It was concluded that LC neurons have a calcium current flowing into the cell at membrane potentials close to threshold for action potential generation. This inward current is voltage dependent, being small at −75 mV and increasing with depolarization; it activates and deactivates rapidly when the membrane is depolarized or hyperpolarized.

Other experiments indicated the presence of potassium currents contributing to spike repolarization; these included a fast 4-AP-sensitive component, the calcium-activated potassium current, and perhaps other "delayed rectifier" currents.

Williams *et al.* (1984) offered the following unifying hypothesis about the mechanisms involved in generation of the pacemakerlike activity of LC neurons. We begin the description of a cycle at the peak of the action potential, a point

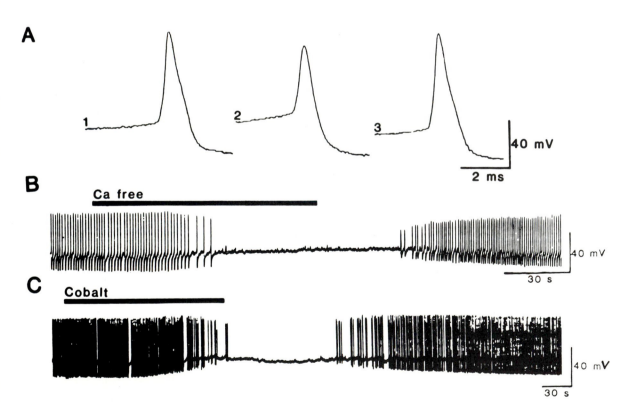

Figure 12. The locus coeruleus action potential (AP) recorded *in vitro* is composed of calcium and sodium spikes. A: Part 1 shows a control spontaneous AP. Part 2 is after addition of 2 mM cobalt; note the persistence of a smaller spike. Part 3 is recovery after washout of cobalt. B and C: In TTX (1 μm), spontaneous action potentials persist but are reversibly abolished by calcium-free solutions (B, with 10 mM magnesium) or by cobalt (2 mM). Modified from Williams *et al.* (1984).

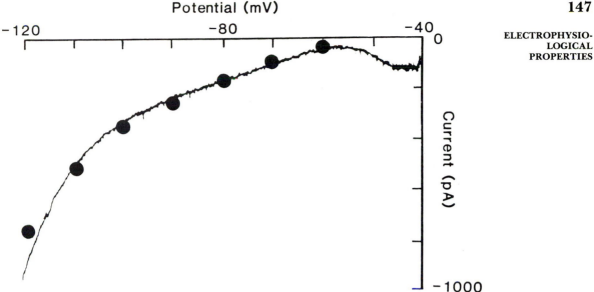

Figure 13. Steady-state I/V characteristics of a locus coeruleus neuron recorded *in vitro*. The continuous line was plotted directly on an $X–Y$ plotter using a ramp depolarization from -120mV to -40 mV. The filled circles indicate the currents evoked by hyperpolarizations from a holding potential of -60 mV. Modified from Williams *et al.* (1988a).

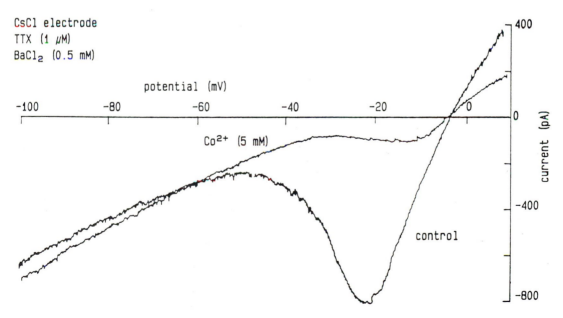

Figure 14. Blockade of calcium current by cobalt abolishes the negative-slope conductance in the I/V plot of a locus coerulus neuron recorded *in vitro*. Graph constructed from ramp depolarizations of a neuron impaled with a CsCl-filled recording electrode. Control I/V plot is in medium with 1 μm TTX and 0.5 mM BaCl$_2$. Note strong negative-slope conductance beginning at about -50 mV that is almost totally abolished by addition of cobalt. This calcium current was also sensitive to dihydropyridines. Figure courtesy of J. T. Williams and R. A. North.

with a high calcium conductance and a consequent rapid increase in internal calcium concentration. Action potential repolarization is dependent on voltage- and calcium-activated potassium conductances; these outward currents bring the membrane potential to -75 mV, at which level the calcium and sodium conductances are near zero. The slow depolarization that follows may be primarily mediated by a progressive reduction in the outward current through a reduction in free intracellular calcium. As the membrane potential moves from -75 mV to less negative values, the 4-AP-sensitive outward current may slow the return to the AP threshold potential. Then, as the membrane potential approaches -55 mV, the slow inward calcium current develops with increasing magnitude. This leads to the initial slow rising phase of the AP. At about -45 mV there is a large increase in the TTX-sensitive sodium channels, leading to the action potential proper. The cycle then repeats itself.

This hypothesis, which the authors caution needs further testing with better voltage-clamp resolution, offers a plausible explanation for the pacemaker activity observed in LC neurons and agrees with data on the origin of spontaneous activity in invertebrate neurons (Smith *et al.*, 1975; Gorman *et al.*, 1982; Smith and Thompson, 1987). It is useful also to underline the distinction between the slowly or noninactivating calcium conductance important in pacemaker activity and the transient, inactivating calcium conductance of the LTS, whose rapid inactivation would not make it a reasonable mechanism to generate the LC pacemaker cycle.

5.3.2. Dorsal Raphe Neurons

As discussed in Chapter 4, there is ample evidence indicating that serotonergic dorsal raphe (DR) neurons have widespread projections and a role in modulating the excitability of the large numbers of postsynaptic neurons. Serotonergic neurons, like LC aminergic neurons, show a dramatic state-related modulation of discharge *in vivo;* they join the LC population in slowing and virtually ceasing discharge with the advent of REM sleep, and, as discussed in Chapter 11, the arrest of their discharges appears to be closely correlated with the onset of the pontogeniculooccipital waves of REM sleep. Thus, the intrinsic membrane properties contributing to their discharge pattern is of considerable interest to physiologists interested in control of behavioral state alterations and in general features of control of excitability in target neurons, such as hippocampus. We discuss two intrinsic inwardly rectifying potassium conductances of DR neurons in Chapter 6, together with the serotonin-controlled inwardly rectifying potassium conductance.

The intracellular *in vitro* data on DR neurons described in this section are from the work of Aghajanian and collaborators (VanderMaelen and Aghajanian, 1983; Aghajanian and Lakoski, 1984; Aghajanian, 1985; Burlhis and Aghajanian, 1987), work that followed the initial *in vitro* extracellular dorsal raphe recordings of Mosko and Jacobs (1976) and Trulson *et al.* (1982). Aghajanian and co-workers utilized 300- to 450-μm-thick frontal (coronal) slices from albino rats that were mounted in a modified Haas chamber (not submerged in perfusate). Viewed through a binocular microscope the DR nucleus was easily visualized, lying ventral to the central aqueduct and dorsal to the medial longitudinal fasciculus and decussation of the brachium conjunctivum. Neurons were classified as serotonergic on the basis of long-duration action potentials (2 msec), large AHPs, and pacemaker potentials; these were characteristic of neurons identified as serotonergic by an *in vivo* double-labeling technique (Aghajanian and VanderMaelen, 1982b).

Input resistances of these presumptive serotonergic neurons recorded *in vitro* were described as 40–230 MΩ (mean 94 MΩ) in the initial study (Vander-Maelen and Aghajanian, 1983) and >150 MΩ, usually 200–300 MΩ, in later studies from this group (e.g., Aghajanian, 1985; Freedman and Aghajanian, 1987). These input resistances were higher than those recorded *in vivo* (Aghajanian and VanderMaelen, 1982a), as is typical for *in vivo* versus *in vitro* input resistance measurements, but other characteristics of the neurons were the same as in the *in vivo* sample.

Extracellular and intracellular recordings of neurons in the slice showed the presence of a spontaneous slow, regular discharge rhythm also characteristic of *in vivo* recordings of these neurons. As shown in Fig. 15, the action potential was

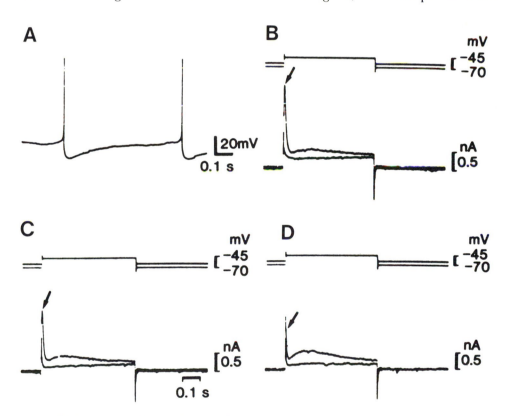

Figure 15. *In vitro* recordings of dorsal raphe serotonergic neurons. Presence of a transient outward current suppressed by 4-AP. A: Spontaneous spikes of a typical serotonergic neuron in the dorsal raphe slice preparation. Note the large AHPs followed by a rapid phase of depolarization and then a plateau period before the subsequent spike. B: Voltage clamp at −70 mV in 1 μM TTX to eliminate sodium spikes; top traces are voltage, bottom are current; outward currents are upward going. A step depolarization to −45 mV elicits a transient outward current (arrow), which peaks 8 msec after the depolarizing step; superimposed traces show the virtual absence of a transient outward current which the holding potential is −60 rather than −70 mV. C: Ten minutes after the addition of 1 mM 4-AP, the transient outward current (arrow) is reduced by about 30%. D: Twelve minutes after the 4-AP has been increased to 2.5 mM, the transient outward current is reduced by more than 60%. Modified from Aghajanian (1985).

followed by an afterhyperpolarization, then a rapid phase of depolarization followed by a long plateau of very slow depolarization, and then the rapidly rising phase of a spike, which typically had a "shoulder" during the repolarization phase (not visible at the recording speed of the figure, but closely resembling that of the LC neuron in Fig. 11). The cycle then repeated; of particular note was the absence of evidence for PSPs that might drive the depolarization, both in the *in vivo* and in the *in vitro* recordings, thus suggesting a true pacemaker organization.

As illustrated in Fig. 15 (Aghajanian, 1985), these neurons showed an early transient outward current with the characteristics of A current (see Sections 5.1 and 5.2). Single-electrode voltage-clamp studies revealed the presence of a transient outward current when depolarizations were made from holding potentials of -70 mV in TTX-containing perfusate but not when holding potentials of -60 mV were used for the same depolarizing pulse. Perfusion with 1 mM 4-AP also greatly reduced this transient outward current.

Activation of this presumptive A current from a holding potential of -80 mV first occurred with a voltage step to -60 mV, with progressive increases in current up to a voltage step to -40 mV. At a holding potential of -40 mV, the current was inactivated; deinactivation occurred only with hyperpolarizations below -60 mV and was maximal at about -90 mV.

Burlhis and Aghajanian (1987) recently demonstrated the presence of an LTS conductance in the serotonergic DR neurons. This conductance was blocked in the presence of nickel and other divalent cations known to block calcium conductances (Fig. 16), was deinactivated at low voltages in a time- and voltage-dependent manner, and was differentiated from an HTS conductance by the failure of the latter to be blocked by nickel. Single-electrode voltage-clamp studies using electrodes filled with cesium (to suppress A current and other potassium conductances) showed a negative-slope conductance from -60 to -50 mV, indicating the presence of an inward current (the LTS current) in this voltage range. The LTS conductance was not directly altered by phenylephrine or serotonin.

These workers suggested the following hypothesis for the sequence of events underlying generation of rhythmic activity in DR serotonergic neurons. With the occurrence of a fast sodium spike, there is entry of calcium through HTS channels. This calcium activates a calcium-dependent potassium current (the AHP current), which hyperpolarizes the neuron to the region of deinactivation for the A current and for the LTS current. As the internal free calcium concentration decreases, the membrane potential depolarizes to the voltage (about -60 mV) where the LTS current is activated, and this current acts to bring the membrane potential to the threshold for the fast sodium spike, and the cycle is repeated.

It will be noted that the inward, depolarizing LTS current is counteracted by the A current, and the relative strength of these two currents may determine the presence and frequency of rhythmic discharge in serotonergic neurons. For example, the pacemaker plateau period occurs between -60 and -50 mV, precisely the range in which both the LTS and the A current become activated. When activated, the outward (hyperpolarizing) A current may thus diminish the frequency of discharge and be responsible for the long plateau period. As is discussed in Chapter 6, this A current is also important because it is decreased by norepinephrine and α_1 agonists and is thus an important pacemaker system component that may be modulated by input from other neurons.

In commenting on this model of the DR rhythmic activity, we underline the fact that both the A conductance and the LTS conductance are transient in the sense of rapidly inactivating. Data presented indicate they both should be inactivated within 200 msec and thus do not, in our opinion, appear to be kinetically suitable conductances for modeling the rhythmic activity of DR neurons. The plateau potential typically lasts severalfold longer than the inactivation time for these conductances and thus could not be caused by them (see Fig. 15A for illustration of relevant kinetics). Voltage-clamp studies of persisting rather than transient conductances and of their kinetics and voltage sensitivity appear to be needed.

5.4. Thalamic Neurons

The intrinsic properties of thalamic neurons allow them to function in two different modes in two distinct types of behavioral states: a *bursting* mode, associated with depressed transfer function during EEG-synchronized sleep; and a *tonic* discharge pattern during both EEG-desynchronized states (wakefulness and REM sleep), accompanied by enhanced and accurate synaptic transmission of incoming information from the outside world during the adaptive waking state (see details in Chapter 8). Although the study of electrical responsiveness of

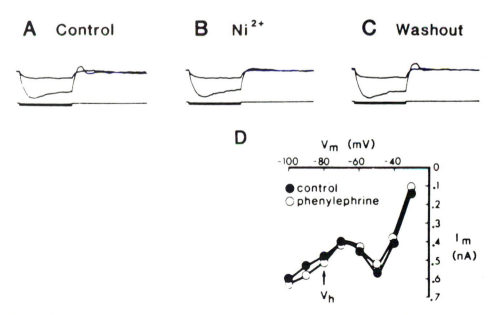

Figure 16. *In vitro* recordings of serotonergic dorsal raphe neurons. Upper panel: Block by nickel of low-threshold current following hyperpolarizing pulse. A: Control, in 1 μM TTX. B: Current is abolished by 100 μM nickel. C: Current returns on washout. Lower panel: D: Single-electrode voltage-clamp data on I/V relationship, showing region of negative-slope conductance. Note that I_m units are tenths of nA. Modified from Burlhis and Aghajanian (1987).

LG thalamic neurons in slices has been attempted since the mid-1970s (Yamamoto, 1974), and postsynaptic potentials (PSPs) in rat and cat LG neurons have been investigated *in vitro* during the late 1970s (Kelly *et al.*, 1979), the discovery of major intrinsic properties of thalamic neurons and of their ionic conductances started in 1982 (Llinas and Jahnsen, 1982; Jahnsen and Llinas, 1984a,b). In the same years, intracellular studies *in vivo* disclosed that relay and intralaminar thalamic neurons possess intrinsic properties similar to those investigated *in vitro* and put them in the context of the oscillatory and relay modes that typically characterize behavioral states of light sleep and wakefulness (Deschênes *et al.*, 1982, 1984; Roy *et al.*, 1984; Steriade and Deschênes, 1984). More recent *in vitro* studies added a series of data related to the various components of the long-lasting hyperpolarization in LG thalamic neurons (Crunelli *et al.*, 1987a–c, 1988; Hirsch and Burnod, 1987). *In vitro* studies mainly related to transmitter actions are discussed in Chapter 6.

The complex series of sodium, calcium, and potassium conductances of thalamic neurons, other than the conventional currents that generate the fast action potential, are reviewed elsewhere (Llinás, 1988; Steriade and Llinás, 1988). Here, we briefly discuss some currents, mainly those that appear to be critical in the patterning of spindle oscillations, the peculiar feature of thalamic neurons during EEG-synchronized sleep. We emphasize that although the intrinsic properties of thalamic neurons endow them with the ability to oscillate, the synchronized oscillations in thalamocortical neurons, as they appear during natural sleep, require a synaptic network with a driving force for the coordination of individual oscillations. The importance of synaptic networks including the RE thalamic nucleus, the pacemaker of spindling, in synchronizing thalamic rhythmicity becomes evident when considering the absence of spindle rhythms in thalamocortical neurons deprived of inputs from RE nucleus despite their having identical intrinsic properties as RE-connected thalamocortical cells (see details in Chapter 7).

5.4.1. The Persistent (Noninactivating) Sodium Conductance

The voltage-dependent, noninactivating (or very slowly inactivating) sodium conductance is also termed persistent and is referred to as $g_{Na(noninact.)}$ or $g_{Na(P)}$. It was first described in cerebellar Purkinje cells, where it generates a slow TTX-sensitive depolarizing response (Llinás and Sugimori, 1980; Fig. 17A). It is located at the soma and has a lower activation threshold and slower kinetics than those generating the fast action potential. In the thalamus, $g_{Na(P)}$ was demonstrated *in vitro* (Jahnsen and Llinás, 1984a; Fig. 17B) and was found to be important in cell oscillation, as it counterbalances g_K to generate a rebound excitation. *In vivo* studies have shown the crucial role of $g_{Na(P)}$ in the patterning of spindle oscillations by means of inactivation of sodium channels through intracellular injection of quaternary derivatives of local anesthetics such as QX314 (Mulle *et al.*, 1985). Figure 18 shows that after QX314 injection in VL thalamic neurons, the spontaneous and evoked hyperpolarizations become exceedingly long-lasting (because of the dominance of potassium currents unopposed by the slow sodium conductance), and rhythmic postinhibitory rebounds disappear.

The calcium-dependent low-threshold spike (LTS) was first described in inferior olive neurons (Llinás and Yarom, 1981) and was thereafter found in guinea pig thalamic neurons *in vitro* (Llinás and Jahnsen, 1982) and cat thalamic neurons *in vivo* (Deschênes *et al.*, 1982). As discussed in the first section of this chapter, the LTS is inactive at rest and is deinactivated with membrane hyperpolarization (Fig. 19A). On the average, deinactivation to allow the necessary level of regenerative response is attained at about −65 mV. The LTS is prevented by calcium blockers such as cobalt or cadmium, and it underlies a burst of fast sodium-dependent action potentials that can be blocked by TTX (Fig. 19B).

At the normal resting membrane potential, the thalamic cell's response to a depolarizing pulse is tonic repetitive firing, and the response to an excitatory synaptic input is an EPSP that may trigger single spikes, whereas each of these stimuli applied to the cell hyperpolarized by a few millivolts from resting membrane potential elicits an LTS crowned by a burst of fast action potentials (top and middle panels in Fig. 20A). The LTS and the superimposed burst may also

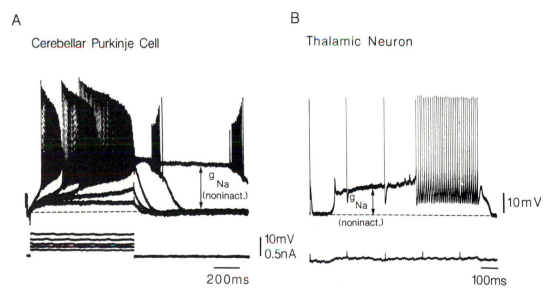

A

Cerebellar Purkinje Cell

B

Thalamic Neuron

g_{Na} (noninact.)

10mV

g_{Na} (noninact.)

10mV
0.5nA

200ms

100ms

Figure 17. Plateau depolarization generated by noninactivating (persistent) sodium conductance, $g_{Na(noninact)}$. A: Direct activation of an intracellularly recorded cerebellar Purkinje cell *in vitro*. Voltage-dependent calcium conductance was blocked by additon of cadmium chloride to the bathing solution. Transmembrane current steps (lower trace) depolarized cell to threshold for spike initiation. Activation consisted of action potentials firing repetitively on a slowly rising depolarizing response that terminates on a plateau potential and spike inactivation. Highest two stimuli generate plateaus that outlast stimulus duration. A fast burst of spikes is seen as plateau depolarization returns to resting membrane potential. This plateau is generated by an equilibrium state between g_K and $g_{Na(noninact)}$. B: Similar set of responses as in A but for a thalamic neuron. A very small depolarizing current step is given, which triggers a rapid depolarization of the thalamic cell and a plateau that lasts for several seconds. This plateau is partly produced by $g_{Na(noninact)}$, and part of voltage is produced by outward current pulse. However, the latter component is small, and $g_{Na(noninact)}$ is responsible for much of the plateau amplitude. Superimposed on this plateau are short-lasting depolarizing pulses that generate single spikes and, as plateau reaches a steady level, general repetitive firing. For thalamic neurons, $g_{Na(noninact)}$ is powerful enough to generate a plateau response without blockage of voltage-dependent calcium conductances. A, unpublished data from R. Llinás and M. Sugimori. B, modified from Jahnsen and Llinás (1984a).

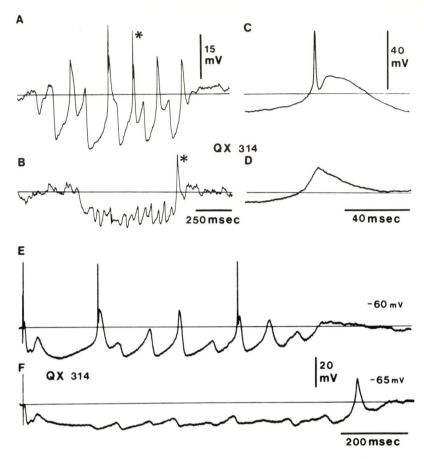

Figure 18. Effect of intracellular injection of QX314, a quaternary derivative of lidocaine that blocks sodium spike electrogenesis and $g_{Na(noninact)}$, on thalamic spindle oscillations. Intracellular recording of a ventrolateral thalamocortical cell in cat under barbiturate anesthesia. A and B: Polygraphic recordings of spontaneous spindle oscillations 2 min (A) and 12 min (B) after impalement with a pipette containing 0.1 M QX314. Spikes are truncated. Asterisks in A and B indicate LTSs that are expanded in C and D, respectively. The LTS in C triggers a sodium action potential. Note, in B, the effect of QX314; abolition of spindle-related rhythmic LTS rebounds and production of a single LTS at the end of the long-lasting hyperpolarization. E and F: Same cell, with spindle oscillations triggered by stimulation of the motor cortex (in E, 2 min after impalement) and the abolition of cortically evoked spindles as an effect of QX314 (in F, 15 min after impalement). Modified after Mulle *et al.* (1985).

be triggered at the break of a hyperpolarizing current pulse (bottom panel in Fig. 20A). These intracellular data indicate that the LTS is the basis of the high-frequency bursts that characterize the activity of thalamocortical neurons during EEG-synchronized sleep, when they become hyperpolarized (see details in monograph by Steriade *et al.*, 1989b).

The LTS is located at the soma of thalamocortical neurons. Indeed, hyperpolarizing currents that leave intact the antidromically elicited initial segment (IS) spike are sufficient to trigger the LTS, but when the antidromic invasion fails, the LTS cannot be induced (Deschênes *et al.*, 1984; Fig. 21).

As shown both *in vitro* and *in vivo*, the deinactivation of the LTS is not only voltage dependent, but also time dependent. Indeed, hyperpolarizing pulses of increasing duration produce graded deinactivation, and short-lasting hyperpolarizing current pulses subthreshold for rebound excitation can sum and trigger overt LTSs (Fig. 22A–C; Steriade *et al.*, 1985). When periodic hyperpolarizing current ramps are injected at a frequency of 12.5 Hz, rhythmic burst discharges are observed at a frequency of about 2.5 Hz (Fig. 22D). This frequency transformation suggests that temporal integration of short hyperpolarizations in normal conditions could lead to production of rhythmic LTSs in thalamic neurons (Steriade *et al.*, 1985).

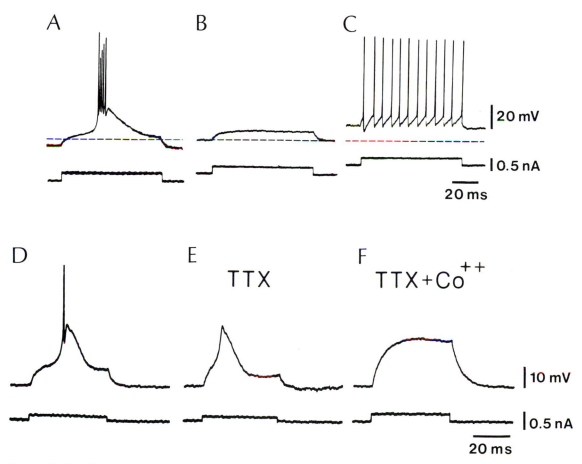

Figure 19. Two firing levels in thalamic neurons and ionic basis for low-threshold spike (LTS) in *in vitro* studies of guinea pig thalamus. A: Cell was directly excited while being hyperpolarized by a constant-current injection. Outward current pulse induces an LTS that triggers a burst of fast action potentials. B: Same current pulse produces a subthreshold depolarization if superimposed on a slightly depolarized membrane potential level. C: After further de-polarization by a direct current, pulse produces a train of action potentials. D: LTS generated by direct stimulation from a slightly hyperpolarized neuron. E: Blockage of g_{Na} by TTX removes fast spike but leaves LTS unmodified. F: Addition of cobalt to the bath abolishes LTS even when current pulse is increased in amplitude by 2.5 times, demonstrating that LTS is generated by low-threshold g_{Ca}. Modified from Llinás and Jahnsen (1982).

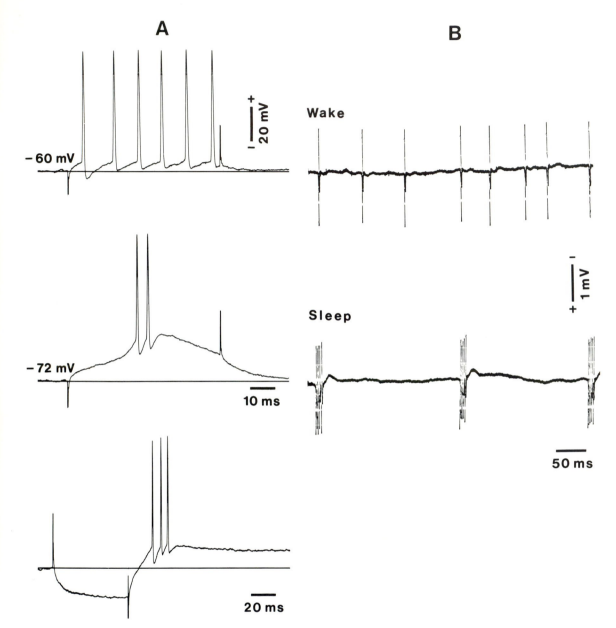

Figure 20. Two firing modes in cat thalamic neurons investigated intracellularly *in vivo* and extracellularly in chronically implanted behaving preparation. A: Effect of membrane potential level on firing modes of anteroventral (AV) thalamic neuron. Top: Tonic firing induced by a depolarizing pulse at resting membrane potential (−60 mV). Middle: The same pulse triggers an LTS crowned by a burst of fast action potentials during hyperpolarization of cell membrane at −72 mV. Bottom: A rebound burst at the break of a hyperpolarizing pulse. B: Tonic firing of a rostral intralaminar thalamic neuron during waking, and burst firing of the same neuron during EEG-synchronized sleep. A, modified from Paré *et al.* (1987). B, unpublished data by M. Steriade and L. L. Glenn.

5.4.3. High-Threshold Calcium Conductance

Presumed intradendritic recordings in thalamic cells studied *in vitro* (Jahnsen and Llinás, 1984b) and *in vivo* (Roy *et al.*, 1984) revealed a voltage-dependent high-threshold calcium conductance that triggers depolarizing responses followed by the activation of a calcium-dependent potassium conductance, $g_{K(Ca)}$. In cortically evoked responses of thalamic neurons *in vivo*, the disclosure of this high-threshold conductance requires an increase in stimulus strength (as compared to the primary EPSP) or the facilitatory action of two or three shocks. This conductance is reflected in the depth of the early IPSP as repetitive fast-rising depolarizations with or without superimposed spike discharges (Fig. 23; Steriade, 1984), and it corresponds to component c in Fig. 24. This high-threshold

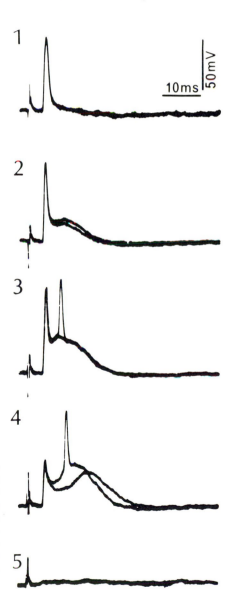

Figure 21. Somatic location of LTS in cat ventrolateral (VL) thalamic neurons *in vivo*. Triggering of LTS by the antidromically elicited (from motor cortex) initial segment (IS) and somatodendritic (SD) action potentials. The VL cell was hyperpolarized by continuous-current injection of increasing intensity from trace 2 to trace 5. In 5, the antidromic response failed, and the LTS disappeared. Resting membrane potential: −62 mV in 1 and −70 mV in 4. From Deschênes *et al.* (1984).

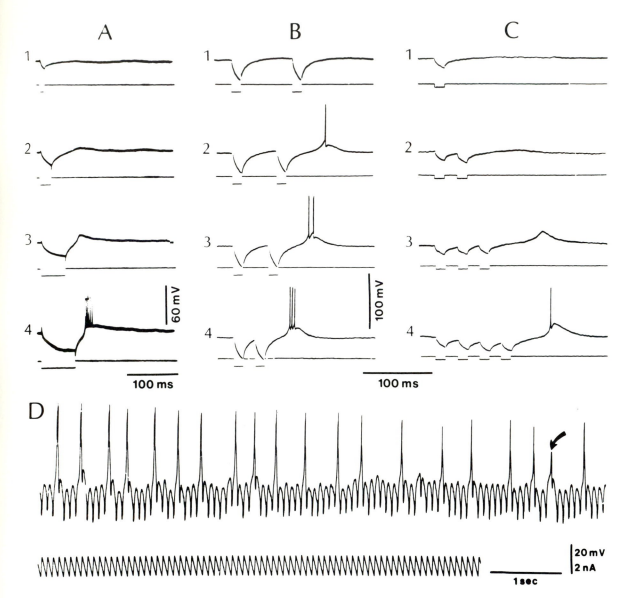

Figure 22. Time dependence of LTS deinactivation in cat thalamic neurons *in vivo* (barbiturate anesthesia). A, and B–D: Two different thalamocortical neurons. Graded deinactivation produced by hyperpolarizing pulses of increasing duration (A), by temporal pairing of two short-lasting current pulses (B), and by a train of short subthreshold hyper- polarizing pulses (C). D: Polygraphic recording showing rhythmic bursting at 2.5 Hz induced by repetitive injection of hyperpolarizing current ramps at a frequency of 12.5 Hz. Arrow: Isolated LTS; amplitude of fast spikes is truncated. Resting potential: −58 mV in A and −63 mV in B–D. From Steriade *et al.* (1985).

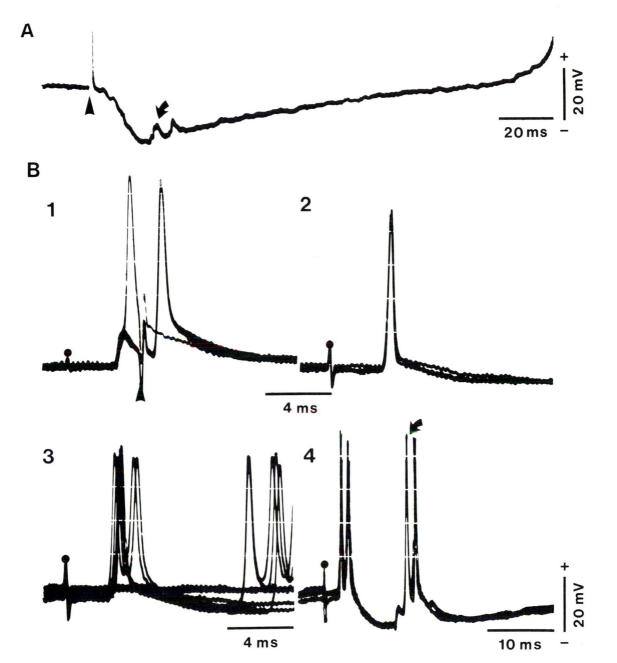

Figure 23. Secondary excitation (see component c in Fig. 24) in cat thalamocortical neurons. Intracellular recordings under barbiturate anesthesia. A: Response of a ventrolateral (VL) thalamocortical cell to cortical precruciate area 4 stimulation (arrowhead); the secondary excitation appears as two rapidly rising depolarizing events (arrow) with a latency of about 25 msec in the deep portion of the early IPSP. B: Response of a ventrobasal (VB) thalamocortical cell to stim-

ulation of the medial lemniscus in the medulla (dot) and antidromic response to stimulation of the primary somatosensory cortex (arrowhead in 1); note collision of cortically evoked antidromic spike with a preceding orthodromic discharge in 1. In 1–4, increasing stimulation intensities to medial lemniscus; note appearance of secondary excitation in 3 and 4 during the early IPSP (arrow in 4). Modified from Roy *et al.* (1984) and Steriade (1984).

secondary excitation was identified *in vivo* as a dendritic calcium conductance on the basis of intracellular injections of ethyleneglycoltetraacetic acid (EGTA), a substance that binds free calcium. This treatment prevents the development of the subsequent $g_{K(Ca)}$. Consequently, the EGTA injections in presumed dendrites of thalamic neurons lead to the appearance of long-lasting plateaus and prolonged spike discharges (Roy *et al.*, 1984).

Some of the fast prepotentials (FPPs) seen in thalamic cells (Maekawa and Purpura, 1967a; Deschênes *et al.*, 1984; Paré *et al.*, 1989) probably represent dendritic spiking since they can be blocked in an all-or-none manner by hyperpolarizing currents. Intracellular injections of QX314 in thalamic neurons (see Section 5.4.1) lead to the appearance of very numerous FPPs because the dendritic conductance dominates the cell's behavior when somatic sodium channels are blocked (Mulle *et al.*, 1985). The main role of dendritic spiking is to assist the neuron in the transfer of EPSPs from distal portions of dendrites toward the somatic spike trigger zone (Steriade and Deschênes, 1984).

5.4.4. Voltage- and Calcium-Dependent Potassium Conductances

There are at least four voltage-dependent potassium conductances in thalamic neurons: (1) the M current activated by depolarization; (2) the A current that is responsible for the slow return to base line following hyperpolarization; and (3 and 4) two anomalous (inward) rectifiers. For details on A current, see Section 5.1.

Among the $g_{K(Ca)}$ currents, the AHP potential (see Section 5.1.3) is a rate-limiting factor. This is demonstrated by the different duration of AHP in two

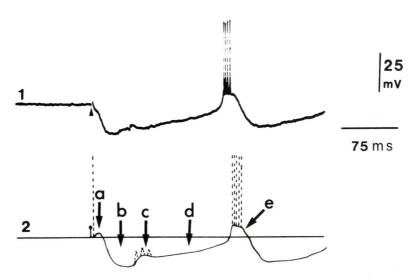

Figure 24. The archetypal response sequence of a thalamocortical cell to cortical stimulation. Intracellular recording of a cat ventrolateral thalamic neuron under barbiturate anesthesia (1) and diagrammatic representation of five components in the excitatory–inhibitory response sequence (2). Components are: a, primary EPSP associated or not with antidromic spike (dotted line); b, early Cl-dependent IPSP; c, secondary excitation; d, late part of the long-lasting hyperpolarization; and e, postinhibitory rebound. See further explanations in text. Modified from Roy *et al.* (1984).

distinct classes of thalamic neurons: the thalamocortical cells have AHPs of about 70 msec, whereas in RE neurons the AHP terminates after 8–10 msec (Mulle *et al.*, 1986). Accordingly, the firing rates of thalamocortical neurons in behaving animals do not generally exceed 7–10 Hz during EEG-synchronized sleep, whereas RE neurons display discharge frequencies of about 20 Hz during the same behavioral state, and, on arousal, RE neurons may reach firing rates between 50 and 100 Hz, which are not seen in thalamocortical neurons (Steriade *et al.*, 1986).

The calcium dependency of the late phase of the hyperpolarization (component d in Fig. 24) was demonstrated by its abolition following intracellular injections of EGTA (a calcium chelator) in thalamic neurons (Roy *et al.*, 1984). The late phase of the long-lasting hyperpolarization leads to a rebound LTS (component e in Fig. 24) and to cyclic oscillations within the frequency range of spindle waves.

5.5. Basal Forebrain Neurons

The intrinsic membrane properties of acetylcholinesterase-positive, presumably cholinergic basal forebrain neurons recorded from the diagonal band (DB) nuclei and ventral part of the medial septum (MS) of guinea pig have been recently studied *in vitro* by Griffith (1988). Three types of neurons were described as displaying slow AHP (duration of about 600 msec) or fast AHP (5–50 msec) of smaller amplitudes; a small proportion (7%) of cells fired in a burst pattern. The slow AHP neurons have been tentatively regarded as corresponding to some slowly firing cholinergic basal forebrain projection neurons, whereas the characteristics of fast AHP elements resembled those of fast-spiking cortical local-circuit cells.

6

Neurotransmitter-Modulated Ionic Currents of Brainstem Neurons and Some of Their Targets

This chapter discusses the actions on target neurons of projections from chemically identified neurons within the brainstem. The actions of brainstem chemical transmitters are discussed primarily on the basis of intracellular investigations *in vitro*, although some intracellular and extracellular *in vivo* data are included. Needless to say, data from *in vitro* experiments are the most reliable since they can be obtained after blockage of synaptic transmission, and the concentrations of agents can be precisely specified, in addition to the greater stability of recording conditions. One should, however, also emphasize the necessity of reproducing the effects of agent application by stimulation of the appropriate pathway. It is also unlikely that the complex conditions of behavioral states, and even the mechanisms underlying just one physiological correlate of states of vigilance, will be found to be attributable to one synaptic transmitter. Thus, the data presented here should be considered as a prologue to future studies that will also explore transmitter interactions, including synergetic or competitive actions of colocalized transmitters, and will more deeply probe second messenger actions.

A general discussion of the criteria to be met in assigning any substance a role as a neurotransmitter, the methods of drug application, the synaptic mechanisms of action, presynaptic and postsynaptic receptors, and correspondences or mismatches between transmitters and receptor localizations may be found in monographs and reviews by Phillis (1970), Krnjević (1974), North (1986a,b), Siggins and Gruol (1986), and Herkenham (1987). The synaptic effects exerted on the same central neurons by stimulating the nuclei giving rise to chemically coded projections are discussed in some sections to allow comparisons between the pure actions of the neurotransmitter and those induced by stimulating the synaptic pathway.

Each section concerning a given transmitter is organized according to projection targets, save for the hippocampus, which has been extensively reviewed elsewhere and hence will be compared and contrasted *en passant* in some sections. For a number of neurotransmitters, a common theme appears to be medi-

163

ation of agonist-induced effects by changes in potassium conductances. For many hyperpolarizing effects, the potassium conductances are inwardly rectifying; i.e., there is increased conductance at more hyperpolarized membrane potential levels. Because of the prevalence of ligand-induced alteration of potassium currents, we also discuss certain intrinsic potassium currents in this chapter in addition to those discussed in Chapter 5.

6.1. Acetylcholine

6.1.1. Brainstem

6.1.1.1. Medial Pontine Reticular Formation

The importance of brainstem cholinergic systems for control of neuronal excitability during the sleep–wake cycle has been the subject of recent intense investigation, and their role in sleep cycle control is discussed in detail in Chapters 11 and 12. From the standpoint of REM sleep it has been known for several years that *in vivo* microinjections of cholinergic compounds into the pontine reticular formation furnish the only phenomenologically adequate pharmacological model of this state. Depending on the injection site, these compounds can reproduce all of the phenomena of REM sleep (Amatruda *et al.*, 1975; see review in Baghdoyan *et al.*, 1985), even extending to the membrane potential alterations found in spinal motoneurons (Morales *et al.*, 1987).

In Chapter 4 we described recent anatomic results that greatly strengthened the argument that cholinergic compounds may play a role in the natural induction and/or maintenance of REM sleep. There are projections from the cholinergic laterodorsal and pedunculopontine tegmental nuclei to the pontine reticular formation, the site of cholinergic REM induction.

An additional essential component of cholinergic hypotheses of REM sleep control is the demonstration that cholinergic compounds directly excite medial pontine reticular formation (mPRF) neurons, an investigation necessitating the synaptic isolation and control of bathing media feasible only with an *in vitro* preparation. Further, it is essential to demonstrate that the direct cholinergic actions on mPRF include those known to occur in natural REM sleep. This section outlines data indicating that cholinergic agonists applied to synaptically isolated mPRF neurons produce powerful muscarinic excitatory effects that parallel the electrophysiological membrane changes seen in natural REM sleep.

Unless otherwise specified the data in this section are taken from work by Greene, Gerber, and McCarley (1989a) and Greene and McCarley (1989). The *in vitro* preparation and methods for mPRF recordings were the same as described in Chapter 5. Drugs were usually bath applied except for a few experiments in which carbachol was applied by a puffer pipette with tip submerged in medium but above the surface of the slice. All neurons maintained robust and stable electrophysiological properties throughout the washin (2–5 min) and washout (10 min) periods.

Neurons in the giant-cell field portion of mPRF were exposed to carbachol at concentrations of 0.5–1.0 μM in the bath or 1–10 mM in puffer electrodes.

Sixty-five percent of neurons responded to carbachol with a depolarization of 16 mV associated with a 20% increase in input resistance (Fig. 1A). Carbachol evoked a hyperpolarization associated with a decrease in input resistance in 20% of the neurons (see Fig. 3A), and a biphasic response of a shorter duration hyperpolarization followed by depolarization was present in 10% of neurons. Only 5% of neurons did not respond to carbachol.

These were direct, nonsynaptically mediated effects, as indicated by their presence during bath application of tetrodotoxin (1 μM), which prevents sodium action-potential-dependent synaptic activity. These carbachol effects were seen

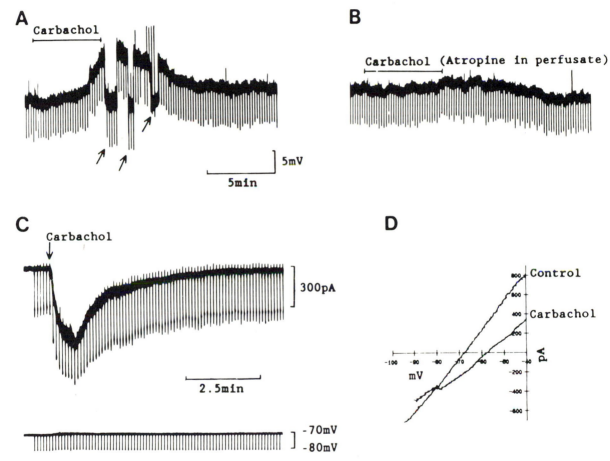

Figure 1. Carbachol depolarization response of mPRF neurons *in vitro* is mediated by a decrease in a voltage-insensitive conductance and is blocked by atropine. A: Chart record of a typical depolarizing response of an mPRF neuron to bath application of carbachol (0.5 μM during time indicated). Downward deflections are caused by intracellular current pulses (400 msec, 200 pA) applied to assess input resistance. At arrows, membrane potential was returned to the baseline potential of −74 mV by D.C. hyperpolarizing current to avoid voltage-sensitive changes of the membrane resistance not specific to carbachol. B: Atropine (0.5 μM) blocks the depolarizing response to carbachol (same neuron as in A).

C: Decreased membrane conductance during puffer application (arrow, 1 sec, 3 p.s.i.) of carbachol (1 mM) is indicated by the decreased amplitude of downward deflections in the upper current record in response to 10-mV, 400-msec membrane potential shift commands (lower record) in a neuron under voltage-champ control. D: *I/V* plot generated by a constant depolarization of the membrane potential (1 mV/200 msec) from −100 mV to −50 mV during control conditions and during exposure to 0.5 μM carbachol in the perfusate. Note the voltage insensitivity of the carbachol current. Modified from Greene *et al.* (1989a).

on each of the two main types of mPRF neuron, the low-threshold burst (LTB) neurons and the nonburst (NB) neurons (see Chapter 5), and the percentages of the types of carbachol responses did not differ in NB and LTB neurons.

Depolarizing Response. The addition of atropine to the perfusate resulted in complete blockade of the carbachol-evoked depolarization (Fig. 1B), indicating its muscarinic nature. This response, studied under voltage-clamp control, was associated with a reduced outward current (a net inward current) and a decrease in membrane conductance (Fig. 1C). The inward current evoked by carbachol was voltage insensitive, having a constant I/V plot slope (Fig. 1D). The reversal potential was -98 ($[K^+]_o = 3.25$ mM), compatible with a reduction primarily in potassium permeability, and with recent studies showing a Nernstian relationship of reversal potential with varying extracellular potassium concentration (Gerber *et al.*, unpublished data).

The depolarization response evoked by carbachol was accompanied by an increase in neuronal excitability, since identical amplitude and duration depolarizing current pulses (Fig. 2A,B) elicited from 1.3- to fourfold as many action potentials during carbachol application as compared with control. To determine if the steady-state reduction in outward current elicited by carbachol was alone sufficient to account for the increased excitability, carbachol application was combined with intracellular injection of a hyperpolarizing D.C. current to return the membrane potential to control level. In this condition, excitability was not increased (Fig. 2C).

The effects of carbachol on postsynaptic potentials (PSPs) elicited by stimulation of the contralateral pontine reticular formation were also examined, since it is known that reticular stimulation during REM sleep produces enhanced PSPs as contrasted with stimulation in EEG-synchronized sleep (Ito and McCarley, 1984). Stimulation of the contralateral mPRF with bipolar double-barrel glass electrodes filled with perfusate evoked depolarizing PSPs (Fig. 2D). These evoked PSPs were enhanced in the presence of carbachol-elicited depolarization, and this enhancement was blocked by atropine.

With respect to the mechanism of depolarization, it should be noted that a similar depolarizing response to muscarinic activation has been reported in neurons of the hippocampus (Madison *et al.*, 1987) and the medial and lateral geniculate thalamic nuclei (McCormick and Prince, 1987d), and in both cases this was mediated by reduction of a potassium conductance active at all membrane potentials, with an apparent lack of inactivation and a reversal potential more negative than -90 mV. This conductance is similar to the S current, modulated by neurotransmitters in invertebrate neurons (Brezina *et al.*, 1987; Pollock *et al.*, 1985; Siegelbaum *et al.*, 1982).

Hyperpolarizing Response. The hyperpolarizing response to carbachol was blocked by atropine and was associated with increased outward current and decreased input resistance (Fig. 3). There was a nonlinear current–voltage relationship (examined between -100 and -50 mV) of this carbachol-evoked current in the presence of 1 μM TTX (Fig. 3). Inward rectification was present; i.e., slope conductance was greater at membrane potential levels negative to the reversal potential, a feature reported to be characteristic of the anomalous rectifier current (Katz, 1949; Hagiwara and Takahashi, 1974). At membrane potentials between −65 mV and −50 mV (currents at potentials depolarized to −50 mV were not examined), the slope conductance was less than 2.5 nS, so that the outward current evoked by carbachol was nearly constant over this range. This was in contrast to a slope conductance of 12 nS over the range of −100 to −80 mV.

As is discussed later in this chapter, cholinergically evoked hyperpolarizations have been observed in both the brainstem (Egan and North, 1986a) and the reticular thalamic nucleus (McCormick and Prince, 1986b), although voltage

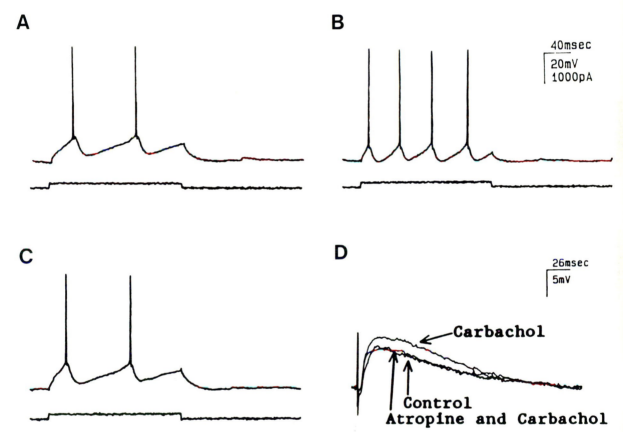

Figure 2. Carbachol elicits an increase in mPRF neuronal excitability *in vitro* and in the amplitude of excitatory postsynaptic potentials (PSPs). A: Control conditions. Two oscilloscope traces of neuronal membrane potential response (upper) to intracellular depolarizing current injection of 400 msec duration and 150 pA (lower). Base-line membrane potential is −65 mV. B: Same stimulus conditions and neuron as in A, but with puffer application of carbachol (10 mM, 0.5 sec, 1.5 p.s.i.). The membrane potential depolarized 6 mV, and the number of spikes increased. C: Same neuron with same stimulus and carbachol application parameters as in B, but with D.C. hyperpolarizing cur- rent injection to return the membrane potential to the con- trol level. Note the number of action potentials is the same as in A. D: Three superimposed oscilloscope traces from an mPRF neuron of a PSP elicited by stimulation of the con- tralateral mPRF (stimulation artifact is the first biphasic positive–negative deflection). Topmost trace is during bath perfusion with carbachol (0.5 μM), and bottom traces are during the control condition and during bath perfusion with both carbachol and atropine (0.5 μM). Note the 20% in- crease of PSP amplitude in the presence of carbachol com- pared to control and carbachol/atropine conditions. Modi- fied from Greene *et al.* (1989a).

sensitivity has not been analyzed. Hyperpolarizations resulting from an enhancement of an inwardly rectifying potassium conductance have been reported in locus coeruleus and submucosal neurons in response to opioid agonists (North *et al.*, 1987; see Section 6.2 of this chapter) and in cultured striatal and hippocampal neurons in response to adenosine (Trussell and Jackson, 1985) or serotonin (Yakel *et al.*, 1988). In cardiac cells, muscarinic cholinergic agonists elicit an

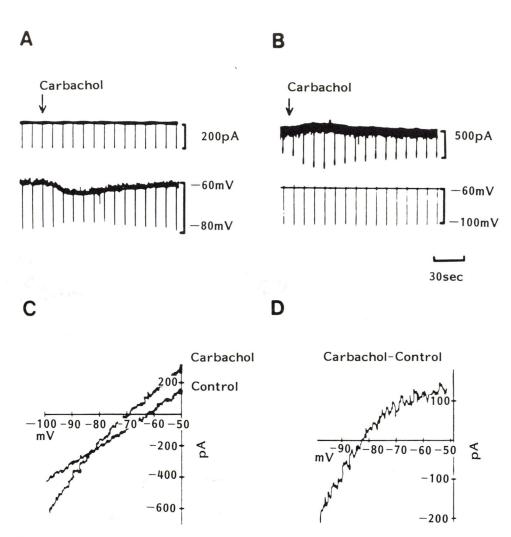

Figure 3. The hyperpolarization elicited by carbachol in mPRF neurons *in vitro* is mediated by an increase in an inwardly rectifying conductance. A and B: Records of current (upper record) and membrane potential (lower record) obtained in current-clamp (A) and voltage-clamp (B) conditions during puffer application of carbachol at arrow (1.0 mM carbachol, 10 sec, 5 psi). In A, downward deflections result from current injection (400 msec), and in B from a membrane potential shift command (400 msec). Following carbachol ejection there is an increase in chord conductance observable in A and B. C: I/V plot from another neuron generated by a constant depolarization of the membrane potential from -100 to -50 mV (1 mV/400 msec) before and during exposure to carbachol ($[K^+]_0 = 5.0$ mM). D: I/V plot of the current elicited by carbachol constructed by subtraction of the control plot from the carbachol plot. Note that the slope conductance of the outward (positive) current is less than that of the inward current, indicative of inward rectification. Modified from Greene *et al.* (1989a).

increase in potassium conductance (Noma and Trautwein, 1978; Sakmann *et al.*, 1983) similar in its inwardly rectifying voltage sensitivity to the responses observed in mPRF neurons and also in amphibian parasympathetic neurons (Hartzell *et al.*, 1977). In vertebrate cells the inwardly rectifying potassium conductance was coupled by GTP-binding proteins (Andrade *et al.*, 1986; Breitwieser and Szabo, 1985; Pfaffinger *et al.*, 1985; Trussell and Jackson, 1987), and in invertebrate neurons, cAMP has been reported to mediate this transmitter-evoked effect (Drummond *et al.*, 1980).

Recent data by Gerber *et al.* (1989b) have suggested that neither the hyperpolarizing nor depolarizing responses of mPRF neurons to cholinergic agonists has the characteristics of M_1 receptor mediation since, as shown in Fig. 4, the pirenzepine sensitivity expected in M_1 receptors was not present. Further work is required to define whether the receptor characteristics are those of an M_2 or another muscarinic receptor type.

The pharmacological, *in vitro* identification of non-M_1 receptors in the reticular formation is in accord with *in vitro* autoradiographic data that indicated almost exclusive presence of M_2 receptors in the brainstem, including those in the PPT and LDT cholinergic nuclei, in the reticular formation, in locus coeruleus, and in cranial nerve nuclei (see Mash and Potter, 1986, who also provide a review of earlier autoradiographic studies). M_1 receptors were largely confined to telencephalic and diencephalic structures.

In summary, two-thirds of mPRF neurons respond to carbachol with a strong depolarizing response that is associated with an increase in input resistance. There is an increase in excitability as measured by an increased number of spikes to the same depolarizing current and enhancement of PSPs elicited by electrical stimulation of the contralateral pontine reticular formation. Atropine blockade of carbachol effects suggests mediation by a muscarinic receptor. The remaining one-third of neurons respond with either a biphasic hyperpolarization–depolarization or hyperpolarization alone, consistent with microiontophoretic studies of ACh effects on spike rates of identified reticulospinal mPRF neurons (Greene and Carpenter, 1985).

The depolarizing effects of carbachol nicely parallel the phenomenology of naturally occurring REM sleep in medial pontine reticular neurons, i.e., a membrane depolarization of 7–10 mV and enhancement of excitatory PSPs elicited by reticular stimulation (Ito and McCarley, 1984; see Chapter 11). Furthermore, the effects on firing pattern of a carbachol-induced depolarization also parallel those occurring during natural REM sleep (McCarley and Hobson, 1975a) in that no bursting discharge pattern is present in REM sleep, a finding that is also compatible with the presence of depolarization-dependent inactivation of the low-threshold calcium spike responsible for the burst discharge pattern.

Thus, the direct effects of cholinergic muscarinic activation of mPRF neurons *in vitro* are consistent with the presence of cholinergic activation of this zone during naturally occurring REM sleep. At the single-cell level these results provide a mechanism for the action of microinjected muscarinic cholinergic agents in pharmacological production of a REM-sleep-like state.

6.1.1.2. Pedunculopontine Tegmental Cholinergic Neurons

The ACh actions on thalamically projecting PPT cells thought to be cholinergic have been studied in guinea pig slices by Leonard and Llinás (1988,

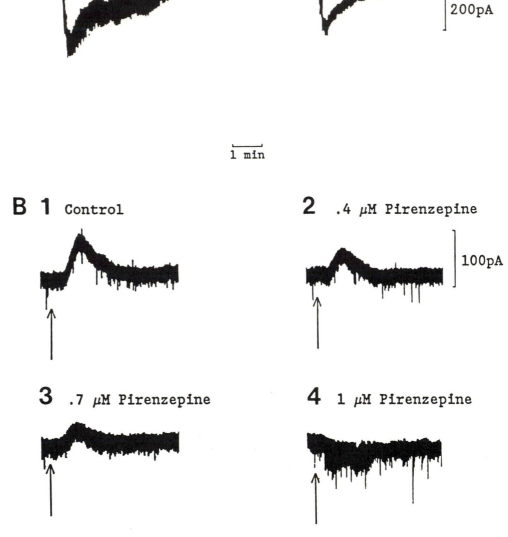

Figure 4. Non-M_1 nature of the *in vitro* mPRF muscarinic response. A: Voltage-clamp recording of the current associated with the depolarizing response elicited by puffer application of carbachol. Note the inward current increase (downward deflection, equivalent to an outward current decrease) in control conditions. Even 1 μM concentrations of pirenzepine did not fully block this response. B: Outward current increase (upward deflection) associated with the hyperpolarizing response; note the failure to block by 400 nM or even 700 nM pirenzepine, although there was blockage at 1 μM. Thus, both the de- and hyperpolarizing responses to carbachol were not blocked by the 200 nM pirenzepine concentration that would have been expected to block an M_1 receptor, given the K_ds of carbachol and pirenzepine for the M_1 receptor (cf. Mash and Potter, 1986). Modified from Gerber *et al.* (1989b).

1989). Figure 5A shows the inhibition of spontaneous firing of a PPT cell associated with hyperpolarization of the membrane by pressure injection of bethanechol from a micropipette positioned above the slice. Superfusion with 20 μM ACh and 20 μM eserine produced a rapid and reversible suppression of neuronal firing and a marked increase in membrane conductance (Fig. 5B). This conductance was probably potassium dependent since it decreased and was reversed by membrane hyperpolarization between −85 mV and −90 mV (Fig. 5D,E), corresponding closely to the potassium equilibrium potential. That this action was direct was demonstrated by blocking spontaneous synaptic potentials by a zero calcium and 2 mM cobalt superfusate (Fig. 6A,B). The hyperpolarizing action of bethanechol was unaffected by this blockage (Fig. 6C,D). The bethanechol-induced hyperpolarization was blocked by the muscarinic anatagonist atropine (Fig. 6F). Leonard and Llinás have obtained preliminary evidence indicating that the muscarinic receptor mediating the hyperpolarization of PPT neurons was not M_1 since high concentrations of pirenzepine were required to block the response.

6.1.1.3. Locus Coeruleus

The presence of cholinergic receptors in locus coeruleus (LC) has been suggested by both acetylcholinesterase staining (Albanese and Butcher, 1980) and *in vitro* autoradiographic techniques (see Mash and Potter, 1986), with the latter study indicating the presence of M_2 but not M_1 receptors. In addition, ChAT immunohistochemical studies indicate the presence of cholinergic fibers in LC (M. T. Shipley, personal communication; Jones, 1989) and the studies of A. Mitani, S. Higo, and R. W. McCarley (unpublished data) also indicate the presence of anterograde LC labeling from PHA-L or WGA−HRP injected in the PPT/LDT cholinergic nuclei.

Egan and North (1985) recorded intracellularly in the *in vitro* rat LC and found that superfusion of ACh (in the presence of neostigmine to prevent degradation) increased the firing rate of LC neurons by depolarizing the membrane. This effect was reduced by antagonists of both nicotinic (hexamethonium) and muscarinic (atropine) types. In this first intracellular recording study defining muscarinic receptor type in single central neurons, they found that the muscarinic action was relatively pirenzepine insensitive, with a mean dissociation constant (K_d) of 233 nM, a value typical of M_2 receptors (Fig. 7). Subsequent experiments (Egan and North, 1986b) showed both the nicotinic and muscarinic actions to be direct, since they persisted in the presence of a zero-calcium/high-magnesium superfusate or in superfusates containing TTX, i.e., solutions blocking synaptic potentials. They further demonstrated that pressure injections of ACh from microelectrodes (puffer electrodes) produced a biphasic depolarization in about half of the neurons; there was a hexamethonium-sensitive (hence nicotinic) initial, rapid component (Fig. 8) and a slower component that decayed slowly over about 30 sec. This late slow component was abolished by atropine. Nearly half the neurons showed only a slow depolarization, requiring 10−20 sec to peak and decaying over 30 sec. Fewer than 10% of the neurons showed only the fast nicotinic response. Voltage-clamp studies indicated the presence of an inward current whose time course paralleled that of the voltage changes. In all types of nicotinic response there was a striking desensitization to nicotine, with a

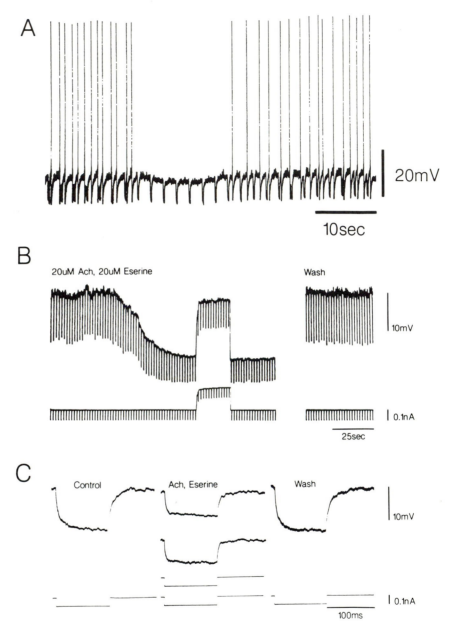

Figure 5. Actions of ACh on guinea pig PPT cholinergic neurons *in vitro.* A: Spontaneous firing is inhibited by pressure ejection of bethanechol from a micropipette positioned above the slice. B: Superfusion with 20 μM ACh and 20 μM eserine in normal Ringer produces a steady, reversible hyperpolarization accompanied by a 50% decrease in input resistance. C: Representative traces from each condition in B displayed at higher sweep speed. D: Bethanechol hyperpolarization elicited by pressure ejection at different membrane potentials. Response is reversed at −95 mV. E: Response amplitude plotted against membrane potential for three neurons. The extrapolated reversal potential is between −85 and −95 mV. Unpublished data by C. Leonard and R. Llinás.

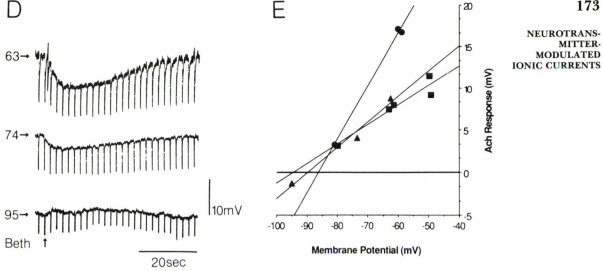

Figure 5. (*Continued*)

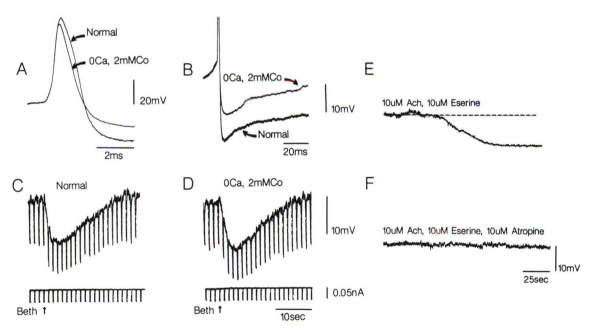

Figure 6. Acetylcholine has a direct muscarinic action on guinea pig PPT cholinergic neurons *in vitro*. A: Action potential (AP) before and after g_{Ca} is blocked by superfusion with 0 mM calcium and 2 mM cobalt. Note the blockade of the calcium-dependent component of the AP. B: Same as A at a slower sweep speed to show the blockade of the calcium-dependent AHP. C: Hyperpolarization of neuron from A and B in normal Ringer produced by pressure ejection of bethanechol. D: Hyperpolarization on neuron from A–C after blockade of calcium conductances (and synaptic transmission). Note that the action of bethanechol is unaffected by calcium conductance blockade. E: Membrane hyperpolarization (another neuron) produced by superfusing 10 μM ACh and 10 μM eserine. F: Membrane hyperpolarization is completely blocked by 10 μM atropine. Unpublished data by C. Leonard and R. Llinás.

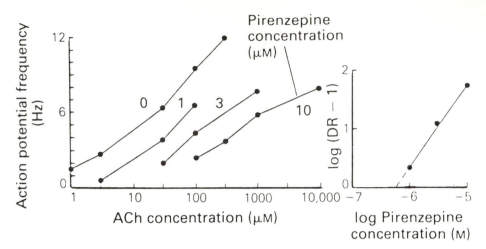

Figure 7. An M_2 receptor mediates muscarinic depolarization of locus coeruleus (LC) neurons *in vitro*. Left panel shows dose–response curve for acetylcholine in terms of LC action potential frequency increase at various concentrations of pirenzepine. The right panel shows a Schild plot of these results. The least-squares line has a slope of 1.1, and the pirenzepine K_d is 288 nM. Modified from Egan and North (1985).

half-time of 30 min for recovery. A practical experimental point is that with superfusion or iontophoresis with ACh, the nicotinic response may be masked by desensitization, as perhaps occurred in Svensson and Engberg's study (1980). It was also of interest that α-bungarotoxin did not block the nicotinic response, suggesting that the LC nicotinic receptor was more like that in sympathetic ganglia than that at the neuromuscular junction.

A final point with respect to ACh and LC is the presence of short-latency EPSPs elicited by electrical stimulation of the slice surface in the LC region (Fig.

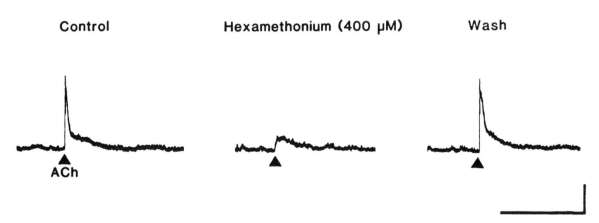

Figure 8. Acetylcholine depolarization of locus coeruleus neurons has fast and slow components. Records are of membrane potential; neurons were held at -75 mV to prevent spontaneous firing. Triangles indicate time of application of a few nanoliters of ACh by pressure injection. Note the presence of a rapid and slow component of the depolarization, with the rapid component being blocked by the nicotinic antagonist hexamethonium (center). The slow component was blocked by muscarinic antagonists (not shown). Modified from Egan and North (1986b).

8). These PSPs were graded with stimulus intensity and abolished by calcium-free solutions and thus likely synaptic, but not blocked by nicotinic antagonists hexamethonium or dihydro-β-erythroidine, arguing against a nicotinic origin of this EPSP. Section 6.4.2 will indicate that this EPSP is mediated by an excitatory amino acid neurotransmitter.

6.1.2. Thalamus

The sources of cholinergic pathways acting on neurons in all thalamic nuclei are in the Ch5 and Ch6 cell groups of the midbrain–pontine reticular formation. For the rostral parts of reticular (RE), mediodorsal (MD), and anteromedial–anteroventral (AV–AM) nuclei, the brainstem cholinergic innervation is supplemented by projections arising in cholinergic neurons in Ch2, Ch3, and Ch4 cell groups of the basal forebrain (see Chapter 4). The understanding of ACh actions on thalamic neurons is of fundamental importance for the concept of ascending reticular activation. Although brainstem cholinergic neurons directly excite thalamocortical neurons, both brainstem and basal forebrain cholinergic neurons hyperpolarize RE thalamic GABAergic neurons, with consequent disinhibition in thalamocortical cells. We discuss the effects of ACh on the three major cell classes in thalamus: thalamocortical, local-circuit, and RE neurons.

6.1.2.1. Thalamocortical Cells

Beginning with the mid-1960s, the excitatory postsynaptic action of ACh has been demonstrated on dorsal thalamic (mainly ventrobasal, VB, and dorsal LG) single neurons recorded extracellularly, some of them identified antidromically as thalamocortical cells (Andersen and Curtis, 1964a,b; McCance et al., 1968a; Phillis, 1971; Duggan and Hall, 1975). Cholinergic facilitation was also selectively observed on the postsynaptic components of evoked mass field potentials in ventroanterior–ventrolateral (VA–VL), VB, and LG nuclei (Marshall and Murray, 1980). The excitatory action of ACh was blocked by both muscarinic (atropine, scopolamine) and nicotinic (hexamethonium, mecamylamine) antagonists (Phillis et al., 1967; Satinski, 1967; Godfraind, 1978). The ACh action is considerably more evident in animals anesthetized with gas than under barbiturate anesthesia (McCance et al., 1968b).

The ACh-induced excitation of VL and ventromedial (VM) thalamic neurons is accompanied by the conversion of the burst response to stimulation of cerebellar afferent pathways into a single-spike response (Marshall and McLennan, 1972; MacLeod et al., 1984). This is similar to the action of a sustained depolarization (see Chapter 5) and much the same as the state-dependent change from passing from EEG-synchronized sleep to wakefulness (see Chapter 8). In fact, ACh-induced excitatory responses of muscarinic type are only observed when the recorded cell is discharging in the single-spike mode associated with EEG desynchronization. The dependency of ACh excitatory action on desynchronized brain electrical activity was observed in VM neurons of acutely prepared animals (MacLeod et al., 1984) and in LG neurons recorded in chronic experiments (Marks and Roffwarg, 1987). In the latter condition, the ACh-elicited facilitation of LG-cell discharges (an action antagonized by scopolamine) was only observed in waking and REM sleep. All these results are congruent with the now established fact that barbiturate anesthesia completely abolishes the excitation by ACh iontophoresis (Eysel *et al.*, 1986) as well as the direct excitation of thalamocortical neurons by stimulating the cholinergic brainstem–thalamic pathways (Hu *et al.*, 1989b).

In vitro studies of medial geniculate (MG) and LG thalamic neurons showed the presence of species differences in ACh effects (McCormick and Prince, 1987a; see also McCormick, 1989a,b).

In the guinea pig, ACh causes a hyperpolarization associated with an increased potassium conductance, followed by a slow depolarization associated with a decreased potassium conductance (Fig. 9). Both these components persist after blockade of synaptic transmission and are mediated by muscarinic receptors.

In the albino rat, unpublished data of the same authors on LG neurons, cited in McCormick and Prince (1987a), indicate that ACh results in the slow depolarization only.

In cat MG neurons and LG neurons recorded from laminae A–A1, some of them identified as thalamocortical cells by intracellular staining or antidromic invasion from the radiation, ACh induces a rapid (nicotinic) depolarization followed by a slow hyperpolarization and a slow depolarization caused by activation of muscarinic receptors (Fig. 10). The nicotinic excitation of LG cells resembles the ACh action on peripheral ganglion cells; corroboratively, the nicotinic receptors in the LG nucleus seem to be of the ganglionic type (Clarke *et al.*, 1985). The hyperpolarization prevails in MG neurons (in keeping with previous extracellular data *in vivo* by Tebecis, 1972). The slow depolarization occurs with equal frequency in MG and LG nuclei. While the fast nicotinic depolarization is associated with an increase in membrane conductance, the slow hyper- and depolarizing events are associated with conductance changes similar to those found in guinea pig (see above). The slow depolarization inhibits the occurrence of burst discharges and promotes single-spike firing, opposite to the action of the hyperpolarization and very similar to the picture seen in transition from sleep to arousal. The fast nicotinic excitation by ACh was also found in medial habenular neurons maintained *in vitro* (McCormick and Prince, 1987b).

6.1.2.2. Local Interneurons

As yet, there are no available data on formally identified local-circuit cells in thalamic nuclei *in vivo*. The ACh effects on these elements have been inferred by investigating the stimulus-specific (or short-range) inhibitions on thalamic relay cells in the LG nucleus (Sillito *et al.*, 1983; Eysel *et al.*, 1986; see a recent review in Sillito, 1987). These studies report that the center-surround antagonism is enhanced by ACh application and conclude there is an excitatory influence of ACh on GABAergic local-circuit cells intrinsic to the LG nucleus. The ACh action seems to be similar to the enhanced discrimination in LG relay neurons on awakening from sleep (Livingstone and Hubel, 1981; see Chapter 8). However, these data are far from definitive because the short-axoned cells should be identified by intracellular staining, and their inhibitory nature has to be demonstrated by immunohistochemistry.

Recently, McCormick and Pape (1988) have identified presumed local-cir-

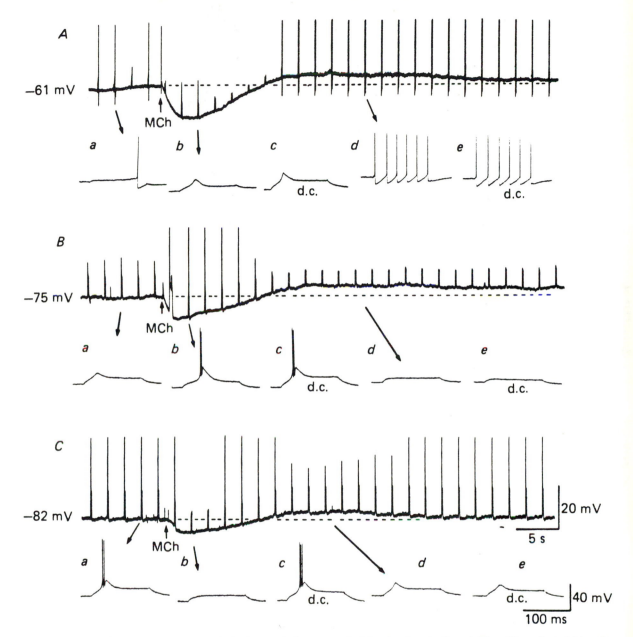

Figure 9. Effect of muscarinic hyperpolarization and slow depolarization on the response of a guinea pig LG thalamic neuron to a depolarizing current pulse. *In vitro* recordings. Responses to three applications of acetylmethylcholine (MCh) are illustrated when the membrane potential was held with D.C. at levels indicated to the left of each segment. The cell was in the single-spike firing mode (A), the burst firing mode (B), and in between (C). Sample traces are ex- panded for detail, as indicated. The effect of mimicking the MCh-induced change in V_m with the intracellular injection of current is indicated by "d.c.". This particular neuron was in the burst firing mode when the membrane potential was around −80 mV. A more typical membrane potential for this type of activity would be between −70 mV and −75 mV. From McCormick and Prince (1987a).

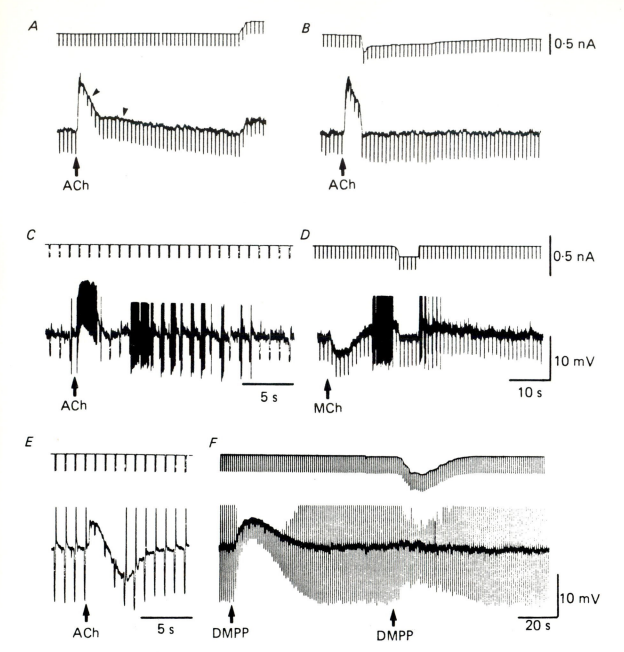

Figure 10. Actions of ACh in the cat LG and MG thalamic neurons *in vitro*. A: Application of ACh to a LG cell in lamina A (resting potential −64 mV). B: Manual voltage clamp of the slow depolarizing component (second arrowhead) of the response to ACh in the neuron in A. C: Application of ACh to another LG neuron in lamina A, depolarized with intracellular injection of D.C. to near firing threshold (−60 mV). D: Application of the muscarinic agonist acetylmethylcholine (MCh) to the neuron of C. E: Application of ACh to an MG neuron. F: Application of the nicotinic agonist DMPP to the MG neuron of E. In all pairs, the top trace is the injected current, and the bottom trace is the membrane potential. Current calibration in E and F as in D. From McCormick and Prince (1987a).

cuit neurons in cat LG slices by their short-lasting action potential, lack of a low-threshold calcium spike (see Chapter 5 for details on LTSs that appear in virtually all thalamocortical cells), and intracellular staining showing a soma-dendritic morphology resembling that of presumed local interneurons (type 3 LG cells), as defined in Golgi studies by Guillery (1966). Acetylcholine was found to hyperpolarize those presumed GABAergic local-circuit cells through an increase in membrane potassium conductance, an action mediated by the M_2 subclass of muscarinic receptors. The locally ramifying axon and the GABAergic nature of those presumed local inhibitory interneurons remain to be demonstrated. Considering this further accomplishment, the inhibitory action of ACh is difficult to understand in the light of iontophoretic studies demonstrating ACh-induced enhancement of stimulus-specific inhibitory responses of LG relay cells (Sillito et al., 1983; Eysel et al., 1986) and the fact that a long series of experimental data demonstrated the ACh-induced inhibition of the other class of thalamic inhibitory neurons, the RE cells (see Section 6.1.2.3). Thus, both types of progenitors of inhibitory processes in the thalamus seem to be inhibited by ACh in spite of the fact that the same transmitter enhances inhibitory processes in thalamocortical neurons. The possibility remains that there are more than one category of local-circuit cells (in fact, McCormick and Pape have chosen their elements by a priori criteria, namely, short spikes and absence of LTS). More probably, however, the ACh inhibition of somatic activity of local interneurons (what can easily be seen by an intracellular impalement) is not accompanied by an inhibition of intraglomerular dendrodendritic synapses between local-circuit and relay cells, the contacts that are presumably involved in shunting inhibitory processes related to discriminatory functions.

6.1.2.3. Reticular Thalamic Neurons

Extracellular recordings in acute experiments on anesthetized animals showed that ACh application depresses the spontaneous and evoked discharges of neurons recorded from the peri-VB, peripulvinar (PUL) or peri-LG (perigeniculate, PG) sectors of the RE nuclear complex (Ben-Ari et al., 1976; Dingledine and Kelly, 1977; Godfraind, 1978; Sillito et al., 1983; Eysel et al., 1986; Sillito, 1987). The ACh-evoked inhibition of RE neurons is blocked by atropine. As opposed to the ACh-induced excitation of thalamocortical neurons, the ACh inhibition of RE neurons is not abolished by systemic injections of barbiturates (Pape and Eysel, 1988). This is congruent with the barbiturate sensitivity of brainstem-induced excitation of LG cells, as opposed to the persistence under barbiturates of the brainstem-induced depolarizing–hyperpolarizing sequence in PG neurons (Hu et al., 1989a,b; see Chapter 8).

Application of ACh on RE neurons in vitro results in a hyperpolarization and increase in membrane conductance, an effect probably mediated by the M_2 subclass of muscarinic receptors (McCormick and Prince, 1986b). Varying extracellular potassium concentration changes the reversal potential of the ACh-induced hyperpolarization, thus indicating that it is the result of an increased potassium conductance. On the other hand, intracellular iontophoresis of chloride fails to alter the RE-cell response to ACh while dramatically altering the response of the same neurons to GABA (Fig. 11; McCormick and Prince, 1987c).

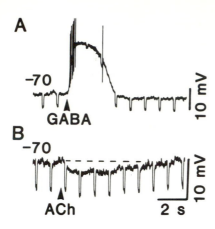

Figure 11. Intracellular injection of KCl dramatically alters the response of a guinea pig RE thalamic neuron to GABA but not to ACh. *In vitro* recordings. A: The fast excitatory depolarizing response of this neuron to GABA after intracellular iontophoresis of chloride. B: Application of ACh to the same neuron as in A results in the typical hyperpolarizing response to ACh, which was subsequently found to reverse at −90 mV. From McCormick and Prince (1987c).

6.1.3. Cerebral Cortex

6.1.3.1. Neocortex

It was initially reported that ACh exerts excitatory actions on neurons of the sensorimotor cortex, that the effects are most clearly seen in cells located relatively deep (below layers II–III), and that they are unambiguously muscarinic in nature (Krnjević and Phillis, 1963a,b; Crawford and Curtis, 1966). The deep cortical location of ACh-excited neurons was confirmed by antidromic identification of pyramidal tract and corticothalamic neurons in layers Vb and VI of rat somatosensory cortex (Lamour *et al.*, 1982, 1983). Whereas more than 50% of corticothalamic or pyramidal tract neurons are cholinoceptive, only 16% of callosally projecting cells are sensitive to ACh (Lamour *et al.*, 1982). The latter investigations on rat showed that the ACh effects on long-axoned cortical cells are most frequently mediated by muscarinic receptors; however, partial suppression of ACh effects by mecamylamine, a nicotinic antagonist, was also observed (see also McLennan and Hicks, 1978, for nicotinic excitation of cortical cells). More recent studies have identified ACh excitatory effects on neurons recorded from both superficial (layer II–III) and deep layers in the visual, cingulate, and somatosensory cortices (Sillito and Kemp, 1983; McCormick and Prince, 1986b; Donoghue and Carroll, 1987).

The ACh-induced muscarinic excitation of cortical neurons *in vivo* is slow in onset and may outlast the ACh application by tens of seconds. Data obtained by Krnjević and his colleagues (1971) indicated that the ACh-induced depolarization occurs through a reduction in potassium conductance and is associated with a rise in membrane resistance (Fig. 12). As in the case of thalamocortical neurons (see Section 6.1.2.1), the ACh excitatory effect is particularly susceptible to depression by barbiturates.

In vitro studies by McCormick and Prince (1985, 1986a; see also McCormick's reviews, 1989a,b) on cingulate, sensorimotor, and visual neurons of guinea pig revealed that before the muscarinic excitation of pyramidal-shaped neurons, those elements display a short-latency inhibition associated with a decrease in input resistance. The initial inhibition of pyramidal cells appears to be mediated by a rapid muscarinic excitation of local GABAergic interneurons,

since (1) it has a reversal potential similar to the hyperpolarizing response produced by GABA and (2) ACh application on elements identified by intracellular
staining as aspiny or sparsely spiny interneurons (cf. McCormick *et al.*, 1985)
results in a short-latency excitation associated with a large decrease in input
resistance, an excitatory response whose duration is similar to the ACh-induced
initial inhibition in pyramidal neurons (Fig. 13; McCormick and Prince, 1985).

The ACh excitation of formally identified cortical interneurons in McCormick and Prince's studies is partially congruent with extracellular data on visual
cortex neurons by Sillito and Kemp (1983). They showed that, in addition to its
facilitatory effect, ACh strikingly increases the stimulus specificity of the response without any loss in the selectivity and suggested that inhibitory inter-

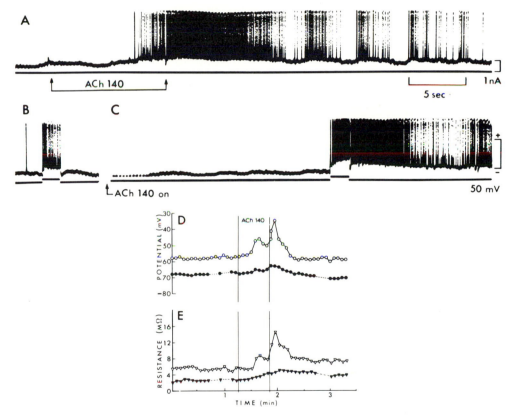

Figure 12. Facilitatory action of ACh in cat cerebral cortex. *In vivo* recordings. A: Intracellular
record from neuron in motor cortical area shows delayed depolarizing effect and prolonged firing
evoked by iontophoretic application of ACh (140 nA). B: Brief and instantly reversible depolarization and strong firing of the same neuron caused by short intracellular current injection (monitored
on lower trace). C: Same neuron depressed after treatment with dinitrophenol no longer fired in
response to application of ACh (as in A). However, during continued ACh application, identical
intracellular current injection (cf. B) now induced particularly powerful and prolonged discharges.
The ACh thus greatly facilitates and prolongs any depolarizing input received by the same cell. D
and E: Magnitude and time course of changes in potential and resistance induced by ACh. Open
circles, resting potential; note slow and prolonged depolarizing effect. Open triangles, resting resistance; note marked increase in resistance synchronous with depolarization. Closed symbols, corresponding data recorded during IPSPs; they show relatively little change except some possible reduction of inhibitory effect. Modified from Krnjevíc *et al.* (1971).

neurons outside layers III–IV are facilitated by ACh. Sillito and Kemp (1983) postulated that another class of cortical interneurons, located in layers III–IV, may be inhibited by ACh, with disinhibitory consequences on pyramidal cells.

The slow muscarinic excitation of pyramidal neurons is mainly mediated by a decrease in a voltage-dependent potassium current (M current; cf. Brown and Adams, 1980) and is associated with a rise in input resistance (McCormick and Prince, 1985, 1986a), in keeping with the earlier *in vivo* studies by Krnjević *et al.* (1971). The ACh-induced slow depolarization of cortical pyramidal neurons is very effectively blocked by pirenzepine, a muscarinic antagonist with a selectivity for M_1 receptors (cf. Bradshaw *et al.*, 1987).

It was hypothesized that cyclic guanosine 3',5'-monophosphate (cGMP) may play a second messenger role in the muscarinic actions of ACh on pyramidal tract and some unidentified neurons in rat and cat cerebral cortex (Stone *et al.*, 1975; Stone and Taylor, 1977; Woody *et al.*, 1978, 1986; but see Krnjević *et al.*, 1976, and Benardo and Prince, 1982b).

The ACh-induced dramatic facilitation and prolongation of any depolariz-

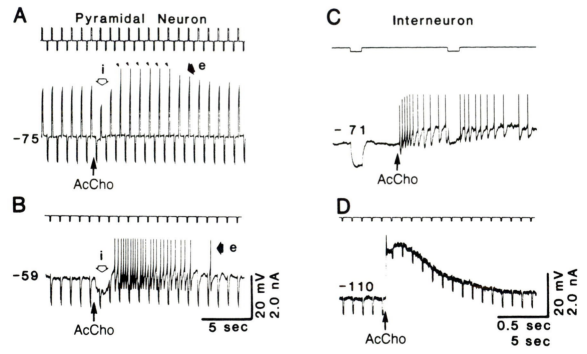

Figure 13. Effects of ACh on identified pyramidal cells and interneurons in guinea pig cerebral cortex. *In vitro* recordings. A: Application of ACh to a typical pyramidal cell at resting membrane potential (−75 mV) initially caused a decrease in the response to the current pulse (i) followed by a selective potentiation of the depolarizing responses without affecting resting membrane potential or the response to the hyperpolarizing pulses (e). The potentiated depolarizing pulses reached firing threshold and evoked action potentials (downward arrowheads). B: Application of ACh to the neuron from A after depolarization to near firing threshold (−59 mV) caused inhibition at a short latency (i) and was followed by a slow depolarization and action potential generation (e). C: Application of ACh to a typical interneuron at resting membrane potential (−71 mV) caused robust excitation at short latency. D: Application of ACh to the interneuron from C after hyperpolarization to −110 mV evoked a large depolarization with a short onset latency. The top trace in each set is the current monitor. The intracellular current pulses were 120 msec in duration and were applied at 1 Hz. Action potential amplitudes are truncated. Time calibration is 0.5 sec for C and 5 sec for other parts. From McCormick and Prince (1985).

ing input received by the same cortical cell (Krnjeviéc *et al.*, 1971; Woody *et al.*, 1978; see Fig. 12) underlies the potentiating effects produced by the modulatory agent ACh released by basal forebrain neurons on phasic specific inputs of thalamic origin received by cortical neurons. This ACh action may be one of the bases of long-term enhancement in cortical responsiveness, such as that involved in the acquisition of responses during some forms of learning and memory.

Studies on cat visual cortex neurons show that although ACh produces an increase of background firing in only 20% of tested cells, it alters the responses to visual stimuli in more than 90% of neurons (Sillito and Kemp, 1983). Acetylcholine permits long-term (from several minutes to over 1 hr) enhancement of somatosensory cortical responses to tactile stimulation of the receptive field or to glutamate application (Metherate *et al.*, 1987). The somatosensory cortical cholinoceptive cells are more likely than noncholinoceptive cells to be driven by ventroposterolateral (VPL) thalamic stimulation, and ACh selectively alters certain properties of the neuron rather than acting as a general excitant (Metherate *et al.*, 1988a). For example, whereas glutamate application results in an uniform decrease of the threshold for activation throughout the receptive field, the ACh effect is more selective and decreases the threshold of activation in only a limited part of the receptive field. Often, the ACh-induced alterations in cellular excitability last for prolonged periods of time. When somatic stimuli are used, about a third of the ACh-induced increases in excitability last more than 5 min (Metherate *et al.*, 1988b).

The enhancement in cortical cell excitability is state-dependent, as the ACh release from the cerebral cortex is dependent on activated behavioral states (cf. Celesia and Jasper, 1966; Collier and Mitchell, 1967). Indeed, the same cortical somatosensory neuron that is unresponsive to passive touch of the digits displays clear receptive fields on the digit when the monkey grasps food (Iwamura *et al.*, 1985). This state dependency of neuronal responsiveness may be related to similar motivational changes in basal forebrain neurons (Rolls *et al.*, 1986) that provide the bulk of cholinergic innervation of the cortex.

6.1.3.2. Hippocampus

In many respects, the ACh effects on hippocampal neurons are similar to those observed in neocortical cells. Most *in vitro* studies have investigated pyramidal cells in the CA1 field of guinea pig and rat (Dodd *et al.*, 1981; Benardo and Prince, 1982a,b; Halliwell and Adams, 1982; Cole and Nicoll, 1983). Acetylcholine depolarizes CA1 pyramidal neurons with an associated increase in input resistance, blocks a calcium-activated potassium conductance, and blocks accommodation of action potential discharges. These actions are mimicked by stimulation of sites in the slice known to contain cholinergic fibers and are reversed by the muscarinic antagonist atropine (Fig. 14; Cole and Nicoll, 1983). A voltage-clamp analysis showed that cholinergic agents (carbachol, muscarine, bethanecol) turn off the M conductance in CA1 pyramidal cells (Halliwell and Adams, 1982).* The overt effect of the ACh-induced reduction of M current is a tenden-

---

*The voltage-dependent potassium current termed M current undergoes a reciprocal regulation by ACh and the somatostatin-derived peptides. The former reduces this current (see above), but somatostatin augments it, as shown by voltage-clamp and current-clamp studies on CA1 pyramidal cells in the slice preparation of rat hippocampus (Moore *et al.*, 1988). A similarly increased M current by somatostatin was observed in the solitary tract complex (Siggins *et al.*, 1987).

cy to discharge repetitively in response to other depolarizing inputs without necessarily causing significant cell depolarization. Such effects have been indeed elicited *in vivo* by septal stimulation on CA1 and CA3 hippocampal neurons (Krnjević and Ropert, 1981).

In addition to direct excitatory effects on pyramidal hippocampal cells, ACh reduces the inhibitory input that normally prevents or limits pyramidal cell discharges (Ben-Ari *et al.*, 1981). Intracellular recordings from CA1 and CA3 neurons indicate that ACh reduces by about 60% the conductance increase associated with IPSPs evoked by entorhinal or fimbrial stimulation (Ben-Ari *et al.*, 1981). The ACh-elicited reduction in the size of IPSPs suggested either an ACh-induced inhibition of GABAergic interneurons or a depression of transmitter release from inhibitory terminals. These data from *in vivo* experiments are congruent with data obtained *in vitro* (Haas, 1982). However, an ACh-induced initial short-lasting hyperpolarization of pyramidal cells with a conductance increase has also been observed (Benardo and Prince, 1981, 1982a,b), thus suggesting that direct ACh excitation of some inhibitory interneurons may also be occurring.

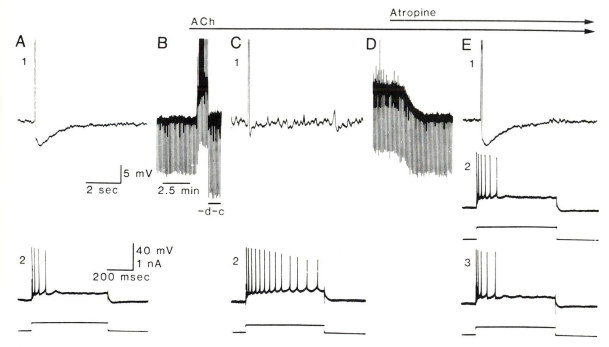

Figure 14. Effects of ACh on rat CA1 pyramidal neurons in hippocampal slice preparation. All responses from the same neuron. A: Chart record of control afterhyperpolarizing potential (AHP) after a 60-msec direct depolarizing current pulse (trace 1) and film record of response to a 600-msec pulse (trace 2). The current record is positioned below the voltage record. B: ACh (200 μM) superfusion depolarized the membrane and increased the cell's input resistance. C: Blockade of the AHP (trace 1) and accommodation (trace 2) in the presence of ACh. D: The addition of atropine (0.5 μM) in the presence of ACh reversed the effects of ACh. E: Atropine also reversed the effects of ACh on the AHP (trace 1) and on accommodation (traces 2 and 3). The current pulse in trace 3 was identical to those in trace 2 in A and C. In trace 2 the current pulse was increased to match the depolarization evoked in the presence of ACh (trace 2 in C). The gain in trace 1 in A applies to trace 1 in C and E, and the time calibration in D is the same as that in B. The calibration for trace 2 in A applies to all the film records. Resting membrane potential, −57 mV. From Cole and Nicoll (1983).

6.1.4. Spinal Cord

185

NEUROTRANS-
MITTER-
MODULATED
IONIC CURRENTS

Spinal cord motoneurons exhibit a slow depolarizing response to ACh, probably because of a reduction in potassium conductance; the slow depolarization is associated with an increase or no change in input resistance and is mediated by muscarinic receptors (Zieglgänsberger and Reiter, 1974). The motoneuronal synapse on an inhibitory Renshaw cell involves a rapid and quickly reversible nicotinic excitation (Curtis and Eccles, 1958; Curtis and Ryall, 1966a), but Renshaw cells also possess muscarinic receptors acting slowly (Curtis and Ryall, 1966b).

6.2. Norepinephrine

Norepinephrine (NE) is recognized as one of the most important neurotransmitters/neuromodulators arising from the brainstem, and the anatomic distribution of afferents and efferents of NE-containing neurons has been described in Chapter 4. Norepinephrine is of great importance to behavior, as an important role for NE has been postulated in almost every behavioral system, including sleep–waking, feeding, thermoregulation, sensory processing, motor activity, and growth and development (see review in Foote *et al.*, 1983).

The early literature on *in vivo* microiontophoresis and systemic injections of NE agonists and antagonists is truly vast. Unfortunately, the absence of control over concentrations, the lack of synaptic isolation, and the inability to manipulate the recorded neuron by injections of current and by voltage clamping render data from this literature less than definitive with respect to receptor type and action. We thus rely on *in vitro* data when available and cite *in vivo* work only where other data are not available or are incomplete. We note also that we do not attempt to cover in any systematic way the large recent literature on second messenger mediation of NE effects.

Electrophysiological responses to NE have been observed following activation of receptors classified as β, α_1, α_2, and also unclassified α receptors in central nervous system (CNS) vertebrate neurons. (We here describe an α receptor as unclassified with respect to subtype when the agonist/antagonist response pattern does not follow that of peripheral receptors; it is an obvious but important point that CNS receptors may not exactly parallel peripheral receptors in structure and sensitivity, and thus the peripheral classification may incompletely describe CNS receptors.) Norepinephrine responses in various CNS neurons have been reported to be mediated by alterations in at least five different types of calcium and potassium conductances (see summary in Table 1). We begin our review with a brief summary of data from hippocampus.

6.2.1. Hippocampus

Norepinephrine effects have been extensively studied in hippocampus, but, since these data have been reviewed extensively elsewhere, we here sketch only a broad outline of effects to serve for comparison with the more detailed exposition of brainstem effects. Hippocampal CA1 neurons respond to NE with a reduction in the calcium-dependent long-duration afterhyperpolarization (AHP) and asso-

Table 1. Adrenergic Receptor Type[a]

	β	α (unclassified)	α₁	α₂
Location	CA1 (β₁), granule cell, in hippocampus; Sensorimotor neocortex (β₁)	Locus coeruleus, PNS, cerebellum	1. Dorsal raphe 2. LC, mPRF neurons, dorsal mtr. vagus, supraoptic nuc.	CA1 (presumptive), locus coeruleus, mPRF neurons, dorsal mtr. vagus, Sub. gelatinosa, sympathetic pregang. neurons
Effects on:				
Membrane potential	↓ AHP (slow), ↓ accommodation	↓ Ca²⁺-dependent action pots. (LC)	1. ↓ Early transient outward rect. 2. Depolarize, ↑ resistance	Hyperpolarization, ↓ resistance
Current	↓ Ca²⁺-dependent K⁺ current	↓ Low- and high-threshold Ca²⁺ current	1. ↓ I_A 2. ↓ K⁺ current	↑ Anomalous rectification (K⁺ current)
Typical agents				
Agonist	Isoproterenol		Phenylephrine	Clonidine
Antagonist	Propranolol		Prazosin	Yohimbine

[a]PNS, peripheral nervous system; mPRF, medial pontine reticular formation; AHP, afterhyperpolarization; rect., rectification. References for antagonists are: yohimbine (Williams *et al.*, 1985; Crepel *et al.*, 1987), prazosin (Aghajanian, 1985; Crepel *et al.*, 1987), propranolol (Madison and Nicoll, 1986a,b). Other references in text, except: sensorimotor cortex (Foehring *et al.*, 1989, who also report a β₁ reduction in a Na⁺-dependent K⁺ current); dorsal motor vagus (Fukuda *et al.*, 1987); supraoptic nuc. (Yamashita *et al.*, 1987); and sympathetic preganglionic neurons (Yoshimura *et al.*, 1987). Note the presence of two types of α₁ effects; the α₁ excitatory effects are developmentally transient in the LC.

ciated accommodation (Madison and Nicoll, 1986a,b), an effect mediated by β₁ receptor activation. This results in an increase in cAMP, which in turn reduces the calcium-dependent potassium current responsible for accommodation and the long-duration AHP. No effect was observed on calcium current in these neurons. Activation of the β receptor also elicits a membrane depolarization in 80% of the neurons, probably as a result of reduction of calcium-dependent potassium current (see Haas and Greene, 1986). In 70% of CA1 neurons, an α-mediated membrane hyperpolarization (possibly α₂) accompanied by a decrease in input resistance was also reported. Recently, activation of an α receptor presynaptic to the CA1 neurons has been reported to reduce IPSP amplitude while increasing the frequency of spontaneous IPSPs (Madison and Nicoll, 1988). In granule cells of the hippocampus, β-receptor activation elicits an increase in calcium current (Gray and Johnston, 1987). As with β effects in CA1 neurons, this may have been mediated by cAMP. Also similar to effects on CA1 neurons, NE was observed to antagonize the long-duration AHP and associated accommodation in granule cells (Malenka *et al.*, 1986; Haas and Rose, 1987).

6.2.2. Locus Coeruleus

One major effect of NE on locus coeruleus (LC) neurons is an α₂-mediated membrane hyperpolarization accompanied by a decrease in membrane resistance similar to the α response observed in the hippocampus. All LC neurons tested by Egan *et al.* (1983) showed a hyperpolarization to puffer electrode or bath application of NE; no depolarizations were observed. The hyperpolarization was attributed to an increase in potassium conductance and is discussed below in detail.

Of great interest in terms of synaptic effects between LC neurons was the response to focal electrical stimulation of the slice in the region of the LC (Egan *et al.*, 1983). As shown in Fig. 15, there was an initial short-duration depolarization followed by a long-lasting hyperpolarization. It was inferred that the de- and hyperpolarization were synaptically mediated since they were reversibly blocked in zero-calcium/high-magnesium superfusates. Both the stimulation- and NE-induced hyperpolarizations showed the same characteristics, namely, a reversal potential of about 110 mV (Fig. 15A), antagonism by bath application of the same concentrations of the α_2 antagonists yohimbine (Fig. 15B) and phentolamine, and potentiation by the NE reuptake blocker desmethylimipramine (DMI). Egan *et al.* (1983) concluded that their data supported the hypothesis that LC neurons can release NE onto the somadendritic membrane of other LC neurons and thereby provide local feedback inhibition. These *in vitro* data support the earlier conclusions of Aghajanian and co-workers (1977) from *in vivo* data on the presence of α_2-mediated LC–LC feedback inhibition.

Subsequent work by Williams *et al.* (1985) has more precisely characterized the receptor type and NE effects. Norepinephrine was found to produce only hyperpolarizations (no depolarizations) in all LC neurons examined. That the mediating receptor was α_2 was supported by reproduction of the effect by the α_2 agonist clonidine but not by the α_1 agonist phenylephrine or β agonist isoproterenol, which at 10 μM had no effects, although higher concentrations (30–100 μM) produced a slight hyperpolarization. The concentration–response curves for clonidine and NE were shifted rightward in a parallel manner by the α_2 antagonists RX 781094, yohimbine, phentolamine, and piperoxan. Figure 16 illustrates the concentration-dependent hyperpolarization of NE and the competitive antagonism of phentolamine.

Recent voltage-clamp recordings by Williams *et al.* (1988a) have clarified the nature of potassium conductances in LC neurons. At membrane potentials more negative than about −60 mV, the steady-state slope conductance increased with successive hyperpolarizations; i.e., inward rectification was present, confirming inferences made by Osmanovic and Shefner (1987). The I/V relationship of the LC neurons in this voltage range was modeled with excellent fit as the result of a voltage-independent potassium conductance and a voltage-sensitive conductance in series. Experimentally the voltage-sensitive conductance had the characteristics of the "classical" inward rectifier (Katz, 1949; Hagiwara and Takahashi, 1974) in terms of rapid kinetics of activation (within 5 msec) and blockage by rubidium, barium (time dependent), and cesium (voltage dependent). This inward rectifier conductance, G_{ir}, was well described by a sigmoid curve with half-maximal conductance centered at about E_K and, as is true for G_{ir} in a number of tissues (Noble, 1985), had a slope dependent on external potassium concentration. Thus, increasing external potassium concentrations shifted the curve to less negative potentials and steepened its slope.

A

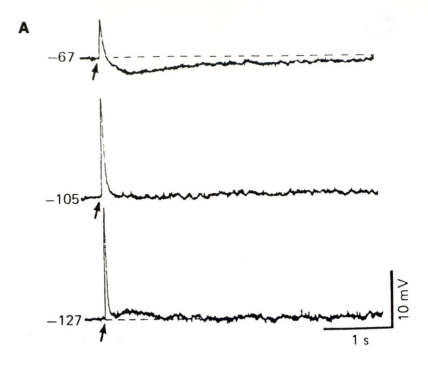

−67

−105

−127

10 mV

1 s

B

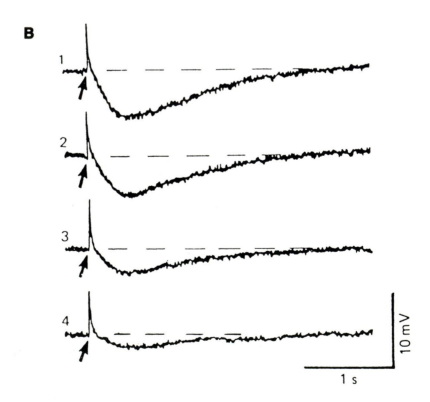

1

2

3

4

10 mV

1 s

6.2.2.1. Potassium Current Changes Evoked by α_2 Adrenoceptor and μ-Opioid Agonists

Both of these classes of agonists increased potassium conductance in LC neurons, and occlusion experiments suggested they acted on the same potassium conductance (North and Williams, 1985; North *et al.*, 1987). Furthermore, the μ and the α_2 agonist-induced shifts in the *I/V* curve were identical (Williams *et al.*, 1988a). Both α_2 and μ agonists produced a voltage-sensitive, inwardly rectifying potassium conductance; the steady-state *I/V* values for an agonist (μ and α_2 agonists gave similar results) are compared with control values in Fig. 17A. The agonist potassium conductance could not be accounted for by a simple increase in the voltage-sensitive potassium conductance, G_{ir}, or its maximum value. Rather, an additional agonist-induced potassium conductance, G_{ag}, with a different voltage sensitivity was present.

Although G_{ag} could be mathematically described by a sigmoid function of the same form as G_{ir}, G_{ag} differed in having a half-maximal value that was approximately -50 mV versus the more negative value (E_K) for G_{ir}; furthermore altering external potassium concentration did not appreciably shift the half-maximal value for G_{ag}, although the slope increased with increasing external potassium concentration. In summary, the μ and α_2 agonist-induced conductance shows inward rectification centered around the resting potential instead of being centered around E_K, as is true for the classical "inward rectifier."

The G_{ag} was similar to the G_{ir} in terms of activation kinetics and sensitivities to blocking agents, leading Williams *et al.* (1988a) to speculate that the same channels were involved but that when they bind G-protein, thought to be activated by μ and α_2 agonists (North *et al.*, 1987), the half-maximal activation point was shifted from close to E_K to close to the resting potential (-55 mV). The functional implication of the agonist conductance curve is that the conductance increase by the agonists is high at the resting potential, and its voltage sensitivity means it continues to increase with further hyperpolarization, and this effect is further amplified by the presence of the G_{ir}. Figure 17B graphs the difference in conductance changes brought about by the agonist and inward rectifier voltage sensitivity compared with a purely linear membrane response, and Fig. 17C shows the membrane equivalent circuit for these potassium currents. Other α-mediated hyperpolarizations have been reported in the spinal cord (North and Yoshimura, 1984; Wohlberg *et al.*, 1986) and the cerebellum (Bloom, 1978).

Figure 15. Reversal potential and yohimbine antagonism of IPSPs in locus coeruleus (LC) neurons elicited by focal electrical stimulation within the LC zone in the rat LC slice preparation. A: Top trace is control condition, showing the stimulation-induced short-duration EPSP and long-duration IPSP. At -105 mV membrane potential, the IPSP is nulled and is reversed at -127 mV. The reduction in duration of both the EPSP and IPSP at -105 and -127 mV is likely caused by membrane rectification at these hyperpolarized potentials. B: Top trace is control condition; subsequent traces show progressive reduction of the IPSP but not EPSP by progressively greater superfusate concentrations of the α_2 antagonist yohimbine at (2) 10 nM, (3) 30 nM, and (4) 100 nM. Text Section 6.4.3 cites evidence that the short-latency EPSP is mediated by an excitatory amino acid neurotransmitter. Modified from Egan *et al.* (1983).

6.2.2.2. Other NE Effects

The second class of locus coeruleus response to NE was an inhibition of the calcium action potential (Williams and North, 1985) mediated by an α receptor of unknown subtype. Neither the α_1 antagonist prazosin nor the α_2 antagonist yohimbine was effective in antagonizing this response. Although an increase in potassium conductance could not be ruled out as the mechanism for inhibition of the calcium action potential, a direct effect on calcium currents was thought to be more probable.

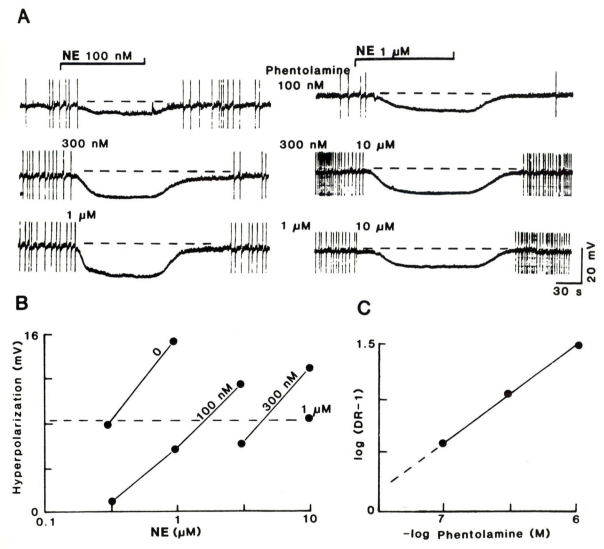

Figure 16. Competitive antagonism of NE by phentolamine on a single *in vitro* LC neuron. A: Left panel shows the concentration-dependent hyperpolarization produced by superfusion of NE (1 μM desmethylimipramine added to block NE uptake), and the right panel shows the antagonistic effect of addition of the indicated concentrations of phentolamine. B: Concentration–response curves for NE in the presence of 0, 100 nM, and 300 nM concentrations of phentolamine. The broken line indicates the effect level selected for the Schild plot, shown in C. The slope is not significantly different from 1.0, and the intercept gives a phentolamine K_e of 19 nM. Modified from Williams *et al.* (1985).

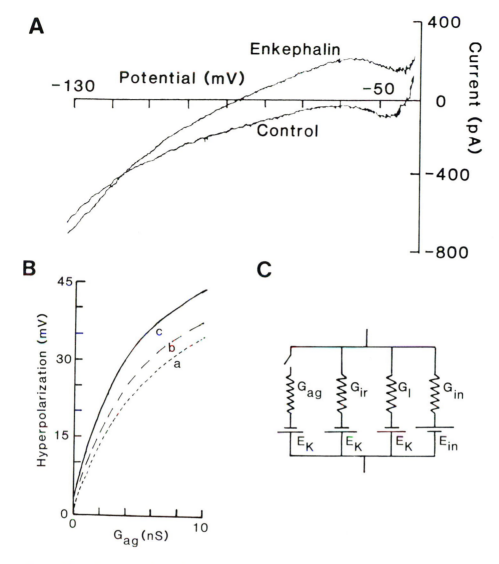

Figure 17. A: Control and agonist steady-state I/V plots for an LC neuron recorded *in vitro*. The agonist generating this plot was [Met]enkephalin (10 μM) in superfusate, but the shape is also characteristic of the I/V plots generated by α_2 agonists (Williams *et al.*, 1988a). Note the voltage sensitivity (inward rectification) for both the control and agonist plots at values more negative than -60 mV. B: Amplification of hyperpolarizing agonist responses by voltage-sensitive LC membrane conductances. The ordinate shows the hyperpolarization caused by a given increase in potassium conductance produced by an agonist (abscissa) under three models. Curve a assumes a linear membrane response: G_{total} = voltage-independent conductance (leak, G_l) + $G_{ag,constant}$. Curve b assumes an inward rectifier membrane, whose voltage sensitivity is indicated by $G_{ir}(V)$: $G_{total} = G_l + G_{ir}(V) + G_{ag,constant}$. Curve c assumes both an inward rectifier membrane and a rectifying agonist conductance, $G_{ag}(V)$: $G_{total} = G_l + G_{ir}(V) + G_{ag}(V)$. Note that for a 1-nS agonist conductance increase, the linear, voltage-insensitive model (curve a) predicts only a 5-mV hyperpolarization while the correct voltage-sensitive model (curve c) indicates a 12-mV hyperpolarization will occur. For these computations, resting conductance at -60 mV is 4.2 nS, and $G_{ir}(V) = $ maximum $G_{ir}/\{1 + \exp[(V_{membrane} - E_K/k]\}$, where $E_K = -116$ mV, k = 15 mV. $G_{ag}(V) = $ maximum $G_{ag}/\{1+\exp[V_{membrane} - V^*)/k]\}$, where $V^* = $ half-max $G_{ag} = -50$ mV. C: Equivalent circuit for modeling potassium conductances in B for LC neuron. G_{ag}, G_{ir}, G_l as in B. G_{in} = nonspecific conductance for all other ions; it and E_{in} were calculated so that there was zero membrane current at -60 mV. Modified from Williams *et al.* (1988a).

In the vertebrate peripheral nervous system, high-threshold calcium currents responsible for high-threshold calcium action potentials have been shown to be antagonized by NE (Dunlap and Fischbach, 1981; Galvan and Adams, 1982; Forscher and Oxford, 1985; Marchetti *et al.*, 1986). A low-threshold calcium current was reported to be antagonized by α-receptor activation in Purkinje neurons of the cerebellum (Crepel *et al.*, 1987). This antagonism was blocked by the α_1-receptor antagonist prazosin but not by the α_2-receptor antagonist yohimbine. A similar NE effect has also been observed in cultured chick dorsal root ganglia neurons and sympathetic neurons recorded with patch-clamp techniques (Marchetti *et al.*, 1986).

α-Receptor activation in Purkinje neurons also resulted in a hyperpolarization, an effect similar to that observed in LC neurons. In marked contrast to the LC, however, the Purkinje neuron hyperpolarization elicited by NE was accompanied by an increase in resistance that was antagonized by the α_1-receptor antagonist prazosin. The mechanism of action for this hyperpolarization and conductance decrease remains to be examined, especially with respect to its sensitivity to calcium channel blockers and alterations in external potassium ion concentrations. Furthermore, the receptor type mediating both this response and the reduction of low-threshold calcium current is not clear, since the α_2 agonist clonidine elicited them and the α_1 antagonist blocked them.

6.2.2.3. Developmentally Transient α_1 Response

In the young rat (8–26 days) slice preparation, Williams and Marshall (1987) observed a depolarizing response to phenylephrine that was antagonized by prazosin, consistent with an α_1 mediation. This response was not present in slices from older animals, where phenylephrine either had no effect or hyperpolarized neurons. This developmentally transient response was consistent with that observed earlier in LC neurons in culture (Finlayson and Marshall, 1986).

This electrophysiological demonstration of a transient α_1 response is paralleled by an *in vitro* autoradiography developmental study in rats utilizing [125I]HEAT [2-β-(4-hydroxyphenylethylaminomethyl)tetralone] as the α_1 ligand. In globus pallidus, HEAT binding sites increased in the first 2 weeks of neonatal life before decreasing to near adult levels at day 35 (Jones *et al.*, 1985b). Unfortunately, this paper did not provide data on changes in brainstem α_1 receptors. The same ligand in adult rats showed a moderate labeling of mesencephalic reticular formation, with increased density in central gray, dorsal and median raphe nuclei, and lateral reticular nucleus (Jones *et al.*, 1985a), but medial pontine and bulbar reticular formation did not label strongly. The HEAT ligand showed a dense labeling of the LC, but it should be cautioned that Young and Kuhar (1980) found little LC binding of another α_1 antagonist, [3H]WB 4101 but did find binding of the α_2 receptor ligand *p*-[3H]aminoclonidine, and the physiological studies cited above suggest α_2 receptors. Young and Kuhar (1980) did not indicate a high density of either α_1 or α_2 receptors in medial reticular formation, but they, as is true of most binding studies, did not take into account the lower "packing density" of mPRF neurons because of the presence of extensive fiber tracks in the reticular formation.

6.2.3. Dorsal Raphe

α_1-Receptor activation in dorsal raphe (DR) neurons was observed to antagonize A current (Aghajanian, 1985; see Chapter 5). Phenylephrine had no direct effect on the low-threshold calcium current (Burlhis and Aghajanian, 1987).

6.2.4. Pontine Reticular Formation

Norepinephrine effects on the medial pontine reticular formation (mPRF) neurons were studied in *in vivo* microiontophoretic experiments by Greene and Carpenter (1985); both reticulospinal and unidentified mPRF neurons were inhibited by NE, although the *in vivo* nature of the experiment precluded analysis of effects on membrane potential, resistance, or specific ionic conductances. Initial data utilizing the pontine reticular formation slice preparation by Greene *et al.* (1989b; see also Chapter 5) have shown that some mPRF neurons respond to bath-applied NE (1–10 μM) in the presence of TTX with a hyperpolarization that reversed with washout of NE, consonant with the *in vivo* work. This response was mimicked by clonidine and accompanied by a decrease in input resistance (Fig. 18B), and may be mediated by an increase in potassium conductance. These effects of NE are consistent with an α_2 inhibitory response.

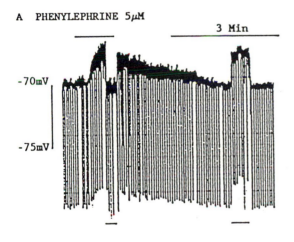

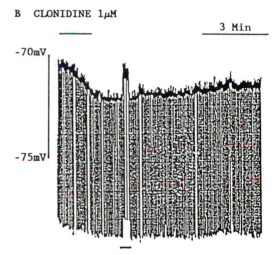

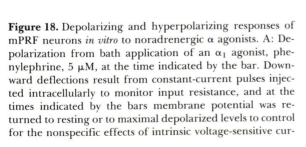

Figure 18. Depolarizing and hyperpolarizing responses of mPRF neurons *in vitro* to noradrenergic α agonists. A: Depolarization from bath application of an α_1 agonist, phenylephrine, 5 μM, at the time indicated by the bar. Downward deflections result from constant-current pulses injected intracellularly to monitor input resistance, and at the times indicated by the bars membrane potential was returned to resting or to maximal depolarized levels to control for the nonspecific effects of intrinsic voltage-sensitive currents on input resistance. Note that phenylephrine produces an increase in input resistance. Note also the increase in PSPs (thickened baseline); KMeSO$_4$ recording electrodes indicated that these were hyperpolarizing. B: Hyperpolarizing response to bath application of the α_2 agonist clonidine, 1 μM. Chart record and downward deflections as in part A; note that clonidine produces a decrease in input resistance. Modified from Greene *et al.* (1989b).

The majority (11/14, 79%) of mPRF neurons in the slice preparation, however, responded to bath-applied NE (1–10 μM) with a depolarization and an increase in input resistance. This was a direct and not a synaptically mediated response since it was seen in the presence of TTX; preliminary data suggest it is mediated by a decrease in potassium conductance. This response was mimicked by phenylephrine (Fig. 18A) and was thus consistent with an α_1 response. An interesting synaptically mediated effect of α_1 agonists on mPRF neurons was to increase the frequency of inhibitory (hyperpolarizing) PSPs, as can be seen in the thickened baseline in Fig. 18.

The presence of α_1 depolarizing effects in a majority of mPRF neurons was somewhat unexpected in view of the *in vivo* results of Greene and Carpenter (1985) showing that NE uniformly produced suppression of firing. It is possible that the *in vivo* firing suppression might have resulted from shunting of excitatory input by the NE-induced inhibitory PSPs or that presynaptic inhibitory effects were prominent. It is also possible that the α_1 depolarizing response found in slices from young rats might be developmentally transient, as was reported for α_1 depolarizing response in LC neurons (see Section 6.2.2). Another possible reason for differences between the cat *in vivo* and rat *in vitro* work is species differences. With respect to the model of REM sleep cycle control presented in Chapter 12 positing an adrenergic suppression of REM sleep, the current *in vitro* data suggest that the primary site of action of inhibitory effects of NE on REM-on neurons should be hypothesized to be on LDT/PPT cholinergic neurons rather than on reticular REM-on neurons, as proposed in the initial version of this model (McCarley and Hobson, 1975b). Further discussion of this issue is in Chapters 11 and 12.

6.2.5. Thalamus

Norepinephrine actions studied *in vivo* were generally described as excitatory in the rat LG and perigeniculate (PG) nuclei (Rogawski and Aghajanian, 1980a,b; Kayama *et al.*, 1982) but mainly depressive on spontaneous and evoked activities of cat LG neurons (Phillis and Tebecis, 1967; Pape and Eysel, 1987). *In vitro* studies of LG neurons of guinea pig and cat showed that NE slowly depolarizes the cell and induces an increase in membrane resistance. The slow depolarization is caused by blockage of a resting potassium conductance (McCormick and Prince, 1988). Thus, NE acts similarly to ACh in blocking the burst firing mode and transforming it into single-spike discharges. Of course, this NE action (namely, that NE activates thalamic neurons synergically with ACh) is only possible during waking, when LC neurons are tonically active. The only sources for thalamic and cortical activation during the other EEG-desynchronized state, REM sleep, are brainstem and basal forebrain cholinergic neurons, which are active during both wakefulness and REM sleep (see Chapter 11).

We do not review here the NE actions on neocortical neurons because systematic intracellular investigations are still lacking. The diversity of results obtained in extracellular recordings *in vivo* (depressive as well as excitatory effects, varying with different anesthetics and cellular types) are discussed in Chapter 8, along with the effects of stimulating the LC nucleus.

6.3. Serotonin

It is now clear from intracellular recordings of *in vitro* preparations of both invertebrate and vertebrate central nervous systems that serotonin (5-HT) elicits a wide variety of changes in ionic conductances.

At least seven different responses to 5-HT have been described in neurons from the molluscan CNS. The first six involve increases in conductance to sodium (fast and slow), potassium, and chloride and decreases in conductance to potassium and in a nonselective cation conductance of sodium and potassium (Gerschenfeld and Paupardin-Tritsch, 1974). The 5-HT-elicited reduction of potassium conductance has been further characterized as a reduction in an outwardly rectifying steady-state current with no threshold for activation (thus distinguishing it from M current). It has been named "S current" and is suggested to mediate the facilitation responsible for sensitization of the tail and siphon–gill withdrawal reflexes (Siegelbaum *et al.*, 1982; Pollock *et al.*, 1985). The increase in potassium conductance by 5-HT results from an increase in the anomalous rectifier potassium current, probably related to an increased number of functional channels (Gunning, 1987). A seventh response was described as an increase in voltage-sensitive calcium conductance (Pellmar and Carpenter, 1980; Paupardin-Tritsch *et al.*, 1986).

In the peripheral nervous system of vertebrates at least four types of 5-HT receptors have been classified (for review, see Richardson and Engel, 1986): 5-HT_{1A}, 5-HT_{1B} (both evoke inhibition), 5-HT_2 (excitatory), and 5-HT_3 (excitatory). There are selective antagonists: spiperone (for 5-HT_{1A}), ketanserin (for 5-HT_2), and ICS205-930 (for 5-HT_3). Agonists are 5-carboxyamidotryptamine (5-CT) for 5-HT_{1A} and 5-HT_{1B}, (+)-s-α-methyl-5-HT for 5-HT_2, and 2-methyl-5-HT for 5-HT_3 receptors. Radioligand binding studies (Peroutka *et al.*, 1981; Pedigo *et al.*, 1981), behavioral models of 5-HT agonist-mediated motor disturbances (Peroutka *et al.*, 1981; Lucki *et al.*, 1984; Goodwin and Green, 1985), microiontophoretic electrophysiological studies (Aghajanian, 1981), and cellular studies of cultured neurons (Yakel *et al.*, 1988) suggest the presence of at least four 5-HT receptors in mammalian CNS. However, classification based on the interaction of the abovementioned agents with electrophysiologically identified serotonergic receptors in *in vitro* preparations is not yet extensive, although current work in these areas is both promising and growing.

6.3.1. Hippocampus

Recordings from hippocampal neurons *in vitro* have revealed that a hyperpolarization mediated by an increase in potassium conductance is evoked by 5-HT. It was not dependent on calcium, but the voltage sensitivity has not been examined (Segal, 1980; Andrade *et al.*, 1986). The inhibitory actions of 5-HT in the hippocampus appear to be mediated by a 5-HT_{1A} receptor, as identified by the use of the agonists 5-carboxyamidotryptamine (5-CT) and 8-hydroxy-2-(di-*n*-propylamine)tetralin (8-OH-DPAT) and the antagonistic actions of spiperone (Beck *et al.*, 1985; Andrade *et al.*, 1986).

6.3.2. Dorsal Raphe Neurons

Application of 5-HT to dorsal raphe neurons *in vitro* produced a hyperpolarization by altering a potassium conductance (Yoshimura and Higashi, 1985); this response was reversibly antagonized by LSD and methysergide and was enhanced by the 5-HT uptake inhibitor imipramine.

Intrinsic and ligand-induced potassium conductances in presumptively serotonergic dorsal raphe (DR) neurons *in vitro* have recently been investigated in some detail by Williams *et al.* (1988b), who described two intrinsic and one 5-HT-induced inwardly rectifying conductances. One intrinsic conductance exhibited the characteristics of the classic inward rectifier and thus was similar to the G_{ir} described for LC neurons (see Section 6.2) in that there was a rapid activation (5 msec), blockage by barium, and with a voltage sensitivity centered about E_K. The second intrinsic inwardly rectifying potassium conductance was seen at potentials negative to -70 mV, where there was a slowly activating (0.3–1 sec), noninactivating, and barium-insensitive but cesium-sensitive inward current. This current thus resembled the Q current described previously (Halliwell and Adams, 1982). The Q-like current had only a minor role in total membrane conductance under conditions of normal potassium concentrations, but the G_{ir} had a relatively prominent role in many neurons. For the DR population as a whole, the slope conductance increase for G_{ir} was about one-half that seen in LC neurons.

The 5-HT$_1$ agonist 5-carboxyamidotryptamine (5-CT) produced a hyper-

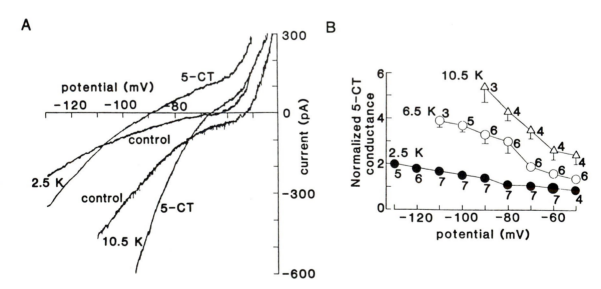

Figure 19. The 5-HT$_1$ receptor-induced increase in potassium conductance in dorsal raphe neurons *in vitro* rectifies inwardly. A: Steady-state current-voltage plots in the presence and absence of the 5-HT$_1$ agonist 5-carboxyamidotryptamine (5-CT) in two concentrations of potassium. Note the reversal potential shifts to a less negative potential in high potassium. B: The 5-CT conductance increases as the membrane potential is made more negative, and the slope increases in high potassium concentrations. (Normalized conductance is expressed in terms of the conductance obtained at -60 mV in 2.5 mM potassium for each of the DR neurons sampled; each point is an averaged value for the given N. Modified from Williams *et al.* (1988b).

polarization by means of an increased potassium conductance that was inwardly rectifying (Fig. 19). The 5-CT-induced hyperpolarization was dose dependent and was blocked by prior treatment with pertussis toxin, suggesting a G-protein link between the 5-HT_1 receptor and the potassium channel. It is of interest that the $GABA_B$ agonist baclofen had parallel effects, both producing the inwardly rectifying potassium conductance and being blocked by pertussis toxin. Further, occlusion experiments suggested that the same channel was affected by both 5-CT and baclofen.

Focal electrical stimulation of the DR produced hyperpolarizing potentials in DR neurons; these were 5–20 mV in amplitude, 1–2 sec in duration, reversed at the potassium equilibrium potential, and were reversibly antagonized by LSD and methysergide and enhanced by the 5-HT uptake inhibitor imipramine, thus suggesting they were caused by synaptic release of 5-HT, presumably from recurrent collaterals of DR neurons (Yoshimura and Higashi, 1985). Williams *et al.* (1988b) further showed that the electrically induced hyperpolarizations were similar to those caused by the 5-HT_1 agonist 5-CT, since they were mediated by an inwardly rectifying potassium conductance with comparable characteristics (see Fig. 20). It might be noted that these data provide strong support for the hypothesis of 5-HT-mediated DR-to-DR feedback inhibition, much as was noted for the LC–LC α_2-mediated feedback inhibition in Section 6.2.2. This postulate is important for the model of sleep cycle control presented in Chapters 11 and 12.

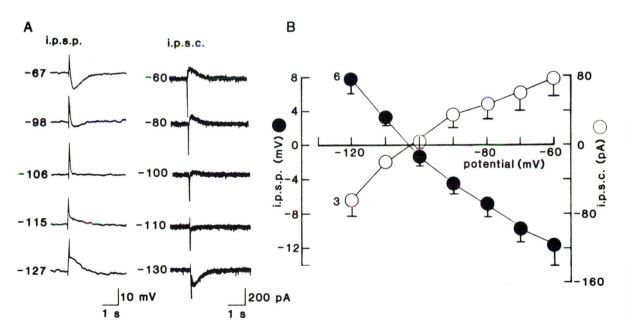

Figure 20. Focal electrical stimulation of the dorsal raphe *in vitro* elicits inhibitory synaptic potentials in DR neurons that is caused by an inwardly rectifying potassium conductance. A: Voltage (left) and current (right) recordings from a single DR neuron held at various membrane potentials. At potentials near resting, the focal stimulation induces a hyper- polarizing response (i.p.s.p.) with outward current (i.p.s.c.). B: The amplitude of the PSP and of the current is a non-linear function of membrane potential, with a marked increase in inward current at negative potentials (inward rectification) comparable to that induced by the 5-HT_1 agonist 5-HC. Modified from Williams *et al.* (1988b).

6.3.3. Pontine Reticular Formation and Facial Motoneurons

Initial data on 5-HT applied to neurons in the pontine reticular formation slice preparation (Stevens *et al.*, 1989) suggest two major serotonin effects. As shown in Fig. 21A, one population of neurons responded with a membrane hyperpolarization and decreased input resistance. This hyperpolarization is mediated by an increase in a voltage-insensitive potassium conductance. This is compatible with a 5-HT_1 response and indeed this hyperpolarizing response is mimicked by the 5-HT_1 agonist 5-CT (D.R. Stevens *et al.*, unpublished data). Still another group of neurons shows a depolarization and increased input resistance, compatible with a non-5-HT_1 response (Fig. 21B). Recent data indicate this response is mediated by a decrease in a voltage-insensitive potassium conductance and is mimicked by the 5-HT_2 agonist α-methyl-5-HT (Stevens *et al.*, unpublished data). Excitatory responses to 5-HT associated with a small decrease in membrane potential and increase in input resistance (probably mediated by a decrease in potassium conductance) have been observed in facial motoneurons recorded *in vivo* (VanderMaelen and Aghajanian, 1980).

6.3.4. Thalamus and Neocortex

Compared to the consistent results from *in vivo* and *in vitro* intracellular studies with ACh application (see Sections 6.1.2 and 6.1.3), extracellular data using 5-HT application report depressive effects on thalamic neurons (Kemp *et al.*, 1982; Pape and Eysel, 1987) and both depressant and excitatory actions on neocortical cells (Reader, 1978; Olpe, 1981), but the receptors and underlying cellular mechanisms of these effects remain to be elucidated.

It is apparent that a rigorous analysis in the mammalian CNS of the electrophysiology and pharmacology of 5-HT effects made technically feasible by *in vitro* preparations is promising but has just begun. The recent availability of more selective agonists and antagonists coupled with the ability to assess 5-HT effects at the cellular level promises greatly to enhance the characterization of mammalian CNS receptors in the next few years.

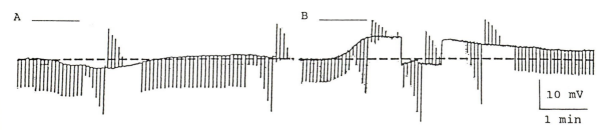

Figure 21. Hyperpolarizing response (A) and depolarizing response (B) of two mPRF neurons recorded *in vitro* to the bath application of 5-HT (10 µM in the presence of 0.5 µM TTX) superfused during the period indicated by the horizontal bar above the trace. Deflections are from constant-current pulses used to measure input resistance. Note the hyperpolarizing response is associated with a decrease in input resistance and the depolarizing response with an increase in input resistance. Modified from Stevens *et al.* (1989).

6.4.1. Summary of Excitatory Amino Acid Receptor Types

As an orientation to excitatory amino acid (EAA) receptor types and physiological characteristics, we summarize previous work on EAA at nonbrainstem sites in Table 2. (We do not present here a detailed, systematic review of possible inhibitory amino acid transmitters of the brainstem, such as GABA and glycine, since extensive *in vitro* work is absent. The existing relevant data are presented in passing in other sections.)

As defined in Table 2 by their specific agonists, three main classes of excitatory amino acid receptors have been described in the mammalian CNS: the NMDA receptor and two non-NMDA receptors, a quisqualate receptor and a kainate receptor (Watkins and Evans, 1981). Characterization of the receptors in terms of their voltage and ionic sensitivities has now been accomplished by voltage- and patch-clamp recordings in cultured mammalian CNS neurons. Channels preferentially activated by the non-NMDA receptors had little voltage sensitivity, were selective for monovalent cations (sodium and potassium), and had reversal potentials of near 0 mV in physiological media. Channels preferentially activated by the NMDA receptor were voltage sensitive and were selectively permeable to divalent (calcium in particular) as well as monovalent cations. Single-channel conductance evaluation showed that each receptor activated a family of conductances ranging from 2 to 50 pS; kainate and quisqualate receptors primarily opened channels with smaller conductances (kainate activation tended toward openings of <5 pS, and quisqualate toward 10–15 pS), and NMDA receptors preferentially activated channels with larger conductances of 45–50 pS (Jahr and Stevens, 1987; Cull-Candy and Usowicz, 1987). The NMDA receptor is of special interest because of its voltage sensitivity, which has been attributed to a voltage-sensitive blockade by magnesium at physiological concentrations (Nowak *et al.*, 1984; Mayer *et al.*, 1984). This blockade is removed by depolarization and endows the NMDA response with some regenerative properties. For example, NMDA may only slightly alter the resting properties of a neuron with membrane potential at rest, but once membrane potential is depolarized past the threshold for removal of the magnesium blockade, NMDA may elicit a large burst of action potentials (Herrling, 1985).

Table 2. Excitatory Amino Acid Receptor Type (Agonist)[a]

Characteristics	NMDA	Quisqualate[b]	Kainate
Voltage sensitivity	+	−	−
Magnesium block	+	−	−
Calcium permeability	+	−	−
Na^+/K^+ permeability	+	+	+
Modulation	Glycine ↑, zinc and opiates ↓	−	−
Antagonist	Kynurenate, CPP, APV	Kynurenate, CNQX	Kynurenate, CNQX

[a]NMDA = N-methyl-D-aspartate; CPP = 3-((+)-2-carboxypiperazin-4-gamma-1)-propyl-1-phosphonic acid; APV = 5-amino-phosphonovaleric acid; CNQX = 2,3-dihydroxy-6-cyano-7-nitroquinoxalone.
[b]Beta-L-ODAP (beta-N-oxalyl-L-alpha, beta-diaminoproprionic acid) binds strongly to the quisqualate class of receptors, less strongly to the kainate class, and only very weakly to the NMDA class.

The calcium conductance activated by the NMDA receptor is of importance and interest because it is of sufficient magnitude to raise significantly the intracellular calcium concentration of the neuron (MacDermott *et al.*, 1986). This likely affects intracellular signal processing and, in fact, has already been implicated as an integral part of the development of long-term potentiation in hippocampal CA1 neurons (Collingridge and Bliss, 1987).

Finally, the NMDA response has been found to be modulated by glycine, zinc, and likely also by opiates (Ascher and Nowak, 1987). Glycine potentiated the NMDA response with maximal effects occurring at such low concentrations (<2 μM, Johnson and Ascher, 1987) that it raises the possibility that NMDA responses are modulated by synaptically released glycine in areas with glycinergic transmission, such as may occur in mPRF (Greene and Carpenter, 1985). Glycine potentiation of NMDA responses was not antagonized by strychnine. Zinc antagonized the NMDA response (Peters *et al.*, 1987; Westbrook and Mayer, 1987). σ-Opiate compounds acted as noncompetitive antagonists to the NMDA receptors, but the electrophysiological effects are still unknown (Cotman *et al.*, 1987).

Antagonists, as summarized in Table 2, include the nonspecific EAA antagonist kynurenate (Perkins and Stone, 1982; Cotman *et al.*, 1986) and the specific NMDA receptor antagonist 3-[(+)-2-carboxypiperazin-4-γ-1]-propyl-1-phosphonic acid (CPP) (Harris *et al.*, 1986).

Recent data (Bridges *et al.*, 1989) indicate that beta-*N*-oxalyl-L-alpha,beta-diaminoproprionic acid (beta-L-ODAP) is a non-NMDA agonist in rat hippocampus. This glutamate analog only weakly interacts with NMDA receptors while having very strong, specific interactions with the quisqualate receptor class and less strong interactions with the kainate class. As also shown in Table 2, CNQX (2,3-dihydroxy-6-cyano-7-nitroquinoxalone) is a potent non-NMDA antagonist (Honore *et al.*, 1987; Blake *et al.*, 1988).

6.4.2. Pontine Reticular Formation and Bulbar Reticular Formation

In vivo studies have shown that excitatory postsynaptic potentials (EPSPs) characterized by a distinctive fast time to peak (<3 msec) were readily evoked in the medial pontine reticular formation (mPRF) by stimulation of all areas of the brainstem reticular formation, including mPRF (see Ito and McCarley, 1987; McCarley *et al.*, 1987). Such types of EPSPs are also present in mPRF stimulation–recording paradigms in the slice. This fast rise time characteristic was mimicked by Greene and Carpenter's (1985) iontophoretic application of glutamate or aspartate. In contrast, no other putative transmitter candidate tested—including ACh, NE, 5-HT, and thyrotropin-releasing hormone—elicited such a mPRF response. Behavioral data also indicate the responsiveness of the reticular formation muscle suppression zone in dorsolateral pons to applications of EAA agonists (Siegel and Lai, 1988). In Chapter 10, we discuss *in vivo* data by Chase and co-workers suggesting that the phasic depolarizations of lumbar α-motoneurons during REM sleep are mediated by non-NMDA receptors; some of these PSPs may be mediated by reticulospinal fibers (see Chapter 4). Data supporting an EAA pathway from the medullary nucleus paragigantocellularis to the locus coeruleus are discussed in the next section. At this point we conclude that it is highly likely, although not yet demonstrated in rigorously controlled *in vitro* studies, that EAA are an important class of excitatory brainstem reticular formation neurotransmitters.

201

NEUROTRANS-
MITTER-
MODULATED
IONIC CURRENTS

6.4.3. Locus Coeruleus

The short-latency excitatory response of LC neurons to focal stimulation of the slice has been illustrated in Fig. 15. In the *in vitro* LC slice preparation, Williams (1988) has recently presented evidence that this fast excitatory EPSP results from activation of an EAA receptor, complementing *in vivo* data indicating an EAA projection from the nucleus paragigantocellularis in medulla (Ennis and Aston-Jones, 1988; see also Chapter 4).

6.4.4. Thalamus and Neocortex

Thalamic and cortical neurons possess both NMDA and non-NMDA receptors (Cotman *et al.*, 1987).

The excitatory responses of LG thalamic cells to optic afferent stimulation are blocked by both NMDA and non-NMDA antagonists (Crunelli *et al.*, 1985). The corticothalamic pathways also use EAA as transmitters since unilateral decortication results in a decline of terminal uptake of aspartate and glutamate in the appropriate ipsilateral thalamic nuclei (Baughman and Gilbert, 1980, 1981), and D-[^{3}H]aspartate injected in various thalamic nuclei is taken up by corticothalamic neurons (Rustioni *et al.*, 1983).

The thalamocortical projections also use EAA as transmitters (Streit, 1980; Ottersen *et al.*, 1983). This was also inferred from the blockade of visually evoked responses of simple neurons in the striate cortex by kynurenic acid, a general EAA antagonist (Tsumoto *et al.*, 1986).

The actions of EAA appear mediated by at least three types of receptors. Aspartate seems to act on NMDA receptor (cf. Watkins and Evans, 1981; Cotman *et al.*, 1987). The other types are non-NMDA receptors, quisqualate and kainate, but their selective blockers are not yet available (cf. Ascher and Nowak, 1987). Glutamate appears to act at both NMDA and non-NMDA receptors. Whereas non-NMDA receptor activation induces a fast-rising EPSP with a short decay time, the NMDA receptor activation produces a depolarization with a long duration (McLennan, 1983; Mayer and Westbrook, 1987; Watkins and Olverman, 1987). The long-term characteristic of the NMDA response probably accounts for NMDA involvement in plasticity processes of the visual cortex (Artola and Singer, 1987) similarly to the long-term potentiation described in the hippocampus (cf. Collingridge and Bliss, 1987).

The striking depolarization produced in cortical cells by EAA is associated with a marked fall in membrane resistance (Krnjević, 1974) like EAA effects on spinal cord (MacDonald and Wojtowicz, 1980) and hippocampal (Dingledine, 1983) neurons. The excitatory effect of EAA on cortical pyramidal-shaped neurons was also studied *in vitro* (Flatman *et al.*, 1983; Thompson, 1986). It was found that the depolarizing response to NMDA is voltage dependent, decreasing in amplitude and duration with membrane hyperpolarization, and it is associated with an apparent increase in input resistance.

7

Synchronized Brain Oscillations and Their Disruption by Ascending Brainstem Reticular Influxes

The physiological bases of the principal EEG synchronized rhythms are summarized here because these rhythms are used to identify objectively waking and sleep states. Most of their alterations are induced by increased or decreased activity in brainstem neurons with thalamic, basal forebrain, hippocampal, and neocortical projections. The knowledge of cellular mechanisms underlying the synchronization of EEG waves is therefore necessary to understand the role played by brainstem modulatory systems.

Synchronization denotes a state characterized by high-amplitude rhythmic EEG waves with different frequencies. The defining feature of all synchronized waves is their relatively large amplitude. Various types of EEG synchronized waves display slow as well as fast frequencies, from less than 1 Hz to more than 40 Hz. The notion of synchronization supposes the coactivation of large neuronal aggregates whose summated synaptic events and/or intrinsic currents reach such a magnitude that they can be recorded with rather gross recording techniques. There is now ample evidence that EEG activity mainly results from extracellular current flow associated with summated excitatory and inhibitory postsynaptic potentials (EPSPs and IPSPs). However, the long-lasting calcium-dependent potassium currents and a series of other intrinsic neuronal properties should also be considered as playing a role in the genesis of various EEG waves.

Conventionally, the term EEG synchronization is used as a label for the quiet sleep state. This is justified by the diffuse occurrence over the neocortical mantle of two major synchronized rhythms, spindles and slow (δ) waves, during the state of sleep preceding REM sleep. However, the synonymity between EEG synchronization and quiet sleep is an oversimplification, since high-amplitude synchronized rhythms may appear in some cortical foci during states of hyper-vigilance, and synchronized θ waves occur in some species during REM sleep and/or active wakefulness.

In what follows, we discuss the frequency characteristics and behavioral connotation of the main types of synchronized EEG activity. To a large extent, the identification of pacemakers and the disclosure of cellular bases have been achieved for spindle waves and θ waves. The mechanisms of other synchronized rhythms, such as α waves, fast oscillations during immobility and hypervigilance, and sleep slow waves, are as yet poorly understood at the cellular level. We first describe in Sections 7.1 and 7.2 two types of synchronized oscillations during the brain-activated states of waking and REM sleep. The few things we know about sleep slow waves are mentioned in Section 7.3. In Section 7.4 we analyze the cellular mechanisms of spindle rhythmicity together with the two types of incremental (augmenting and recruiting) evoked field potentials that mimic spontaneously occurring spindles. Since the α rhythm is usually recorded over the scalp in humans, its cellular bases are not known. We refer to this rhythm in the section devoted to EEG spindling (Section 7.4.1) but only to mark the differences between these two types of oscillations with overlapping frequencies but quite distinct behavioral connotations. Finally (Section 7.5), we discuss the cellular mechanisms of spindle disruption, a major aspect of EEG desynchronizing processes on arousal and during REM sleep.

7.1. Oscillations during Waking Immobility

Synchronized EEG waves within the frequency range of 12–16 Hz have been described during wakefulness associated with complete absence of phasic motor activity. Such oscillations, initially termed the "sensorimotor rhythm" (Roth *et al.*, 1967), have been postulated to reflect active suppressive or inhibitory processes (Sterman and Wyrwicka, 1967). These oscillations are homologous to a similar rhythm described by Gastaut (1952) over the central sulcus in humans, which is also related to the blockage of motor activity. Subsequently, this rhythm was more precisely localized within the somatosensory system, as it was recorded in the ventroposterolateral (VPL) thalamic nucleus and its cortical projection area (Howe and Sterman, 1972).

The patterns of EEG activity during waking immobility (with the exception of occasional eye and tail movements) were analyzed in detail by Rougeul-Buser and her colleagues (1983). They attempted to characterize different frequencies of oscillations while placing the cat in experimental conditions that may be qualified as "hunting" situations. Two distinct behavioral conditions were associated with two different frequencies and cortical locations of oscillations. When the animal was in a position of expectancy, waiting for the unseen mouse to come out through a hole, the rhythms were around 14 Hz and were localized over the anterior limb zone of primary somatosensory area (Fig. 1A). However, when the cat was watching the visible but out of reach mouse, high-frequency (35–45 Hz) rhythms appeared in two foci, one in the pericruciate (motor) cortex, the other in the periansate (parietal association) area (Fig. 1B). Similar fast rhythms have been described in the monkey (Rougeul *et al.*, 1979).

On the basis of macroelectrode recordings and lesions in the cat thalamus, it was hypothesized that the thalamic source of the 14-Hz rhythm is the VPL nucleus, and the medial part of the posterior thalamic complex (POm) was thought to generate the fast rhythms (35–45 Hz) that appear over the pericruciate and periansate cortices (Bouyer *et al.*, 1980, 1981, 1987). A microelectrode exploration revealed that a very limited number (13%) of VPL thalamic cells changed their discharges when the 14-Hz rhythm occurred in the cortex, and those few neurons displayed various firing patterns during cortical oscillations: tonic firing or phasic discharges related to the cortical rhythm (Rougeul-Buser *et al.*, 1983). The spontaneous activity of VPL thalamic neurons fluctuates with the degree of vigilance and with the presence or absence of the cortical 14-Hz rhythm, being higher between the trains of 14-Hz waves than during those trains (Delagrange *et al.*, 1987).

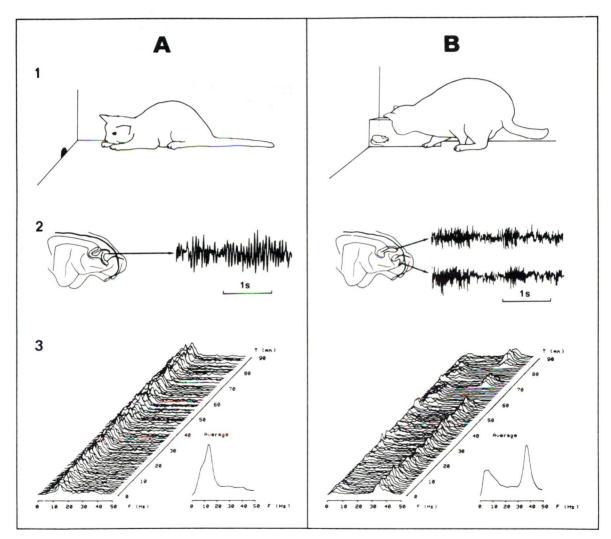

Figure 1. Cortical rhythms during waking immobility in cat. A: Expectancy, rhythm frequency 14 Hz. B: Focused attention, rhythm frequency 36 Hz. See text for behavioral paradigms. In both A and B, 1 illustrates the animal's most common attitudes in the used experimental design. 2 depicts types of rhythmic patterns and their localization: one focus in the primary somatosensory cortex (in A) and one motor and one parietal focus (in B). 3 depicts evolutive spectra taken during 90-min recording time. Each spectrum was computed from 1-min recording. Heights of peaks indicate spectral power (μV^2) in the frequency band 0–50 Hz (resolution/cf = 0.2 Hz). Added to each set of evolutive spectra is the average spectrum computed over the 90-min recording time. From Rougeul-Buser *et al.* (1983).

Recently, fast (40–Hz) oscillations have been described in the primary visual cortex of cat in response to moving light bars (Singer *et al.*, 1988). The active cell populations engaged in the synchronous oscillations of area 17 can extend from 300 μm to 1500 μm (Gray *et al.*, 1988).

Despite some superficial similarities with spindle waves, the rhythms during waking immobility are basically different from spindles. The dissimilarities concern not only the 35 to 45-Hz rhythm that is far beyond the frequency range (7–14 Hz) of spindles but also the slower (14-Hz) "sensorimotor" rhythm. Indeed, sleep spindles are recorded over extensive cortical areas, whereas the 14-Hz oscillations related to expectancy are restricted within a cortical territory that does not exceed 5 mm²; also, cortical spindles are generated by rhythmic high-frequency bursts in thalamocortical neurons (see Section 7.4), which also contrasts with the few thalamic cells found to discharge in phase with the expectancy rhythm. The location of driving forces and the cellular mechanisms of the 14-Hz expectancy rhythm remain to be elucidated.

The fast (35 to 45-Hz) oscillations of pericruciate and periansate cortices are suppressed after bilateral electrolytic lesions of the ventral tegmental area of the mesencephalon, thus suggesting that a dopaminergic mechanism is involved in their genesis (Montaron *et al.*, 1982). Since there are no known dopaminergic projections to the thalamus (see Chapter 4), the cortical origin of such fast oscillations is probable.

7.2.   θ Waves

The θ rhythm consists of high-amplitude regular waves that appear in the septohippocampal system and related subsystems of nonprimate mammals. The θ waves have a frequency of 4 to 7 Hz in rabbit and cat and 6 to 10 Hz in rat. The relationship between θ rhythm and brain-activated states (arousal and REM sleep) is clearly established in rodents. In rat, the animal of choice for the study of θ rhythm in relation to different types of waking behavior, hippocampal θ waves appear during walking, running, jumping, head movements, and manipulation of objects with the forelimbs but not during automatic or simple reflexive behavior such as licking, chewing, or face washing (cf. Vanderwolf and Robinson, 1981). In cat, hippocampal θ is more evident during REM sleep than during alertness.

Initially, the septum was regarded as the pacemaker of θ rhythm,* a nodal relay between the brainstem and hippocampus that transforms the steady flow of impulses from the brainstem reticular core into rhythmic discharges transferred to the hippocampus (Petsche *et al.*, 1965; Gogolak *et al.*, 1968). The brainstem sites whose electrical stimulation induces hippocampal θ are found along the entire longitudinal extent of the reticular formation, as far caudal as

---

*Although almost all evidence points to the septum as a pacemaker of θ waves, experiments on rat hippocampus *in vitro* have shown that application of the cholinergic agonist carbachol in the slice produces θ-like rhythmical waves in the stratum moleculare of the dentate gyrus, a response that could be antagonized by atropine (Konopacki *et al.*, 1987). These results are in line with the demonstration *in vivo* that θ waves can be produced by direct infusion of carbachol into the hippocampal formation (Rowntree and Bland, 1966).

the magnocellular nucleus in the medulla. The frequency and amplitude of θ waves are increased by stimulating progressively more rostral in the brainstem reticular core (Vertes, 1982). Brainstem reticular impulses reach the septum through the medial forebrain bundle. Septohippocampal neurons have been anatomically traced (Segal and Landis, 1974) and antidromically identified (Lamour *et al.*, 1984), and their cholinergic nature is well established (cf. Fibiger, 1982).

The mechanism of θ waves was first investigated intracellularly by Fujita and Sato (1964), who proposed that impulses of septal origin excite hippocampal pyramidal cells that display depolarization–hyperpolarization sequences related to the negative–positive phases of the extracellularly recorded θ. The hyperpolarizing component was ascribed to recurrent collateral excitation of local hippocampal interneurons.

A study of the relations between discharges of different types of CA1 and dentate gyrus neurons (pyramidal cells, granule cells, and interneurons) and focal waves in the behaving rat reached the conclusion that, in addition to the recurrent collateral pathway, hippocampal interneurons are driven directly from septal pacemaker neurons as well as from the entorhinal cortex (Buzsaki *et al.*, 1983). The noncholinergic entorhinal input was required to explain the failure to eliminate hippocampal θ after atropine administration. In fact, after lesions of the entorhinal cortex, atropine completely eliminates θ rhythm (Vanderwolf and Leung, 1983). On the other hand, the direct access of septal cholinergic neurons to hippocampal interneurons is supported by anatomic evidence (Mosko *et al.*, 1973) and by the strong AChE activity coinciding with the distribution of the local-circuit cells in the stratum oriens, radiatum, and the hilus of the dentate gyrus (Mathiesen and Blackstad, 1964; Vijayan, 1979).

The role played by the entorhinal cortex as a local generator of θ waves was investigated by Alonso and Garcia-Ausst (1987a,b), who have demonstrated the presence of rhythmic discharges (time locked with θ waves) of neurons located in layers II and III of this structure. In fact, θ waves can probably be generated within multiple sites of the limbic system. Neurons recorded from the medial subdivision of mammillary bodies display spontaneous oscillations of the membrane potential sustaining rhythmic bursts of discharges; the basic mechanism of these oscillations is a calcium-dependent plateau potential (Alonso and Llinas, 1988) different from the calcium-dependent low-threshold spike (see Chapter 5). Thus, θ rhythm can no longer be viewed as exclusively generated by a unique pacemaker, the septum, but by an interaction between coupled oscillators within the limbic system. In this view, the medial septum is regarded as a tuning element, mediating phase relations between various generators (A. Alonso, personal communication).

There are reports indicating that θ waves recorded from the neocortex may result from hippocampal volume conduction. However, at least for the cingulate cortex, the intracortical generation of θ was suggested by neuronal firing at the θ frequency (Holsheimer, 1982; Leung and Borst, 1987) and by persistence of θ rhythm (even with increased amplitude) after lesions of medial septum that produced abolition of hippocampal θ (Borst *et al.*, 1987). The origin of the cingulate θ in the absence of the septohippocampal and direct septomammillary systems, which are generally thought to transmit θ waves to the cingulate cortex through a prior relay in the anterior thalamic nuclei, is not known.

7.3. Sleep Slow Waves

Slow (δ) waves at 0.5–4 Hz prevail during the late stage of EEG-synchronized sleep, when they are indented by the faster spindle waves. The cortical origin of slow waves was suggested by their persistence in animals with bilateral thalamic destruction (Villablanca, 1974) and their disappearance at subcortical levels after large neocortical ablations (Jouvet, 1962).*

There is no systematic intracellular study of slow waves. Laminar profiles in cat suprasylvian cortex indicate that the generator of slow waves is at a depth between 0.6 and 0.9 mm (Calvet *et al.*, 1964), between layers III and V. Current source-density analyses showed that 4-Hz waves in rabbit visual cortex display dipoles between layers II–III and V, whereas waves within higher-frequency bands are more pronounced in deeper cortical layers (Petsche *et al.*, 1984). The surface-negative component of slow waves reverses abruptly at the upper border of layer V, and the depth-positive wave is typically associated with silence in neuronal firing (Buzsaki *et al.*, 1988). Similar relations between the surface-negative component and deep intracortical inhibitory processes have been reported for pathological slow waves induced by thalamic or midbrain reticular lesions (Ball *et al.*, 1977).

The amplitude of cortical slow waves display oscillations (periods 6 to 12 sec) and increase progressively from the transitional period of drowsiness to fully developed sleep, in close temporal relationship to a progressive decrease in discharge rates of midbrain reticular neurons (Oakson and Steriade, 1982, 1983; Fig. 2). Since midbrain reticular neurons do not have direct cortical projections (see Section 4.2.1), this relationship is presumably transmitted by intercalated neurons. In particular, basal forebrain cholinergic neurons seem to influence the genesis of cortical slow waves since their unilateral destruction produces an asymmetric map of δ distribution, with an increase in the δ band ipsilateral to the lesion (Buzsaki *et al.*, 1988; see Chapter 13, Fig. 8).

7.4. Spontaneous Spindles and Evoked Incremental Waves

7.4.1. Spindle Waves

The appearance of spindle waves on the EEG marks the transitional period from waking to sleep. Spindles are defined as waxing and waning waves between 7 and 14 Hz grouped in sequences that last for 1.5–2 sec and recur with a slow rhythm of 0.1–0.3 Hz (see Fig. 2 of Chapter 1). The slow rhythm of spindle sequences is seen in both naturally sleeping animals and barbiturate-treated preparations (Steriade and Deschênes, 1984).

---

*However, typical high-amplitude slow (0.5–4 Hz) waves are seen in focal recordings from the RE thalamic nucleus after disconnection from the cerebral cortex (Steriade *et al.*, 1987a). Moreover, the same type of slow waves appear in the ventrolateral thalamic nucleus in close time relation with spike barrages in its major source of inputs, the neurons in deep cerebellar nuclei (Steriade *et al.*, 1971). These data suggest that the site of origin of EEG waves within the frequency range of 0.5–4 Hz transcends the cerebral cortex.

Although some authors regard α waves (8–12 Hz) as embryos or congeners of spindles, probably because of the overlapping frequencies of these two rhythms, α and spindle waves must be dissociated because of their dissimilar grouping, cortical distribution, but especially because of their quite different behavioral connotations. Indeed, spindles are characteristically associated with blockage of information transfer through the thalamus and unconsciousness (see Chapter 8), whereas the incidence and amplitude of occipital α waves may increase during some attentional tasks (Creutzfeldt *et al.*, 1969; Ray and Cole,

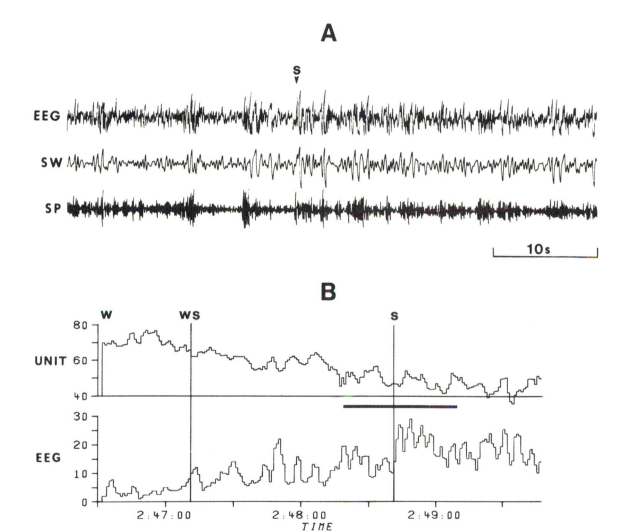

Figure 2. Discharge of a neuron in midbrain reticular formation (MRF) and simultaneously recorded EEG rhythms during transition from wakefulness (W) to EEG-synchronized sleep (S) in chronically implanted cat. WS, transitional period between W and S. A: Pericruciate neocortical EEG (upper trace) of a WS–S transition, with filtered slow waves (SW, 0.5–4 Hz, middle trace) and filtered spindle waves (SP, 7–9 Hz, lower trace). B: MRF unit discharge (spikes/sec, upper trace) and relative EEG slow-wave amplitudes (lower trace) for entire transition. Note gradual lowering of firing rate and signs of rate rhythmicity as transition progresses, accompanied by increased EEG synchronization with rhythmic fluctuations in amplitude. Horizontal bar in B indicates segment of transition displayed in A. Both traces were smoothed by a three-bin nonweighted moving average. Modified from Oakson and Steriade (1983).

1985). Besides, spindles are transmitted over the cortex by thalamocortical neurons, whereas α waves are thought to propagate mainly through surface-parallel intracortical connections (Lopes da Silva *et al.*, 1980; Lopes da Silva, 1987).

After the demonstration that spindles originate in the thalamus, as they are recorded in the intralaminar nuclei after decortication and high brainstem transection (Morison and Bassett, 1945), the mechanisms of spindle genesis have been investigated intracellularly. The main events underlying spindles under barbiturate anesthesia or occurring naturally in the *encéphale isolé* preparation are long-lasting (70–150 msec) hyperpolarizations in thalamocortical neurons, occasionally interrupted by rebound bursts of high-frequency spikes (Andersen and Eccles, 1962; Andersen and Sears, 1964; Maekawa and Purpura, 1967a,b). The hyperpolarizations could be reversed by current and chloride injections (Deschênes *et al.*, 1984), thus indicating that they are imposed on thalamocortical neurons by synaptic actions from thalamic inhibitory elements.

Two main theories emerged in relation to the thalamic networks involved in spindle genesis.

The theory elaborated by Andersen and Andersson (1968) postulated that spindle oscillations are generated in intranuclear circuits involving thalamocortical neurons, their hypothesized recurrent axonal collaterals, and inhibitory local-circuit neurons. No particular nucleus was assumed to play the role of a general pacemaker; synchronization of spindles throughout the thalamus was ascribed to spread of oscillations from one nucleus to another by means of "distributor" neurons. This theory was challenged by (1) the absence of intranuclear recurrent collaterals of thalamocortical axons in most nuclei, including the ventrobasal complex where Andersen's experiments were conducted (e.g., Yen and Jones, 1983; Kita and Kitai, 1986; Yamamoto *et al.*, 1986; Harris, 1987), and (2) the absence of connections between most thalamic nuclei (cf. Jones, 1985).

The other theory (Steriade *et al.*, 1985, 1987a) points to the reticular thalamic (RE) nucleus as the spindle pacemaker on the basis of following experimental evidence.

During spindling, the discharge patterns of rostral, rostrolateral, and perigeniculate (PG) neurons of the RE nuclear complex are inverse images of those in thalamocortical neurons. The spindle-related oscillations of RE neurons occur on a slowly growing and decaying depolarization with superimposed spike barrages, whereas thalamocortical neurons simultaneously exhibit long-lasting cyclic hyperpolarizations that occasionally deinactivate brief rebound bursts (Fig. 3). The ionic conductances involved in the patterning of spindle oscillations of RE and thalamocortical neurons (namely, the persistent sodium current, the low-threshold calcium rebound spike, and various voltage- and calcium-dependent potassium currents) are discussed in Chapter 5. The high-frequency bursts of thalamocortical neurons are transferred to the cerebral cortex, where they trigger rhythmic depolarizing events within the frequency of spindle waves in pyramidal neurons (Fig. 3). These are the cellular bases of spindling in thalamocortical systems.

Since RE neurons are GABAergic (Houser *et al.*, 1980) and project to virtually all thalamic nuclei (cf. Jones, 1985; Steriade *et al.*, 1984a), the hypothesis was advanced that the spindle-related hyperpolarizations of thalamocortical neurons are induced by the inhibitory actions of rhythmic spike barrages in RE

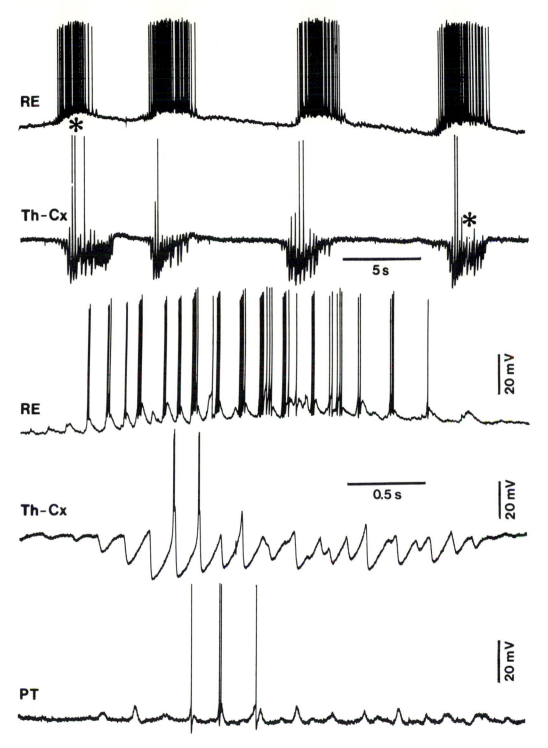

Figure 3. Intracellular aspects of spindling oscillatory activities in reticular thalamic (RE), thalamocortical (Th-Cx; recorded from the ventrolateral nucleus), and pyramidal tract (PT; recorded from precruciate gyrus) neurons of cat under barbiturate anesthesia. Resting potentials over −55 mV. The spindle sequences marked by asterisks in top traces of RE and Th-Cx neurons are depicted below at higher speed. Modified from Steriade and Deschênes (1988).

neurons. This hypothesis implied that those thalamic nuclei that were experimentally disconnected from the RE nucleus or are naturally devoid of RE inputs would not display spindle rhythmicity. This idea was tested, and the results are briefly summarized below.

After thalamic transections in acute experiments that disconnected the dorsal thalamic nuclei from the RE neuronal sheet, or after chemical lesions of RE perikarya in chronic experiments, spindling was abolished in RE-deprived thalamic nuclei. The abolition of spindling was associated with replacement of long-lasting (70–150 msec) hyperpolarizations in thalamocortical neurons by short-duration (12–20 msec) IPSPs displaying no rhythmicity (Fig. 4A; Steriade *et al.*, 1985). Moreover, the spindlelike cyclic hyperpolarization–rebound sequences elicited in intact thalamocortical neurons by cortical stimulation were replaced, after destruction of RE perikarya, by a *single* phase of hyperpolarization, eventually followed by a rebound spike (Fig. 4B; Steriade and Deschênes, 1988). Therefore, both spontaneous and cortically evoked spindling activities disappear in thalamocortical neurons disconnected from the RE neurons.

The anteromedial–anteroventral (AM–AV) and lateral habenular (LH) thalamic nuclei are among the very few thalamic nuclei that do not receive afferent connections from the RE nuclear complex (Steriade *et al.*, 1984a; Paré *et al.*, 1987; Velayos *et al.*, 1989). Despite their possessing intrinsic properties similar to other thalamic neurons (see Fig. 6), neither AM–AV nor LH neurons display spindle rhythms. The AM or AV single neurons were simultaneously recorded with dorsal thalamic cells that are known to receive powerful inputs from the RE nucleus, and the lack of spindle oscillations in the former stood in clear contrast with the spindle oscillations and related rhythmic spike bursts in the latter (Figs. 5 and 6; Paré *et al.*, 1987). This same phenomenon is found in LH neurons; these have ionic conductances similar to other thalamic neurons (Wilcox *et al.*, 1987). However, instead of spindles, the LH nucleus displays θ waves within the range of 5–7 Hz, in synchrony with hippocampal θ, during activated behavioral states (M. J. Gutnick, personal communication).

These results indicate that the afferent connections from the RE nucleus are a necessary condition for the occurrence of spindles in target thalamic nuclei.

Figure 4. Abolition of spontaneous and evoked spindle oscillations in thalamocortical neurons disconnected from the RE thalamic nucleus. Intracellular recordings. A: Spindle oscillations in intact preparation (the two traces represent ink-written recording at the top and oscilloscopic recording at the bottom) and, below, after thalamic transections that disconnected dorsal thalamic nuclei from the RE nucleus. In transected preparation, spindle-related rhythmic long-lasting hyperpolarizations are abolished. In 1 of the transected preparation (ink-written recording), polarizing currents (arrows) were passed through the cell membrane to reveal the presence of numerous low-amplitude IPSPs (for comparison, the speed of recording was identical to that in top trace of the intact preparation). In 2, left part shows ink-written recording of IPSPs at higher speed, and right part depicts the same events in oscilloscopic recordings; note the depolarizing hump of the short-lasting IPSP. B: Absence of evoked spindlelike oscillatory response in thalamocortical neurons after kainic lesion of RE perikarya. 1: Typical oscillatory response of a ventrolateral (VL) thalamocortical cell to cortical stimulation in an intact preparation. 2: Response of a VL thalamocortical cell to cortical stimulation after RE kainic lesion; note absence of oscillations and the presence of a single period of hyperpolarization followed by a low-threshold rebound spike (arrow). See the histology of thalamic transections and kainate-induced lesions of the RE nucleus in Steriade *et al.* (1985). Modified from Steriade *et al.* (1985) and Steriade and Deschênes (1988).

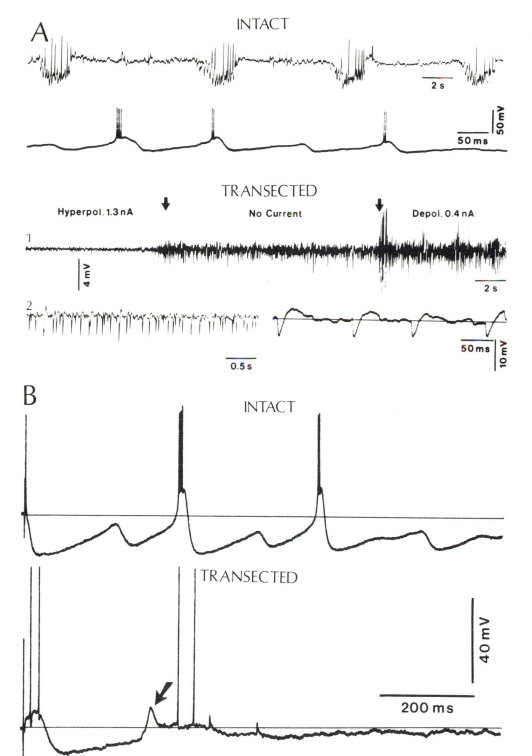

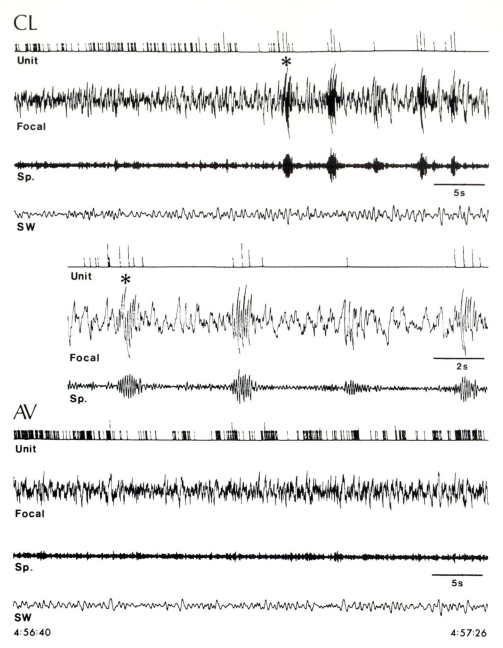

Figure 5. Absence of spindle oscillations in the anterior thalamic nuclei, a group devoid of inputs from the RE thalamic nucleus. Simultaneous recordings of a centrolateral (CL) thalamic neuron and an anteroventral (AV) thalamic neuron. Real time of recording indicated at bottom. Unanesthetized *cerveau isolé* preparation. Unit discharges were used to deflect a pen of the ink-writing machine; each deflection exceeding the common level of single spikes represents a burst of high-frequency spikes. Focal thalamic waves, simultaneously recorded by the same microelectrodes in CL and AV nuclei, are shown in three different ways: as recorded (Focal), after passage through a 7- to 14-Hz bandpass filter to depict spindles (Sp), and after passage through a 1- to 4-Hz band-pass filter to depict slow waves (SW). The epoch including the asterisk-marked spindle sequence in the CL recording, together with the concomitant unit discharges and filtered focal spindles, are depicted at a faster speed in the middle of this figure. Note activity changes of the CL neuron (from a tonic to bursting discharges) with the appearance of spindle oscillations. By contrast, the discharge pattern of the AV neuron did not change, and there were no spindles in the focal recording. From Paré *et al.* (1987).

The crucial evidence that RE neurons are pacemakers of spindle rhythmicity is that focal spindle oscillations and related spike barrages of single neurons can be recorded in the RE nucleus deafferented by transections from its major, thalamic and cortical, input sources (Fig. 7; Steriade *et al.*, 1987a).

The concept of causal relations between rhythmic bursts of GABAergic RE thalamic neurons and cyclic hyperpolarizations of thalamocortical neurons underlying spindle oscillations is supported by *in vitro* studies in which stimulation was applied to the RE nucleus at the periphery of the slice and relay cells in

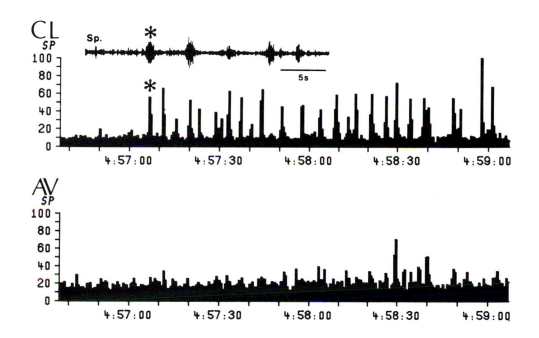

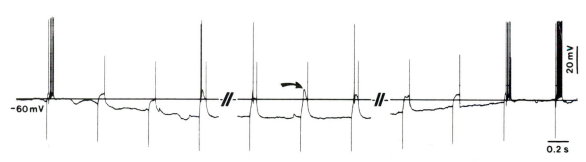

Figure 6. Digitized aspects of focal waves simultaneously recorded in CL and AV thalamic nuclei, as depicted in Fig. 5 (top part), and intrinsic membrane properties of anterior thalamic neurons of cat (bottom part). Top part: Computer-generated graphs represent amplitudes of spindle (SP) waves filtered at 7–14 Hz. First spindle sequence in CL recording is marked by asterisk; inset depicts an ink-written recording at higher speed. Abscissas indicate real time. Bottom part: Effect of membrane potential on firing mode of an anteromedial thalamic cell. Tonic firing induced by a depolarizing pulse at rest (−60 mV) developed into an LTS and spike burst under steady hyperpolarization when membrane potential reached −72 mV; recovery of tonic mode at right; oblique arrow indicates LTS in isolation. Compare with similar intrinsic properties of other thalamic neurons discussed in Chapter 5. Modified from Paré *et al.* (1987).

adjacent thalamic nuclei were recorded intracellularly (Thompson, 1988a). The chloride-mediated IPSPs in thalamocortical cells generated by train of pulses to the RE nucleus give rise to postinhibitory rebounds (Fig. 8A). In contrast to the absence of self-maintained oscillations after current pulses in thalamocortical cells, membrane potential oscillations within spindle frequencies were observed after long trains of IPSPs induced by stimulation of the RE nucleus (Fig. 8B). It is

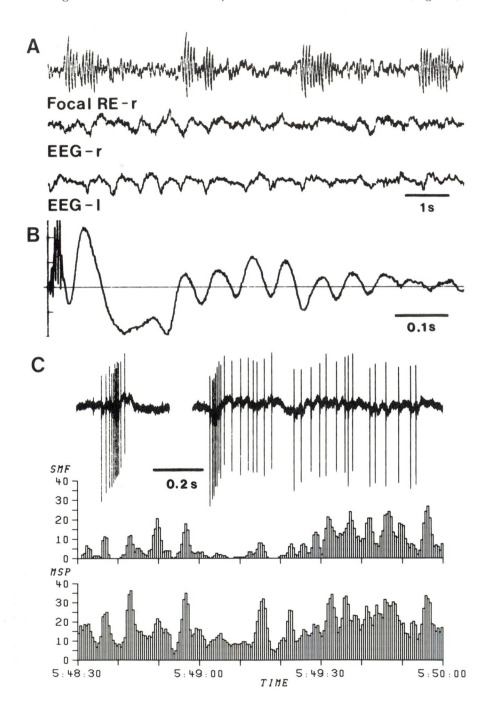

worth mentioning that the most effective frequency of RE stimulation for inducing self-maintained oscillations in thalamocortical neurons was around 160 Hz, that is, within the range of usual intraburst frequencies of RE neurons during spindling in naturally sleeping animals (Domich *et al.*, 1986; Steriade *et al.*, 1986).

7.4.2. Incremental (Augmenting and Recruiting) Responses

Cortical responses to thalamic stimulation grow in size during the pulse train when low-frequency (7–14 Hz) stimuli are used. The most dramatic change occurs from the first to the second response in the train (see Figs. 9 and 10). After a few responses with increased amplitudes, the evoked potentials have a tendency to wane.

This phenomenon was initially described by Morison and Dempsey (1942), who distinguished two types of incremental thalamocortical responses as a function of the stimulated site. (1) Augmenting responses were elicited from cortically projecting lateral thalamic nuclei and were recorded as surface-positive potentials in appropriate, quite circumscribed cortical territories. (2) Recruiting responses were evoked by stimulating intralaminar and some medial thalamic nuclei, appeared as surface-negative responses, and, compared to augmenting responses, had a relatively longer latency and appeared on more widespread cortical territories. In their paper, Morison and Dempsey referred to a personal communication by Lorente de Nó who helped to explain the "specific" augmenting responses with restricted cortical distribution and the "nonspecific" recruiting responses with broad distribution. In particular, the recruiting responses to intralaminar thalamic stimulation were attributed to "cell groups, not ordinarily thought of as projection nuclei, [that] send fibers to the cortex which make more diffuse connections than do the specific projection fibers, and may be especially rich in association areas" (Morison and Dempsey, 1942, p. 291). This interpretation is supported by investigations using modern tracing techniques (see Section 7.4.2.2).

7.4.2.1. Augmenting Responses

Depth-profile analyses (Spencer and Brookhart, 1961a) indicate that the surface positivity of the augmenting response results from excitatory thalamo-

---

Figure 7. The deafferented RE thalamic nucleus of cat generates spindle rhythmicity. For histology of transections that created an isolated island containing the rostral pole of the RE nucleus, see Figs. 1 and 2 in Steriade *et al.* (1987a). A: Normal cyclic recurrence of spindle sequences in the rostral pole of the RE nucleus recorded by means of a microelectrode; absence of spindle rhythms (but persistence of slow waves) on cortical EEG recordings following thalamic transections. B: Oscillations within spindle frequency evoked in the rostral pole of the RE nucleus by stimulating (five-shock train) the white matter overlying the caudate nucleus (50 averaged traces). C: Slow rhythm of spindle sequences and related cell burst oscillations in the rostral pole of the RE nucleus deafferented by thalamic and corona radiata transections. Discharges of a single RE neuron were simultaneously recorded with focal spindle oscillations by the same microelectrode. Sequential mean frequency (SMF) of the neuron is depicted with the normalized amplitudes of focal waves filtered for spindle waves (MSP). Abscissa indicates real time. At top, two (short and long) bursts from the same period. Modified from Steriade *et al.* (1987a).

cortical inputs that create sinks mostly in midlayers (IV—III), with current flow along the vertical core conductors represented by the apical dendrites of pyramidal neurons. The basic mechanism of augmenting responses is an increased secondary depolarization and an attenuation of hyperpolarizing potentials beginning with the second stimulus in the pulse train (Purpura *et al.*, 1964; Creutzfeldt *et al.*, 1966).

The increased amplitude of the depth-negative secondary excitatory component is associated, during the augmenting process, with a decreased amplitude of the primary excitatory component (Fig. 9; Morin and Steriade, 1981). Such a differential evolution of focal waves in the cortical depth is paralleled by an increased number of spike discharges superimposed on the secondary (augmented) field potential. Simultaneously there is a decreased probability of unit discharges associated with the primary thalamocortical excitation. This phenomenon was observed in both somatosensory and parietal association cortices

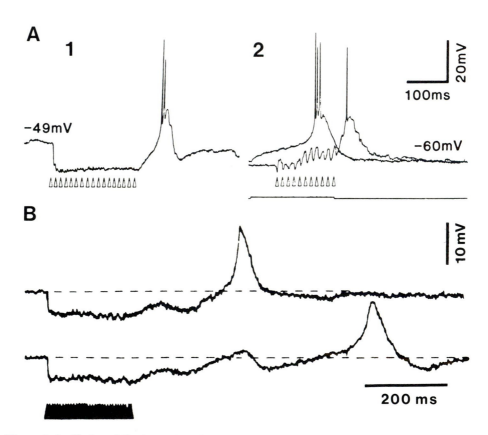

Figure 8. Oscillations following trains of IPSPs induced in rat thalamic neurons studied *in vitro* by stimulating the RE nucleus. A, left: Low-threshold spike (LTS) evoked in dorsal thalamic cell by trains of hyperpolarizing IPSPs induced by stimulation of RE nucleus in the slice; stimulation artifacts indicated by arrowheads. A, right: Same cell; comparison between LTS induced by a depolarizing current pulse and LTS following RE-evoked depolarizing IPSPs from a more negative membrane potential. Resting membrane potentials are indicated. B: A high-frequency (160 Hz) train of RE-evoked IPSPs evokes oscillations in dorsal thalamic neuron. Modified from Thompson (1988a).

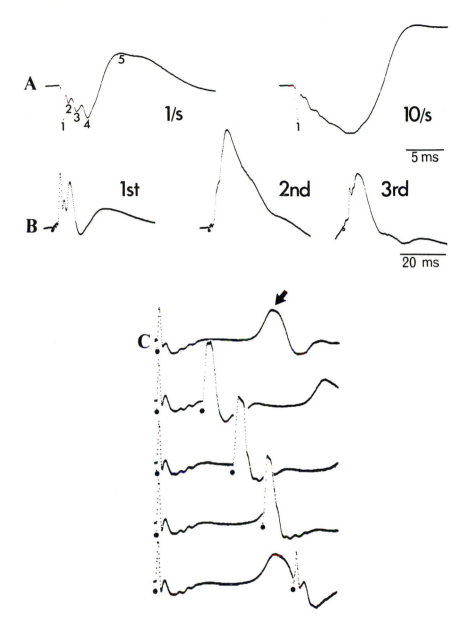

Figure 9. Primary and augmenting responses of primary somatosensory (S1) cortex by stimulating the ventroposterior (VP) thalamic complex in the *encéphale isolé* cat; 50 averaged traces. A: Surface recording of responses evoked by 1/sec and 10/sec VP stimulation; responses consist of five components (numbered 1 to 5); note unchanged presynaptic (1) component. B: Another preparation; depth (0.7 mm) recording of the first, second, and third responses to a shock train at 10/sec; presynaptic deflection was not evident in this case; note, during augmentation, reduced amplitude of early postsynaptic rapid components and protracted duration of the slow negative wave. C: Depth (0.5 mm) recording of responses to single VP shock (first trace) and to paired VP shocks separated by 60, 100, 140, and 180 msec. Rebound component (peak latency 150 msec) indicated by arrow on the first trace. See text. Modified from Morin and Steriade (1981).

(Fig. 10; Steriade, 1978; Morin and Steriade, 1981). That the incremental augmenting potential develops simultaneously with a reduced-amplitude primary response was confirmed in an analysis of augmentation in the visual cortex (Ferster and Lindström, 1986).

Since maximal augmentation develops when the second stimulus is delivered at time intervals of 60–120 msec following the first stimulus (see Fig. 9C), i.e., at a time when cortical neurons are in a hyperpolarized state after the initial excitation induced by the first shock, the augmented wave may well reflect a summation of low-threshold rebound spikes (LTS) deinactivated by hyperpolarization (see Chapter 5). In support of this assumption, (1) the second stim-

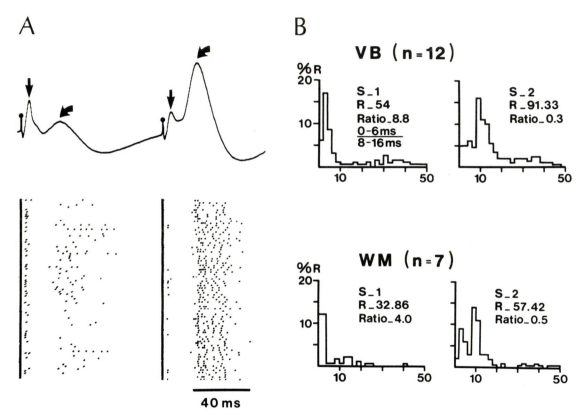

Figure 10. Increased secondary excitation during thalamocortical augmenting responses in *encéphale isolé* cats. A: Neuron recorded from parietal association cortex, simultaneously with focal waves. Two 100-msec delayed shocks applied to the lateral posterior (LP) thalamic nucleus. Top 50 averaged traces of focal waves; bottom, 50-sweep dotgram (each dot represents one action potential). Note that the response to the second shock had decreased amplitude of the early slow depolarizing field potential (right arrows) and, relatedly, decreased probability of firing in the first part of the unitary response, whereas the second depolarizing field potential (oblique arrows) increased in amplitude, and there was an increased number of repetitive discharges. B: Augmentation phenomenon in primary somatosensory (S1) cortex by stimulating at 10/sec the ventrobasal (VB) thalamic complex and the white matter (WM) underlying S1 cortex after destruction of the VB complex. Poststimulus histograms (2-msec bins) of unit discharges pooled on a bin-by-bin basis in a group of 12 VB-driven units and seven WM-driven units. Testing VB and WM stimuli applied at time 0 on the abscissa. S, stimulus number (first stimulus in the train and second stimulus delayed by 100 msec). R, responsiveness (total number of discharges to 100 shocks). Ratios indicate the probability of evoked discharges in the 0–6 msec bins (primary excitation) over the probability of discharges in the 8–16 msec bins (secondary excitation). Modified from Steriade *et al.* (1978) and Steriade and Morin (1981).

ulus in the train fails to elicit an augmenting potential when delivered after the postinhibitory rebound potential induced by the first stimulus (see Fig. 9C) because of the refractory phase of the LTS, and (2) the depth profiles of the rebound component and of the augmented wave are almost identical to and very different from that of the primary thalamocortical component (see Fig. 6 in Morin and Steriade, 1981).

Although inhibitory-rebound phenomena at the thalamic stimulated site may play a role in cortical augmentation, the cerebral cortex has the required circuitry to generate augmenting responses in the absence of the thalamus. This was shown by eliciting augmenting responses in the somatosensory cortex to direct stimulation of radiation axons in preparations with destruction of ventrobasal thalamus (Morin and Steriade, 1981). Similarly, the visual cortex may display augmenting responses by antidromic activation of corticogeniculate axons after destruction of the lateral geniculate nucleus (Ferster and Lindström, 1986).

7.4.2.2. Recruiting Responses

The initial negativity at the cortical surface that distinguishes the recruiting from the augmenting responses arises from the superficial projection over cortical layer I of those thalamic nuclei whose stimulation characteristically induces recruiting. This applies to the three main recruiting systems: (1) the centrolateral–paracentral (CL-PC) rostral intralaminar nuclei (Cunningham and LeVay, 1986), (2) the ventromedial (VM) nucleus (Herkenham, 1979; Glenn et al., 1982), and (3) the ventroanterior (VA) nucleus (Oka et al., 1982). Although CL-PC intralaminar and VM nuclei project diffusely over the cerebral cortex, the projection of VA nucleus is more restricted and primarily directed to the anterior parietal region (cf. Jones, 1985).

The surface negativity of the VM-evoked recruiting response and its superficial (0.25–0.3 mm) reversal, together with the reduction in amplitude of the surface-negative wave by cortical superfusion with manganese, indicated that direct depolarizing actions of VM–cortical axons are exerted on apical dendrites reaching layer I (Glenn et al., 1982). Similar superficial depolarizing actions are postulated for CL–cortical (Foster, 1980; Jibiki et al., 1986) and VA–cortical (Sasaki et al., 1970, 1975; Steriade et al., 1978; Jibiki et al., 1986) recruiting systems.

Obviously, both augmenting and recruiting responses are artificial events, as they are produced by electrical brain stimulation. However, they are useful physiological processes to mimic naturally occurring spindle waves and to investigate their mechanisms in the cerebral cortex.

Indeed, laminar analyses show that augmenting thalamocortical potentials are homologous with type I (surface-positive) cortical spindles, whereas recruiting responses are homologous with type II (surface-negative) spindles (Spencer and Brookhart, 1961b). The mixed pattern of waves within spindle sequences, with both type I and II components, results from afferent connections to cortical areas from multiple thalamic nuclei that project to midlayers IV–III and to the superficial layer I. For example, the parietal association area 5 of cat receives thalamocortical axons from three main nuclei: the lateroposterior (LP) nucleus projecting mainly to midlayers IV–III, the VA nucleus projecting to layer I, and

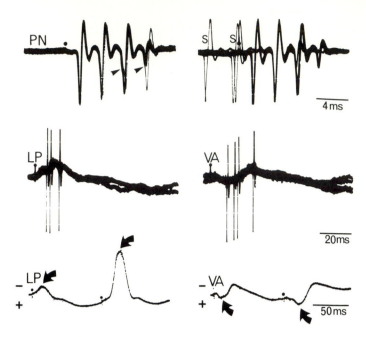

Figure 11. Synaptic excitation of a corticopontine neuron from two thalamic nuclei inducing augmenting and recruiting responses in the parietal association cortex of chronically implanted cat. Top: Antidromic responses of cortical neuron by stimulation of pontine nuclei (PN) with four-shock train (only the first shock is marked by dot). Arrowheads in left superimposition indicate break between initial segment (IS) and somatodendritic (SD) spikes. Right superimposition depicts collisions of responses to the first shock with two spontaneously (S) occurring discharges. Middle: Synaptically evoked discharges of the same neuron by stimulating the lateral posterior (LP) and ventroanterior (VA) thalamic nuclei. Bottom: Fifty averaged sweeps of field potentials evoked by LP and VA thalamic stimulation with two shocks separated by 100 msec. Unit discharges were cut off. Note depth-negative augmenting responses induced by LP stimuli (reflecting the prevalent mid-layer termination of LP–cortical axons) and depth-positive recruiting responses induced by VA stimuli (reflecting the prevalent termination of VA axons in the superficial cortical layers). Modified from Steriade (1978).

the intralaminar CL nucleus projecting to both layers I and VI. In the same corticopontine neuron recorded from cat area 5, LP-evoked discharges are superimposed on augmenting (depth-negative) potentials, whereas VA-evoked discharges are superimposed on recruiting (depth-positive) potentials (Fig. 11; Steriade, 1978).

The similarity between incremental evoked potentials and spindle waves is also clearly demonstrated by their similar alterations under brainstem reticular stimulation and across the natural sleep–waking cycle (see Section 7.5).

7.5. The Blockage of Synchronized Spindle Waves and of Incremental Thalamocortical Responses by Ascending Brainstem Reticular Influxes

It is known that natural arousal or brainstem reticular stimulation readily blocks spontaneous or evoked spindle waves and transforms the oscillatory mode in thalamocortical systems into a relay functional mode, with tonically increased firing rates and enhanced cellular excitability (cf. Steriade and Llinás, 1988). In addition to the two factors represented by the pacemaking reticular (RE) thalamic neurons that generate spindles and some intrinsic properties of thalamocortical neurons that contribute to the patterning of oscillations, spindles appear as a consequence of dampening activities in brainstem reticular neurons with thalamic projections. Midbrain reticular neurons significantly decrease their firing rates during the transitional period from waking to sleep and reliably slow or completely stop their discharges about 1 sec in advance of the first spindle sequence and in repeated transitions from EEG-desynchronized to spindling periods during the drowsiness state (Fig. 12; Steriade, 1980).

In view of the cyclic hyperpolarizations that underlie spindles (see Fig. 3), the occurrence of spindles after the arrest of discharges in brainstem–thalamic neurons may be ascribed to rhythmic hyperpolarizations resulting from disfacilitation processes in the thalamocortical target neurons of brainstem reticular neurons. The excitatory cholinergic brainstem projections to the thalamus are discussed in Chapters 4 and 6. The disfacilitation in the brainstem–thalamic pathways is one of the possible mechanisms, but it only accounts for focal spindles in localized thalamic territories. The generalized spindle rhythmicity is under the control of RE thalamic cells, and the mechanism of diffuse spindle disruption by brainstem ascending influxes, as is the case on natural arousal, should be sought at the very site of spindle genesis, the RE thalamic nucleus. As shown below, the basic mechanism of generalized spindle desynchronization is probably a decoupling in the RE network caused by a cholinergic hyperpolarization of brainstem reticular origin.

The blockage, during natural EEG desynchronization or brainstem reticular stimulation, of spindle-related rhythmic sequences of inhibition and postinhibitory rebound bursts was reported for thalamocortical neurons recorded extra- and intracellularly from the lateral geniculate (LG) (Singer, 1973; Hu *et al.*, 1989a), lateroposterior (LP) (Steriade *et al.*, 1977b), ventrolateral (VL) (Steriade *et al.*, 1971; Steriade, 1984), and intralaminar centrolateral (CL) (Glenn and Steriade, 1982) nuclei. In lightly anesthetized or unanesthetized (brainstem-transected or chronic) preparations, the brainstem-induced blockage of spindle sequences is associated with tonic firing of thalamocortical neurons, which may outlast the stimulation period. Under barbiturate anesthesia, however, spindling is blocked without the occurrence of any tonic discharges in thalamic relay cells, and a single rebound spike terminates the aborted spindle sequence (Fig. 13A,B). It is known that barbiturate anesthesia prevents the direct cholinergic excitation of thalamocortical neurons by brainstem reticular stimulation (see Chapter 6). Thus, the replacement of oscillatory mode by a tonic discharge pattern in thalamocortical neurons occurs in chronically prepared animals or require the use of unanesthetized acute preparations.

The origin of spindle disruption in thalamocortical cells by brainstem reticular stimulation is the blockage of spindles at the site of their generation, the RE nucleus. Short pulse trains to the cholinergic peribrachial (Ch5) cell group at the midbrain–pontine junction prevent the occurrence of spindles in the perigeniculate (PG) sector of the RE nuclear complex or block ongoing spindle sequences (Hu *et al.*, 1989a). The direct peribrachial–PG cholinergic pathway is documented in Fig. 8 of Chapter 4.

As is known, spindle oscillations of RE cells develop on a depolarizing envelope (See Fig. 3). The brainstem peribrachial stimulation induces a large hyperpolarization that blocks the spindles in PG neurons (Fig. 14A). Measurements of conductance changes associated with the hyperpolarizing response of PG neurons showed an increased conductance of about 40–50% (Fig. 14B).

Since the peribrachial-induced hyperpolarization of RE neurons is abolished after administration of the muscarinic blocker scopolamine (see Chapter 6), the main mechanism of the spindling blockage by brainstem reticular stimula-

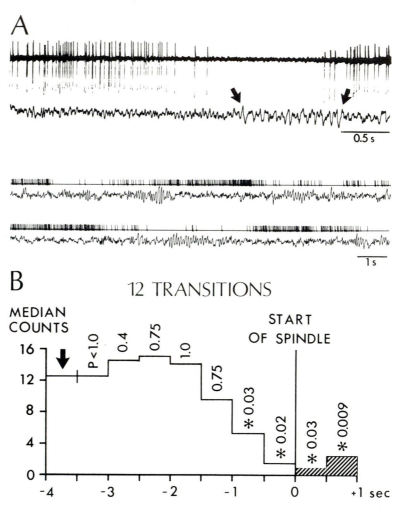

Figure 12. Midbrain reticular formation neuron with antidromically identified projection to the intralaminar thalamus decreases discharge rate in advance of the first spindle sequence during transition from waking (W) to EEG-synchronized sleep (S) in cat. A: Top two traces depict original spikes and EEG waves simultaneously recorded on oscilloscope. First spindle sequence in W–S transition indicated between arrows. Bottom traces: Same activities during repeated EEG desynchronization–synchronization transitions (ink-written recordings). B: Twelve transitions of unit firing with respect to start of EEG spindle (time 0). Arrow at left, level of discharge (median rate) during W; asterisks, bins with significant (<0.05) decrease in firing rate compared with median rate during W. Significantly decreased firing rate occurred 1 sec before spindle onset. Modified from Steriade (1980, 1984).

tion seems to be a cholinergic hyperpolarization. This assumption is further supported by the fact that data similar to those depicted in Fig. 14 were also obtained after amine depletion in reserpine-treated animals (Hu *et al.*, 1989a). The conductance increase associated with the hyperpolarization of RE neurons by brainstem peribrachial cholinergic stimulation is probably mediated by a potassium current, as ACh application *in vitro* hyperpolarizes RE neurons by increasing a potassium conductance (McCormick and Prince, 1986b; see details in Chapter 6).

We dealt in Section 4.2 with the projection from cholinergic and GABAergic basal forebrain neurons to the rostral pole and rostrolateral districts of the RE nucleus and with the projections from brainstem reticular core to basal forebrain neurons. The existence of these circuits indicates that whenever brainstem reticular stimulation is applied, the spindle blockage may arise from an inhibition of spindle genesis in the RE nucleus from the brainstem–RE neurons as well as from the parallel activation of the basal forebrain structures. The latter circuit is not responsible for data reported in the perigeniculate zone of the RE nucleus (see Fig. 14), since there are no basal forebrain projections to that caudal part of the RE nucleus. However, for most dorsal thalamic nuclei that receive powerful projections from the rostral pole and rostrolateral zones of the RE nucleus, one should consider that basal forebrain neurons play a role in spindle blockage. In keeping with this idea, Buzsaki *et al.* (1988) have shown in the rat that chemical lesions of basal forebrain perikarya are followed by a statistically significant increase in the incidence of spindle activity and that a decrease in discharge rates

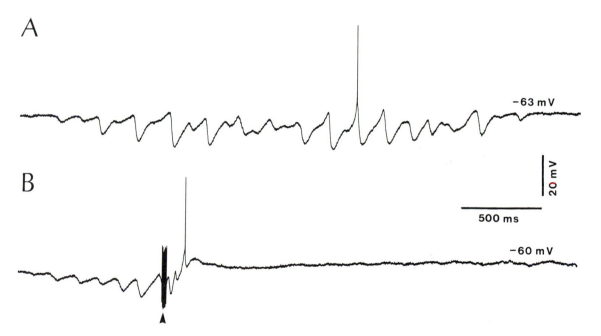

Figure 13. Blockage of spindle oscillations in thalamic relay neuron by stimulating the brainstem peribrachial (PB) area in cat. Intracellular recording from a cell in the dorsal lateral geniculate (LG) nucleus. Resting potential is indicated. A–B: Spontaneous spindle sequence (A) and disruption of a spindle sequence by PB stimulation (arrowhead in B). Modified from Hu *et al.* (1989a).

of basal forebrain neurons is associated with spindle oscillations in thalamocortical systems. These data suggest that a dampening activity in basal forebrain cholinergic and/or GABAergic neurons is a permissive factor for spindle genesis in the RE nucleus and corroborate similar results concerning the actions of thalamically projecting brainstem reticular neurons (see above, Fig 12). The

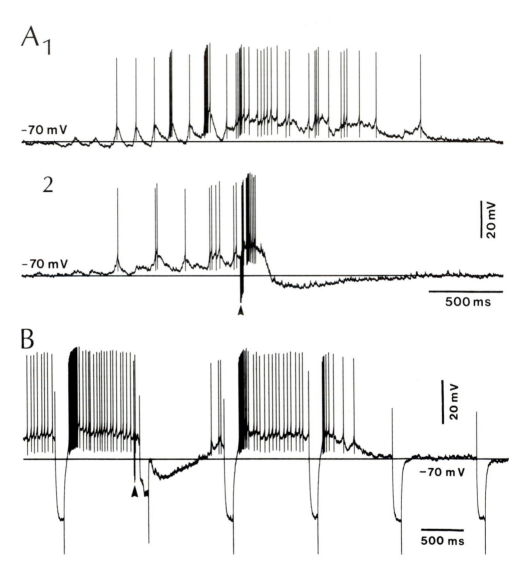

Figure 14. Blockage of spindles at the very site of their genesis, the (RE) thalamic nuclear complex, by brainstem peribrachial (PB) stimulation in cat. Intracellular recordings of two (A and B) neurons from the perigeniculate (PG) sector of the RE nuclear complex. Resting potential is indicted. A: An expanded spindle sequence is shown in 1, and another spindle sequence was aborted by PB stimulation (arrowhead in 2). B: Change in membrane resistance induced by PB stimulation in a PG thalamic cell. Current pulse intensity, 2 nA. In the right part of the trace, a sustained hyperpolarizing current was injected to estimate the amount of anomalous rectification in the conductance change observed during the response. Note that in spite of anomalous rectification, the drop in membrane resistance was of the order of 50%. Modified from Hu *et al.* (1989a).

powerful inhibition exerted by ACh and GABA, the probable synaptic transmitters of basal forebrain neurons with RE projections, are discussed in Chapter 6.

In conclusion then, the blockage of spindle rhythms during EEG desynchronization results from a decoupling in the synaptic networks of RE nucleus by brainstem and basal forebrain axons.

Similarly to the brainstem-induced blockage of spindles, incremental (augmenting and recruiting) thalamocortical responses are blocked during upper brainstem reticular stimulation and are transformed into responses of a primary type. This effect occurs through selective obliteration of the secondary excitatory component, which is typical for the augmentation process (Fig. 15A; Steriade, 1970). The same reduction in the amplitude of augmenting field potentials is observed during behavioral states of wakefulness and REM sleep, both compared with EEG-synchronized sleep (Fig. 15B). The augmented discharges of cortical somatosensory neurons to 10/sec ventrobasal thalamic stimuli consist of spike trains at latencies of 10–20 msec. These discharges are blocked during brainstem reticular stimulation and replaced by primary, single-spike excitation at 2–4 msec (Steriade and Morin, 1981). This transformation results from the brainstem-induced diminution of the long-lasting hyperpolarization in cortical neurons. Consequently, the second stimulus in the 10/sec train is delivered

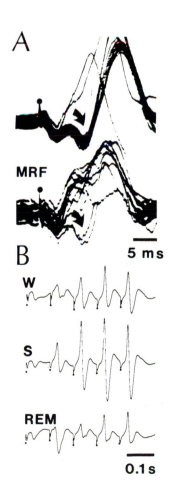

Figure 15. Reduction of augmenting thalamocortical responses during EEG-desynchronized states in cat. A: Superimposed augmenting field potentials evoked at motor cortical surface by 10/sec stimulation of the ventrolateral (VL) thalamic nucleus (oblique arrow points to the augmented component) and dramatic reduction of the augmented component during high-frequency stimulation of the midbrain reticular formation (MRF). B: Augmenting field potentials (50 averaged sweeps) at depth of 0.7 mm in cortical area 5 during 5–10/sec stimulation of lateral posterior (LP) thalamic nucleus during waking (W), EEG-synchronized sleep (S), and EEG-desynchronized sleep (D). A, modified from Steriade (1970); B, modified from Steriade (1981).

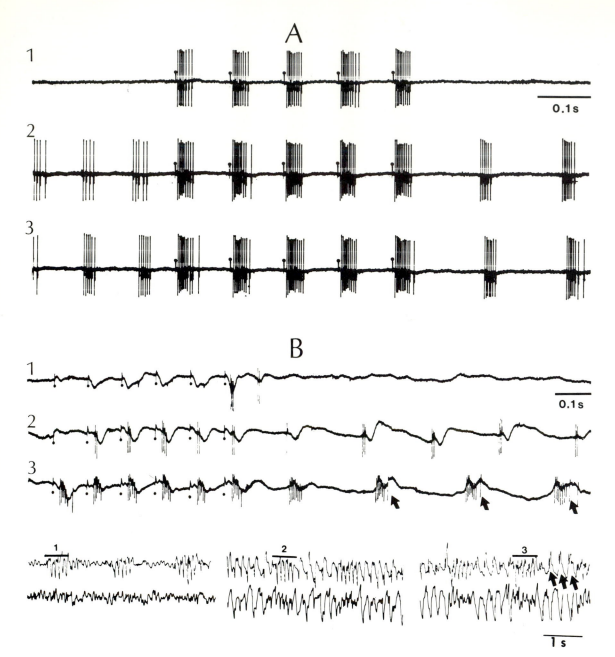

Figure 16. Cortically evoked responses in bursting thalamic neurons of *encéphale isolé* cats, leading to self-sustained spike-and-wave (SW) complexes. A: A ventrolateral (VL) thalamic cell driven by motor cortex stimulation with five shocks at 10/sec (in 1) delivered every 2 sec. Note appearance of "spontaneous" bursts resembling the evoked ones at a late stage of stimulation (in 2 and 3). B: Effects of stimulation of the suprasylvian area 7 with trains of six shocks at 10/sec (as in 1) on a bursting cell recorded from the lateral posterior (LP) thalamic cell. Beginning with the 12th shock train, the cell was regularly driven and displayed self-sustained rhyth- mic bursts at 5/sec between cortical shock-trains. In 3 (28th shock train), self-sustained SW complexes appeared (ar- rows). Below, the two ink-written traces represent focal waves in the LP nucleus recorded by the same micro- electrode used for unit recording (upper trace, negativity upward) and EEG rhythms from the surface of the suprasyl- vian gyrus (bottom trace). Figures (1–3) on the EEG record- ings correspond to the periods of stimulation depicted with the same figures in oscilloscopic recordings. The three SW complexes are indicated by arrows on oscilloscopic trace 3 and EEG recordings. Modified from Steriade *et al.* (1976).

following the completion of the postinhibitory rebound, thus leading to obliteration of the augmenting component because of the refractory phase of the rebound (see details about the common nature of the rebound and the augmented wave in Section 7.4.2.1 and Fig. 9).

Augmenting thalamocortical responses within the frequency range of spindle oscillations may be followed by self-sustained epileptic activity of the spike-and-wave (SW) type (Steriade, 1989). Similar events occur in thalamic neurons by stimulating corticothalamic pathways within the same low-frequency (7–14 Hz) range (Steriade *et al.,* 1976). The appearance of self-sustained SW epileptic activity is related to resonance phenomena in reciprocal thalamocorticothalamic loops, characterized by the occurrence of "spontaneous" burst responses during periods free of stimuli and having the same patterns and frequency as the evoked responses (Fig. 16).

The development of augmenting responses into self-sustained SW epileptic complexes is particularly pronounced during drowsiness in chronically implanted monkey (Steriade, 1974) and periods of EEG synchronization in the *encéphale isolé* preparation (Steriade and Yossif, 1974). This propensity to self-sustained activity during EEG-synchronized epochs is in line with the development from spindling to SW complexes in the feline generalized epilepsy model (cf. Gloor and Fariello, 1988). It was also demonstrated that a time-ordered relationships exists between an increased number of petit-mal attacks with SW complexes in humans and the spindle stage of slow-wave sleep, whereas an abrupt attenuation of SW epileptic activity occurs in those patients on awakening (Kellaway, 1985).

A common mechanism was proposed to account for the obliteration of spindle oscillations, augmenting thalamocortical responses, as well as their consequences, the SW epileptic complexes, on natural arousal or midbrain reticular stimulation (Steriade, 1989). This mechanism is the drastic shortening in duration of the long-lasting hyperpolarization of thalamocortical neurons on brainstem reticular stimulation (see Chapter 8). The consequence for the augmenting responses is that the postinhibitory rebound to the first stimulus in a series of 7–14 Hz is completed with a decreased latency, the second stimulus falls after the completion of the rebound, and cortical augmentation is thus prevented (see Fig. 9C).

8

Brainstem Ascending Systems Controlling Synaptic Transmission of Afferent Signals

We now examine the state dependency of thalamic and cortical neuronal responses to afferent signals and the underlying mechanisms of the enhanced excitability in those neurons during the EEG-desynchronized states of wakefulness and REM sleep compared to EEG-synchronized sleep. Data showing the striking electrophysiological similarities between two behavioral states that were initially considered as two poles of the waking–sleep cycle led to the conclusion that both waking and REM sleep are brain-activated states, notwithstanding great differences in their mental content and despite the fact that central motor commands are blocked at the spinal motoneuronal level during REM sleep. During waking, the increased neuronal responsiveness is associated with an increased efficacy of sculpturing inhibition involved in discriminatory tasks. We examine the control exerted by brainstem ascending systems and their neurotransmitters on both excitatory and inhibitory processes in the thalamus and neocortex. Inhibitory processes have not yet been systematically investigated during REM sleep, and this promising avenue of research may eventually substantiate, at a cellular level, some of the basic psychological differences between the two brain-activated states, otherwise similar from various electrophysiological points of view.

We first discuss the mechanisms of enhanced synaptic excitability in thalamic and cortical neurons to peripheral or central stimuli during the state of generalized arousal. In this context, we examine the direct excitation of thalamocortical cells by brainstem cholinergic and norepinephrinergic systems and the generalized disinhibition of thalamocortical neurons resulting from the inhibition of GABAergic reticular thalamic neurons by brainstem and basal forebrain cholinergic systems (Sections 8.1 and 8.2). Thereafter, we deal with investigations of selective attention from studies using field potentials in humans and unit activities in primates (Section 8.3). Recent data on electrophysiological processes mediated by two GABA receptors are discussed in Section 8.4; these data may explain the blockage of long-lasting cyclic inhibitions on awakening, with preservation of short-range inhibitory processes involved in center–surround antagonism and other feature detection properties of central neurons. The thalamic transfer of the internally generated signals during dreaming sleep is discussed in Chapter 9.

8.1. Generalized Increase in Excitability of Thalamocortical and Corticofugal Neurons

The thalamus is the first station here synaptic transmission is facilitated during diffuse arousal and where blockade of incoming messages occurs from the very onset of drowsiness. This was first shown by recording photically evoked field responses with enhanced amplitudes in the dorsal lateral geniculate (LG) thalamic nucleus during EEG desynchronization produced by midbrain reticular stimulation in spite of no change in responses simultaneously recorded from optic tract fibers (Steriade and Demetrescu, 1960). Subsequent studies, using extra- and intracellularly recorded neuronal responses to peripheral or central stimuli, have confirmed and expanded the notion that an enhanced responsiveness in the thalamus on arousal does not depend on modifications of excitability in prethalamic relays of specific sensory and motor pathways. To a large extent, what goes on in the cerebral cortex depends on fluctuations in thalamic excitability, and minimal increases in thalamic output may generate marked enhancement in cortical responses.

Data presented below derive from experiments employing both peripheral sensory stimulation and electrical stimuli applied to central pathways. Although the latter are abnormally synchronous, they allow analytical investigations of changes in excitability in thalamic neurons (with testing stimuli to prethalamic axons) or in cortical neurons (by stimulating radiation axons), thus avoiding unknown modifications at multiple intercalated synapses, as is the case with natural sensory stimulation.

8.1.1. Two Modes of Spontaneous Firing during EEG-Desynchronized and EEG-Synchronized Behavioral States

The potentiation of synaptic transmission during the two EEG-desynchronized states of waking and REM sleep is associated with a relative depolarization of thalamic and cortical neurons in both states that is reflected in their modes of spontaneous firing. We have discussed in Chapter 5 that the tonic repetitive firing at a relatively depolarized level of membrane potential develops into burst firing when the membrane potential is hyperpolarized (see Figs. 19 and 20 in Section 5.4.2). The burst of thalamic neurons is an intrinsic property of thalamic cells uncovered by the state of hyperpolarization, and the number of spikes within a burst is not related to any feature of an incoming message. In other words, the bursting mode is associated with a low or null transfer function. Conversely, the tonic firing mode during waking and REM sleep allows neurons faithfully to follow quite rapid rates of stimuli and to insure an accurate transfer of incoming messages on their route toward the cerebral cortex.

Hubel (1960) was the first to show the LG thalamic neurons discharge high-frequency spike bursts during EEG-synchronized sleep, a pattern that is not accompanied by similar alterations in the activity of afferent optic tract axons. The independence of bursting firing mode of thalamic neurons on the activity in prethalamic afferents was also shown by unchanged interspike interval distribution of burst discharges in ventrolateral (VL) thalamic neurons after destruction of their input sources, the deep cerebellar nuclei (Steriade *et al.*, 1971). The rhythmic spike bursts of thalamocortical neurons during EEG-synchronized sleep, compared to the tonic firing patterns during waking and EEG-desynchronized sleep, are illustrated in Fig. 1. The spindle-related rhythmicity of these bursts was documented by autocorrelogram analysis (Steriade *et al.*, 1985). The structure of thalamic bursts was quantitatively analyzed in studies of LG (McCarley *et al.*, 1983), intralaminar (Glenn *et al.*, 1982), and other cortically projecting thalamic nuclei (Domich *et al.*, 1986; see details on burst structure in monograph by Steriade *et al.*, 1989b). The LG thalamocortical neurons are hyperpolarized by about 7–10 mV in EEG-synchronized sleep; this is the necessary level to deinactivate the low-threshold spike crowned by high-frequency discharges (see Chapter 5) as was demonstrated in the behaving animal by Hirsch *et al.* (1983).

8.1.2. Evoked Potential Studies

The advantage of using the method of field potentials evoked by central stimuli (Fig. 2) is that one can monitor the magnitude of the incoming volley by measuring the amplitude of the presynaptic (or tract, t) deflection and, thus, ascertain whether changes in the postsynaptic (or relayed, r) components of the response are intrinsic to the explored structure or depend on changes in afferent pathways. In this way, it has been demonstrated that EEG desynchronization elicited by stimulation of the midbrain reticular formation (MRF) or natural awakening from EEG-synchronized sleep is accompanied by an increased amplitude of the monosynaptic thalamic response evoked by prethalamic stimulation, without any measurable change in the presynaptic component (Steriade, 1970; Fig. 2A1,B). The idea that the arousal-related enhancement in thalamic excitability does not depend on activity in prethalamic relays is supported by absence of excitability changes in bulbothalamic somatosensory neurons from sleep to wakefulness (Carli *et al.*, 1967).

The increased thalamic output on arousal results in an increased amplitude of simultaneously recorded cortical responses (Fig. 2A1). However, cortical facilitation is not merely caused by facilitation of synaptic transmission through specific thalamic relays, since a significant potentiation of cortical responses occurs on MRF stimulation even when testing stimuli are applied to the white matter just beneath the recorded cortical area or to deep cortical layers (Steriade, 1969, 1970; Fig. 2A2,3). Since there are virtually no direct MRF–cortical projections in cat (see Section 4.2.1), two intermediate relays of brainstem ascending influxes (other than specific thalamic nuclei) account for the facilitation at the cortical level.

One circuit involves the cholinergic and noncholinergic neurons of the basal forebrain and their widespread cortical projections. Much remains to be done toward the understanding of neurotransmitters and physiological actions in the circuit between the brainstem core and the basal forebrain (Semba *et al.*, 1988). Furthermore, besides some extracellular data reporting excitatory responses of cortical neurons to stimulation of peripallidal and basal forebrain areas (Edstrom and Phillis, 1980), the synaptic actions in this projection and their suppres-

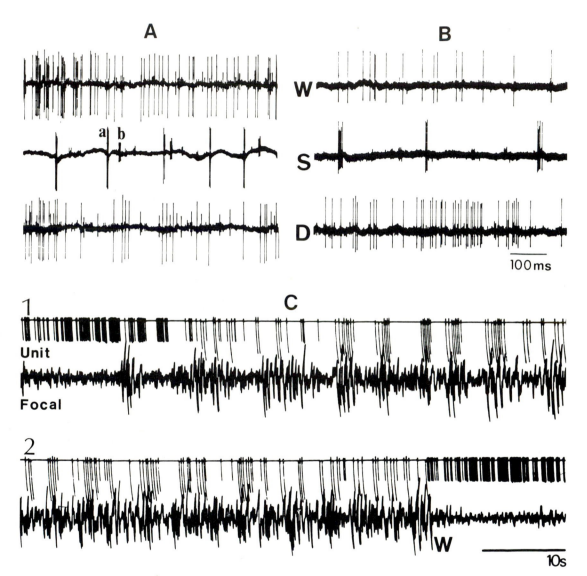

Figure 1. Tonic and bursting firing of thalamocortical neurons during EEG-desynchronized and EEG-synchronized behavioral states in the cat. A and B: Rostral intralaminar CL-PC neurons. Note high-frequency spike bursts in EEG-synchronized sleep (S) and their replacement by sustained discharges in both behavioral states of waking (W) and EEG-desynchronized sleep (D). C: Neuron in the VL thalamic nucleus. Ink-written recording: VL unit spikes were used to deflect a pen of the EEG machine (each deflection exceeding the common level represents a group of high-frequency, >250 Hz, spikes); focal waves simultaneously recorded by the same microelectrode are also depicted. Note close time relation between groups of spike bursts and high-amplitude spindles; EEG desynchronization is associated with tonic firing and increased discharge rates. Modified from (A and B) Steriade and Glenn (1982) and (C) Steriade *et al.* (1971).

sion by various cholinergic antagonists also await elucidation at the intracellular level. What has been investigated is the action of muscarinic and nicotinic blockers on the brainstem-induced potentiation of electrically evoked field responses in the visual cortex. This led to contradictory results. The facilitation of the cortical response to an optic tract stimulus by brainstem reticular stimulation was found unaltered (Bremer and Stoupel, 1959) or blocked (Singer, 1979) by systemic administration of atropine. The blockage could have been exerted either

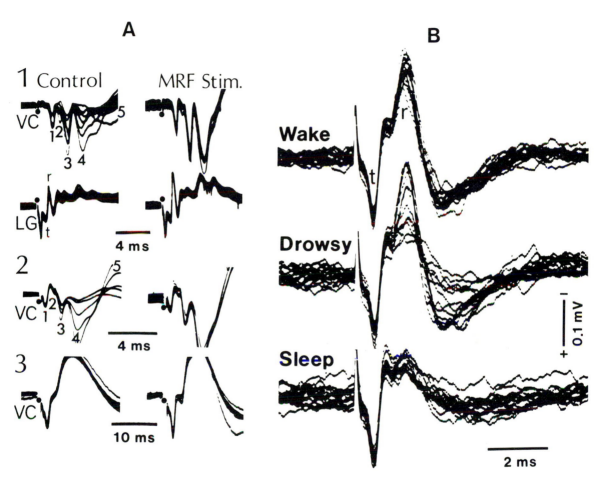

Figure 2. Effects of midbrain reticular formation (MRF) stimulation and natural states of vigilance on thalamic and cortical field responses in cat. A: Evoked potentials in control periods with EEG synchronization (left column) and effects of MRF stimulation (right column). In 1, simultaneous recording of field potentials evoked in the LG thalamic nucleus and at the surface of the visual cortex (VC) by optic tract stimulation. The LG response consists of a presynaptic (tract, t) component and a monosynaptically relayed (r) component. Different components of the VC response are numbered from 1 to 5. Note, during MRF stimulation, enhancement of the monosynaptically relayed LG response without alteration in the presynaptic deflection; also note the increased amplitude of the VC response. In 2 and 3, same MRF-induced potentiation of the VC response with testing stimulation applied to the underlying white matter or to deep layers in the VC, respectively. B: Blockade of synaptic transmission in the thalamus of sleep onset in the chronically implanted behaving cat. Field potentials evoked in the VL thalamic nucleus by stimulation of cerebellothalamic fibers. Note progressively diminished amplitude of monosynaptically relayed (r) wave during drowsiness up to its complete disappearance during EEG-synchronized sleep in spite of lack of changes in the afferent volley monitored by the presynaptic t component. A, modified from Steriade (1970). B, unpublished data.

at the LG thalamic level (see Section 6.1.2.1) or at the cortical level. Adams *et al.* (1988) have reinvestigated this problem by applying testing stimuli for eliciting visual cortex responses to either optic tract (OT) or optic radiation (OR) in order to distinguish between the thalamic and cortical levels of brainstem cholinergic potentiation. Atropine did not alter the facilitation of electrically evoked cortical responses by brainstem reticular stimulation. Mecamylamine, a nicotinic antagonist, reliably reduced the brainstem-induced facilitation of the OT-evoked cortical response by about 50%, and it reduced the brainstem-induced potentiation of the OR-evoked cortical response by 70%. The nicotinic mediation of the cortical cholinergic effect was thus postulated. However, since lesions of intralaminar thalamic nuclei significantly reduced the brainstem-induced potentiation of cortical response (Adams *et al.*, 1988) and an intralaminar thalamic relay of the brainstem-induced cortical potentiation seems demonstrated (see below), it is also possible that mecamylamine acted at the brainstem–thalamic synapses.

The other circuit consists of the excitatory projections from the upper brainstem reticular core to rostral intralaminar thalamic nuclei (Steriade and Glenn, 1982), which, in turn, have excitatory cortical projections (Endo *et al.*, 1977) to large territories, including primary sensory areas (see Fig. 5 of Chapter 2 and Section 4.2.2.4). Indeed, stimulation of intralaminar thalamic nuclei potentiates visual cortex responses (Steriade and Demetrescu, 1960), and lesions of those nuclei reduce the MRF-induced facilitation to no more than 50% of the control values (Adams *et al.*, 1988).

The increased responsiveness in thalamic nuclei and cortical areas is at least as high during REM sleep as during wakefulness, both compared to EEG-synchronized sleep (Steriade *et al.*, 1969).

The field potentials have also been used to investigate, during waking and sleep states, the fluctuations in amplitudes of different components recorded across various cortical layers in monkeys and over the scalp in humans. In monkey, the amplitude of the early surface positivity evoked in the primary somatosensory cortex by a cutaneous stimulation (P1, latency around 12 msec) varies solely as a function of stimulus intensity, whereas the amplitude of the surface negativity (N1) that peaks at a latency of 50 msec predicts the behavioral discrimination response (Kulics *et al.*, 1977; Kulics, 1982). Current-source-density analyses and multiunit activities showed that the excitatory events that characterize the monkey's N1 component during waking are replaced during EEG-synchronized sleep by a period of inhibition, with large current sources through layer III (Cauller and Kulics, 1988). In humans, the early cortically generated components of the somatosensory field potentials (see Section 8.1.3) are indented by multiple fast-frequency (40–50 Hz) potentials that are markedly attenuated or totally disappear when the subject is in stages II to IV of EEG-synchronized sleep; these fast potentials return to waking values in REM sleep (Emerson *et al.*, 1988; Yamada *et al.*, 1988). Although the generation mechanism of fast potentials remains unknown, these data, along with the similar morphology of the somatosensory evoked potentials in neonates during waking and REM sleep (Desmedt *et al.*, 1980), are in line with the demonstrated similarity between waking and REM sleep as far as the electrophysiological processes of the thalamus and cerebral cortex are concerned.

In general, the results of studies using extracellular recordings of thalamic and cortical cells are congruent with those obtained by means of field potentials, discussed above.

The synaptic excitability of cortically projecting neurons recorded from relay and intralaminar thalamic nuclei, tested with central stimuli, is enhanced during both EEG-desynchronized behavioral states of waking and REM sleep as well as during MRF stimulation (Sakakura, 1968; Steriade *et al.*, 1977a,b; Glenn and Steriade, 1982). The state-dependent transfer properties of thalamic neurons have been mainly studied in the LG nucleus by using different forms of visual stimulation. The transfer ratio of an LG cell was determined in "quasi-intracellular" recordings (that allowed estimations of ratios between actions potentials, as output, and "EPSPs," as input) and was found to be twice as high during wakefulness as in EEG-synchronized sleep (Coenen and Vendrik, 1972). During behavioral and EEG signs of wakefulness in the midpontine pretrigeminal preparations, the oscillation of firing rate of LG neurons is a perfect replica of the sine-wave photic stimulation, whereas this relationship disappears during EEG-synchronized sleep even with a threefold increase in the intensity of testing stimulation (Maffei *et al.*, 1965a–c).

The potentiation of thalamic cells' excitability can be elicited by setting into motion two modulatory (cholinergic and norepinephrinergic, NE) systems. The cholinergic nature of the effects induced by stimulating the upper brainstem reticular core was shown by Francesconi *et al.* (1988; see also intracellular data in Section 8.1.4). Stimulation of locus coeruleus was reported to increase the spontaneous firing as well as the responses of LG thalamic cells to optic tract stimulation (Kayama *et al.*, 1982), a response mediated by α-adrenergic receptors (Rogawski and Aghajanian, 1982). Whereas cholinergic excitation was reported in virtually all thalamic nuclei so far investigated, the facilitatory effects of locus coeruleus stimulation and NE application are more controversial. In cat's LG cells, NE iontophoresis resulted in inhibitory effects of 91% of tested LG cells (Pape and Eysel, 1988). Opposite, facilitatory effects were obtained *in vitro* by McCormick and Prince (1988; Section 6.2.5). Locus coeruleus stimulation was also reported to inhibit the spontaneous firing and the evoked responses of ventrolateral thalamic neurons (Rivner and Sutin, 1981).

The increased probability of monosynaptic thalamic responses on arousal or MRF stimulation occurs simultaneously with a decreased probability of spike bursts appearing at a longer (5–12 msec) latency (Filion *et al.*, 1971; Steriade *et al.*, 1971; MacLeod and James, 1984; MacLeod *et al.*, 1984). This change in response pattern is explained by the depolarization of thalamocortical neurons during arousal, a state that inactivates the low-threshold burst response of thalamic cells (see Section 5.4.2).

As also observed with field-potential recordings, the facilitation of antidromically or synaptically evoked cortical discharges on arousal or MRF stimulation (Steriade *et al.*, 1974a) is not merely a result of an enhanced output from thalamic neurons, since the potentiation at cortical level may be observed even when no change is detected in recordings from thalamocortical axons just beneath the cortex (Gücer, 1979) and when testing stimuli are applied to the radiation axons after destruction of the appropriate thalamic nuclei (Steriade and Morin, 1981). The circuits subserving this potentiation that bypasses thalamic relay neurons are discussed in Section 8.1.2).

8.1.4. Intracellular Recordings

Under barbiturate anesthesia, MRF stimulation facilitates the synaptic transmission of the specific afferent inflow through the dorsal lateral geniculate

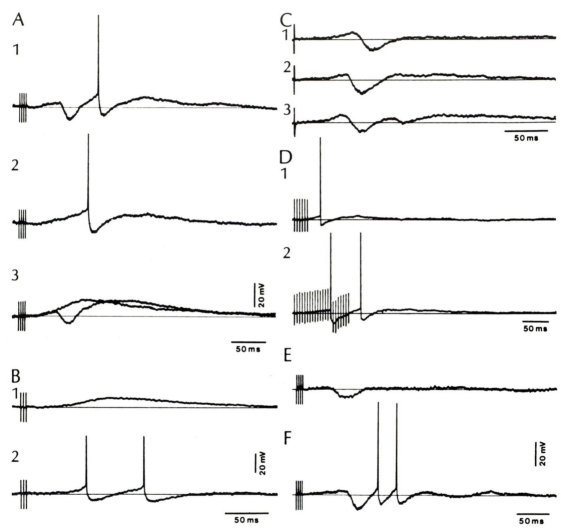

Figure 3. Sample of brainstem PB-evoked responses in LG thalamic relay cells of cat. Intracellular recordings. A: Typical response obtained under urethane anesthesia after reserpine treatment. In A3, the cell was slightly hyperpolarized to prevent spike discharges. Note the all-or-none character of the IPSP. Responses in B and C were recorded from two LG neurons in a reserpine-treated animal with bulbospinal transection and deafferentation of trigeminothalamic pain pathways. Note in C the occasional occurrence of a second IPSP and the shift in latency of the first IPSP. Responses in D were recorded in a deafferented cat without reserpine treatment. Note the smaller amplitude of the response even when a long stimulus train was used (D2). Traces F and F show the responses of two different cells recorded in the same animal under urethane anesthesia. Traces E and F were recorded, respectively, 30 min and 5 hr after reserpine administration. Voltage calibration in F also applies in C, D and E. From Hu *et al.* (1989b).

(LG) thalamic nucleus without, however, exerting direct depolarizing effects on LG cells (Singer, 1973). Singer's (1977, 1979) conclusion was that the brainstem-induced facilitation of synaptic transmission through the thalamus, hypothesized to be cholinergic in nature, occurs exclusively by a global disinhibition of thalamocortical neurons through the inhibition of both reticular (RE) thalamic and local-circuit inhibitory neurons.

It is now known that the excitatory effects of ACh on thalamic relay neurons are extremely sensitive to low doses of barbiturates (see Section 6.1.2.1). On the other hand, brainstem reticular stimulation induces a direct powerful excitation

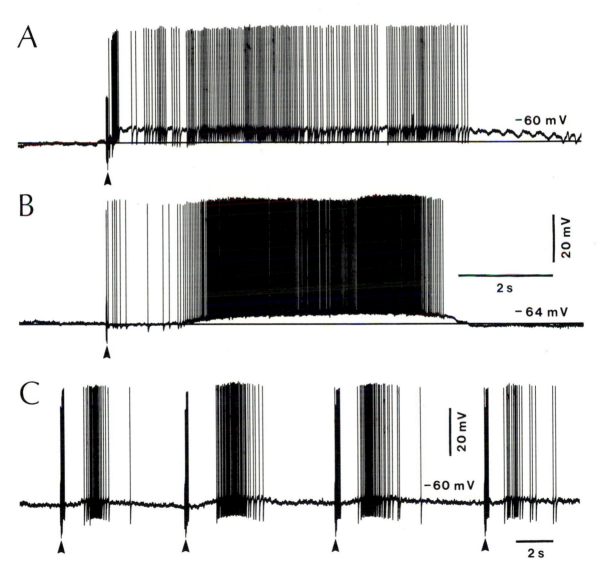

Figure 4. Direct excitation of LG relay neurons of cat by stimulating the brainstem PB area. Intracellular recordings in unanesthetized, brainstem-transected preparations with deafferentation of trigeminothalamic pathways. A and B: A few shocks to the PB area (arrowheads) elicited a short-latency excitation followed by a long-latency (1–1.5 sec) and prolonged (1.5–2.5 sec) excitation. C: A series of successive PB-evoked responses (early and late excitations) at a lower speed. Modified from Steriade and Deschenes (1988).

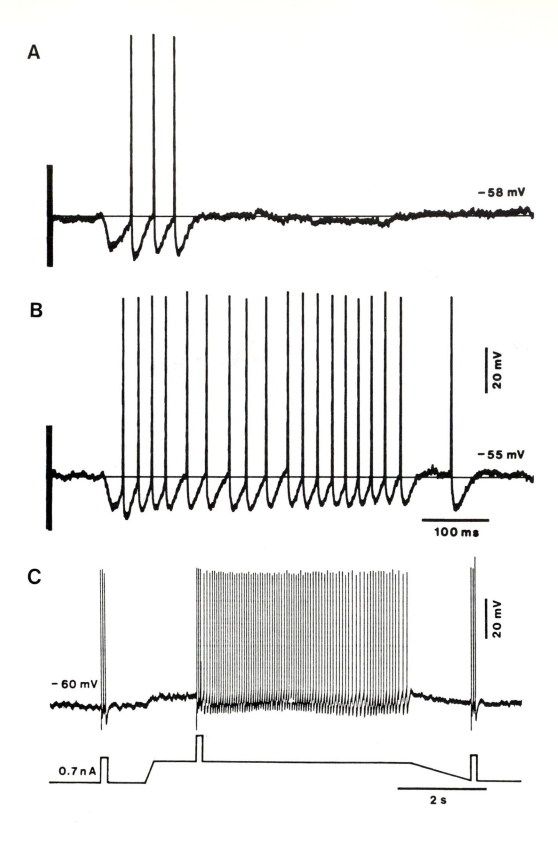

A
−58 mV

B
20 mV

−55 mV

100 ms

C
20 mV

−60 mV

0.7 nA

2 s

of RE thalamic neurons in unanesthetized intact animals (see Section 8.2), and local-circuit inhibitory neurons also seem to be excited by ACh application, as inferred from the analysis of short-term inhibitory processes in relay cells (Sillito *et al.*, 1983; Sillito, 1987; see Section 8.3). These data are hardly reconcilable with the hypothesis of global disinhibition of thalamocortical neurons on brainstem reticular stimulation and arousal.

The effect of stimulating the brainstem cholinergic peribrachial (PB) area (or Ch5 group) on intracellularly recorded LG neurons in unanesthetized cats (brainstem-transected preparations with trigeminal deafferentation) provided evidence for direct excitation of LG thalamic relay neurons from the brainstem reticular core (Hu *et al.*, 1989b; see retrograde transport and immu-nohistochemical data on the cholinergic PB–LG pathway in Section 4.2.2.1). The brainstem-induced excitation is direct, as it was obtained in animals deprived of their retinal and visual cortex inputs.* The coactivation of passing fibers issuing from the locus coeruleus or other monoaminergic cell aggregates was avoided by pretreating the animals with reserpine (in fact, the brainstem–LG depolarization was enhanced after monoamine depletion; see Fig. 3E,F).

Two types of responses are seen in LG relay neurons after brainstem PB stimulation. (1) An early transient depolarization appears with a latency of 20–30 msec, has a duration of 150–300 msec, and is interrupted by a short-duration unitary IPSP (Fig. 3). This response is the intracellular counterpart of the field pontogeniculooccipital (PGO) wave in the thalamus (see Section 8.2). (2) The occurrence of a longer-latency (1–2 sec), long-lasting (2–5 sec) depolarization usually requires more than a single PB stimulus (Fig. 4; Steriade and Deschênes, 1988). The long-lasting depolarization was subsequently detected in other thalamic nuclei and was closely associated with EEG desynchronization (R. Curro Dossi, D. Paré, and M. Steriade, manuscript in preparation).

The late depolarization depicted in Fig. 4 was quite labile, and its nature is not yet completely elucidated. Contrariwise, the constancy of the early de-polarization interrupted by a unitary IPSP allowed a detailed investigation.

At rest (−60 mV), PB stimulation triggers a 5- to 8-mV depolarizing re-sponse, transiently interrupted by an IPSP and giving rise to a few spike dis-charges (Fig. 5A). The same stimulation leads to long periods of tonic discharges when the membrane potential is kept slightly depolarized (Fig. 5B). This pro-longed activation reflects a voltage-dependent inward current (probably the persistent sodium current described in thalamic neurons; see Section 5.4.1),

---

*It was also reported (Kayama *et al.*, 1986b) that the rate of spontaneous discharges of LG thalamic relay cells increases on repetitive stimulation of the cholinergic laterodorsal tegmental nucleus (Ch6 group). However, long latency of the response (0.2–1 sec) and the fact that visual cortex was not ablated cast doubt about a direct brainstem–LG effect in those experiments. Intracellular data (Hu *et al.*, 1989b) reported above show that the brainstem–LG depolarizing response occurs with a latency of about 20 msec.

Figure 5. Effect of subthreshold depolarizing currents on brainstem PB-evoked responses of LG thalamic neurons of cat. Same neuron from A to C, recorded in a nonreserpinized animal under urethane anesthesia. The control response in A was transformed into a longer-duration tonic bar-rage (B) by a subthreshold outward current of 0.4 nA. Tonic discharges appear to result from the activation of a persistent inward current since they could also be generated by short-duration current pulses when the membrane potential was set just below the spike trigger level (in C). From Hu *et al.* (1989b).

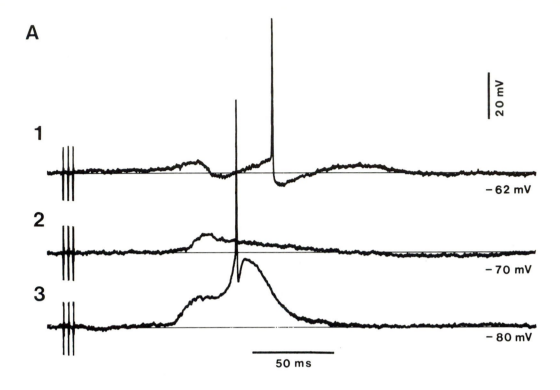

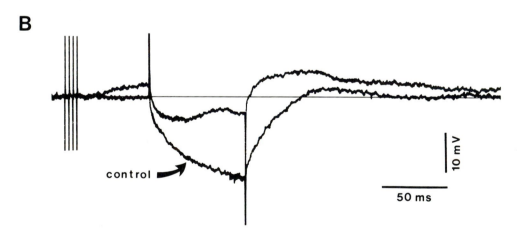

Figure 6. Brainstem PB-evoked response in intracellularly recorded LG thalamic neurons of reserpine-treated cat under urethane anesthesia. A: Effect of membrane hyperpolarization. At rest, the response consisted of a slow depolarization interrupted by an IPSP, which was followed by a single spike discharge. On hyperpolarization, the depolarizing component increased, the IPSP amplitude decreased, and a delayed low-threshold spike was triggered. B: Increase in membrane conductance during the PB-evoked response in another LG cell. Modified from Hu *et al.* (1989b).

since current pulse injections produce similar protracted firing when delivered on a background of slight depolarization (Fig. 5C).

The amplitude of the depolarization and its rate of rise increase with membrane hyperpolarization, eventually triggering a low-threshold rebound spike when the membrane potential is sufficiently negative (Fig. 6A). The early depolarization is associated with a marked drop in input resistance (Fig. 6B). This conductance change is similar to that associated with the fast nicotinic excitation observed with ACh application on cat LG neurons *in vitro* (see Section 6.1.2.1).

The IPSP that interrupts the early depolarization is a chloride-mediated event, and the reversed response by chloride injection is made by a series of depolarizing wavelets, suggesting that a bursting element is at the origin of the IPSP (Hu *et al.*, 1989b). Since in these acute experimental conditions, the brainstem-evoked early depolarization of GABAergic perigeniculate (PG) neurons does not usually lead to spike discharges (see Section 8.2), it is postulated that the short-duration IPSP evoked in LG relay cells by PB stimulation originates in GABAergic intra-LG elements, activated in parallel by the cholinergic brainstem–LG projection.

The conclusion of this work (Hu *et al.*, 1989b) is that a nicotinic excitation underlies the early response of LG thalamocortical neurons to brainstem PB stimulation and that a parallel activation affects at least one category of LG local interneurons (see Section 8.4). It must be emphasized, however, that other transmitters or modulators are colocalized in cholinergic brainstem reticular neurons and that the identification of the role of all these substances in synaptic transmission is impossible at this time, since there are no tools to decipher their individual actions and their competitive or synergistic interactions. Suffice it to mention that the late and very prolonged excitation in LG relay cells depicted in Fig. 4 may well be caused by the action of peptides that were found in brainstem cholinergic neurons by Vincent *et al.* (1983, 1986).

8.2. The Dual Response of Reticular Thalamic Neurons

High-frequency stimulation of rostral brainstem reticular formation in acutely prepared animals under different anesthetics depresses the spontaneous firing and evoked discharges of reticular (RE) thalamic neurons (Schlag and Waszak, 1971; Yingling and Skinner, 1975, 1977; Dingledine and Kelly, 1977). The brainstem-induced blockade of RE-cell activities was interpreted as a cholinergic effect, as ACh application results in a powerful hyperpolarization of RE cells (see Section 6.1.2.3). However, large applications of atropine are ineffective against the early phase of the brainstem-induced inhibition of RE neurons and weakly antagonize only a late phase of inhibition (Dingledine and Kelly, 1977).

In unanesthetized behaving animals recorded in chronic experiments, brainstem reticular stimulation was applied in the rostral midbrain or in the PB area of the pedunculopontine nucleus after chronic bilateral lesions of locus coeruleus to allow anterograde degeneration of axons passing through the stimulated focus (Steriade *et al.*, 1986). In those conditions, brainstem reticular stimulation induces a short-latency (5–10 msec) excitation, followed by a longer period of suppressed firing, in neurons recorded from the rostral pole and

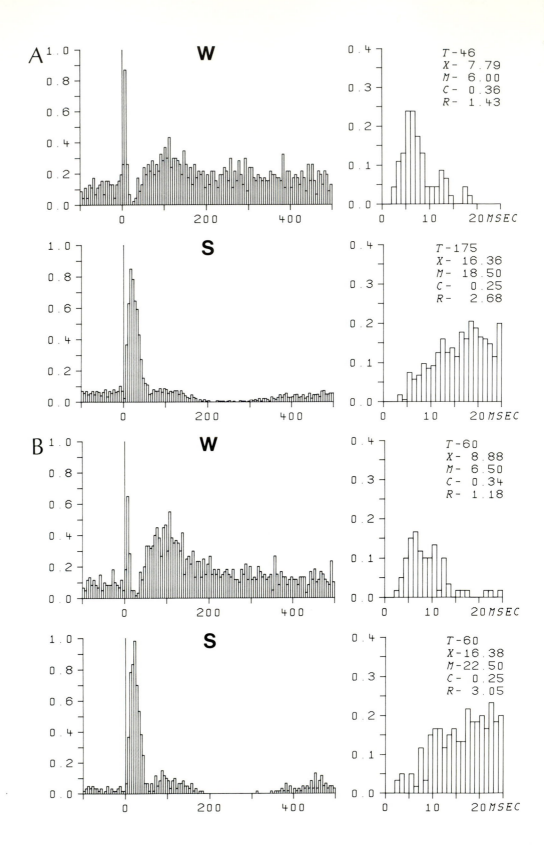

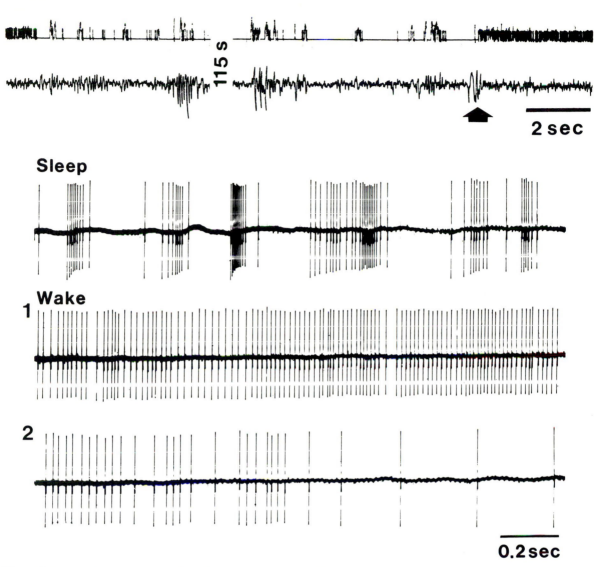

115 s

2 sec

Sleep

Wake

1

2

0.2 sec

Figure 8. Increased firing rates of RE thalamic neurons on natural arousal in chronically implanted cat. Top: Ink-written recording (unit firing and EEG waves; arrow points to arousal). Below: Oscilloscopic recordings display typical RE cell's barrages during EEG-synchronized sleep and tonic firing at onset of awakening (1) and toward the end of waking state, just before the appearance of EEG synchronization (2). Modified from Steriade *et al.* (1986).

Figure 7. Short-latency excitation followed by firing suppression, elicited by brainstem reticular (PB) stimulation in rostral RE thalamic neurons of cat after chronic bilateral lesions of locus coeruleus. See histology of locus coeruleus lesions in Steriade *et al.* (1986). Extracellular recordings in chronically implanted, behaving preparation. In both (A and B) neurons, two 3-msec-delayed shocks were applied at time 0 (stimulus artifacts deleted from peristimulus histograms, PSHs). For both neurons, two PSHs are depicted in behavioral states of waking (W) and EEG-synchronized sleep (S): left PSH with 5-msec bins; right PSH with 1-msec bins. Symbols: *T*, number of trials; *X*, mean latency (in msec); *M*, latency mode; *C*, coefficient of variation; *R*, sum of all bin responsiveness. Description in text. From Steriade *et al.* (1986).

rostrolateral districts of the RE nuclear complex. Both components of the response are state dependent (Fig. 7). During wakefulness, the latencies of short bursts of RE neurons are grouped between 5 and 10 msec, with modes around 6 msec; a secondary excitation occurs between 50 and 150 msec. During EEG-synchronized sleep, the latency mode of the early excitation lengthens to 15–20 msec, and the duration of the evoked burst increases, reaching 50 msec. The histograms of Fig. 7 suggest that the underlying EPSPs have a much shorter rise time and duration during waking than during EEG-synchronized sleep. The period of suppressed neuronal firing is much longer during sleep than during wakefulness. The initially excitatory effects of brainstem reticular stimulation on RE thalamic cells are consistent with the tonically increased firing rates of the same neurons on arousal from quiet sleep (Fig. 8; Steriade *et al.*, 1986).

The two components, excitatory and inhibitory, of the RE-cell response to brainstem reticular PB stimulation were further substantiated in intracellular recordings from the rostral pole and the perigeniculate (PG) sectors of the RE nucleus (Hu *et al.*, 1989a).

The depolarizing response started at a latency of 8–10 msec, lasted up to 200 msec, and was followed by a long-lasting hyperpolarization (Fig. 9). The early brainstem-evoked depolarization can be considered a direct excitatory effect on rostral RE or PG neurons. The following experimental precautions were taken to ensure that the early depolarization was not caused by costimulation of noradrenergic fibers coursing through the stimulated brainstem focus, that it was not transmitted by prior excitation of LG relay cells or other thalamocortical cells, and that it was not relayed by corticofugal pathways projecting to various sectors of the RE nuclear complex. Our experiments (Hu *et al.*, 1989a) were conducted on reserpine-treated animals with cortical ablation, and the direct depolarization of rostral RE or PG cells was also obtained under barbiturate anesthesia (see Fig. 9B,C), a condition that is known to block the brainstem-induced excitation of thalamic relay neurons (see Section 8.1.4). In addition, the latency of brainstem–PG depolarizing response was shorter (8–10 msec) than that (>20 msec) of the brainstem–LG excitation.

The amplitude of the hyperpolarizing response decreased with hyperpolarizing current injections or when the cell hyperpolarized spontaneously (Fig. 9C), and was associated with a conductance increase of the order of 40–50% (see Fig. 14B in Section 7.5). The cholinergic nature of this component was demonstrated by its abolition after scopolamine administration, a condition that prolonged the early depolarization and led to repetitive discharges (Fig. 10).

Figure 9. Effects of brainstem peribrachial (PB) stimulation on intracellularly recorded reticular (RE) thalamic neurons in the cat. A: Unanesthetized deafferented preparation. Three PB shocks evoked a series of fast depolarizations followed by a long period of hyperpolarization. B: Cell recorded under barbiturate anesthesia in the rostral part of the RE nucleus. The response to PB stimulation was also characterized by a depolarizing–hyperpolarizing sequence. Note, however, the shorter duration of the depolarizing envelope. The right-hand inserts show in greater detail the early part of the response evoked in each cell. C: Effect of membrane potential on the PB-evoked hyperpolarization in perigeniculate (PG) neurons. Cell recorded under barbiturate anesthesia. In C1, the cell displayed a depolarizing shift of its membrane potential during a spindle sequence. The membrane potential was hyperpolarized to −70 mV by a long PB pulse train. During the interspindle lull (in C2), when the membrane potential was already at −70 mV, no net hyperpolarization resulted after the PB stimulation; note the plateauing of the PB-evoked depolarization during the pulse train. Modified from Hu *et al.* (1989a).

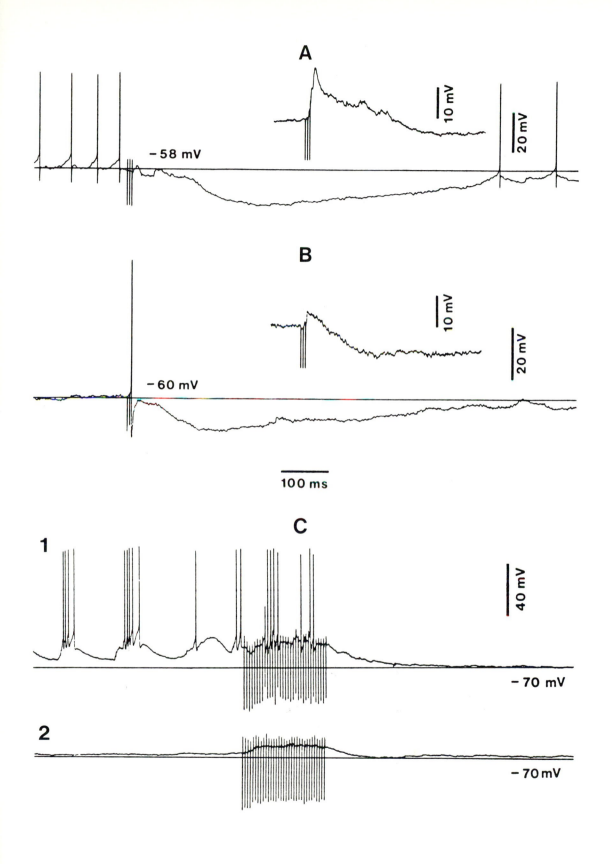

A

− 58 mV

10 mV

20 mV

B

10 mV

20 mV

− 60 mV

100 ms

C

1

40 mV

− 70 mV

2

− 70 mV

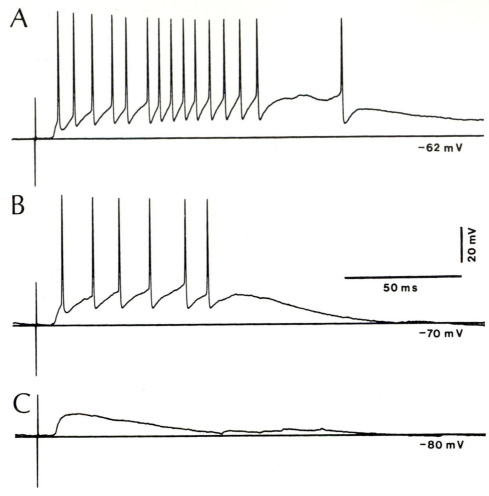

Figure 10. Absence of brainstem PB-evoked hyperpolarization in a rostral reticular (RE) thalamic neuron recorded under barbiturate anesthesia after i.v. injection of scopolamine (1 mg/kg). After scopolamine, the PB stimulus triggered a prolonged burst (A), which was eventually reduced to a subthreshold EPSP by hyperpolarizing the cell membrane (B, C). From Hu *et al.* (1989a).

The above results (Steriade *et al.*, 1986; Hu *et al.*, 1989a) indicate that brainstem reticular stimulation induces a dual response in rostral RE and PG thalamic neurons. Both excitatory and inhibitory components of the response sequence are dependent on the behavioral state (see Fig. 7), and both are direct. This is shown for the excitatory component by its latency (8–10 msec), which fits with the slow conduction velocities of PB–PG axons (Ahlsén, 1984). The hyperpolarization is also direct and starts almost simultaneously with the depolarization. This is indicated by PB-induced depression of PG cells' burst discharges evoked by optic tract stimulation, even when the optic tract stimulus is delivered during the PB-evoked early depolarization (Fig. 11; Hu *et al.*, 1989a). This result strongly suggests that the mechanism of PB inhibition in PG or other RE thalamic cells involves a large drop in membrane input resistance that renders those neurons transparent to synaptic currents.

Whereas the hyperpolarization depends on muscarinic receptors, as it is abolished by scopolamine, the nature of the early excitation remains to be elucidated. It may be induced by an unknown transmitter colocalized in brainstem cholinergic cells, or it may be mediated by a nicotinic receptor. The failure to observe a nicotinic response in RE neurons maintained *in vitro* (McCormick and Prince, 1986a) could well be attributed to the mode of ACh application leading to a rapid desensitization of the response. Nicotinic receptors have been mapped within the RE thalamic nucleus of monkeys (Jones, 1985) and rats (Clarke *et al.*, 1985).

The difference between the two types of experiments, one conducted in behaving animals (Steriade *et al.*, 1986) and the other under acute experimental conditions with anesthetics or with brainstem transection and trigeminal deafferentation (Hu *et al.*, 1989a), is that in the latter studies the brainstem-induced early depolarization does not induce tonic firing in RE thalamic neurons. Most likely, this is ascribable to the difference in the level of membrane polarization between an anesthetized/deafferented preparation and an intact unanesthetized animal. The dramatic increase in tonic discharges of RE neurons on arousal from sleep (see Fig. 8) results from the depolarizing pressure exerted by thalamo-RE and cortico-RE neurons that discharge tonically in an intact vigilant animal and thus create favorable conditions for overwhelming the concomitant inhibition arising in the cholinergic neurons of the brainstem core. These conditions result in an increased spontaneous and evoked firing of RE cells, as is the case during natural awakening (Steriade *et al.*, 1986).

Until the recent discovery that brainstem reticular neurons with ascending axons (but yet undetermined transmitters) directly excite RE thalamic neurons, only the second part of the dual brainstem–RE response (namely, the long-lasting hyperpolarization of RE cells) was taken into consideration. The brainstem-induced cholinergic inhibitory effect on GABAergic RE neurons was commonly regarded as the basis of generalized disinhibition of thalamocortical neurons on arousal. Such an interpretation obviously reflects only one aspect of the more complex reality. Indeed, since RE thalamic neurons discharge quite rapidly and are highly responsive to brainstem and cortical volleys during waking (Steriade *et al.*, 1986), the parallel increase in spontaneous firing rates and synaptic excitability of both RE neurons and their presumed inhibited targets, the thalamocortical neurons, raises difficult questions that remain to be answered. The suggestion that, on arousal, RE-induced inhibition of thalamocortical cells may be overwhelmed by disinhibition (via inhibitory contacts between RE and local-circuit inhibitory neurons) was substantiated by the occurrence of very numerous and short IPSPs in thalamocortical neurons following disconnection from the RE nucleus (Steriade *et al.*, 1985). Although such a disinhibition would increase the transfer ratio in thalamocortical neurons, it would also deprive them of local-circuit inhibitory cells subserving discrimination tasks. This aspect was not yet elucidated. We discuss in Section 8.4 the basic circuits of inhibitory processes in the thalamus and suggest some possibilities that await experimental testing.

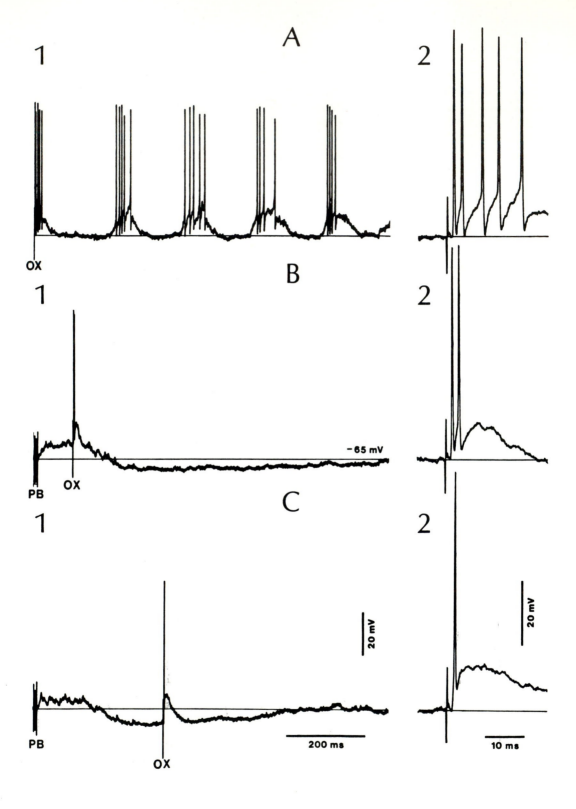

8.3. Selective Increase in Cortical Excitability during Attentional Tasks

The above two sections (Sections 8.1 and 8.2) dealt with the diffuse excitability enhancement in thalamic and cortical neurons during both EEG-desynchronized states of waking and REM sleep. In those studies, the term "waking" state was used rather globally, since experimental animals were not submitted to tests of selective attention. We now briefly turn to investigations using scalp-recorded evoked potentials in humans and extracellular unit recordings in monkeys that employed sophisticated experimental paradigms to distinguish focused attention from diffuse arousal.

8.3.1. Event-Related Potentials in Humans

A warning stimulus gives rise to a slow negative shift recorded from the scalp, termed *expectancy wave* or *contingent negative variation* (CNV; Walter *et al.*, 1964), which is followed by an imperative stimulus that evokes an event-related potential (ERP). The amplitude of CNV increases when more attention is required or when there is greater incentive for prompt action (cf. Hillyard and Picton, 1987, for a review). The CNV was thought to originate in diffusely projecting brainstem systems, and a corticofugal feedback control was hypothesized to suppress irrelevant response tendencies (Lang *et al.*, 1983). The ERP consists of various subcortically and cortically generated components whose latencies signal the arrival of input through different relays and may differ from one sensory modality to another.

The early components of peripherally elicited ERPs, up to a latency of 20 msec, reflect far-field events originating in the spinal cord, brainstem, and thalamic nuclei. For example, in the somatosensory system, all components of the ERP up to and including P14 (a scalp-recorded positive wave with 14-msec peak latency) are believed to be generated below the thalamus (Fig. 12A; Desmedt and Bourguet, 1985) because wave P14 can be recorded in patients with thalamic lesions (Mauguière and Courjon, 1983). Cortically generated components begin with N20, which occurs over the parietal scalp contralateral to the stimulus, and P22, which appears in the prerolandic field (Desmedt and Bourguet, 1985). It seems that subcortically generated potentials in the somatosensory and auditory modalities do not vary with the attentional state (Picton *et al.*, 1977, 1978; Schulman-Galambos and Galambos, 1979; Desmedt, 1981). It is, however, possible that the absence of changes in components that precede the entry of the afferent volley in the cerebral cortex reflects difficulties in recording discrete alterations of distant events over the scalp. Future investigations by

Figure 11. Decreased responsiveness of RE thalamic neuron after a conditioning brainstem PB stimulation in cat. Intracellular recording of a PG cell under urethane anesthesia. The control response to optic chiasm (OX) stimulation is shown in A1. The first part of the response is expanded in A2. In B and C, the same OX stimulus was delivered at different intervals after a short PB pulse train. The respective responses are depicted in B2 and C2. Note that the cell responsiveness to OX stimulus was already decreased in B during the early depolarization induced by PB stimulation. From Hu *et al.* (1989a).

A

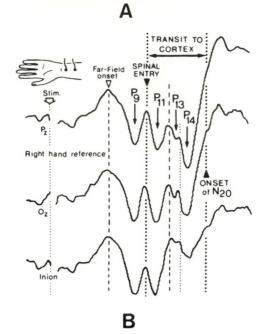

B

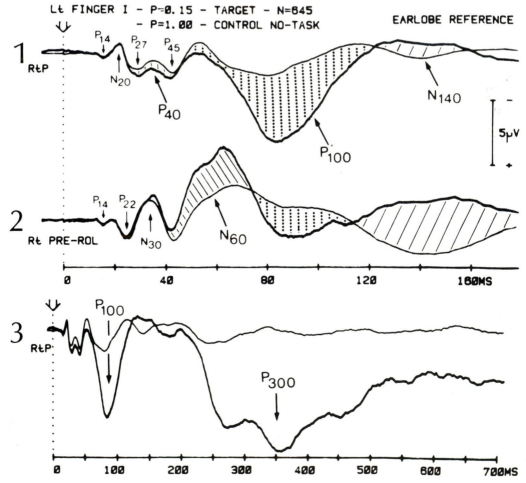

means of deep electrodes should explore the possibility that thalamic neurons are capable of discriminatory processes.

The cortically generated components of ERPs are enhanced during selective attention tasks. Desmedt *et al.* (1983) investigated subjects who were instructed to attend an infrequent somesthetic stimulus (for example, to the left thumb) designated as target and to press a button as quickly as possible (with the right index finger) for each such target. In such conditions, ERP changes consist of increased amplitudes of waves P40, N60, and especially P100 and P300 (Fig. 12B). Whereas P40 and N60 are confined to the contralateral parietal and prerolandic areas, respectively, P100 is distributed bilaterally with a contralateral predominance, and P300 is a generalized event like the CNV. Desmedt and his colleagues propose that P40 and N60 are the signs of "priming" for infrequent signals, that P100 is the electrical index for identification of input signals, and that P300 reflects a nonspecific postdecision closure related to the diffuse control of brainstem modulatory systems on the telencephalon. The changes in auditory ERPs with selective attention are fully summarized in Hillyard and Picton (1987).

The understanding of mechanisms underlying the amplitude fluctuations of ERP components while attending a stimulus or not will probably come with animal models of ERPs that would allow combined field potential and unit analyses in cortical and thalamic structures. Attempts at identifying the homologues of P300 wave were made in squirrel monkey (Neville and Foote, 1984; Pineda *et al.*, 1988) and macaques (Arthur and Starr, 1984). Although the significance of P300 is still debated, earlier attention-sensitive components, such as N170, were found to be similarly enhanced in unitary neuronal recordings in monkeys (Wurtz *et al.*, 1980) and in human ERPs (Galambos and Hillyard, 1981; Fig. 13).

8.3.2. Neuronal Recordings during Set-Dependent Tasks in Monkeys

Hebb's (1972) model of set includes the possibility of different responses to an identical sensory stimulus, depending on prior instructions. It is generally

---

Figure 12. Cognitive components of somatosensory evoked potentials (SEPs) in humans. A: Far-field SEPs. Stimulation of the left median nerve indicated by the vertical dotted line at left. Negativity upward. Active electrode at the parietal midline (Pz), occipital midline (Oz), and 2 cm above the inion. Onset of first far-field potential indicated by white arrowhead and vertical interrupted line. B: SEPs to electrical stimuli delivered to the left thumb. The thicker SEP traces were averaged in runs when the thumb stimuli are infrequent ($P = 0.15$) targets to which the subject has to respond by pressing a microswitch with the right index finger. Thicker traces were obtained by redrawing the same trace three times. These SEPs are superimposed on control SEPs averaged in other runs of the same experiment when identical thumb stimuli were delivered alone ($P = 1.0$) at the same intervals and not mixed with any other stimuli. 1: Right parietal scalp derivation. 2: Right prerolandic scalp derivation. 3: Same trace as 1 displayed on a lower time base. The vertical dotted line on the left side indicates the time of delivery of the thumb stimulus. The small arrows identify standard early SEP components, namely, the P14 far-field, the parietal N20–P27–P45, and the prerolandic P22–N30. Cognitive components identified through divergence of the superimposed traces are indicated by the following symbols: P40 (vertical lines), N60 (oblique lines), P100 (vertical rows of dots), N140 (widely spaced oblique lines). Vertical calibration, 5 μV. Horizontal calibration in milliseconds. Negativity of the active scalp electrode registers upward in all traces. Modified from Desmedt *et al.* (1983) and Desmedt and Bourguet (1985).

assumed that the site of this behavioral flexibility is the cerebral cortex, which would explain why cellular studies are overwhelmingly conducted in the cerebral cortex of monkeys. The cerebral cortex is probably not the unique site of flexible decisions, and this should be further assessed. Various methods used to study the switching mechanisms involved in the flexible control of input–output information processes are described in Evarts *et al.* (1984).

In general, the macaque receives an instruction consisting of a sensory cue (relevant stimuli are differentiated from irrelevant ones) signaling what type of motor response must be executed after a waiting period in order to receive a reward. It must be noted that usually cortical neurons are recorded without precise knowledge of their direct inputs and targets, as one could ascertain by standard electrophysiological procedures of monosynaptic and antidromic activation. Notable exceptions are Evarts and his colleagues (Evarts and Tanji, 1976; Tanji and Evarts, 1976), who have recorded identified pyramidal tract (PT) neurons in the primary motor cortex. Instructions to push or pull a handle elicited increases or decreases in activity of the same PT cell; and when the monkey responded incorrectly, the neuronal activity corresponded to the animal's motor preparation rather than the sensory nature of the instructive stim-

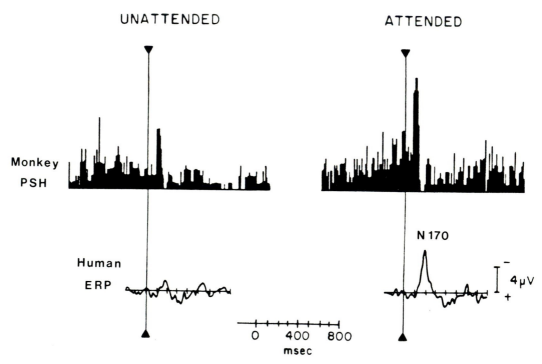

Figure 13. Effects of visual attention on unit activity in posterior parietal cortex of a rhesus monkey and on event-related potentials (ERPs) recorded from the parietal scalp in a human subject. Two peristimulus histograms (PSHs) are depicted in the monkey experiment, comparing conditions when the testing flash of light was not attended and when it was attended. Note similar modulation of flash-evoked activity with similar enhancement when testing stimulus was attended in the two species. Monkey experiment from Wurtz *et al.* (1980). Human experiment from Galambos and Hillyard (1981).

ulus (Fig. 14A). Similar conclusions, namely, that activity changes are specifically related to the state of motor preparation, were drawn from studies on premotor cortical neurons (Fig. 14B; Wise *et al.*, 1983).

The differentiation between the effects of diffuse activation and those of selective attention leading to initiation of movements was emphasized in studies of primary visual and posterior parietal cortices (see Mountcastle *et al.*, 1984; Wurtz *et al.*, 1984). In the primary visual cortex, neurons increase their firing rates by diffuse arousal but not by selective attention (Wurtz and Mohler, 1976).

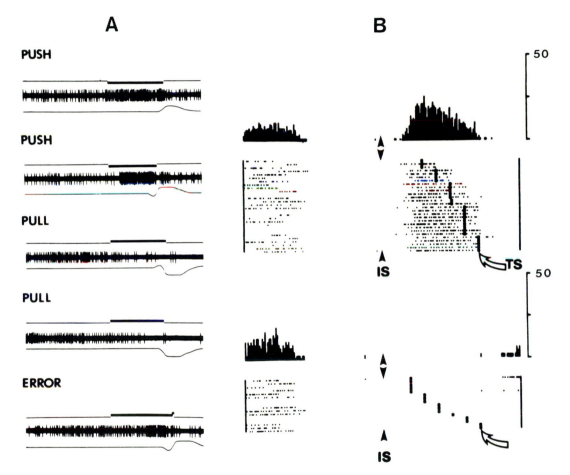

Figure 14. Set-related neuronal activity in primary motor (A) and premotor (B) cortices of monkey. A: Time of instruction presentation is indicted by the thickening of the horizontal bar above each electrode trace; the instruction delivered is indicated above each trace. Below each electrode trace is an indication of the animals' arm position. Push instructions lead to increases in activity, and pull instructions lead to decreases. Note that in the bottom record the monkey responds incorrectly (he was instructed to pull but instead pushed the handle) and in this case the activity re- sembles other trials in which the monkey ultimately pushes the handle. Thus, the activity appears to reflect the animal's (inferred) motor set regardless of the instruction. B, top: Trials in which the monkey is instructed (IS) to make an arm movement in a certain direction and later is given a trigger- ing stimulus (TS) that allows him to execute the movement. In the bottom raster and histogram, the same cell shows no activity when an identical visual stimulus instructs him to withhold movement. Modified from Tanji and Evarts (1976, A) and from Wise *et al.* (1983, B).

This fact suggested that striate cortical cells are not committed in a given circuit but are used for subsequent processing stages (Wurtz *et al.*, 1984), such as those involving the posterior parietal cortex and frontal eye fields, where saccadic movements are initiated. Mountcastle *et al.* (1981) used three types of behavioral conditions in their studies on light-sensitive neurons recorded from the posterior parietal cortex; (1) a no-trial state, that is, a state of quiet waking with no involvement in a behavioral task; (2) a trial state, that is, a condition of attentive fixation of a target during which the monkey is engaged in a dimming detection task; and (3) an intertrial mode, which alternates with the trial mode. The light-sensitive neurons of the posterior parietal cortex significantly increase their excitability in the trial mode compared to both no-trial mode and the intertrial state, with the conclusion that the enhanced synaptic excitability is specifically related to the directed visual attention to the target light and is not merely related to changes in generalized arousal.

8.4. Two Inhibitory Phases in Thalamic and Cortical Neurons and Their Differential Alterations during Brain-Activated States

However efficiently brainstem reticular stimulation and natural arousal obliterate the *long-lasting* phase of inhibition and its cyclic repetition, these conditions do not eliminate the early *short-lasting* period of inhibition during which spontaneous and evoked discharges are suppressed. This statement (Steriade *et al.*, 1977b) was based on extracellular recordings of thalamocortical neurons in the lateral posterior nucleus. Since that time, this notion was expanded at the intracellular level.

The emphasis on a differential action exerted by brainstem reticular arousing systems on the two phases of thalamic inhibitory processes is of importance since, during the 1960s, arousal was regarded as an "inhibition of inhibition" (Purpura *et al.*, 1966), and until quite recently activation phenomena elicited by brainstem reticular stimulation or ACh application were thought to be associated with a global blockade of thalamic inhibitory processes through inhibition of both GABAergic thalamic cell classes, namely, the RE and local-circuit neurons (Singer, 1977; Ahlsén *et al.*, 1984; McCormick and Prince, 1986b; McCormick and Pape, 1988). The idea of a global blockade of inhibitory mechanisms on awakening was supported by some data reporting an increase in receptive-field diameter of LG thalamic neurons during "arousal" in acutely prepared unanesthetized animals (Godfraind and Meulders, 1969; Meulders and Godfraind, 1969). These and similar results were regarded as embarrassing (Steriade *et al.*, 1974b) and perplexing (Livingstone and Hubel, 1981) because loss of center-surround antagonism and other feature-detection properties that assist thalamic and cortical neurons in their discrimination tasks would be difficult to conceive during the adaptive state of wakefulness.

It is now demonstrated that the long-lasting period of hyperpolarization elicited in thalamic neurons by a synchronous testing stimulus to the prethalamic or corticofugal pathways consists of two distinct components mediated by $GABA_A$ and $GABA_B$ receptors, to which a calcium-dependent potassium conductance is added. Similar aspects are found in neo- and allocortical neurons.

The first indication that, after the early chloride-dependent IPSP, a late bicuculline-resistant IPSP follows in hippocampal CA1 pyramidal neurons belongs to Newberry and Nicoll (1984). The same sequence was reported in neurons recorded from the sensorimotor neocortex (Avoli, 1986). Recently, two studies conducted on LG thalamic neurons of rat have described two types of IPSPs evoked by stimulation of optic tract axons (Hirsch and Burnod, 1987; Crunelli *et al.*, 1988). (1) The early IPSP appears with a latency shorter than 5 msec, lasts for 25–35 msec, is associated with a 75% decrease in input resistance, and is thought to be mediated by $GABA_A$ receptors since it is chloride dependent and is blocked by bicuculline. (2) The late IPSP appears with a latency of 35–45 msec, lasts for 250–300 msec, is associated with a less marked decrease (45%) in input resistance, and is thought to be $GABA_B$ mediated because it varies in an Nernstian fashion with the extracellular potassium concentration, is mimicked by baclofen, a $GABA_B$ agonist, and is selectively blocked by phaclofen, a $GABA_B$ antagonist (see Soltesz *et al.*, 1988). The two receptors implicated in

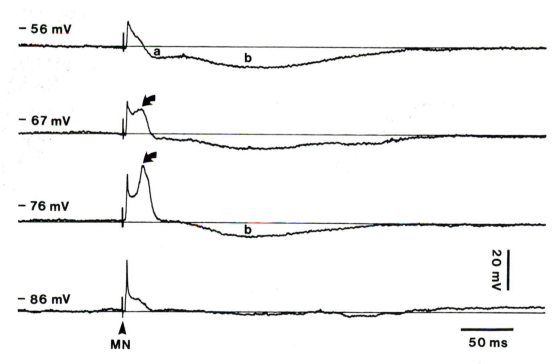

Figure 15. Two types of IPSPs evoked in cat's anteroventral thalamic neuron by stimulation of the mammillary nucleus (MN). At resting membrane potential (−56 mV), MN evoked a primary EPSP (stimulus intensity adjusted below the threshold of action potential) and a long-lasting hyperpolarization that consisted of two (a and b) components. Under steady hyperpolarization (−76 mV), the EPSP increased in amplitude, a low-threshold spike was triggered (arrows), and the early chloride-dependent IPSP was reversed. The reversal of the late (b), probably potassium-mediated, component was at −86 mV. Unpublished data by D. Paré and M. Steriade.

the genesis of these two thalamic IPSPs have been identified in autoradiographic studies (Bowery *et al.*, 1987) that emphasized that GABA$_B$ receptors may even outnumber GABA$_A$ receptors in some thalamic nuclei.

The progenitors of the two IPSPs in thalamic neurons are not yet determined. In studies with deliberate exclusion of the perigeniculate sector of the RE nuclear complex from the thalamic slice (Hirsch and Burnod, 1987; Crunelli *et al.*, 1988), the only possible source for both of these inhibitory components is GABAergic local-circuit cells in the LG nucleus. *In vivo* studies of anterior thalamic nuclei, a group that is naturally devoid of RE inputs (Steriade *et al.*, 1984a), also demonstrated the presence of two IPSPs evoked by mammillary stimulation in anterior thalamic cells (Fig. 15; D. Paré and M. Steriade, unpublished data). The early IPSP (component a in Fig. 15) was reversed at −76 mV, whereas the late long-lasting IPSP (component b), probably potassium mediated, was reversed at −86 mV.

Although these data point to local-circuit cells as generators of both IPSPs, RE thalamic neurons are also involved in their genesis. That stimulation of the peripherally located RE nucleus in the thalamic slice induces chloride-dependent GABA$_A$-mediated IPSPs in dorsal thalamic neurons was demonstrated by Thompson (1988a). Direct evidence for the participation of RE neurons in the long-lasting GABA$_B$-mediated IPSP is still lacking, but available evidence suggests that RE neurons are prevalently implicated in the genesis of this component. Indeed, after disconnection of cortically projecting thalamic nuclei from the RE thalamic complex by transections or chemical lesions of RE perikarya, thalamocortical neurons no longer display their long-lasting hyperpolarizations

---

Figure 16. Effects of midbrain reticular formation (MRF) stimulation and natural arousal on inhibitory processes of thalamocortical and corticospinal neurons in cat and monkey. A: Encéphale isolé cat. 1: Dotgram showing periods of suppressed firing (a, b, c) and postinhibitory rebound excitations elicited during EEG-synchronized epochs by single-shock stimulation (arrow) of cortical area 5 in a thalamocortical neuron of lateral posterior thalamic nucleus. 2: Reduction of cortically evoked cyclic periods of suppressed firing (with preservation of the first inhibitory phase) and replacement of burst firing mode by tonic firing mode after MRF stimulation (a 100-msec shock train at 300 Hz preceded cortical stimulation; not depicted). B: Intracellular recording of a thalamocortical cell in ventrolateral (VL) nucleus of cat. 1: Cyclic hyperpolarizations within frequency range of spindle waves elicited by a shock (arrowhead) to motor cortical area. 2: A preceding shock train to MRF facilitated antidromic invasion and transformed cyclic hyperpolarizations into a single hyperpolarization. C, left column: Method of testing recurrent inhibition acting on antidromic discharges elicited in cat pyramidal tract (PT) neuron. Conditioning (C) volley was delivered at 13 V, which was the minimal voltage required to elicit inhibitory effects on testing (T) response induced by shock at 5 V, which was the minimal voltage required to evoke 100% antidromic invasion. At paired C–T stimulation, complete inhibition of T response or spike fragmentation (arrow). Graph depicts much longer inhibition with three antidromic (pes peduncular, PP) conditioning stimuli than with single shock. With both conditioning procedures (1 PP and 3 PP), recovery of antidromically elicited spike was slower in EEG-synchronized sleep (S) than during waking (W). Note deep but short inhibition in W. Right column in C: Inhibition of synaptic discharges evoked by stimulation of posterior part of the thalamic VL nucleus in precentral PT neuron of chronically implanted macaque monkey. Top part: Field positive (inhibitory) wave evoked by first VL stimulus and facilitation (during W) of evoked discharges by second stimulus at 75-msec interval toward the end of inhibition. Bottom part: Percentage responsiveness of discharge evoked by first stimulus (time 0) and by second stimulus at three time intervals (15 msec, 27 msec, and 75 msec) during W and S. Modified from Steriade *et al.* (1977b, A), Steriade and Deschênes (1988, B), and Steriade and Deschênes (1974, C).

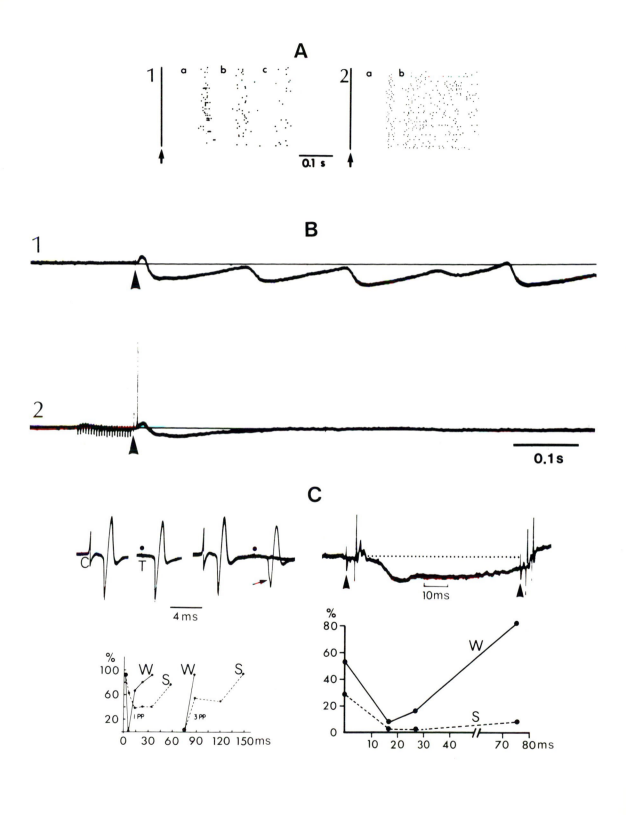

A

1 a b c

2 a b

0.1 s

B

1

2

0.1s

C

C T

4 ms

10ms

%
100
60
20
W S
W S
1 PP 3 PP
0 30 60 90 120 150ms

%
80
60
40
20
W
S
10 20 30 40 70 80ms

as seen in intact animals, but they exclusively exhibit quite short (15–20 msec) bicuculline-sensitive IPSPs (Steriade *et al.*, 1985). Such IPSPs originate in the other source of thalamic inhibition, the local-circuit neurons. The disappearance of the long-lasting phase of hyperpolarization after disconnection from the RE nuclear complex suggests that RE neurons are particularly involved in the genesis of this late IPSP. The role played by each of the two sources of thalamic inhibition (RE and local-circuit neurons) in the two IPSPs of thalamocortical neurons is difficult to assess because RE neurons have access not only to thalamocortical neurons but also to local-circuit cells. Further experiments should be conducted on neurons located in nuclei deprived of RE inputs to selectively study the role of local-circuit cells (see Fig. 15) and in nuclei deprived of local-circuit cells, such as the ventrobasal complex of rat, to investigate the role of RE thalamic neurons.

The progenitors of inhibitory processes and their circuitries in the thalamus and cerebral cortex are dissimilar (see details for the visual thalmocortical system in Steriade *et al.*, 1989d). In spite of these notable differences, inhibitory events in thalamocortical and corticofugal neurons of cats and monkeys are similarly altered during brainstem reticular stimulation or natural arousal. In thalamocortical neurons, the cortically evoked cyclic repetition of the long-lasting inhibitory periods and postinhibitory rebound bursts are blocked by midbrain reticular stimulation, but the first inhibitory phase is left intact (Steriade *et al.*, 1977b). This was observed with both extracellular (Fig. 16A) and intracellular (Fig. 16B) recordings. In corticospinal neurons too, the recovery of responsiveness follow-

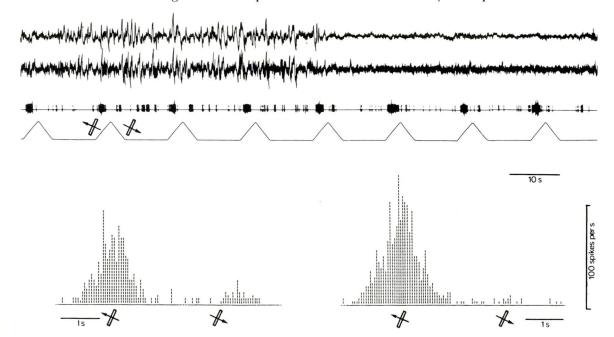

Figure 17. Effects of arousal from slow-wave sleep on responses and response selectivity of a cell in layer II of striate cortex in cat. About half way through the 2-min record, the cat is aroused by a noise. An optimal split ½°/3°, oriented 25° clockwise to vertical, evokes a response (third trace) that is much greater to movement up and to the left than down and to the right. Arousal results in a moderate increase in the response to leftward movement and a virtual elimination of the response to rightward movement (see histograms). Arousal also produces suppression and smoothing of the spontaneous firing. From Livingstone and Hubel (1981).

ing inhibition evoked by antidromic or synaptic volleys is twice as long during EEG-synchronized sleep compared to waking, but the early phase of inhibition (15–25 msec) is preserved or even enhanced during wakefulness (Fig. 16C; Steriade and Deschênes, 1974). These results were interpreted as subserving accurate discrimination of incoming information during waking and are supported by more recent data indicating an improvement of response specificity and directional selectivity on arousal from EEG-synchronized sleep (Fig. 17; Livingstone and Hubel, 1981) and an arousal-induced potentiation of cortical inhibition induced by visual or LG thalamic stimulation (Swadlow and Weyand, 1987).

The idea of preservation of the early IPSP under brainstem reticular stimulation was strengthened by recording intracellularly the two distinct IPSPs in LG relay neurons and by stimulating the cholinergic peribrachial area (Fig. 18A; Hu *et al.*, 1989b). Only the late, presumably potassium-mediated IPSP was blocked, and the early chloride-dependent IPSP was left intact. A similar picture may be found in previous results from extracellular recordings of somatosensory cortical neurons (Steriade and Morin, 1981) showing the brainstem-induced

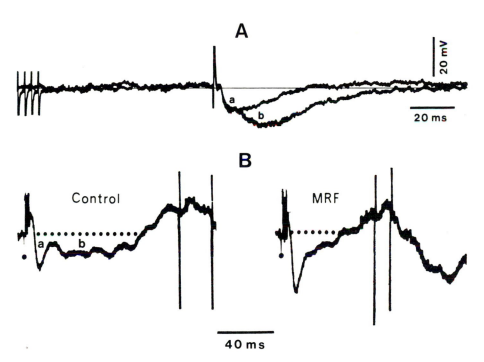

Figure 18. Two inhibitory phases and their differential alteration on midbrain reticular stimulation in cat. A: Intracellular recording of a LG thalamic relay cell in cat under urethane anesthesia and reserpine treatment. The parameters of the optic chiasm (OX) stimulus (middle of the trace) were adjusted to enhance the separation of the two (a and b) IPSPs. When preceded by a pulse train to the brainstem peribrachial area, component b was blocked, but component a persisted. B, control: A testing ventrobasal (VB) shock (dot) induced an inhibitory field potential positivity in the primary somatosensory (S1) cortex, consisting of two (a and b) components. Right part depicts the effects of a preceding shock train to the midbrain reticular formation on the VB-evoked activity in S1. Note enhanced amplitude of the first inhibitory component and great reduction in the second component. Modified from Hu *et al.* (1989b, A) and Steriade and Morin (1981, B).

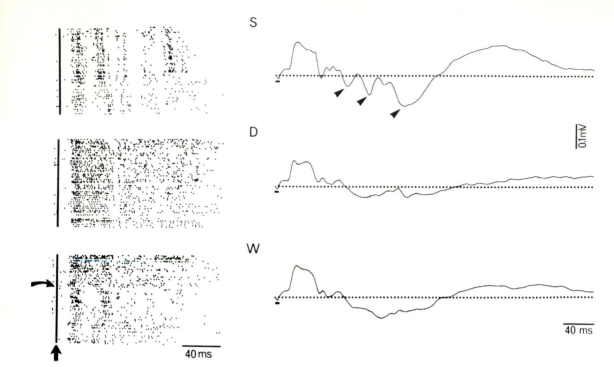

Figure 19. Flash-evoked activities in cortical area 7 of cat during the sleep–waking cycle (S, EEG-synchronized sleep; D, EEG-desynchronized sleep; W, wakefulness). Discharges of a single neuron (dotgrams at left) and focal slow waves simultaneously recorded by the same microelectrode (right: 50 averaged traces, positivity downward) evoked by a 5-msec flash (indicated in dotgrams by upward arrow and uninter- rupted lines and in averaged field potentials by a horizontal line at extreme left of traces). Arousal from D marked by oblique arrow in dotgram. Note rhythmic positive waves (arrows) associated with periods of suppressed firing in S and clear inhibitory period after the initial excitation on arousal from REM (D) sleep. Unpublished data by M. Steriade.

blockade of the late long-lasting inhibitory field potential, although the early inhibitory phase was simultaneously enhanced (Fig. 18B).

The inhibitory processes have not yet been systematically investigated during REM sleep. The light-evoked inhibition in cortical association neurons is much less conspicuous during REM sleep than during other states of vigilance, and inhibition sculptures again the initial response on awakening from REM sleep (Fig. 19; M. Steriade, unpublished data). The study of inhibitory processes may open new avenues for differentiating at the cellular level the two EEG-desynchronized behavioral states.

9

Brainstem Genesis and Thalamic Transfer of Pontogeniculooccipital Waves

Pontogeniculooccipital (PGO) waves are stigmatic events of REM sleep, the sleep stage when dreaming episodes occur. PGO waves are generated in different neuronal groups of the brainstem reticular core and are transferred to many thalamocortical systems in addition to the visual one where they were originally thought to be confined. Interest in the PGO waves stemmed from the discovery that eye movement direction may be related to gaze direction in dream imagery, coupled with data from animal experiments showing that saccadic REMs are often coincident with PGO events (Dement and Kleitman, 1957; Jouvet, 1972). These observations led to the thesis that PGO waves are physiological correlates of brain activation during dreaming sleep, a major part of "the stuff that dreams are made of."

In this chapter we first discuss data on PGO wave genesis in the brainstem (Section 9.1). Thereafter (Section 9.2), we deal with the thalamic responses to the brainstem-generated PGO signals, as revealed by intracellular studies of reserpine-induced PGO waves and by extracellular recordings of neurons in the dorsal lateral geniculate–perigeniculate (LG–PG) thalamic complex in naturally sleeping animals.

9.1. Brainstem PGO-on Neurons

A long series of experimental evidence, including stimulation, lesion, reversible cooling, and recordings of cellular activities, have established that neurons that transfer the brainstem-generated PGO waves to the thalamus are located in and around the PPT cholinergic nucleus (for recent reviews, see Sakai, 1985a; Hobson and Steriade, 1986). That these thalamically projecting brainstem neurons are cholinergic is an assumption resulting from the demonstration that systemic (Ruch-Monachon *et al.*, 1976) and iontophoretic applications of nicotinic antagonists into the LG thalamic nucleus (Hu *et al.*, 1988) abolish the thalamic PGO waves. Recent experiments have indeed shown that at chronic

263

stages after chemical lesions of PPT cholinergic perikarya, PGO waves are largely suppressed during REM sleep (Fig. 1; Webster and Jones, 1988; see Chapter 12, Section 4 for further discussion of these lesions).

The electrophysiology of neurons implicated in the brainstem–thalamic transfer of PGO waves is at its beginnings. Since the late 1970s, it was reported that some PPT neurons (alternatively termed peribrachial or PB neurons) discharge groups of three to five spikes, reliably preceding by 10–25 msec the LG–PGO wave (McCarley *et al.*, 1978; Sakai and Jouvet, 1980; Nelson *et al.*, 1983). Antidromic identification of PGO-on burst cells was achieved by stimulating the intralaminar thalamic nuclei (Sakai, 1985a). There is a three-way correlation among eye movement direction and the discharge of PB burst neurons related to the LG–PGO wave: rightward eye movements are associated with PB neuronal discharge that leads to predominantly right LG–PGO waves (Fig. 2; Nelson *et al.*, 1983). In addition to short-lead (10–25 msec) PB burst neurons, longer-lead (50–150 msec) PGO-on neurons have been recorded from the medial pontine reticular formation and the tegmental reticular nucleus (Fig. 3; McCarley and Ito, 1983). This zone and the prepositus hypoglossi nuclei, which send projections to PPT (Higo *et al.*, 1989a), may furnish eye-movement-related information to PPT for eye-movement-gated PGO waves.

It should be mentioned that PGO-on bursting cells recorded from the PPT nucleus merely represent <5% of the sampled brainstem population (Nelson *et al.*, 1983). The question then arises: How does the vast majority of thalamically projecting PPT neurons behave during PGO waves? Another unsolved question concerns the discharge patterns of PGO-on neurons during the waking–sleep continuum, including periods of REM sleep free of PGO waves. In particular, do PGO-on neurons selectively discharge spike bursts temporally related to PGO waves, or do they also display other types of activity during wake–sleep states? Until quite recently, the only indication was that some of the PGO-on bursting cells also displayed short bursts (Sakai and Jouvet, 1980) or single spikes (Nelson *et al.*, 1983) in association with eye movement potentials (EMPs) during the waking state.

Since the thalamus is the major site where PGO waves are usually recorded, and the PGO thalamic response is a nicotinic event (see above), the assessment of the role played by PGO-on brainstem neurons should start with the antidromic identification of brainstem-–thalamic cells recorded within the limits of cholinergic pedunculopontine tegmental (PPT) and laterodorsal tegmental (LDT) nuclei. These identification procedures are shown in Fig. 3 of Chapter 11. The extracellular data reported below, related to brainstem PGO-on elements, resulted from analyses of such neurons.

A recent study of PGO-on cells recorded from the cholinergic PPT and LDT nuclei and antidromically activated from thalamic nuclei was conducted during natural REM sleep of behaving cats and in acutely prepared cats with PGO waves induced by reserpine treatment. This study revealed various PPT and LDT cell classes discharging single spikes, trains of tonic single spikes, or spike bursts with different patterns preceding the negative peak of PGO field potential recorded from the LG thalamic nucleus (Steriade *et al.*, 1989a).

In chronic experiments, some PPT/LDT neurons discharged single spikes preceding by 15–25 msec the negative peak of the LG–PGO field potential. Intracellular recordings of similar neurons in reserpine-treated preparations

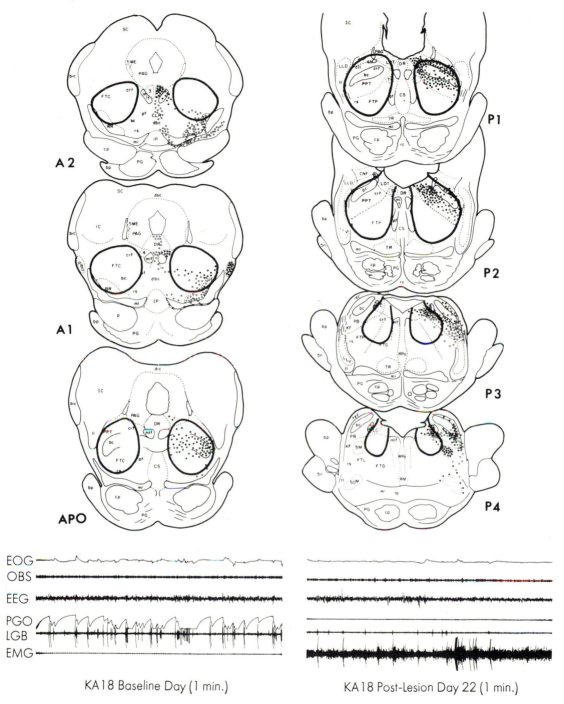

Figure 1. Kainate-induced destruction of PPT cholinergic neurons is followed by PGO suppression during REM sleep of chronically implanted cat. The frontal brainstem sections show encircled territories of cell loss after kainic acid injections. Filled circles indicate ChAT-positive cells, and empty circles indicate tyrosine hydroxylase (TH)-positive cells as revealed in normal animals (see Fig. 1 of Chapter 4). At bottom, control polygraphic record of cat KA18 before kainic injection and 22 days after the injection; note disappearance of PGO waves in the LG thalamic nucleus. In the entire sample of 11 cats, ChAT-positive cells were reduced by 59% and PGO wave spike rate in REM sleep was reduced by a mean of 73% (28 days after the injection). Modified from Webster and Jones (1988).

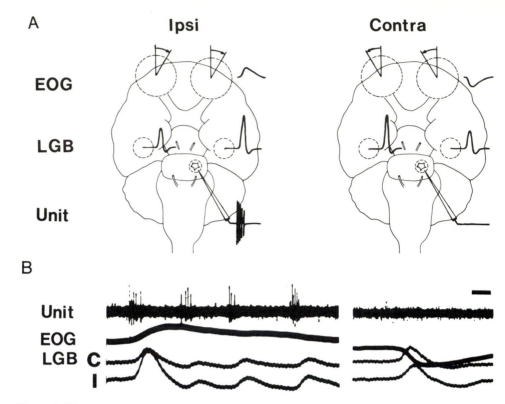

Figure 2. Three-way correlation among PGO burst cell discharge, eye movement directionality, and primary PGO waves in the cat. A: Two dorsal-view drawings of the brain schematize eye movement direction (EOG), laterality of amplitudes of dorsal LGB PGO waves, and a PGO burst cell being extracellularly recorded by a microelectrode. The left diagram (Ipsi) shows an eye movement toward the side of the recorded burst cell in the pons; the EOG trace is upward, the larger (primary) PGO wave is in the ipsilateral dorsal LGB, and there is a burst of spikes in the unit recording. In contrast, the right diagram (Contra) shows that with an eye movement away from the side of the recorded neuron, there is no burst of spikes, and the larger (primary) PGO wave is in the contralateral dorsal LGB. B: Filmstrips show the raw data from which the diagrammatic conclusions in A were drawn. LGBi is PGO wave recording in the dorsal LGB ipsilateral to the unit recording. Upward EOG traces indicate eye movements toward the side of the recorded neuron. Calibration, 50 msec. From Nelson *et al.* (1983).

disclosed that these single spikes rose from large composite EPSPs whose amplitudes grew with membrane hyperpolarization (D. Paré and M. Steriade, unpublished data).

Another cell class discharged tonic trains of single spikes whose onset preceded by 100–200 msec the thalamic PGO wave. The tonic discharge patterns of these PGO-on neurons are substantiated by interspike interval histograms of cellular activity taken during the period of PGO-related increased neuronal firing, indicating the presence of medium (10–25 msec) intervals and the virtual absence of short (<8 msec) intervals that would reflect spike bursts (Fig. 4).

The class of PGO-on bursting neurons comprises a series of different neuronal types displaying spike bursts with quite different structures.

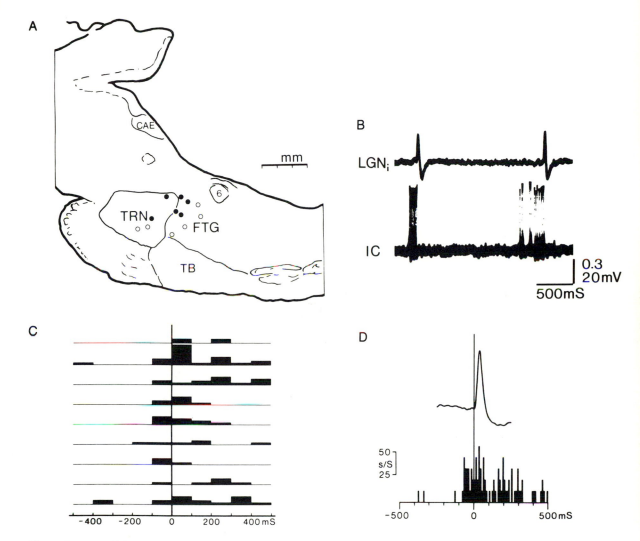

Figure 3. Intracellularly recorded long-lead PGO-on neurons in the cat medial pons. A: Brainstem schematic at 0.8 mm lateral showing location of intracellularly recorded long-lead PGO-on neurons (closed circles) and neurons with lesser PGO wave correlation and/or no phase-leading relationship (open circles). Abbreviations: CAE, locus coeruleus; TRN, tegmental reticular nucleus (of Bechterew); FTG, gigantocellular tegmental field; 6, abducens nucleus; TB, trapezoid body. B: Intracellular record (IC) of an mPRF long-lead PGO-on neuron in the transition period showing phase-leading discharge prior to primary PGO waves (upper trace) in the LGN ipsilateral to recording site. C: Raster display showing that long-lead PGO-on neuronal discharges began prior to time of onset (0 msec) of eight of nine (89%) ipsilateral dorsal LGN primary PGO waves. The height of each black bar is proportional to the number of discharges in each 100-msec bin; scale is provided by the bin in the second row from top with maximal number of discharges. N = 10 (= rate of 100 spikes/sec). Note consistency of discharge–PGO wave relationship. (Different neuron than in B.) D: PGO wave–discharge cross-correlogram, same neuron as in part C. Top is average waveform of nine PGO waves (peak voltage is 400 μV); below is the associated discharge level of the long-lead PGO-on neuron in spikes per second. Note marked acceleration of discharge rate at 80 msec prior to PGO wave onset (bin width = 10 msec). From McCarley and Ito (1983).

Some neurons discharged a group of three to five spikes, as reported in previous investigations (see above and Fig. 2). However, the intraburst frequency in those neurons (130–170 Hz) is well below the frequency generated by a typical low-threshold somatic spike, which usually ranges above 250 Hz (see Chapter 5). Further intracellular studies should test the possibility that such PGO-on bursts of PPT/LDT neurons originate at the level of their dendrites. It is known that the spike bursts of reticular thalamic neurons have lower frequencies (160–170 Hz) than those (>250 Hz) of thalamocortical cells (Steriade *et al.*, 1986; Domich *et al.*, 1986). Correlatively, the rebound bursts of the former neurons originate in dendrites, whereas the rebound bursts of the latter neurons

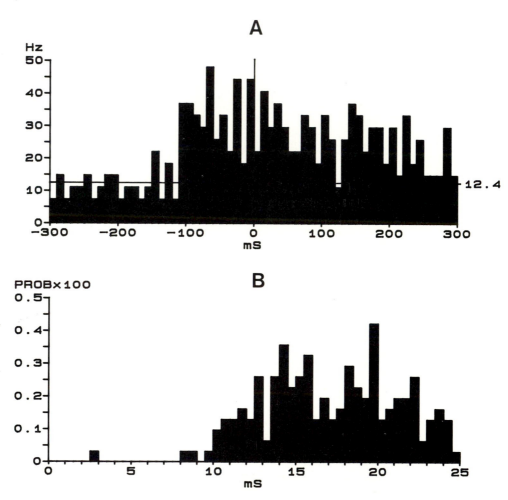

Figure 4. PGO-on PPT cell with tonic discharge patterns during REM sleep of chronically implanted cat. A: Peri-PGO histogram (10-msec bins) of PPT-cell's discharges. Time 0 is the negative peak of the PGO wave recorded from the ipsilateral LG thalamic nucleus. Note increased firing about 110 msec before the thalamic PGO wave. The level of spontaneous discharge during REM sleep (12.4 Hz) is indicated. B: Interspike interval histogram (0.5-msec bins) of cell's activities during the period of increased firing rate around time 0. Note medium intervals (10–25 msec) and virtual absence of short interval (below 8 msec) that would reflect presence of spike bursts. Unpublished data by M. Steriade, S. Datta, G. Oakson, and D. Paré.

originate at the soma (cf. Steriade and Llinás, 1988). The mechanism underlying stereotyped spike bursts, like those displayed during REM sleep by such brainstem PGO-on bursting cells, is probably the deinactivation of a low-threshold spike by membrane hyperpolarization (see Chapter 5). If so, the hypothesis that postulates that the genesis of these particular PGO-on bursts involves a disinhibition of brainstem cholinergic neurons consequent to the suppressed activity in monoaminergic elements should be revised. Instead, the possible sources of inhibition acting on this type of PPT/LDT neurons should be sought. It is during their hyperpolarization that impulses of different origin may trigger the low-threshold spike and the superimposed bursts of fast action potentials. One of the likely sources of inhibition acting on PPT cells is substantia nigra pars reticulata, which consists of GABAergic neurons that project directly to PPT. This hypothesis (Steriade and Paré, 1989) should be tested.

Other PPT neurons discharged high-frequency (500–600 Hz) spike bursts in close temporal relation with thalamic PGO waves. However, distinct from what has been reported, these bursts occurred on a background of tonically increased discharge rates during REM sleep (Fig. 5; Steriade *et al.*, 1989a). These data raise the intriguing possibility that high-frequency bursts may be generated at a depolarized level, at variance to what is expected for a common low-threshold calcium spike.

Still another type of PPT/LDT neurons discharged tonically, at high rates (>30 Hz), during epochs of REM sleep without PGO events and stopped firing prior to and during thalamic PGO waves (Fig. 6). The behavior of these PGO-off cells is unexpected for cells located within the limits of brainstem cholinergic nuclei and is the functional counterpart of the heterogeneity of PPT/LDT nuclei. The admixture of cholinergic and monoaminergic neurons in the cat PPT nucleus was already discussed (see Section 4.1.2), but such PGO-off cells are obviously not aminergic in the light of the virtual silence of aminergic neurons during REM sleep (see Chapter 11). The discovery of GABAergic neurons within brainstem cholinergic nuclei (Kosaka *et al.*, 1987) raises the possibility that PGO-off neurons, such as that illustrated in Fig. 6, are GABAergic and that their silenced firing prior to and during PGO waves could disinhibit adjacent neurons with tonically increased discharges during PGO waves, as depicted in Fig. 4.

These investigations in behaving animals reveal the organizational complexity of PPT/LDT nuclei, which defies simplistic statements on the properties of neurons that transfer PGO waves to the thalamus. The disclosure of these neuronal properties in the behaving animal should be followed by intracellular studies on reserpine-induced PGO waves in simplified preparations.

9.2. Thalamic Transfer of Brainstem-Generated PGO Waves

Thalamic PGO waves are spiky, biphasic (initially negative) field potentials that are usually recorded in the LG thalamic nucleus, where they display their maximum amplitudes because of the LG laminated structure. Other thalamic nuclei that exhibit PGO waves include especially the associational visual (pulvinar and lateral posterior), rostral intralaminar, and the anterior nuclear group (unpublished data). This diffusion throughout the thalamus of a phenomenon

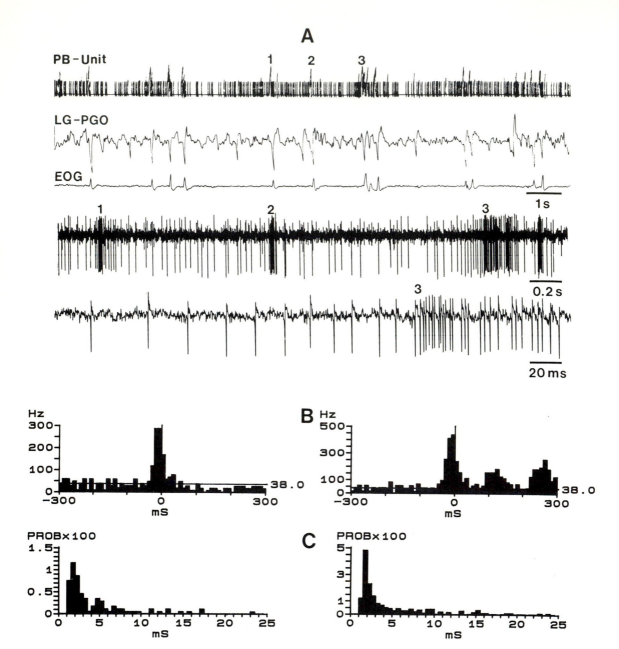

Figure 5. Activity of PGO-on burst neuron in the PPT nucleus during REM sleep of chronically implanted cat. A: Polygraphic ink-written Qecord (unit discharges: deflections exceeding the common level represent high-frequency spike bursts; LG-PGO waves; and EOG) and original spikes with two different speeds, showing three (1 to 3) PGO-related bursts as indicated on the first trace of the ink-written records. B: Peri-PGO histograms (10-msec bins) of PPT cell's discharges (time 0 is the negative peak of the LG–PGO wave) for single and clustered PGO waves (left and right panels, respectively). The level of overall spontaneous discharges in REM sleep (38 Hz) is also indicated. C: Interspike interval histograms (0.5-msec bins) of PPT cell's activity during the period of increased firing rate around the PGO events for single and clustered PGO wave (left and right panels, respectively). Note very short intervals (<3 msec) reflecting high-frequency bursts. Unpublished data by M. Steriade, D. Paré, S. Datta, R. Curro Dossi, and G. Oakson.

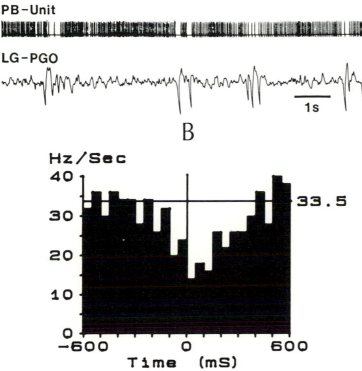

Figure 6. Neuron in the PPT nucleus diminishing its rate of firing or ceasing its discharges prior to and during PGO waves during REM sleep of chronically implanted cat. A: Ink-written recording with unitary discharges and LG–PGO waves. B: Peri-PGO histogram (50-msec bins) showing decreased firing rate beginning about 300 msec prior to the negative peak of the LG–PGO wave. The level of overall spontaneous discharges during REM sleep (33.5 Hz) is also indicated. Unpublished data by M. Steriade, S. Datta, R. Curro Dossi, D. Paré, and G. Oakson.

that was initially regarded as restricted to the geniculostriate system is not surprising, since brainstem cholinergic neurons that give rise to PGO waves project to virtually all relay, associational, and intralaminar thalamic nuclei (see Section 4.2.2).

The PGO waves herald REM sleep by about 30 to 90 sec, appearing as high-amplitude isolated events that precede the other key signs of REM sleep (EEG desynchronization, muscular atonia, and ocular saccades), and they continue throughout the state of REM sleep as clustered waves with lower amplitudes (see Fig. 3 in Chapter 1). Thus, the thalamic transfer of brainstem-generated PGO signals has to be considered in two distinct stages: (1) the transitional period between EEG-synchronized and EEG-desynchronized sleep during which PGO waves appear over the background of a fully synchronized EEG (panels 1 and 2 in Fig. 3 of Chapter 1 up to EEG desynchronization), a period termed *pre-REM;* and (2) the REM sleep associated with EEG desynchronization. Besides the change from high-amplitude isolated PGO waves to clustered PGO waves with lower amplitudes, pre-REM and REM sleep should be dissociated because thalamic neurons display opposite firing modes during behavioral states associated with EEG synchronization versus states accompanied by EEG desynchronization: they are hyperpolarized during the former and tonically depolarized by 7–10 mV during the latter (see Sections 5.4 and 8.1). These two distinct stages have not been analyzed in previous works dealing with the PGO-related neuronal activity in the thalamus (for a review of those early studies, see Steriade and Hobson, 1976).

We shall discuss the thalamic transfer of PGO on the basis of recent experiments using intracellular recordings of LG relay cells in acute experiments on reserpine-treated cats (see Jouvet, 1972, and Hobson and Steriade, 1986, for reviews of monoamine depletors leading to the appearance of REM sleep signs) and extracellular recordings of LG neurons in chronically implanted, naturally sleeping cats.

9.2.1. Cellular Mechanisms of Reserpine-Induced Thalamic PGO Waves

The intracellular studies on reserpine-induced thalamic PGO waves (Deschênes and Steriade, 1988; Hu *et al.*, 1989c) were carried out in cats under urethane anesthesia because the brainstem–thalamic PGO response is a cholinergic event (see below) and the cholinergic activation of thalamocortical neurons is blocked by very low doses of barbiturates (see Section 6.1.2.1). The animals were acutely deprived of retinal and visual cortex inputs to prevent massive synaptic bombardment and to avoid activation of LG neurons through circuitous pathways involving cortical neurons. In such simplified experimental conditions, the intracellular response of LG cells to "spontaneous" PGO waves occurring under reserpine treatment are quite stereotyped, and they resemble the LG response to stimulation of brainstem peribrachial area, which contains the neurons of the final common path transferring brainstem-generated PGO waves to the thalamus. The thalamic field PGO waves obtained in these restricted acute experimental conditions are almost identical to those described in chronically implanted, naturally sleeping animals (Brooks and Gershon, 1971; Steriade *et al.*, 1989c); namely, they start with an initial focal negativity followed by a longer-duration positivity that may have a negative notch on its rising phase or may be followed by a second full negative component whose peak follows the peak of the first negativity by about 80 msec (see Figs. 7A and 8). Thus, the total duration of PGO waves varies between 200 and 500 msec, depending on the time course of the positive phase.

The intracellular events of LG relay thalamic neurons associated with the PGO field potential recorded in the vicinity of the micropipette can be summarized as follows. Each PGO field potential is associated in the intracellular recording with a depolarizing potential interrupted by a short-lasting (50–60 msec) hyperpolarization whose initiation lags the onset of the depolarizing component by 40 to 80 msec (Fig. 7). The total duration of the depolarization is about 200–300 msec, and firing may occur during the early phase (second and third PGO waves in Fig. 7A) or after the completion of the hyperpolarizing component (sixth PGO wave in Fig. 7A and first PGO wave in Fig. 9A1).

The expanded intracellular records in Fig. 8 show that (1) the field negativity

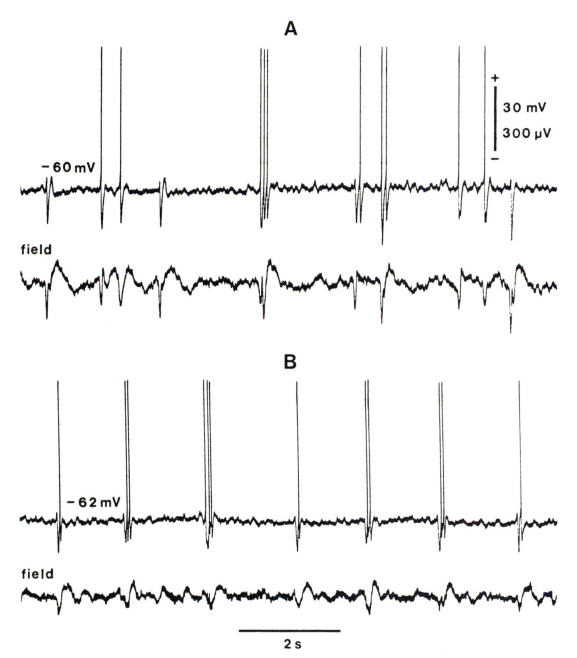

Figure 7. Simultaneous recordings of spontaneous PGO waves and intracellular events in two LG thalamic relay neurons of cat. Traces in A were recorded under urethane anesthesia, and those in B in a brainstem-transected cat. Both animals were treated with reserpine (1 mg/kg, i.p.) 24 hr before the recording sessions. From Hu *et al.* (1989c).

is associated with a purely depolarizing potential (A1 and B1), (2) a positive-going upswing deflection correlates with a transient hyperpolarization (A2), and (3) a second positive upswing in the field potential is associated with a second hyperpolarization (B3). On passage of hyperpolarizing currents, the amplitude of the depolarizing potential increases, whereas the amplitude of the hyperpolarization decreases (Fig. 9A2). When PGO waves occur in doublets, the first wave is made of a depolarization followed by a hyperpolarization, whereas the second one consists of a pure depolarization (Fig. 9B1). On hyperpolarization by 8 mV, the depolarization becomes larger (B2), and further hyperpolarization reaching 12 mV from the resting membrane potential triggers a low-threshold spike (B3); simultaneously, the hyperpolarizing component becomes smaller and eventually is no longer visible. The membrane conductance increases by 25–40% during the PGO wave, and this is observed even when the hyperpolarizing event is not detectable (Hu *et al.*, 1989c).

Iontophoresis of nicotinic blockers (mecamylamine or hexamethonium) in the LG thalamic nucleus strongly depresses the unit activity related to "spon-

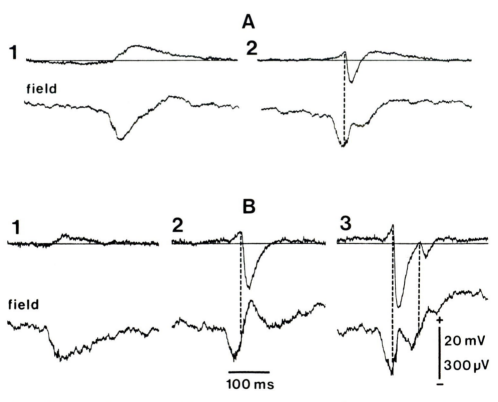

Figure 8. Sample of spontaneous PGO waveforms with their intracellular counterparts taken from two LG thalamic neurons (A and B) in cats under urethane anesthesia and reserpine treatment. Negative PGO waves showing a smooth return toward the baseline were usually correlated with pure depolarizing events in LG neurons (A1 and B1). When the negativity was interrupted by a positive-going deflection, a prominent IPSP was always present in the intracellular traces (A2, B2, B3). Double-notched PGO waveforms were correlated with the appearance of a second IPSP in the traces (B3). Vertical lines indicate the IPSP onset and emphasize the close time relationship between IPSPs and the positive upswing in the field potentials. All cells were slightly hyperpolarized to prevent spike discharges. From Hu *et al.* (1989c).

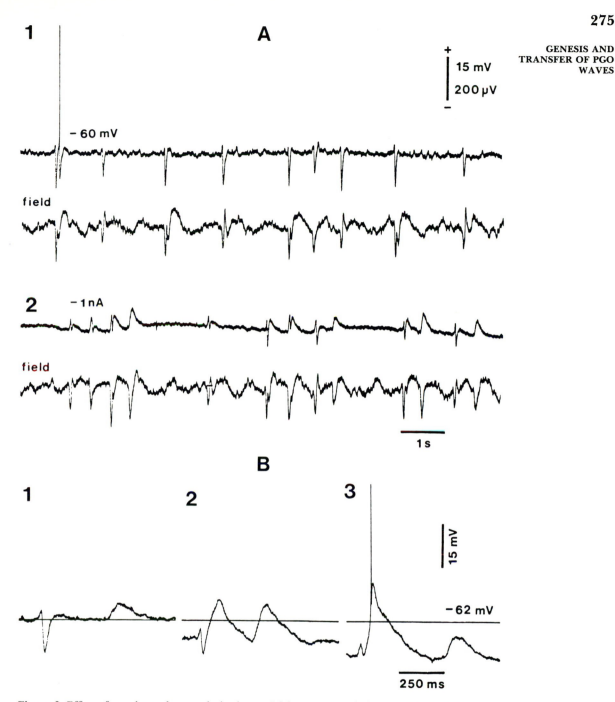

Figure 9. Effect of membrane hyperpolarization on PGO waves recorded intracellularly in LG neurons of reserpinized cats under urethane anesthesia. Spontaneous PGO waves were recorded at rest (A1) and during a sustained injection of inward current (A2). Note that the depolarization increased in amplitude as the size of IPSPs decreased. In the other example (B), the cell displayed at rest a stereotyped PGO activity consisting of doublets: a biphasic PGO wave followed by a monophasic one. Membrane hyperpolarization to −68 mV (B2) increased the size of the depolarization, and when the membrane potential reached −74 mV (B3), a low-threshold response with a fast action potential was triggered by the first PGO event. From Hu *et al.* (1989c).

taneous" PGO waves under reserpine or to PGO waves evoked by brainstem peribrachial stimulation, whereas the muscarinic blockers (scopolamine) have no significant effect on PGO-related unit activities (Hu *et al.*, 1988). These data are in line with earlier results obtained by means of systemically injected mecamylamine (Ruch-Monachon *et al.*, 1976).

In conclusion, the thalamic PGO wave involves a direct nicotinic excitation of LG relay cells by brainstem cholinergic neurons and an activation of intra-LG inhibitory interneurons that is reflected in the PGO-related IPSP seen in LG relay cells. In fact, presumed LG interneurons display an initial depolarization during PGO field potentials that may reach firing, which is closely coupled with the IPSP onset in LG relay cells (see Fig. 9 in Hu *et al.*, 1989c). Although the GABAergic neurons in the perigeniculate (PG) sector of the reticular (RE) thalamic nucleus are also activated during PGO waves in the chronically implanted behaving animal (Steriade *et al.*, 1989c), the PG neurons do not fire in response to the brainstem peribrachial volley in the restricted acute experimental conditions involving visual cortex ablation (Hu *et al.*, 1989c), probably because their discharges require a certain depolarizing pressure from corticofugal fibers. Thus, in the acute intracellular recordings reported above, the only source for the IPSPs observed in LG relay cells is the pool of intra-LG GABAergic interneurons.

9.2.2. PGO-Related Neuronal Activities in the LG–PG Thalamic Complex during Natural Sleep

By contrast with reserpine-induced PGO waves in acutely prepared animals, which do not exhibit fluctuations in behavioral states (so-called state-independent PGO waves), the naturally sleeping animal provides the advantage of studying the cellular correlates of thalamic PGO waves during two different stages of sleep cycle: the pre-REM transitional epoch accompanied by EEG synchronization (see Fig. 3 of Chapter 1) and the full-blown REM sleep associated with EEG desynchronization. Data discussed in Section 5.4 and at the beginning of Section 8.1 emphasized that thalamic neurons operate in two distinct modes during states associated with EEG synchronization as opposed to EEG-desynchronized states. During EEG-synchronized sleep, almost 50% of interspike intervals of LG-cells' spontaneous discharges are grouped between 2 and 3 msec, thus reflecting the high intraburst frequencies (>300 Hz) characteristic of this stage of sleep, and the relationship between LG thalamic bursts and spindle waves at 7 Hz is reflected by a late mode at 120–160 msec in the interspike interval histogram, representing the silent periods between 7-Hz bursts (see top panel in Fig. 10). On the other hand, during REM sleep, the proportion of intervals within the 2- to 3-msec class is negligible, betraying the inactivation of bursts through the tonic depolarization of LG relay cells (bottom panel in Fig. 10). The pre-REM stage is intermediate between the EEG-synchronized sleep and REM sleep.

Figure 10. Interspike interval histogram (ISIH) of a LG thalamic relay cell during slow-wave sleep (SWS), pre-REM stage, and REM sleep in chronically implanted cat. In each state, two ISIHs are shown, with 1-msec bins (left) and 10-msec bins (right). Symbols: N, number of intervals; X, mean interval (msec); M, interval mode (msec); C, coefficient of variation; E, proportion of intervals in excess of the depicted time range. Since the percentages of intervals exceed the ordinate maximum in first bins of right panels, the real percentages are indicated. From Steriade *et al.* (1989c).

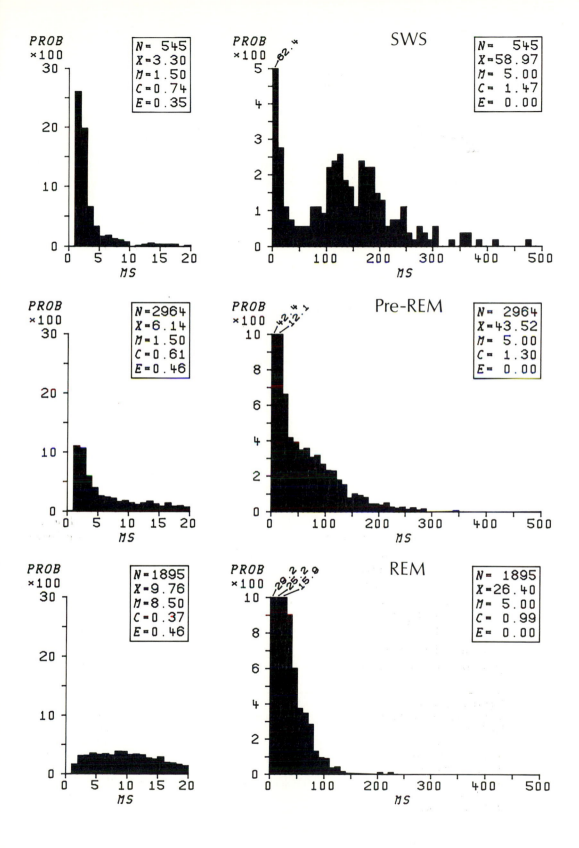

What is then the thalamic response to the brainstem-generated PGO volley during the pre-REM stage when thalamocortical neurons are hyperpolarized by about 7–10 mV and during REM sleep when the same neurons are tonically depolarized? And how do these possibly different responses of LG neurons influence the signal-to-noise ratio in the visual channel, i.e., the ratio between the neuronal activity related to the PGO signal and the background firing of the same cell? Because PGO waves are commonly regarded as physiological correlate of dreaming, the last question may give clues to the vivid imagery during the pre-REM stage as compared to REM sleep. These topics have been recently investigated in the chronically implanted, behaving cat (Steriade *et al.*, 1989c).

The activity of LG neurons related to PGO field potentials, simultaneously recorded with the same microelectrode, is quite different during pre-REM and REM sleep. During pre-REM, the activity of LG relay cells starts with a short (7–15 msec) high-frequency (300–500 Hz) spike burst coinciding with the initial negativity of the PGO wave and continues with a train of single spikes at 50–80 Hz, lasting for 200–400 msec (Fig. 11, top panel). During REM sleep, the rate of LG-cells' spontaneous firing is 1.5- to threefold higher than in pre-REM, the peak-to-peak amplitudes of PGO waves are two to three times lower, and the PGO-related activity of LG neurons lacks the initial high-frequency burst that is characteristic for the pre-REM stage (Fig. 11, bottom panel). The peri-PGO histograms of neuronal activities in the two LG elements depicted in Fig. 12 show that the signal-to-noise ratio reaches values of about 6 to 7 during the pre-REM epoch, whereas the ratio values during REM sleep are between 1.5 and 2.5. Less dramatic but consistent effects are seen when examining the pooled signal-to-noise ratio in all analyzed LG neurons, with values of 2.4 during pre-REM and 1.6 during REM sleep (Fig. 13).

The stereotyped features of the burst that starts the PGO-related activity of LG neurons during the pre-REM stage indicate that it is probably a low-threshold calcium spike crowned by high-frequency sodium action potentials, as described in Section 5.4.2. Further evidence for this assumption comes from the peri-PGO burst occurrence, showing a markedly decreased probability of bursts for 300–400 msec after the PGO wave (Fig. 14). It is known that the relative refractory period of the low-threshold spike in thalamic neurons may reach 200–300 msec (cf. Steriade and Llinás, 1988). The hypothesis then emerged that the much larger amplitude of spiky PGO field potentials during the pre-REM stage, as compared to PGO waves during REM sleep (see averaged PGO field potentials in Fig. 12), is caused by synchronous bursts in pools of LG neurons.

The greater signal-to-noise (PGO-to-spontaneous discharge) ratio in the geniculostriate channel during the pre-REM stage than during REM sleep suggests that the vivid imagery associated with dreaming sleep may appear well

Figure 11. PGO-related activity of a LG relay cell during pre-REM epoch and REM sleep in chronically implanted cat. Ink-written records depict unit discharges (deflections exceeding the common level of single spikes represent high-frequency spike bursts), focal waves recorded by the same microelectrode, electrical activity in the contralateral LG nucleus recorded by a coaxial electrode, eye movements (EOG), and cortical EEG. In both pre-REM and REM, PGO-related unit activity is depicted with original spikes below each ink-written recording. Note the tonically increased firing rate in REM, the smaller amplitudes of PGO field potentials in REM (compared with pre-REM), and the absence of PGO-related spike bursts in REM (contrasting with their presence, arrows, in pre-REM). From Steriade *et al.* (1989c).

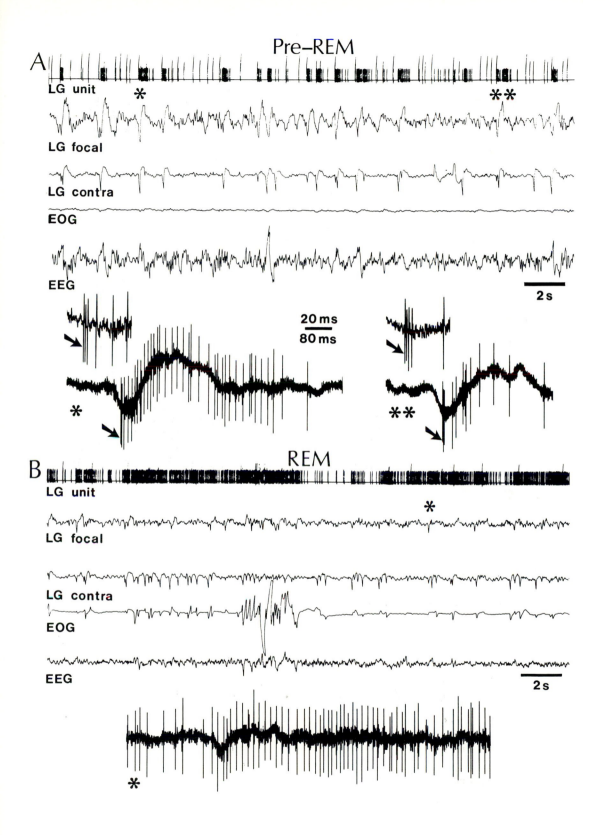

Pre-REM

A

LG unit

LG focal

LG contra

EOG

EEG

20 ms
80 ms

2 s

REM

B

LG unit

LG focal

LG contra

EOG

EEG

2 s

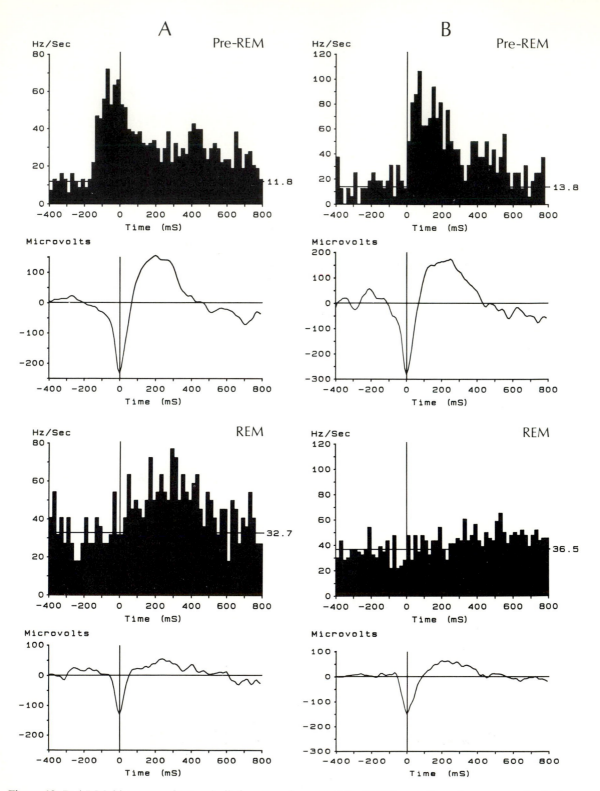

Figure 12. Peri-PGO histogram of LG unit discharges and averaged focal PGO waves from the same epochs during pre-REM and REM sleep in chronically implanted cat. A and B, two LG neurons. The average level of spontaneous discharges (11.8 Hz, etc.) is also indicated in each histogram. A, 19 PGO events in pre-REM, 23 PGO events in REM sleep. From Steriade *et al.* (1989c).

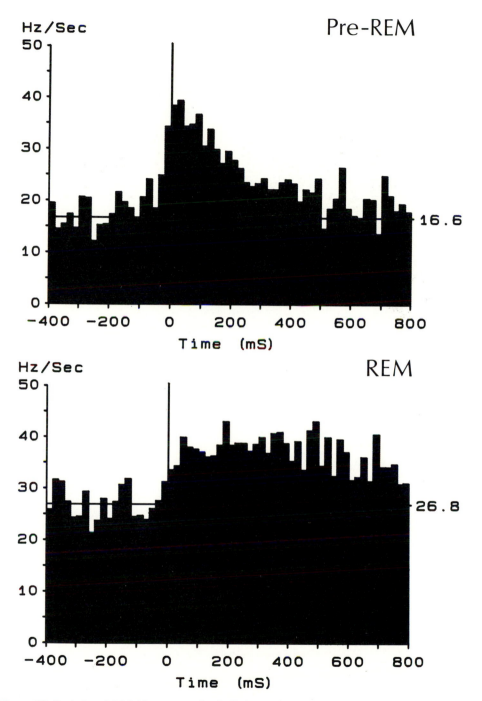

Figure 13. Pooled peri-PGO histograms of unit discharges in a sample of 15 LG neurons during pre-REM and REM sleep in naturally sleeping cats. Time 0 taken at the same point as in Fig. 12. Level of spontaneous firing (16.6 and 26.8 Hz) is also indicated. From Steriade *et al.* (1989c).

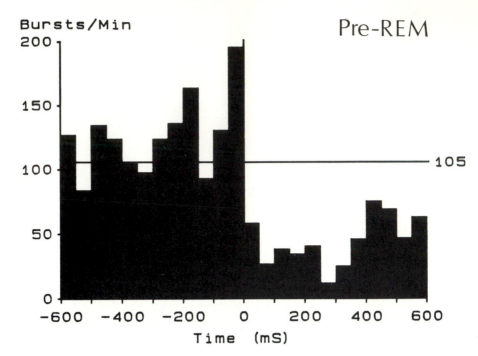

Figure 14. Probability of high-frequency spike bursts before and after pre-REM PGO waves in a sample of 11 LG neurons. Time 0 is the peak of the negative PGO wave (as in two preceding figures). For criteria of bursts and their computer detection, see Methods in Steriade *et al.* (1989c).

before REM sleep, during a period of apparent EEG-synchronized sleep. As to whether or not one may speak about dreaming behavior when discussing results obtained in animal studies, a positive answer is provided by experiments in which a behavioral repertoire typical for dreaming mentation was obtained after muscular atonia had been prevented by adequate lesions of certain brainstem structures (see Section 1.2). The idea that PGO waves with greater amplitudes during the pre-REM stage may reflect more vivid imagery during that epoch than even during REM sleep (Steriade *et al.*, 1989c) corroborates earlier data by Dement *et al.* (1969), who studied the rebound (or compensation) phenomenon after REM sleep deprivation in cats. Instead, however, of the standard deprivation of REM sleep, Dement and his colleagues interrupted sleep immediately after the occurrence of the first PGO wave (during the period we term pre-REM) and eliminated about 30 sec of the EEG-synchronized sleep that precedes fully developed REM sleep. The comparison between the standard REM sleep deprivation and "PGO deprivation" led to the conclusion that "the crucial factor in the so-called REM-sleep deprivation–compensation phenomenon is the deprivation of phasic events." And the increase in total REM time after deprivation was regarded "as a response to an accumulated need for phasic events rather than a response to the loss of REM sleep per se" (Dement *et al.*, 1969, pp. 310–311). The observation that some of the dream reports from EEG-synchronized sleep are indistinguishable from those obtained from REM-sleep awakenings (cf. Hobson, 1988) suggests that such dreams occur during the pre-REM stage and invites researchers to explore the dreaming imagery during the period immediately preceding REM sleep in humans.

Motor Systems

The Brainstem Oculomotor System and Mechanisms of Motor Atonia in REM Sleep

The first seven sections of this chapter review the brainstem oculomotor system, and the last sections review mechanisms involved in production of the muscle atonia of REM sleep. With respect to the oculomotor system, conjugate eye movements include saccades, pursuit movements, and the eye movements associated with optokinetic and vestibular nystagmus. In this chapter we review in some depth the brainstem role in production of one of these conjugate eye movements, saccades, since these play such a prominent role in both waking and REM sleep, and much has been learned about their brainstem mechanisms.

10.1. Saccadic Eye Movements

Saccades are rapid eye movement comprised of a rapid acceleration to peak velocity and a deceleration that brings the eye to its final position. Primate saccades usually last 15–100 msec and may have peak velocities of more than 500 degrees/sec. All saccades are thought to share a common generator, and it is this common brainstem generator that has been the subject of intense and productive work over the last 20 years (Fuchs *et al.*, 1985). We adopt an "outside in" approach and describe the system beginning at the oculomotor motoneurons and then move centrally. The anatomic locus of the various neuronal types involved in saccade generation will be described in conjunction with the physiology. It is worth emphasizing that the somewhat vague term "paramedian pontine reticular formation" (PPRF) used in early papers to describe the locus of reticular neurons participating in saccade generation can, in most cases, be replaced by more precise anatomical terms.

10.1.1. Physiological Properties of Oculomotor Neurons

During visual fixation, oculomotor motoneurons discharge tonically at a fixed rate proportional to the degree of muscle tension required to maintain the fixation. Hence, rate is maximal at the extreme "on" direction of the controlled muscle, such as extreme leftward fixation for the left abducens motoneurons. Threshold for the onset of this tonic discharge is usually within 10–20° in the "off" direction, i.e., rightward fixation for left abducens motoneurons. Between threshold and maximal rate each neuron has its own constant of proportionality, termed K, relating firing rate and fixation change in degrees. Typical K values range from 1 to 12 spikes/sec per degree.

For saccadic changes in position in the "on" direction, there is a rapid acceleration of firing rate some 8 msec prior to saccade onset, then a slight decrease in frequency during the saccade, with a rapid deceleration and cessation of discharge some 10 msec prior to saccade end (Fig. 1). The duration of this heightened firing rate codes saccade duration, which in turn determines the magnitude of eye position change. The convention in the oculomotor literature is to refer to the heightened firing rate as a "burst" and to designate neurons with a firing pattern consisting of short-term or phasic discharges as "burst" neurons. Because this convention is so well entrenched, we use it, but the reader is warned that the term "burst" pattern would, in our opinion, be better rendered as "phasic" pattern so as to reserve the term "burst" for truly stereotyped clusters of spikes such as those seen with calcium spikes in brainstem reticular and thalamic neurons (Chapter 5). It is of interest from the point of view of intrinsic properties of neurons that abducens neuronal discharge frequencies during a saccade are frequently 400 spikes/sec and may peak at 800 spikes/sec.

However only the first three to five spikes have shorter interspike intervals than the steady-state level, which is always reached within 50 msec, shorter than the usual burst (Grantyn and Grantyn, 1978). Thus, although it is indeed possible that the initial spikes might reflect a pattern determined by intrinsic mem-

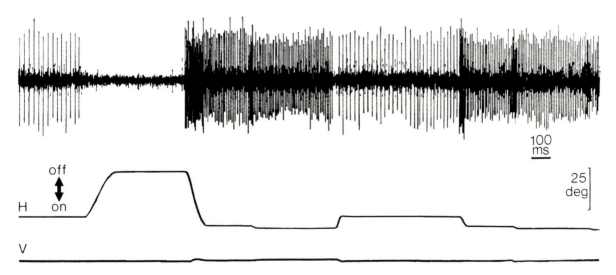

Figure 1. Discharge pattern of an identified motoneuron in the abducens nucleus of the monkey. The arrow above the horizontal channel (H) indicates the "on" and "off" directions of this motoneuron. From Fuchs *et al.* (1985).

brane properties (see discussion of true burst discharge in Chapter 5), the entire run of clustered spikes characteristic of an oculomotor system "burst neuron" is too long for this explanation. Thus, other characteristics of motoneuron firing during saccades are determined by input from afferent neurons. It is thought that in general the "tonic" and "phasic" components are coded separately. Special cases are medial and lateral rectus motoneurons, which receive inputs from the contralateral abducens and from the prepositus hypoglossi, respectively, that have combined "tonic–phasic" information.

10.1.2. Afferents to Oculomotor Motoneurons: Lesion Studies

That the site of afferent input generating the saccade-related discharge of motoneurons was the nearby reticular formation was suggested by early electrolytic (Goebel *et al.*, 1971) and later kainic acid lesions (Lang *et al.*, 1982; Henn *et al.*, 1984b) placed in the pontine reticular formation region rostral to abducens and bounded dorsally by MLF and ventrally by nucleus reticularis tegmenti pontis. Unilateral lesions in this reticular zone produce an enduring paralysis of horizontal eye movements toward the side of the lesions. Vertical eye movement deficits are produced by unilateral lesions in the rostral interstitial nucleus of the MLF (riMLF, a portion of midbrain reticular formation) in the monkey (Büttner-Ennever and Büttner, 1978) and of the homologous nucleus of the prerubral field in the cat (Graybiel, 1977b). More recently reversible lesions of vertical saccades have been produced by microinjections of muscimol, a GABA agonist, into riMLF (Vilis *et al.*, 1986). Bilateral kainic acid lesions, even small ones, in caudal PRF lead to a severe disruption of rapid eye movements in all directions (Henn *et al.*, 1984b; see Fig. 2). These studies suggest, of course, that a

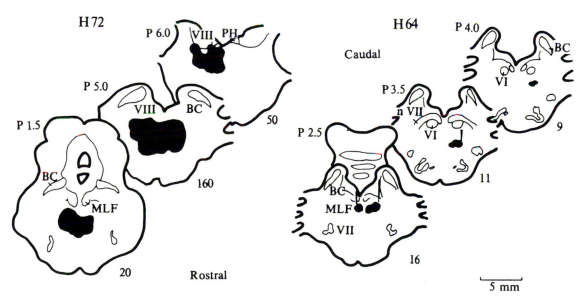

Figure 2. Bilateral kainic acid lesions in the caudal PPRF of two monkeys (H72 and H64) that disrupted saccades in all directions, even when the lesions were small (H64). Numbers above drawings of sections indicate stereotaxic planes of coronal sections. BC, brachium conjunctivum; MLF, medial longitudinal fasciculus; PH, nucleus prepositus hypoglossi; VI, abducens nucleus; VII, facial nucleus; n VII, facial nerve. From Henn *et al.* (1984b).

population of neurons important for horizontal eye movements is present in the rostral pontine reticular formation and that a population important for vertical eye movements is present in the midbrain reticular formation, whereas the caudal PRF may be important for all saccades. Anatomic studies described below have more specifically implicated these and other portions of brainstem reticular formation as projecting to abducens and other oculomotor nuclei.

10.1.3. Efferent Projections of Abducens Neurons

In addition to neurons innervating the lateral rectus and the projections of internuclear neurons to the group of medial rectus motoneurons in the oculomotor complex, there are projections to other oculomotor structures. About one-third of the internuclear neurons have axon collaterals that extend caudal to the abducens nucleus (Highstein *et al.*, 1982), where they may innervate the nucleus prepositus hypoglossi and parts of the vestibular complex (Baker and McCrea, 1979). There is also a population of abducens neurons that projects directly to the flocculus of the cerebellum (e.g., Alley *et al.*, 1975; Langer *et al.*, 1985). Thus, the abducens neurons have a much larger function than simple contraction of the lateral rectus muscle.

Physiological studies have described three types of brainstem neuron with discharge patterns linked to saccades. These are "burst" neurons, "omnipause" neurons, and "tonic" neurons and are discussed in that order.

10.2. Burst Neurons

10.2.1. Burst Neuron Physiology

Short-lead burst neurons is the term used to designate the reticular neurons whose discharge commences about 8–10 msec prior to saccades and continues until near saccade offset (Fig. 3). Originally these neurons were called "medium lead" to distinguish them from motoneurons, but short lead is now in general use. The term "short lead" is used in contradistinction to *"long-lead" burst neurons,* whose discharge onset may occur 100 msec or more prior to saccade onset. (Figure 4 schematizes the discharge patterns of the various types of burst neurons described in this section.) Although the short- and long-lead burst neurons were originally described as separate by Luschei and Fuchs (1972), they now appear to be on a continuum, since intermediate lead times have now been described in cat (Kaneko *et al.*, 1981) and monkey (Scudder *et al.*, 1982). Most pontobulbar burst neurons discharge most vigorously and earliest for ipsilateral horizontal saccades, although these neurons also show some discharge for vertical saccades. A smaller population of pontine neurons have near-vertical on directions, and still fewer have oblique on directions.

There are two subclasses of burst neurons.

Excitatory burst neurons (EBN) make monosynaptic excitatory connections with the ipsilateral abducens nucleus (Sasaki and Shimazu, 1981) and are localized to the ipsilateral dorsal pontine reticular formation in both cat and monkey, as is more fully described below (Langer *et al.*, 1986). Keller (1974) described these neurons as most dense within 2.0 mm of the midline in the cat. Both short- and long-lead burst neurons are found in this region, although in monkey long-lead burst neurons tend to occur more rostrally in the non-giant-cell portion of pontine reticular formation (Luschei and Fuchs, 1972; Hepp and Henn, 1983).

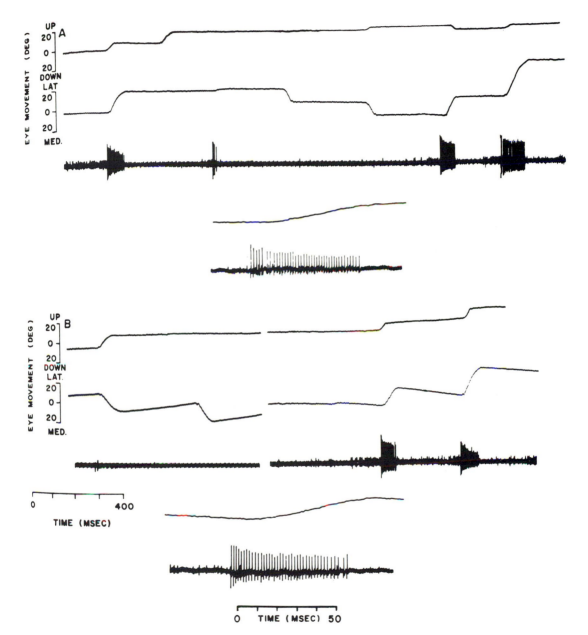

Figure 3. Activity of an ipsilateral short-lead burst unit in the cat during saccadic eye movement (A) and the quick-phase movements of rotationally induced vestibular nystagmus (B). In A and B upper trace is vertical and middle trace is horizontal eye position. The time calibration for both is shown below B. Insets in A and B are high-speed records of one horizontal rapid eye movement and associated unit activity; inset time calibration is shown below B, and eye movement calibration is the same as in low-speed records. From Keller (1974).

Inhibitory burst neurons (IBN) (Hikosaka *et al.*, 1978) monosynaptically inhibit contralateral abducens neurons and are located in the dorsomedial pontobulbar reticular formation caudal and ventromedial to the abducens nucleus (see below) and consist of both short- and long-lead burst neurons in both cat (Kaneko and Fuchs, 1981) and monkey (Scudder *et al.*, 1988).

Burst neurons with vertical on directions have been recorded in the rostral interstitial nucleus of the medial longitudinal fasciculus (riMLF; Büttner and Henn, 1977; King and Fuchs, 1979). They resemble pontine short-lead burst neurons but have shorter lead times. Within this area are both excitatory and inhibitory burst neurons (Nakao and Shiraishi, 1983).

Most short-lead burst neurons have nearly horizontal or vertical preferred directions, and this may reflect coding either along the pulling planes of the extraocular muscles (Büttner *et al.*, 1977) or along the planes of the semicircular canals (Robinson and Zee, 1981). One approach to decoding saccade generation has been to evaluate certain parameters of short-lead burst neuron discharge as determining saccade duration, peak velocity, and saccade size (Luschei and Fuchs, 1972; Keller, 1974; Kaneko and Fuchs, 1981; van Gisbergen *et al.*, 1981; Yoshida *et al.*, 1981).

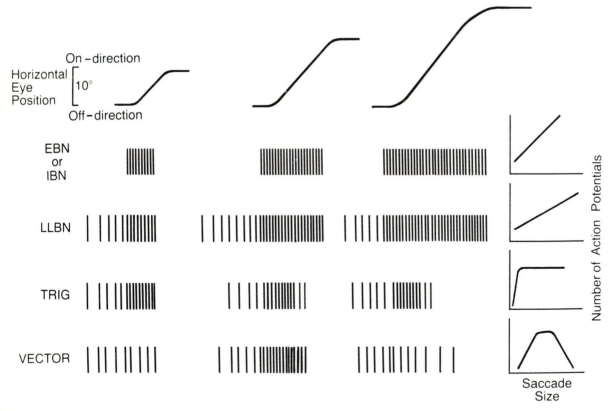

Figure 4. Schematic discharge patterns of the different types of burst neurons for three sizes of horizontal on-direction saccades. To the right, the number of action potentials in the burst is plotted as a function of saccade size for each unit type. The units are an excitatory (EBN) or an inhibitory (IBN) burst neuron, a long-lead burst neuron (LLBN), a trigger burst neuron (TRIG), and a vector burst neuron (VECTOR). From Fuchs *et al.* (1985).

Another approach has been to consider saccades as vectors, with both angle and magnitude encoded by properties of pontine reticular neurons (Henn and Cohen, 1976; Hepp and Henn, 1983). Henn and colleagues suggest, as do other workers in the field, that short-lead burst neurons are the "predominant final common pathway for all rapid eye movements." Targets are initially centrally coded not in retinal but in head (spatial) coordinates. This centrally available target information is processed into a neuronal signal encoding an *eye displacement vector* to the target in the superior colliculus and the frontal eye fields (see below for discussion of these zones). The transformation of this spatial coding to the temporally coded discharges of short-lead burst neurons has been the object of study by Hepp and Henn (1983), who quantitatively analyzed the rapid eye movement parameters of long-lead burst neurons in monkey pontine reticular formation (PRF) in relationship to the corresponding firing patterns of short-lead burst neurons. These workers found that burst neurons in rostral PRF have predominantly *spatially coded* movement fields, whereas in the caudal PRF there is *temporal coding* of burst strength in the pulling directions of extraocular eye muscles (near horizontal or near vertical). Both rostral and caudal PRF populations have ipsilateral on directions and contain long-lead burst neurons. The temporally coded long-lead bursters, termed "direction bursters or D-burster" have discharge patterns similar to short-lead burst neurons save for earlier "on" latencies and some preferences for small or large oblique saccades. The new feature postulated by these workers is that "the spatially coded burst neurons form a *motor map of saccadic vectors*." These spatially coded long-lead neurons are called "vector bursters or V-bursters" and discharge only for saccades to a limited region of the visual field, which they term the cell's "motor field."

They postulate the following signal transformation sequence. Superior colliculus projects to V-bursters in spatial coding (head coordinates). The V-bursters project to D-bursters in both PRF and mesencephalic reticular formation (MRF), and it is this projection that effects the transformation from head coordinates to eye position coordinates. It is proposed that D-bursters in PRF project to one population of horizontal short-lead burst neurons and D-bursters in MRF to one population of vertical short-lead burst neurons, with relative projection strength being proportional to the relative proportion of horizontal and vertical movement to be effected. Section 10.6 below discusses evidence other workers have found for an important role of the superior colliculus in the transformation of spatial to eye movement motor coding.

10.2.2. Anatomic Connectivity of Burst Neurons

10.2.2.1. Anatomy of Pontobulbar Reticular Projections to Abducens

Pontine reticular formation projections to abducens were first shown in anterograde tracing experiments in the cat (Büttner-Ennever, 1976; Graybiel, 1977a). A recent HRP study by Langer *et al.* (1986) using the more sensitive TMB method has confirmed the presence of quite substantial reticuloabducens projections (Fig. 5), whose extent was not seen in earlier HRP studies using a less sensitive chromogen (Maciewicz *et al.*, 1977; Gacek, 1979). In the region rostral to the abducens in the monkey, neurons projecting to the abducens are confined

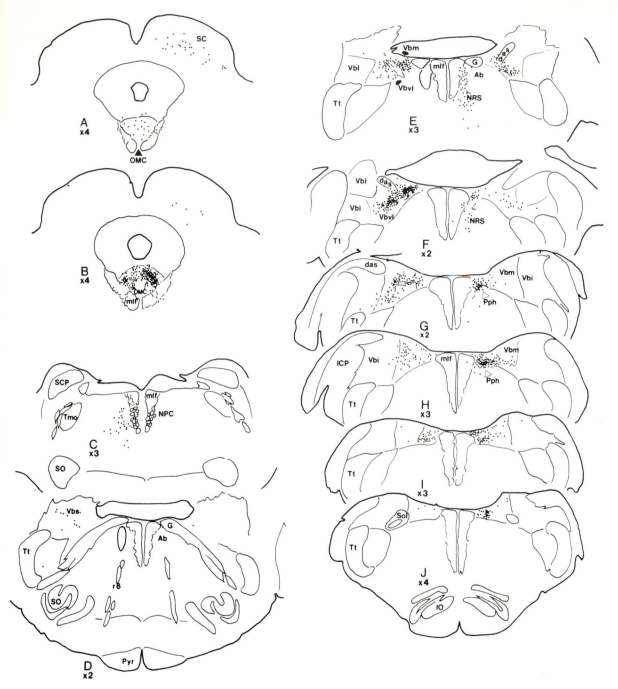

Figure 5. Distribution of retrogradely labeled neurons after HRP injection in cat right abducens nucleus. The ellipsoid shape just to the left of MLF in sections E and D indicates the injection site. Each dot represents one retrogradely labeled neuron. The numbers under the section letters indicate the number of histological sections that were compressed into the illustrated section. Ab, abducens nucleus; SC, superior colliculus; OMC, oculomotor complex; NPC, nucleus reticularis pontis caudalis; G, genu of VII; Vb, vestibular nuclei; i,l,m,s, inferior, lateral, medial, superior, respectively; NRS, nucleus reticularis supragigantocellularis (a non-giant-cell zone dorsal to the FTG); Pph, prepositus hypoglossi. From Langer *et al.* (1986).

almost entirely to the *ipsilateral* region dorsomedial or medial to the large-cell regions of the rostral and caudal medial pontine reticular formation, whereas in the cat they are somewhat more dispersed and mingled with the large neurons of this region. These neurons undoubtedly correspond to the physiologically defined excitatory burst neurons.

In the cat just at and slightly caudal to the level of abducens is another cluster of neurons in a *contralateral* region just lateral to the MLF but medial to the lateral border of abducens and extending dorsoventrally from the ventral border of abducens approximately to the same level ventrally as the MLF. This region is devoid of giant cells, being both somewhat dorsal to the giant-cell zone and also in the pontomedullary junction portion of PFTG and BFTG that is without giant cells. In the monkey the abducens projecting neurons occupy approximately the same contralateral non-giant-cell region as in the cat. These contralaterally situated neurons correspond to the physiologically defined group of inhibitory burst neurons. In the monkey but not the cat, a few contralateral neurons are seen in reticular core rostral to the rootlets of the abducens nerve, also in accord with physiologically defined burst neurons that fire before contralateral saccades (Luschei and Fuchs, 1972; Henn and Cohen, 1976).

10.2.2.2. Nonreticular Brainstem Projections to Abducens

In both the cat and the monkey, Langer *et al.* (1986) found the largest source of abducens afferents to be bilateral projections from the ventrolateral vestibular nucleus and the rostral pole of the medial vestibular nucleus. This suggests that the heavy vestibular labeling found by the Stanton and Greene (1981) HRP study resulted from HRP deposition in the abducens nucleus and not in the pontine reticular formation, which, by contrast, was shown to have only relatively sparse afferents from vestibular nuclei in the Shammah-Lagnado *et al.* (1987) study. Large numbers of abducens-projecting neurons are also found in the ventral margin of the nucleus prepositus hypoglossi in the cat and the common margin of this nucleus and the medial vestibular nucleus in the monkey. The prepositus–medial vestibular complex and projection to oculomotor neurons may be the source of the "neural integrator"; these neurons show burst–tonic discharge patterns (see discussion below). In the monkey large numbers of neurons are present in contralateral medial rectus subdivision of oculomotor complex, whereas in the cat large numbers of retrogradely labeled neurons are seen in a small periaqueductal gray nucleus just dorsal to the caudal pole of the oculomotor complex. Both species have a few contralateral superior colliculus neurons projecting to the abducens. The monkey but not the cat has abducens-projecting neurons in the nucleus reticularis tegmenti pontis and in the ipsilateral riMLF and bilateral interstitial nucleus of Cajal.

10.2.2.3. Superior Colliculus and Frontal Eye Field Projections to Reticular Formation

The paramedian pontine reticular region involved in saccade generation receives important input from higher centers. The contralateral superior colliculus provides a monosynaptic excitatory input to medial pontobulbar reticular formation in both cat (Grantyn and Grantyn, 1976) and monkey, consistent with anatomic data; recordings in alert monkeys indicate that this short-latency input is to long-lead burst neurons and to omnipause neurons (see below) but not to short-lead burst neurons (Raybourn and Keller, 1977). The likely cellular source of this superior colliculus input has been recently identified by Moschovakis and co-workers (1988a,b), who intraaxonally labeled squirrel monkey superior colliculus neurons whose saccadic parameters had been defined in the alert animal. One type of tectal efferent neuron morphologically identified as the T group was found to send axonal projections to the contralateral predorsal bundle (Fig. 6A), whose targets include the pontine nuclei reticularis pontis oralis and caudalis (Harting, 1977). Axonal collaterals also contact eye-movement-related areas of mesencephalic reticular formation as well as other tectal neurons. These neurons discharge with intense bursts beginning about 20 msec before spontaneous saccades within their movement field (see Fig. 6B) and hence were termed "vectorial" bursters. This wiring is compatible with the notion of the superior colliculus as transforming retinal error signals into motor commands and transmitting them to preoculomotor structures (see discussion below in Section 10.6).

In addition to a frontal eye field to superior colliculus projection (Segraves and Goldberg, 1987), there is a direct frontal eye field (prearcuate frontal cortex) to paramedian pontine reticular formation projection (Leichnetz *et al.*, 1984).

10.3. Omnipause Neurons

Omnipause neurons (OPNs, Fig. 7) are characterized by pauses that begin shortly before saccades in all directions (latency of 13–16 msec; Raybourn and Keller, 1977; Evinger *et al.*, 1982) and are thought to exert a tonic inhibition on the short-lead burst neurons of the medial pontine reticular formation. The arrest of the high-frequency firing of omnipause neurons (100–200 Hz) releases the short-lead burst neurons, whose activity, in turn, directly and indirectly excites the extraocular muscle motoneurons and leads to saccades. The OPNs likely also project to riMLF (Büttner-Ennever, 1977).

In the monkey Büttner-Ennever *et al.* (1988) have recently described a new nucleus, which they have named the nucleus raphe interpositius (rip), as the anatomic locus of the omnipause neurons. The rip lies in the midline area at the same rostrocaudal level as the descending sixth nerve rootlets, i.e., in caudal pons and including the most rostral portion of bulb. The rip is ventral to the raphe pontis.

Büttner-Ennever and co-workers used extracellular recordings to define units with omnipauser characteristics, and the recording area so marked with a

---

Figure 6. Camera lucida reconstruction of initial axonal system of a centrally located tectal long-lead burst neuron. Solid triangle in the reticular formation points to origin of the commissural (C) branch from one of the ascending fibers. X in circle indicates the point of descent to pons in the predorsal bundle (PDB). Bottom: Plot of the number of spikes in burst (N_b) for the neuron shown above as a function of amplitude of horizontal and vertical displacement of the eyes. Axis labels indicate number of degrees displacement. Modified from Moschovakis *et al.* (1988b).

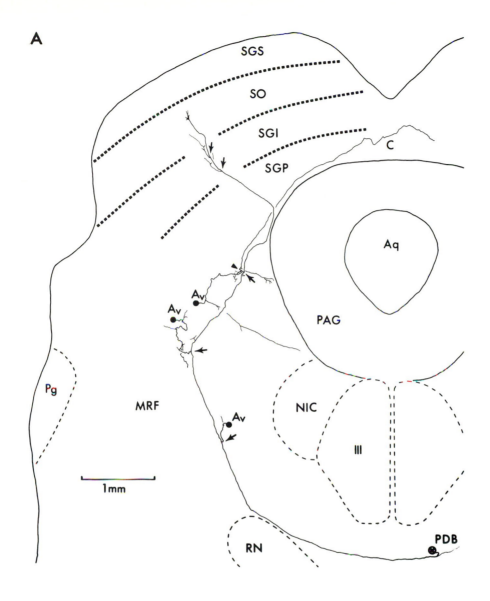

A

SGS

SO

SGI

C

SGP

Aq

Av

Av

PAG

Av

Pg

MRF

NIC

III

1mm

RN

PDB

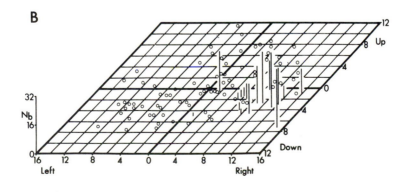

B

12

Up

8

4

32

Nb

0

16

4

8

0

Down

16   12   8   4   0   4   8   12   16   12

Left   Right

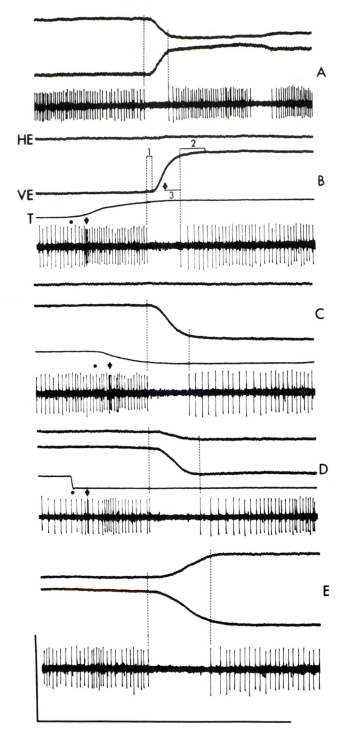

Figure 7. Discharge patterns of OPNs during spontaneous (A,E) and visually elicited (B–D) saccades. In B–D, the onset of the target movement (T) is indicated by a dot, and the downward arrows point to the visual response. In B, period 1 is the interval from the beginning of the pause to the beginning of the saccade, period 2 is from the end of the saccade to the end of the pause, and period 3 is from maximum velocity (upward arrow) to the end of the pause. Calibration is 25° and 500 msec. From Evinger *et al.* (1982).

single electrolytic lesion per animal has a quite distinct morphology compared with the more ventral and rostral pontine raphe pontis. As shown in Fig. 8, rip neurons in the monkey are arranged in a distinctive, narrow, orderly band on either side of the midline; these neurons have very large horizontally oriented dendritic trees that cross the midline. A similar morphology is found in the human, while in the cat and rat similar cell types are present but are not arranged in two distinct, bilateral groups. The rip is distinguished from raphe pontis by the presence in the latter nucleus of clustered neurons without large dendritic fields and, in cytochrome oxidase stain, a darkly staining neuropile. Also in contrast to raphe pontis, anterograde tritiated leucine studies indicate a direct projection from deep layers of superior colliculus, primarily crossed, to rip in contrast to no direct connectivity to raphe pontis and magnus. The rip also receives a direct input from the frontal eye field (Stanton *et al.*, 1989).

10.4. Tonic Neurons

We have previously discussed the saccade-related burst neuron input to the oculomotor system motoneurons. These motoneurons not only have a "burst" coding a change in eye position but a steady, tonic firing that codes eye position during fixation. How is the input to motoneurons for the steady fixation generated? As illustrated in Fig. 9, Robinson (1975) proposed that the "burst" discharge of excitatory and inhibitory burst neurons (which codes eye velocity) is integrated over time (in the mathematical sense) by a set of neurons called "the neural integrator" and that this integrator serves all systems using conjugate eye movements, i.e., the saccadic, vestibuloocular, optokinetic, and smooth pursuit systems.

A few units have been found in pontine reticular formation that carried a pure position signal (Luschei and Fuchs, 1972; Keller, 1974) compatible with the output of a neural integrator. However, the PRF lesions by Henn *et al.* (1984b) did not produce neural integration deficits, suggesting that the integrator might lie elsewhere. Recently Cannon and Robinson (1987) have presented kainic and ibotenic acid lesion evidence that the medial vestibular nucleus (MVN) and nucleus prepositus hypoglossi are the loci of the neural integration of horizontal eye movements. Microinjections of these neurotoxins into the prepositus–MVN complex of the monkey produced the characteristic stigmata of a "leaky integrator": saccades were made with accuracy to targets, but the fixation did not hold, and eye position drifted back to a null position with an exponential time constant whose rate of decay reflected the leakiness or damage to the integrator. The dynamism of this lesion is shown in Fig. 10, illustrating progressively more severe effects (parts B → C → D) following injection in the alert monkey. [The kainic/ibotenic acid effects were not permanent, and recovery ensued usually after a few hours or at a maximum of a week. Acute toxic effects in the awake monkey prevented the administration of doses of kainic acid higher than 2–4 μg/ul (with 1-μl doses to avert spread). There was very little neuronal damage save for the immediate area of the cannula tip, thus suggesting that acute effects resulted from depolarization sufficient to cause action potential blockade but not sufficient to kill the neurons.] As predicted for a common integrator system, the

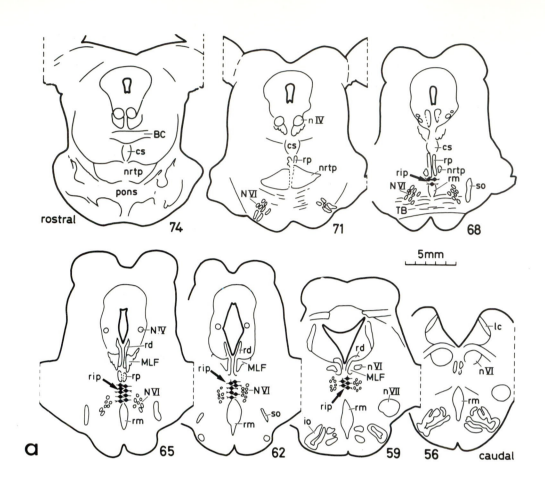

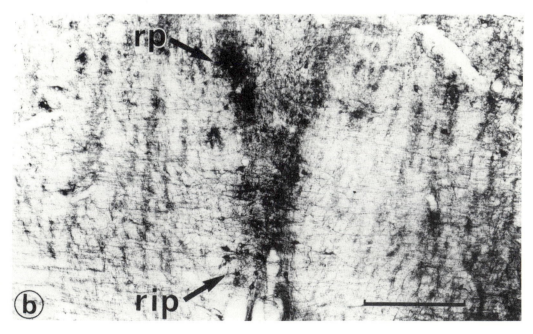

vestibuloocular reflex, optokinetic responses, and smooth pursuit were also affected. Independent and simultaneously obtained data from Cheron and collaborators (1986a,b) indicate that electrolytic lesions of the propositus hypoglossi in the cat also cause a complete loss of the neural integrator.

10.5. Saccade Generation: Interaction of Neurons in the Circuit

Figure 11, from Fuchs *et al.* (1985), summarizes the known and postulated connectivity of the horizontal saccade generator. During fixation OPNs fire at high rates, inhibit EBNs and IBNs, and prevent saccades. For saccade generation an excitatory signal proportional to the desired saccade size is fed to the appropriate EBNs while at the same time an inhibitory trigger signal is given to the OPNs. Note that the excitatory signal to EBNs derives from input from superior colliculus that reflects the horizontal distance of the target from the current foveal position and is fed through the long-lead burst neurons. The EBNs are disinhibited when OPNs cease firing; they then respond to the excitatory input and drive ipsilateral motoneurons to produce the burst component of their discharge. The EBNs also excite IBNs, which in turn inhibit the OPNs for the duration of the saccade—this feature means the saccade continues even if initiated by a transient trigger signal.

Some comment on the postulated anatomic underpinnings of portions of this sketch is useful. In Robinson's model (1975) the EBNs project to tonic neurons, which both lesion data (Cannon and Robinson, 1987) and recent electrophysiological recordings (McFarland and Fuchs, personal communication) have suggested may be localized to the medial vestibular–prepositus complex. These tonic neurons might be part of a network that integrates the EBN signal to yield an eye position signal. The "trigger" input to OPN may come from superior colliculus, directly and/or through a relay involving the long-lead burst neurons, and the frontal eye field is yet another possible input source.

Both superior colliculus and the frontal eye fields could provide excitatory inputs into the burst generator since stimulation of either evokes short-latency saccades and both project to PRF. In particular, the saccade-related cells of deep and intermediate layers of superior colliculus that discharge only during saccades are particularly appealing sources since physiological data suggest they project to long-lead burst neurons, which in turn may project to EBNs (although proof of this latter projection is still lacking). The frontal eye fields, which project directly to PRF, are also postulated to initiate saccades via projections to long-lead burst neurons.

Figure 8. The brainstem of a macaque monkey drawn from cresyl-violet-stained sections, cut in the stereotaxic plane, to show the location of the cell group nucleus raphe interpositus (rip). The cells of rip are indicated by arrows and drawn diagrammatically. Consecutively numbered sections are 240 μm apart. Bottom: Cytochrome-oxidase-stained section. Note the darkly stained cell bodies of rip around the midline and their extensive horizontally oriented dendritic fields. Calibration, 1 mm. Abbreviations: cs, nucleus centralis superior; rp, nucleus raphe pontis; nrtp, nucleus reticularis tegmenti pontis; rm, nucleus raphe magnus. Modified from Büttner-Ennever *et al.* (1988).

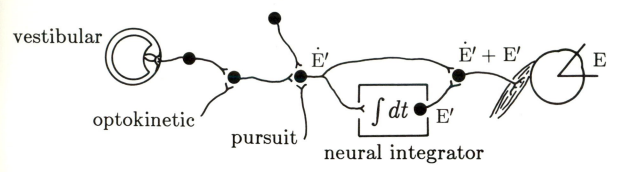

saccades and
quick phases

vestibular

Ė′

Ė′ + E′

E

optokinetic

pursuit

∫ dt

E′

neural integrator

Figure 9. The final common integrator hypothesis. All eye movement commands are initiated as eye-velocity encoded signals, Ė′, which then enter the neural integrator to provide the eye-position encoded signal, E′, present on the motoneuron. The arrangement is schematic and is only intended to show that all eye-velocity signals are passed directly to the motoneurons along with the integrated eye-position signals and is not intended to represent neurons actually involved in this process. From Cannon and Robinson (1987).

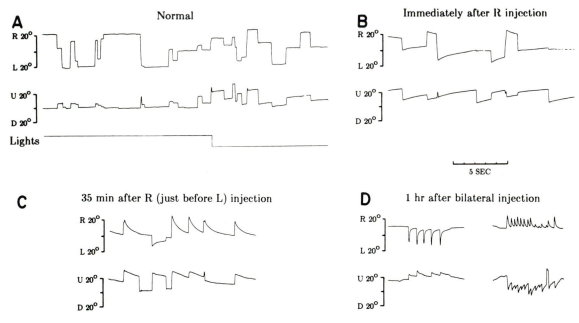

A Normal

R 20°
L 20°

U 20°
D 20°

Lights

B Immediately after R injection

R 20°
L 20°

U 20°
D 20°

5 SEC

C 35 min after R (just before L) injection

R 20°
L 20°

U 20°
D 20°

D 1 hr after bilateral injection

R 20°
L 20°

U 20°
D 20°

Figure 10. Saccadic eye movements before and after ibotenate injection in prepositus hypoglossi. Horizontal eye position is on upper trace, vertical on lower. A: Target-directed and spontaneous saccades recorded from a normal monkey. In the first half of the record the fixation target was alternated between right and left 20°. For the second half, spontaneous eye movements were recorded in total darkness. Notice that even in total darkness horizontal gaze holding is steady. The upward drift in darkness is a form of downbeat nystagmus found in many normal rhesus monkeys. B–D: Each panel shows spontaneous saccades recorded in total darkness from the same monkey as in A at various times after the injection of 30 μg ibotenate in right (R) and left (L) prepositus hypoglossi. The records in D are two excerpts from a continuous record to demonstrate that eye position drifts centripetally after both leftward and rightward saccades. The time constant of the horizontal drift decreases progressively from 2 to 0.6 to 0.2 sec in B–D. A–D were recorded at the same time scale as indicated. R, L, U, D are right, left, up, and down. From Cannon and Robinson (1987).

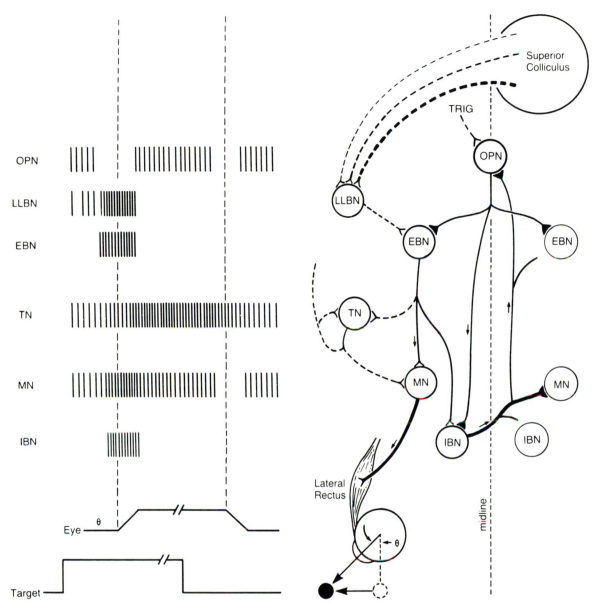

Figure 11. The discharge patterns and connections of neurons in the horizontal burst generator. Left: Firing patterns for an on-direction (first vertical dashed line) and off-direction (second dashed line) horizontal saccade of size θ to a target step (schematized in the eye and target traces below). Right: Excitatory connections are shown as open endings, inhibitory connections are shown as filled triangles, and axon collaterals of unknown destination (revealed by intracellular HRP injections or postulated in models) are shown without terminals. Connections known with certainty are represented by thick lines, uncertain connections by thin lines, and hypothesized connections by dashed lines. A description of the behavior of this neural circuit is found in the text. The abbreviations identify excitatory (EBN) and inhibitory (IBN) burst neurons, long-lead burst neurons (LLBN), trigger input neurons (TRIG), omnipause neurons (OPN), tonic neurons (TN), and motoneurons (MN). From Fuchs *et al.* (1985).

10.5.1. Role of Superior Colliculus in Saccades

Cells in the intermediate layer of superior colliculus discharge before saccadic eye movements. As illustrated in Fig. 6, each cell has its own movement field and discharges only before saccades with a particular range of directions and amplitude. Most superior colliculus neurons increase their discharge rate before saccades made under any condition (to visual targets, spontaneously, in the light or in the dark). Cells in the intermediate layers of the superior colliculus are organized so that their movement fields form a topographic map that is congruent with a visual map in the superficial layers. Electrical stimulation in the superior colliculus elicits saccadic eye movements in all mammals thus far studied, including monkey (Schiller and Stryker, 1972), cat (Hyde and Eason, 1959), and rodent (McHaffie and Stein, 1982). Microinjections of muscimol, a GABA agonist, into the monkey superior colliculus selectively suppress saccades to the movement field of the cells near the injection site (Hikosaka and Wurtz, 1985a). Muscimol produces both a striking decrease in velocity of saccades to visual targets and markedly distorted trajectories of remembered saccades, findings consistent with the initiation of saccadic vectors by superior colliculus and with an inhibitory role of GABA. By contrast the GABA antagonist bicuculline caused "irrepressible saccades" initially specific to the movement field at the injection site. Subsequent injections of muscimol and bicuculline into the pars reticulata of substantia nigra (SNPR) showed that the GABAergic projection was presumably via action on the GABA-receptive neurons of SNPR (Hikosaka and Wurtz, 1985b). (Because GABA is inhibitory to SNPR and the SNPR $\rightarrow$ SC input is inhibitory, bicuculline in SNPR acts like muscimol in SC, whereas muscimol in SNPR acts like the bicuculline in SC.) It is to be noted that in similar SNPR injections in rats there is a circling behavior to the side contralateral to the injection, suggesting that the SNPR may control all orienting movements, which are more eye-oriented in the fovea-dominant monkey and more body-oriented in the rat.

10.5.2. Saccade Trajectories: Mutable or Immutable?

An early assumption was that the burst generator was controlled by a retinal error signal (position of the target relative to the fovea) and that the course of saccades was immutable once initiated. Newer data suggest that, in fact, there is internal feedback control in terms of eye position. Monkeys viewing a quick sequence of two targets whose presentation is terminated before any saccade onset make successive and accurate saccades to the first and then to the second target. This is true despite the fact that the "retinal error signal" at the time of presentation of the second target is not equivalent to the size and angle of the saccade that moved the fovea from target 1 to target 2. ("Retinal error signal" is the difference between foveal position and either of the targets.) This consequently suggests that current eye position is used in conjunction with retinal error to generate saccades (Mays and Sparks, 1980). Target position in space (see definition below) rather than retinal error may be the driving signal for saccades.

In 1975 Robinson proposed an enormously influential and useful model that incorporated the above findings and that has been of great impetus to research. He suggested that the EBNs are driven by a signal proportional to (target position in space) − (eye position) (see Fig. 12):

TIS = target position in space = (neural representation of eye position, from integration of EBN output by tonic neurons) + (retinal error signal)

Since this signal is delayed by 0.2 sec, the neural representation of the target position in space does not change in the course of a normal saccade. Also, the neural representation of eye position is subtracted by the EBN to produce a motor error signal in retinal coordinates. Note that the initial motor error for single saccades is exactly equal to retinal error. However, before the second saccade in the above double-step paradigm the initial motor error will be:

dynamic motor error = (target position in space) − (current eye movement)

Note also that as the eye approaches the target, the dynamic motor error declines and reaches zero, leading to a zero net drive to EBNs and silencing them, thus terminating the saccade. The control is not ballistic, since the feedback loop will correct for an unexpected perturbation and allow the eyes to reach the target. This feedback control is supported by Sparks and Mays's (1983) experiment showing that stimulation of the superior colliculus in the middle of a targeting saccade, thereby perturbing the system by altering eye position, led to a subsequent new saccade that compensated for this perturbation. Other groups have also stimulated OPNs during an ongoing saccade; the interrupted saccade accurately reached the target (see Fuchs *et al.*, 1985).

Several modifications to the original Robinson model have now been proposed, and we present one of these to give the flavor of the kind of modifications being made. Scudder (1988; see Fig. 12B) suggests a more realistic representation of superior colliculus influence in that the LLBNs receive a topographically weighted output (represented by lines of different strength) of the superior colliculus (SLBN do not receive direct superior colliculus input). The eye position (motor) error feedback in this model is on the LLBN and is via an inhibitory recurrent projection from an IBN, whose discharge pattern is essentially identical to that of an EBN. [Keller (1980) has proposed that the neural replica of eye position is sent to the superior colliculus, where it is compared with target position to generate motor error.] When the number of spikes added by the colliculus equals the number of spikes subtracted by the IBN feedback (note that the LLBN is connected to perform as an integrator), there is a cessation of LLBN discharge, the EBN ceases firing, and the saccade ends. In addition to the absence of any documented SC → SLBN input, the colliculus already encodes initial motor error (= desired saccade size) in the topographic distribution of its neurons. Another feature of the Scudder model is that there is a nonspecific SC

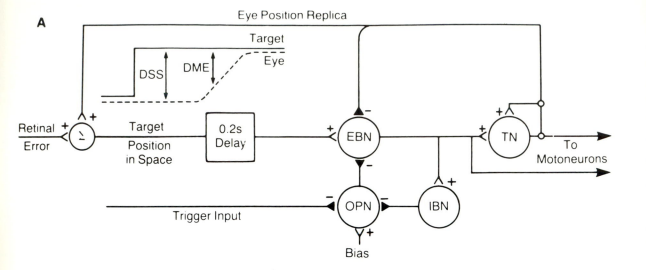

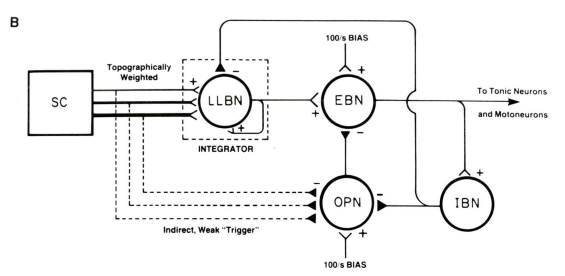

Figure 12. Models of the saccade generator. A: The Robinson model, in which a neural replica of eye position is added to retinal error to create target position in space and later subtracted to generate motor error at the EBN membrane. The physical variables that exist as neural replicas in the model include (inset) target and eye position relative to the head, desired saccade size (DSS, the motor error that exists before the saccade begins), and dynamic motor error (DME, the motor error that exists while the saccade is in progress). The bias signal to the OPN produces its steady firing between saccades. B: The Scudder model. The model uses local (i.e., neural) feedback, but unlike the Robinson model,

it matches change in target position (the output of the colliculus) with change in eye position (the output of the IBN). Topographical weighting of the colliculus projection is symbolized by the lines of different thickness. The unweighted and indirect inhibitory projection from the SC to the OPN is symbolized by the dotted lines of constant thickness. The LLBN is wired to integrate its two inputs as symbolized by the recurrent positive feedback with a gain of 1.0. The EBN projects to the IBN as shown and is also assumed to project to the tonic neurons and motoneurons (not shown) as in the Robinson model. Modified from Fuchs *et al.* (1985) and from Scudder (1988).

trigger output to OPNs assisting in saccade initiation, although the degree of OPN inhibition and hence its role in saccade initiation is less critical in this model.

As a sample of the kinds of experiments the Robinson model's conceptualizations have promoted and of the current state of confirmation/nonconfirmation, it is useful to review Sparks and co-workers' recent study (1987) of the effect of pontine reticular stimulation in the monkey on eye movements. They reasoned that if a copy of the motor command is used as a feedback signal of eye position (note feedback loop in the Robinson model), then failure to compensate for stimulation-induced movements would indicate that stimulation occurred at a site distal to (e.g., closer to the motoneurons) the point from which the eye position signal was derived. Thus, in the sketch in Fig. 11, stimulation would occur at a point nearer to the motoneurons than the takeoff point of the feedback signals. It is known, for example, that animals do not compensate for direct stimulation of the trochlear nerve or of sites close to the abducens nucleus. Briefly, the results were that animals compensated for stimulation at about one-half of all pontine sites where SLBN have been reported. Only the compensation is predicted by Robinson's model. (This of course assumes that the electrical stimulation is indeed a fair test of SLBN activation, since activation of fibers of passage with unknown effects would complicate the interpretation.) An unexpected finding was that pontine stimulation at times prematurely triggered impending visually directed saccades. The time course of this effect suggested that the build-up of input to saccadic generator circuits occurs over an epoch of some 100 msec. A further point of theoretical importance was that the "saccade trigger signal" was dissociated from the signal providing the metrics of the upcoming saccade.

In concluding this portion of the chapter it is again useful to emphasize the important role of formal modeling in making explicit the assumptions of various hypotheses of neural control and processing. Although the pure empiricist may object to the "postulation" of more circuitry than is known, and to the substitution of simplified schemes for the full complexity of neural circuitry and physiological actions, we suggest the history of the development of knowledge about the oculomotor system provides one of the best "case examples" of the usefulness of models for the experimental neurophysiologist.

10.6. Gaze Control

The previous sections have discussed control of eye movement, considered independently of movements of the head directed toward visual targets. It is, however, apparent that control of gaze, defined as cooperative movements of both eye and head in targeting, is also an important topic, although one that has been less intensely investigated. Bender *et al.* (1964) had observed that stimulation of caudal PRF led to ipsilateral head and eye movements, and Sirkin *et al.* (1980) found that electrolytic lesions of this zone eliminated ipsiversive head movements as well as the ipsilateral quick phases of ocular nystagmus. Because these lesions could have involved fibers of passage, more reliable information appears in more recent studies using intraaxonal recordings and HRP labeling.

Grantyn and colleagues recorded intraaxonally in the caudal pons in alert, head-restrained cats and found, among the many axons sampled, a small group of neurons ($N = 5$) whose soma location could be determined and that met the criteria of antidromic activation from ipsilateral cervical spinal cord and monosynaptic activation from ipsilateral superior colliculus (Grantyn and Berthoz, 1987; Grantyn *et al.*, 1987). Soma location was determined either by HRP labeling ($N = 2$) or by the presence of attenuated PSPs ($N = 3$), indicating axonal recordings near the soma. The somas so localized were in caudal pons rostral to abducens, and three of the five neurons had a discharge pattern that led to their description as "eye–neck" reticulospinal neurons (EN-RSN). The EN-RSN had discharge patterns correlated with ipsiversive eye movements, eccentric eye fixations, and the EMG profile of ipsilateral neck muscles in the course of the behaviors of spontaneous visual scanning or tracking of objects presented in the visual field. These neurons were silent when the eyes were deviated contralaterally (beyond the vertical meridian), and the ipsilateral neck muscles were

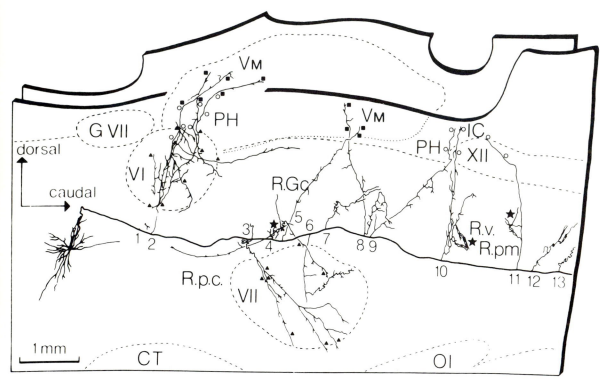

Figure 13. Parasagittal plane reconstruction of an intraaxonally HRP-stained eye–neck reticulospinal neuron in the cat. Physiologically this neuron was characterized by a monosynaptic response to contralateral superior colliculus stimulation and antidromic invasion from stimulating electrodes in C2. The axon courses 0.8–0.9 mm lateral to the midline and ventral to the MLF, although the soma is about 1.3 mm lateral to midline. Collateral projections are widespread but are clustered in particular target zones rather than being diffusely distributed throughout the rhomben- cephalon. Symbols denote portions of collaterals restricted to the abducens (VI) or facial (VII) nuclei (filled triangles); to the prepositus hypoglossi (PH) and nucleus intercalatus Staderini (IC, open circles); and to the medial (Vm) vestibular nucleus (filled squares). Other abbreviations: R.p.c, nucleus reticularis pontis caudalis; GVII, genu of VII; R.Gc., R.v., R.pm, nucleus reticularis gicantocellularis, ventralis, and paramedianis, respectively; IC, nucleus intercalatus. Adapted from Grantyn *et al.* (1987).

relaxed. However, they became phasically active before saccades terminating close to the vertical meridian or further in the ipsilateral hemifield, with the onset and time course of activity correlating with ipsilateral neck EMG activation. Overall discharge rate was approximately proportional to the eccentricity of gaze shift in this "head-fixed" condition, although with prolonged eccentric eye fixation discharge rate declined, thus suggesting a predominant role in phasic components of gaze. The functional inference is that, at eye positions in the ipsilateral hemifield, targets located still further (ipsi-) laterally in the visual field would demand a neck movement to bring the target on the fovea. The firing pattern of EN-RSN neurons was distinct from that of excitatory burst neurons (see previous discussion), although the EN-RSN were located in the same caudal PRF region just rostral to abducens (pontine FTG region) as excitatory burst neurons.

In two neurons intraaxonal HRP labeling was sufficiently complete to label the axon course as far as the medullary pyramidal decussation and also to label its extensive collaterals (Grantyn *et al.*, 1987), and Fig. 13 shows a camera lucida parasagittal section reconstruction of one. Its axonal collateral distribution pattern and a bouton density analysis indicated extensive projections to abducens, seventh nerve nucleus, prepositus hypoglossi, vestibular nucleus (especially medial), and bulbar reticular formation, especially the giant-cell field.

This neuron is of interest also in terms of reticular neuronal morphology. Its axonal pathway in the bulbar reticular formation (ventral and lateral to the MLF and neighboring associated fiber tracts, see Chapter 4) labels it as an iBRF neuron in the reticular neuronal axonal classification scheme derived from the larger sample study of descending PRF neurons described in Chapter 4 (Mitani *et al.*, 1988a,b), which found that only iBRF neurons were collateralized. Further, the two HRP-labeled neurons in the Grantyn *et al.* study had soma diameters of 45 and 55 μm, similar to the 47-μm soma size of the iBRF neuron illustrated in Fig. 25 of Chapter 4 that had both abducens and BRF projections. The reticular and nuclear projection zones of the EN-RSN neurons targeted those areas demonstrated to be involved in control of eye, ear, and axial movements, making the point that although reticular formation neurons may have widespread projections, it is, at least in the case of these two neurons, misleading to call the projections diffuse. It was of interest that some collaterals and their ramifications in reticular formation show a "segmental" pattern of distribution, e.g., projecting to a "poker-chip shaped" diskoid area suggested by Scheibel and Scheibel (1958) to be the predominant mode of reticular organization; however, many collaterals in the adult cats studied by Grantyn *et al.* did not have this pattern.

10.7. State-Dependent Alterations in Oculomotor System Function

10.7.1. Waking-to-Synchronized Sleep Transitions

The characteristic waking eye movement pattern of fixation, alternating with high velocity saccades, or of slow movements in response to visual or vestibular stimuli is transformed during the transition to sleep. As drowsiness occurs, saccadic velocity and number are reduced, and the transition to light slow-wave sleep is marked by an abrupt change to slow, drifting eye movements. In the transition to slow-wave sleep the discharge activity of brainstem oculomotor system neurons is also characteristically altered. Omnipause neurons suddenly

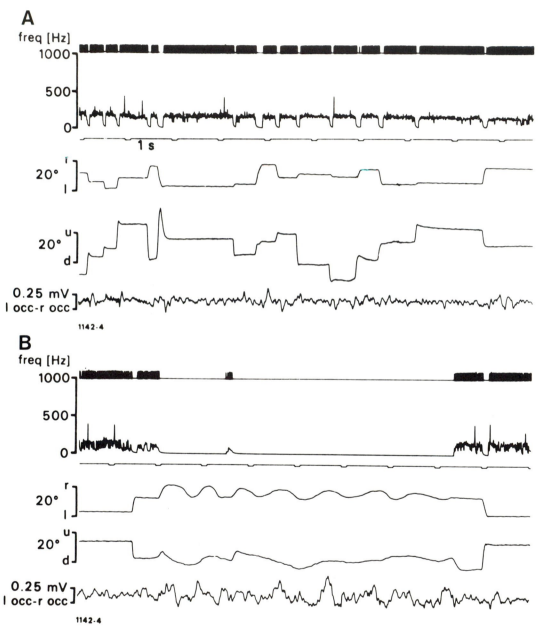

Figure 14. Pause neuron from the monkey pontine reticular formation. A: During alertness there is continuous regular discharge at about 180 Hz, which is only interrupted prior to and during rapid eye movements. B: During a period of light sleep there is cessation of neuronal activity and concomitant irregular continuous eye movements. Traces from above: blips marking the occurrences of spikes, instantaneous firing rate, horizontal and vertical eye position, and EEG traces (either left versus right occipital or left parietooccipital). From Henn *et al.* (1984a).

become silent coincident with the loss of ability to maintain fixation (Raybourn and Keller, 1977; Henn *et al.*, 1984a); they just as suddenly resume their firing on a slow-wave sleep-to-waking transition (Fig. 14). It is of interest that multiunit recordings showed that this omnipauser silence occurs throughout the population and that this "moment of sleep" change is completed in less than 10 msec (Henn *et al.*, 1984a). However, although the degree of latency of responsivity to synaptic input are altered during sleep, omnipause units retain sufficient responsivity to discharge in response to superior colliculus stimulation (Raybourn and Keller, 1977).

During slow-wave sleep both medial rectus and vertical eye movement motoneurons show a decreased amount of tonic firing for a given eye position as compared to the waking state, the decrease reaching approximately 50% in the monkey for longer sleep episodes (Henn *et al.*, 1984a), with similar findings being present in the cat abducens and internuclear motoneurons (Delgado-Garcia *et al.*, 1988a,b); this suggests that coactivation of the extraocular muscles is strongly relaxed during slow-wave sleep.

Short-lead burst neurons in slow-wave sleep show a marked decrease in the sharpness of "bursting," i.e., the occurrence of high peak of firing frequency as the burst begins, and the duration of bursts tends to be prolonged (Henn *et al.*, 1984a: see their Fig. 2). This neuronal activity corresponds to the presence of slow, drifting eye movements during slow-wave sleep as contrasted with the rapid, saccadic eye movements of waking. About one-half of short-lead bursters show tonic activity after waking–sleep transition, but this activity decreases as sleep becomes deeper. In general the distinction between short- and long-lead bursters blurs further as sleep is entered, and both discharge types show increased burst-on latencies. Burst–tonic neurons and vectorial long-lead bursters, like short-lead burst neurons, show decreased peak frequency and increased burst duration. Raybourn and Keller (1977) found that PRF tonic reticular units also became silent during drowsiness and light slow-wave sleep, whereas PRF burst–tonic neurons remained active. In contrast to the disruption in the oculomotor system, activity in vestibular-only neurons in the vestibular nuclei remains unchanged during head rotation in sleep (Henn *et al.*, 1984a). These workers reasoned that the observed sharp drop of vestibulooculomotor reflex (VOR) gain in sleep might consequently be the result of oculomotor system changes (although, it may be noted parenthetically, vestibular-only neurons may not participate in VOR). The sharp wake-to-sleep change in the oculomotor system has been modeled as a nonequilibrium phase transition (Hepp and Henn, 1983). It should be appreciated that the results described here have, in general, been obtained during "light" or initial slow-wave sleep and that the system has not been thoroughly explored in deep slow-wave sleep.

10.7.2. Activity during REM Sleep

The eye movements of REM sleep have been characterized in monkeys by use of the search-coil technique and have been found to differ considerably from those in waking. The first report was by Fuchs and Ron (1968), who found that most (60%) "rapid" eye movements of REM sleep had velocities less than 50 degrees/sec, whereas those with velocities >200 degrees/sec, the usual lower velocity cut-off for waking saccades, accounted for only 14% of eye movements in REM sleep. These REM sleep saccades usually had very short duration with very short intersaccade intervals (often 100 msec), much shorter than seen in waking. In waking with and without targets, eye movement velocities clustered at two extremes: most movements were saccades with velocities between 250 and 1000 degrees/sec, and smooth pursuit movements with velocities <50 degrees/sec were less frequent. In REM sleep about 30% of eye movements had velocities of 50–200 degrees/sec, whereas such velocities were quite rare in waking. Furthermore, records of REM sleep saccades had a "round-shouldered" appearance, indicating the absence of high-frequency components present in waking.

Perhaps the most distinctive difference between waking and REM sleep eye movements was a "loop" pattern observable in REM-sleep eye movements displayed in a two-dimensional format on an oscilloscope (Fig. 15). These loops were composed of both saccadic and slower movements with a usual range of 3–11 movements/loop. Loops occupied almost 30% of the REM period, with each loop lasting an average of 2.5 sec and loops occurring at a "remarkably constant" rate of about 7/min. Often the same starting point would be used for several loops, as seen in Fig. 15B. This loop pattern was in marked contrast to eye movements in waking with and without targets present, where loops were only very rarely present. Similar findings were reported by Bon *et al.* (1980), who used the search-coil technique in the semichronic *encephale isolé* cat and described REM-sleep eye movements as having "loop-shaped trajectories" that frequently returned to the original position, a pattern also not seen in waking in this cat preparation. Saccades in REM, as in waking, consist of conjugate eye movements, as contrasted with the disjunctive movements of slow-wave sleep.

We note that many studies have characterized eye movements in REM sleep using AC coupling of EOG signals; this technique is inferior to the search-coil technique, as it is unable to establish the absolute position of the eyeball. The

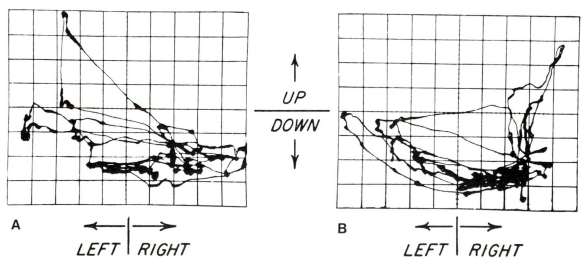

Figure 15. Two-dimensional displays of eye position during (A) a 15-sec and (B) a 30-sec interval within a REM-sleep episode in the monkey. Each small square is 10° on a side. The primary direction of gaze lies at the center of the oscilloscope screen. The trace intensity provides a qualitative measure of eye velocity ranging from dark spots showing fixation points to thin traces indicating a very rapid movement. Note the presence of many loop patterns. From Fuchs and Ron (1968).

technical limitations of earlier studies may have led to the belief that REM sleep eye movements resembled those of waking in the monkey (Weitzman, 1961), in the human (Roffwarg *et al.,* 1962), and in the cat (Jeannerod *et al.,* 1965). This belief, in turn, suggested the plausibility of the "scanning" hypothesis, that the REM sleep eye movements represented a "scanning" of the dream image. This hypothesis is obviously rendered implausible on the basis of the marked differences in animals between REM and waking eye movements described above. In addition, Aserinsky and colleagues (1985) have presented data from humans indicating that the eye movements of REM sleep are considerably slower than waking saccades of comparable amplitude (a finding compatible with the animal data) and that this slowing is greater than that attributable to either eye closure or eye movements in total darkness, thus disputing the earlier findings of Herman *et al.* (1983).

It may be somewhat surprising to the reader that the neuronal activity underlying the distinctive eye movements of REM sleep has not yet been thoroughly described. Unfortunately, laboratories interested in precise characterization of waking eye movements and neuronal activity have not done unit recordings during REM sleep, and laboratories interested in REM sleep neuronal activity have not employed the search-coil or DC recording-electrode techniques necessary for precise characterization of eye movement direction, velocity, and amplitude. Pivik *et al.* (1976) used AC-coupled EOG electrodes and reported an eye movement-associated discharge of neurons extracellularly recorded in various regions of the pontine reticular formation; since direction, velocity, and amplitude of eye movements could not be precisely specified, essentially only discharge latency and intensity relative to eye movement onset were available as data. These data did suggest that among the units recorded were neurons that might be characterized as short-lead and long-lead burst neurons and burst tonic neurons in the oculomotor literature. These units discharged in association with waking eye movements but had markedly reduced discharge in slow-wave sleep; during the rapid eye movements of REM sleep, the eye-movement-correlated firing again appeared, with both similarities and dissimilarities of discharge latency and intensity being present in waking and REM sleep. Many of these units were recorded in the giant-cell field; current data (Chapter 4) make it unlikely that these were giant cells, but the short-lead burst patterns observed may have been derived from recordings from the nongiant neurons in this region that project to abducens (Langer *et al.,* 1986; Mitani *et al.,* 1988b).

10.8. Mechanisms of the Muscle Atonia of REM Sleep: Motoneurons

One of the most striking features of REM sleep is the apparently paradoxical presence of muscle atonia coupled with a high level of activity of central neurons, including those in motor systems. In fact, one of the synonyms for REM sleep, paradoxical sleep, was coined by Jouvet and co-workers as an expression of this feature of REM sleep. The next portion of the chapter discusses cellular mechanisms for production of atonia. As with the oculomotor system, we take an "outside in" approach and discuss REM mechanisms for inhibition of spinal and trigeminal motoneurons before taking up the central mechanisms.

10.8.1. Inhibition and Diminished Excitability of Trigeminal Jaw-Closer Motoneurons during REM Sleep

Chase and co-workers (1980), using intracellular recordings in naturally sleeping cats, first identified jaw-closer motoneurons in the trigeminal motor nucleus by their monosynaptic response to stimulation of mesencephalic trigeminal nucleus and further identified masseter motoneurons by antidromic activation following masseter nerve stimulation. They then tracked membrane potential (MP) and other motoneuron parameters over the sleep–wake cycle. The most dramatic changes in MP occurred on transition from slow-wave sleep (S) to REM sleep, where all neurons underwent a tonic hyperpolarization that lasted throughout REM sleep and was 2–10 mV in magnitude (Fig. 16). On transition to waking the MP invariably depolarized. The MP on transition from waking to slow-wave sleep showed either a slight hyperpolarization or remained the same. Spontaneous discharge activity diminished and usually ceased with the hyperpolarization of REM sleep, with the occasional exception of discharges in association with the rapid eye movements or facial muscle twitches.

It was concluded that active inhibition rather than disfacilitation was respon-

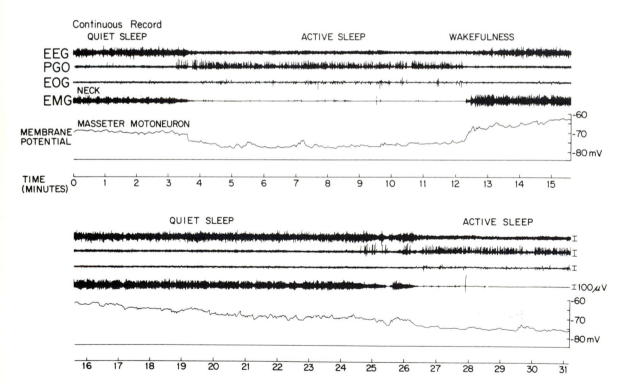

Figure 16. Intracellular recording from a trigeminal jaw-closer motoneuron: correlation of membrane potential and state changes. The membrane potential hyperpolarized rather abruptly at 3.5 min in conjunction with the decrease in neck muscle tone and transition from quiet (SWS) to active sleep (REM sleep). At 12.5 min the membrane depolarized, and the animal awakened. After the animal passed into quiet sleep again, a brief, aborted episode of active sleep occurred at 25.5 min that was accompanied by a phasic period of hyperpolarization. A minute later the animal once again entered active sleep, and the membrane potential increased. EEG trace, marginal cortex; membrane potential band-pass on polygraphic record is D.C. to 0.1 Hz. From Chase *et al.* (1980).

sible for this REM-sleep-specific hyperpolarization (Chandler *et al.*, 1980). In REM sleep, antidromic spikes were either blocked or showed a decrease in spike peak potential, with absolute amplitude also frequently reduced; in addition there was a decrease in amplitude and increased rate of decay of monosynaptic EPSPs from stimulation of the trigeminal mesencephalic nucleus, data all consistent with an increased conductance and hence increased inhibitory rather than decreased excitatory input. (The degree of spike peak potential reduction was not correlated with the degree of MP hyperpolarization that occurred in REM sleep.) Since these effects were less pronounced than those obtainable with inferior alveolar nerve inhibitory input, an input thought to be on the soma, it was concluded that the REM inhibition was likely mediated by synapses not only on the soma but also on more distant sites, i.e., on dendrites (Mariotti *et al.*, 1986). A final feature of the REM-sleep-associated changes was presynaptic inhibition of jaw-closer Ia muscle afferents. This was inferred from a decrease in amplitude of the monosynaptic Ia EPSP without the changes in rise or decay time that would have suggested membrane conductance changes associated with postsynaptic inhibition. Subsequent pharmacological studies (Soja *et al.*, 1987a) using microinjection techniques have suggested that the REM sleep suppression of the masseteric jaw-closer reflex during active sleep is partly but not completely mediated by strychnine-sensitive postsynaptic inhibition, suggesting glycinergic mechanisms of inhibition.

10.8.2. Spinal α-Motoneurons during the Sleep–Wake Cycle

10.8.2.1. Changes in Membrane Potential of Lumbar α-Motoneurons during Waking and Sleep

Morales and Chase (1978, 1981) recorded antidromically identified lumbar motoneurons in naturally sleeping cats using the chronic intracellular recording techniques pioneered by them. The low-pass-filtered record of membrane potential during a sleep–wake cycle is shown in Fig. 17. Mean resting potential in W was −65 mV, and there was a slight hyperpolarization from active W to slow-wave sleep. During the passage from S to REM sleep there was a marked membrane hyperpolarization, averaging 6.7 mV with a range of 4–10 mV; this hyperpolarization was temporally coincident with the loss of nuchal EMG activity. On transition to W the level of polarization decreased. Similar findings have been observed by Glenn and Dement (1981). Overall these data establish the basis of one of the hallmarks of REM sleep, muscle atonia, as a result of motoneuronal hyperpolarization and confirm hypotheses made in earlier extracellular and reflex studies by Pompeiano and co-workers (Pompeiano, 1967a; see review in Chase and Morales, 1985).

Lines of experimentation similar to those described for jaw-closer motoneurons suggested the presence of a tonic increased membrane conductance in REM sleep and hence of increased inhibition, rather than disfacilitation, as the basis of the REM sleep hyperpolarization (Morales and Chase, 1981). During REM sleep there was an increased duration of the IS–SD delay, an increased rheobase not accounted for by hyperpolarization alone, and a directly measured decrease in input resistance from 1.8 to 1.0 MΩ is S as compared with REM sleep. (Input resistance was not measured with the MP returned to the same baseline in S and REM sleep, a manipulation more difficult to accomplish in the chronic preparation.) In addition to the tonic inhibition just described there were phasic episodes of enhanced postsynaptic inhibition of lumbar motoneurons coincident with the occurrence of phasic runs of rapid eye movements (Chase and Morales, 1983). Thus, both phasic presynaptic inhibition (see Section 10.8.1 on trigeminal motoneurons) and postsynaptic inhibition occur during REM sleep.

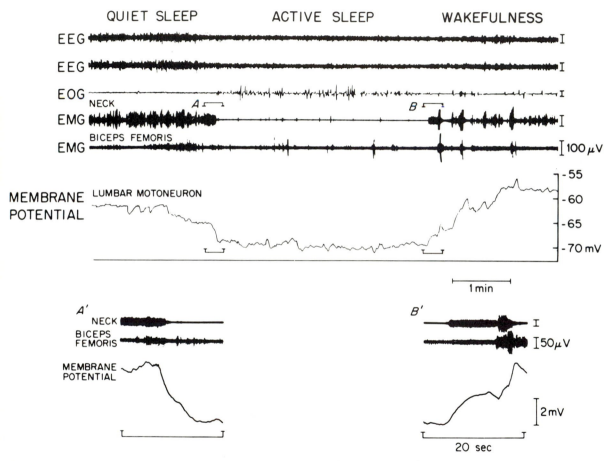

Figure 17. Intracellular record from a lumbar motoneuron during sleep and wakefulness: correlation of membrane potential and behavioral state. This figure highlights the membrane hyperpolarization that accompanies active sleep (REM sleep). Hyperpolarization commenced prior to the cessation of muscle tone, which was accompanied by a further and rather sharp increase in membrane polarization (A, and shown oscilloscopically at higher gain and expanded time base in A'). At the termination of active sleep the membrane depolarized coincident with the resumption of muscle tone and behavioral awakening (B,B'). Note the brief periods of depolarization during active sleep and wakefulness, which were accompanied by phasic increases in muscle activity (i.e., muscular twitches during active sleep and leg movements during wakefulness). Spike potentials often occurred during these periods of depolarization but are not evident in this figure because the D.C. record was passed through a 0.1-Hz high-frequency polygraphic filter. This motoneuron was recorded for 28 min; the traces shown were obtained 12 min after the cell was impaled. The first and second polygraph traces are those of EEG activity recorded from left and right frontal–parietal cortex, respectively. From Morales and Chase (1978).

10.8.2.2. Hyperpolarizing PSPs in Lumbar α-Motoneurons during Waking and Sleep

Subsequent work has examined in detail the spontaneous, discrete IPSPs impinging on lumbar motoneurons (Morales *et al.*, 1987a); these were automatically detected and classified according to amplitude and parameters of rise and decay times. Figure 18 is a high-gain intracellular record showing the presence of distinctive large-amplitude PSPs during REM sleep that are not present during W and S, and Fig. 19 shows that the REM sleep potentials are distinct in that (1) they have larger amplitudes and (2) they have a faster rise time per unit of IPSP amplitude. It was thus concluded that they arose from a distinct set of inhibitory neurons that became active during REM. Recently Chase *et al.* (1989) have reported that the microiontophoretic application of strychnine (but not picrotoxin or bicuculline) onto lumbar motoneurons was effective in abolishing the large-amplitude spontaneous IPSPs of REM sleep, suggesting that glycine is the principal neurotransmitter mediating these potentials in lumbar motoneu-

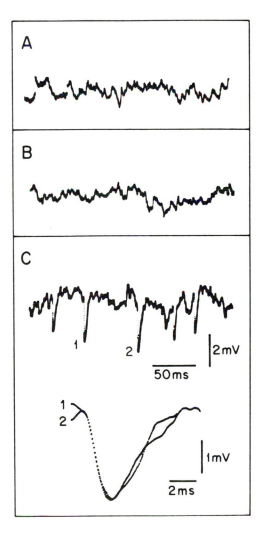

Figure 18. High-gain intracellular recording of the membrane potential activity of a tibial motoneuron during wakefulness (A), quiet sleep (B, SWS), and active sleep (C, REM sleep). Note the appearance *de novo* during AS of large amplitude and repetitively occurring inhibitory postsynaptic potentials. Two representative potentials, which were aligned by their origins, are shown at higher gain and at an expanded time base (C1,2). These potentials were photographed from the screen of a digital oscilloscope. The analog-to-digital conversion rate was 40 μsec/bin. The membrane potential level during these recording during active sleep was −67.0 mV; the antidromic action potential was 78.5 mV. From Morales *et al.* (1987a).

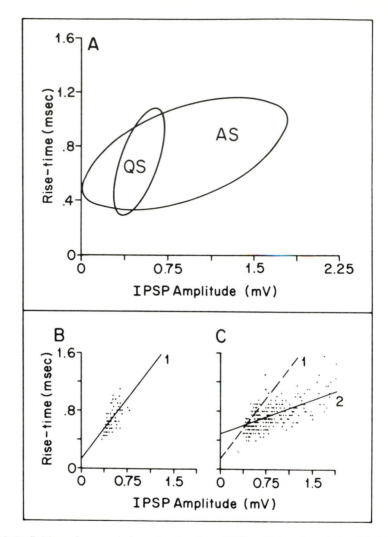

Figure 19. Definition of a population of active-sleep IPSPs utilizing the relationship between the waveform parameters of amplitude and rise time. The two ellipses in A illustrate the 90% confidence region of the data points corresponding to the potentials recorded during quiet sleep (SWS) and active sleep (REM sleep). Note that the ellipse corresponding to the active-sleep episode is shifted to the right (i.e., to the region of potentials of larger amplitude) and that the major axis of the larger active-sleep ellipse has a lesser slope than that of the quiet-sleep ellipse (see text). The original data from which these ellipses were constructed are illustrated in the scattergrams B (quiet sleep) and C (active sleep). Also included in these plots are the regression lines for the correlations B_1 and C_1 (quiet sleep and active sleep, respectively). In both sets of data, there was a direct relationship between rise time and amplitude (data obtained during active sleep: r = 0.69, slope = 0.31, n = 294, $P < 0.01$; during quiet sleep: $r = 0.63$, slope = 1.09, $n = 65$, $P < 0.01$). The regression line in B_1 is also depicted in C in order to illustrate that the large-amplitude active-sleep IPSPs are all situated beneath this line. From Morales *et al.* (1987a).

rons. (Evidence supporting a glycinergic role in the trigeminal motoneuronal inhibition of REM sleep has been described in Section 10.8.1.)

315

MOTOR SYSTEMS

10.8.2.3. Excitatory Activity in Lumbar α-Motoneurons during Waking and Sleep

Chase and Morales (1983) also examined excitatory processes occurring during REM, primarily those occurring at the same time as the runs of rapid eye movements, and found them different from waking (Fig. 20). In waking action potentials usually occurred following a prolonged depolarization (Fig. 20A), whereas in REM sleep the majority of action potentials were observed to occur following a hyperpolarization followed by a depolarizing potential on which rode a burst of two to four spikes, and with an absence of the spike after hyperpolarization typical of waking (Fig. 20B). Chase and Morales interpreted this as indicating simultaneous coactivation in inhibitory and excitatory drives, a pattern not found in waking but distinctive to REM sleep. A possibility not considered when the paper was written in 1983 but raised by us is the presence of a low-threshold calcium spike (see discussion in Chapter 5) that was deinactivated at the hyperpolarized membrane potential of REM sleep and was triggered either as a rebound following a hyperpolarization (compare Figs. 3 and 4 of Chapter 5 with the present Fig. 20B) or following a depolarization. As discussed in Chapter 5, a frequent concomitant of a long-duration calcium spike is a burst of fast (sodium) action potentials riding on it. The picture present in Fig. 20B,F with the presence of a spike burst with a short first interspike interval has strikingly similar morphology to that of calcium spikes and associated sodium spikes in reticular formation neurons (see Chapter 5). It should be noted that not all REM sleep spikes occurred with this particular pattern, and some appeared to arise from depolarizing potentials like those seen in waking (Fig. 20D,E); these spikes did not occur in as bursts. The possibility that calcium spikes may be present in these records is strengthened by a report of Walton and Llinás (1986), who found calcium-dependent low-threshold rebound potentials in lumbar motoneurons in the *in vitro* spinal cord preparation from neonatal rats, although it was not observed in mature motoneurons in this preparation.*

Recent work has indicated that a non-NMDA excitatory amino acid may mediate some of the EPSPs of REM sleep. Soja *et al.* (1988) have reported that the phasic depolarization of lumbar motoneurons occurring during the rapid eye movement portions of REM sleep were blocked by microiontophoretic application of kynurenic acid, a nonselective EAA receptor blocker, but not by 5-aminophosphonovaleric acid (APV), a selective blocker of NMDA receptors (see Chapter 6). In these experiments APV was applied in doses that were sufficient to antagonize the effects of microiontophoretically applied NMDA.

---

*Chase and Morales state that hyperpolarization during waking with depolarizing input did not produce the burst pattern. However, as reviewed in Chapter 5, the calcium spike deinactivation is time and voltage dependent, and the presence of a burst is also dependent on the strength of hyper- or depolarizing input. It is possible that these complex conditions for a calcium spike may not have been satisfied in the *in vivo* waking preparation or that some factor specific to REM sleep may promote this calcium conductance. We thus consider it an open question as to whether calcium spikes could account for these phenomena.

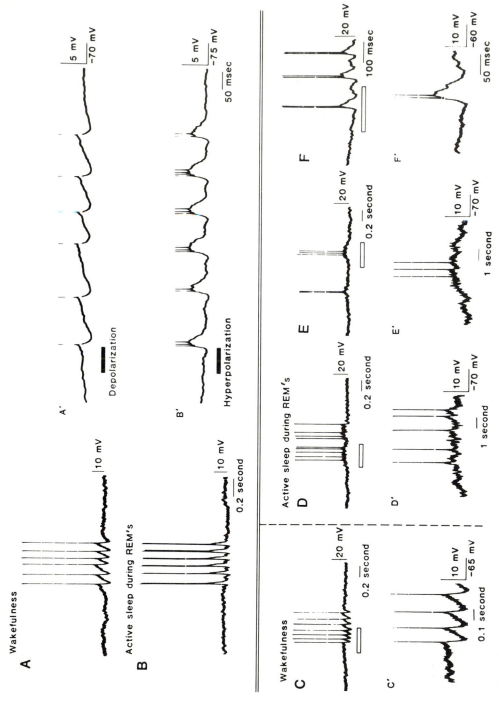

Figure 20. Patterns of spike generation during REM periods of active sleep. A: During wakefulness, depolarization (bar in A′) was the initial membrane potential event. B: During REM periods, each depolarization shift was preceded by hyperpolarization (bar in B′) (see also F and F′). Full-sized spikes developed in both examples; in B doublets, triplets, and quadruplets accompanied each depolarizing shift. The open bars indicate the period of the traces shown in C′–F′. C: spike generation during wakefulness. An irregular pattern of spike activity (D), intermittent bursts (E), and spike doublets (F) is present during REM periods. An increase in hyperpolarizing subthreshold synaptic activity during interspike intervals is present in D′ and E′. A and B are records from a single tibial motoneuron, and C through E from a single peroneal motoneuron; F is from another peroneal cell. From Chase and Morales (1983).

As to the possible source of the hyperpolarization during REM, Chase and co-workers (1986) found that electrical stimulation of the bulbar FTG during REM sleep produced prominent long-latency (28 msec to onset, 43 msec to peak) hyperpolarizing potentials in lumbar motoneurons during REM sleep. That these potentials were IPSPs was indicated by their reversal by chloride injection or by hyperpolarization and by their being abolished on the microiontophoretic application of strychnine (Soja *et al.*, 1987b). These IPSPs were only intermittently present with the same stimulation parameters in W and S. It was of interest that short-latency (5–10 msec) hyperpolarizing potentials did not vary with state. Our interpretation of these data would agree with Chase and co-workers that bulbar RF may be an important source of descending inhibition and add that the long-latency, REM sleep state-specific hyperpolarizing potential may be caused by recruitment of more reticular formation neurons by the stimulus in REM, an effect related to the REM sleep-specific population depolarization of reticular neurons (Chapter 11). Similarly, Chase and co-workers have noted there is a REM-sleep-selective effect of stimulation of the pontine reticular formation (nucleus reticularis pontis oralis) in producing hyperpolarizing potentials in lumbar motoneurons (Fung *et al.*, 1982), an effect not seen in other states and conceptualized by these workers as resulting from more recruitment of reticular neurons in REM sleep by these stimuli; this interpretation is compatible with the data in Chapter 11 indicating REM sleep state-specific activation of reticular neurons and the data for Chapter 5 indicating dense excitatory pontobulbar connectivity.

Finally, in view of the possible role of cholinergic neurons in REM sleep phenomena (Chapter 11), it is of interest that Morales and co-workers (1987b) found that microinjections of carbachol into the pontine reticular formation of decerebrate cats produced postsynaptic inhibitory effects on lumbar motoneurons that were "remarkably similar" to those described above in the chronic cat during natural REM sleep, including changes in input resistance (1.5 to 0.8 MΩ), rheobase (increased 88%), and development of large discrete inhibitory PSPs. That MP was hyperpolarized only 2.2 mV following carbachol versus 6.7 mV in natural REM sleep may at least in part reflect the 3 mV greater baseline hyperpolarization of neurons in the decerebrate cat versus the intact cat in slow-wave sleep.

10.9. Central Mechanisms of REM-Sleep Muscle Atonia

10.9.1. Lesion Data and REM without Atonia

The Lyon group reported that bilateral lesions of the pontine reticular region just ventral to the locus coeruleus (LC), termed by this group the LCα and peri-LCα, and its descending pathway to the bulbar reticular formation abolished the muscle atonia of REM sleep (Fig. 21; Sastre and Jouvet, 1979; Jouvet, 1979). (The projections of this region to BRF and whether they are to magno- or gigantocellular field are discussed in Chapter 4.) This group also reported that not only was the nuchal muscle atonia of REM sleep suppressed but that cats so lesioned exhibited "oneiric behavior" including locomotion, attack behavior, and behavior with head raised and with horizontal and vertical movements "as if watching something."

Morrison and collaborators (Hendricks *et al.*, 1982) confirmed the basic finding of REM sleep without atonia with bilateral pontine tegmental lesions but found that lesions extending beyond the LCα region and its efferent pathway to bulb were necessary for more than a minimal release of muscle tone and to produce the elaborate "oneiric behaviors." They found that particular lesion locations were associated with particular sets of behaviors, e.g., attack behavior with lesions that extended into midbrain and interrupted amygdalar pathways, locomotion with lesions near the brainstem locomotor region, and orientinglike behavior with small, symmetrical dorsolateral pontine lesions (Fig. 22). Finally, the presence of attack and locomotion behaviors in REM without atonia was reported to be associated with an increased incidence of these behaviors in waking, leading to the interpretation that the lesions may have done more than simply counteract a behaviorally nonspecific muscle inhibition during REM sleep: they may have released the particular behaviors appearing in both REM sleep and waking. Chapter 13 discusses the relationship of these "oneric behaviors" in animals to similar phenomena seen in cases of human pathology and their relationship to dreaming.

Recently Holmes *et al.* (1988) have reported preliminary data that quisqualate lesions of bulbar FTG and FTM led to a marked decrease of the muscle

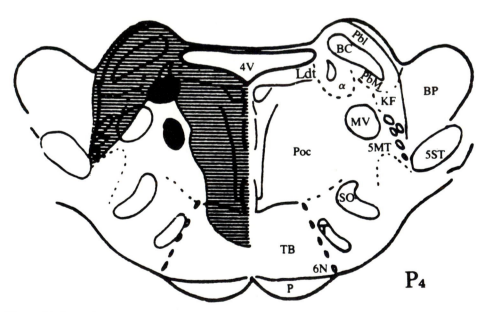

Figure 21. Frontal section of the pons of the cat in the Horsley–Clarke coordinate P4. The solid areas indicate the localization of the lesions that suppress postural atonia during REM sleep. These lesions coincide with the locus coeruleus α (a) or its descending pathway. The horizontal hatching corresponds to lesions that do not suppress postural atonia. Pbl, n. parabrachialis lateralis; Ldt, n. lateralis tegmenti dorsalis; PbM, n. parabrachialis medialis; KF, n. Kölliker–Fuse; Poc, n. pontis caudalis; BP, brachium pontis; 5MT, motor nucleus of trigeminal nerve; 5ST, sensory nucleus of trigeminal nerve; BC, brachium conjunctivum; 4V, fourth ventricle. From Jouvet (1979).

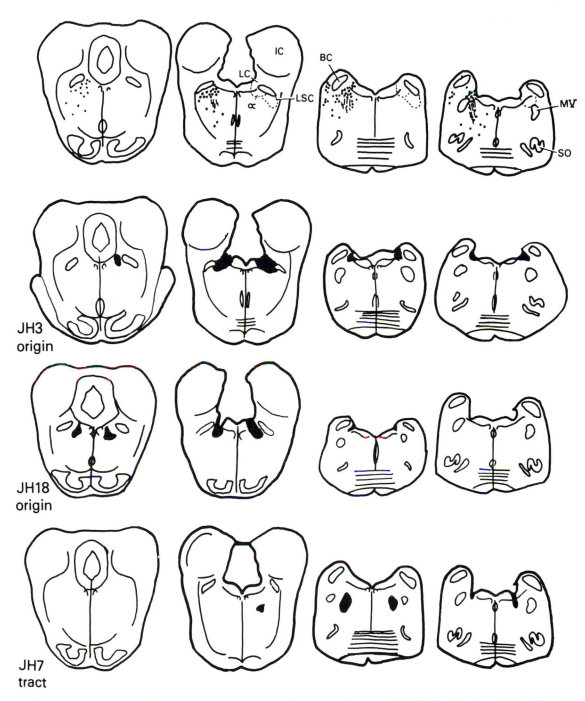

Figure 22. Lesions releasing minimal limb and neck movements, compared with the tegmentoreticular tract. Top row: Coronal sections at levels P1,2,3,4 from left to right. Left side: Cells of origin and projection fibers of tementoreticular tract proposed by Sakai *et al.* (1979) to mediate the atonia of REM sleep. Right side: Dashed lines outline components of the locus coeruleus complex in the terminology of Sakai *et al.* (1979). Second and third rows: Lesions that bilaterally damaged the origin of the tegmentoreticular tract: the medial locus coeruleus α and medially adjacent reticular formation. Fourth row: Lesion placed bilaterally in the projection of the tract as it descends medial to the motor nucleus of the trigeminal nerve. Abbreviations for all figures; α, locus coeruleus, pars α; BC, brachium conjunctivum; IC, inferior colliculus; LC, principal locus coeruleus; LSC, locus subcoeruleus; MV, motor nucleus of trigeminal nerve; SO, superior olive; VII, seventh nerve. From Hendricks *et al.* (1982).

atonia of REM sleep and to the appearance of paddling behavior during this state. The percentages of time spent in REM and non-REM sleep and in waking were not greatly altered. These data further support a role of bulbar FTG/FTM in REM sleep muscle atonia.

10.9.2. Electrophysiological Data and REM Muscle Atonia

With respect to cellular activity in the peri-LCα region, Sakai reported that seven of 19 extracellularly recorded units in this region showed a selective tonic discharge during REM, some but less discharge during deep SWS, and no discharge activity during waking (discharge statistics and further details are not available since only preliminary reports of these data in book chapters and a review have appeared; see Sakai, 1980, 1985a,b, 1986; Sakai *et al.*, 1981). Of these seven REM-sleep-specific neurons, three were antidromically activated from the bulbar magnocellular field. Within the magnocellular reticular formation, Kanamori, Sakai, and Jouvet (1980) have reported the presence of ten REM-specific neurons among the 69 recorded in this zone (Fig. 23). These extracellularly recorded neurons had discharge rates that were virtually zero in W; even in the presence of sensory stimulation and voluntary movements, discharges remained near zero in early SWS, and then in SWS with PGO waves (5–20 sec prior to REM sleep) discharges increased to about 5 spikes/sec and further increased to approximately 30 spikes/sec in REM sleep, with intense acceleration of firing concomitant with runs of PGO waves and eye movements. Electrical stimulation of the peri-LCα resulted in synaptic excitation of two of the ten neurons with latencies of 2 and 4.5 msec; in the data from one neuron that is included in a figure (Fig. 23B), spike latency varies by 1 msec, indicating that this response may not be monosynaptic, and, indeed, Kanamori *et al.* do not claim that their data indicate a monosynaptic peri-LCα to bulbar magnocellular field projection. Two of the ten neurons had antidromic responses to stimulation of the "ventral reticulospinal tract at P16." [P16 is in caudal medulla just rostral to the decussation of the pyramidal tract (Berman, 1978).] It may also be noted that the magnocellular bulbar RF area recorded includes the classic medullary inhibitory zone of Magoun and Rhines (1946) and that Tohyama *et al.* (1979a,b, Fig. 4) have provided data from retrograde labeling of HRP placed in the ventral portion of the lateral funiculus that magnocellular neurons indeed project to this spinal zone.

Sakai (1980) interprets these data as consistent with a hypothesis that non-monoaminergic neurons of the peri-LCα (e.g., reticular neurons) become active just before and during REM sleep and, via tegmentoreticular tract projections to the bulbar magnocellular field, excite neurons in this reticular zone, which, in turn, via projections in the ventrolateral reticulospinal tract, may cause the postsynaptic inhibition of spinal motoneurons. [The data cited by Sakai supporting a role of the lateral reticulospinal tract involvement in the postural atonia mechanisms of REM sleep derive from studies by Pompeiano (1976).]

Our own view of these data is, in general, consistent with the possibility of such an interpretation. However, we think it useful to emphasize the possibility of involvement of other portions of reticular formation. This is because, first of all, Sakai and co-workers tend to call reticular zones "magnocellular" that others label "gigantocellular" (Cf. Chapter 4 discussion), and thus much of the localization question may be purely terminological; another reason is that more sensitive HRP chromogens and even smaller injection zones in cord have indicated the presence of bulbar FTG as well as FTM projections to the ventral portion of lateral funiculus (Cf. Chapter 4 and Mitani *et al.*, 1988a, Fig. 13). Finally, the Rye *et al.* (1988) data indicate projections in the peri-LCα area are primarily to bulbar FTG. With respect to the electrophysiology, the evidence for monosynaptic projections from peri-LCα to FTM is not compelling. Also, although Sakai and co-workers did not find REM-specific neurons outside of the FTM, Netick *et al.*

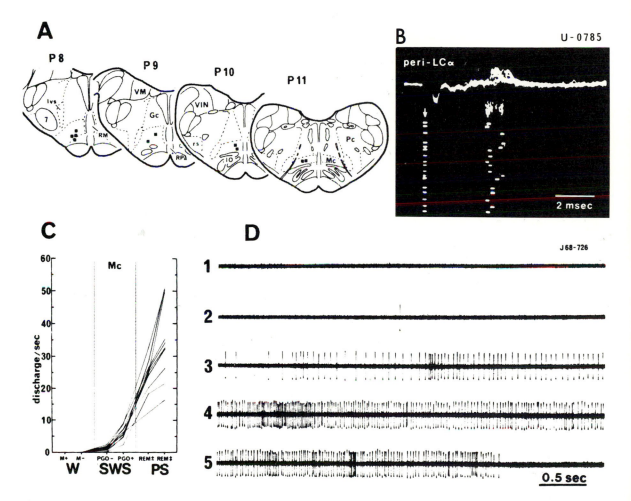

Figure 23. A: Location of the magnocellular (Mc) REM-sleep-specific neurons. B: Effects of stimulation of the peri-LCα (B) on a Mc REM-sleep-specific cell. Superimpositions of several synaptic responses and dotgrams of 17 successive sweeps (the first dot represents the shock artifact) following stimulation of the peri-LCα. C: A summary of neuronal discharge rates of Mc PS-specific cells during the sleep–waking cycle. D: An example of single-unit discharges recorded in the Mc during the actual time epochs of W (1), SWS without PGO waves (2), SWS with PGO waves to REM sleep (3), REM sleep (4), and REM sleep to W (5). Abbreviations: 7, facial nucleus; FLM, fasciculus longitudinalis medialis; Gc, n. reticularis gigantocellularis; IO, inferior olivary complex; Ivs, direct lateral vestibulospinal tract; Mc, n. reticularis magnocellularis; Pc, n. reticularis parvocellularis; RM, n. raphe magnus; RPA, n. raphe pallidus; rs, rubrospinal tract; VIN, inferior vestibular nucleus; VM, medial vestibular nucleus; S, nucleus of the solitary tract. From Kanamori *et al.* (1980).

(1977) have recorded similar cells in head-restrained cats in a small-cell bulbar reticular zone outside the FTM, perhaps in FTL. Chase *et al.* (1984), utilizing extracellular recordings in head-restrained cats, recorded ten neurons in bulbar nucleus gigantocellularis (= FTG), a part of the zone that stimulation experiments in acute cats had implicated in inhibitory projections to jaw-closer motoneurons (see Nakamura *et al.*, 1975). Chase and co-workers describe these neurons as having discharges that increase in a continuum from W to S to REM sleep (Fig. 24), with population mean discharge rates in spikes/sec: W, 3.8; S, 13.1; REM sleep with no eye movements, 38; and REM sleep with EMs, 83. These discharge rates were in a reciprocal relationship with the magnitude of the state-related amplitude of the trigeminal monosynaptic reflex, which is suppressed in REM sleep. Supporting the hypothesis that these neurons may be responsible for the inhibition of trigeminal jaw-closer motoneurons was the fact that two of the ten had spike-triggered averaging data consistent with a monosynaptic inhibitory input to the jaw-closer motoneuron pool.

Finally, with respect to the peri-LCα neurons, it is unfortunate that only seven neurons of the selective REM-on type have been reported. It is somewhat difficult to base a comprehensive theory of REM sleep muscle atonia on this

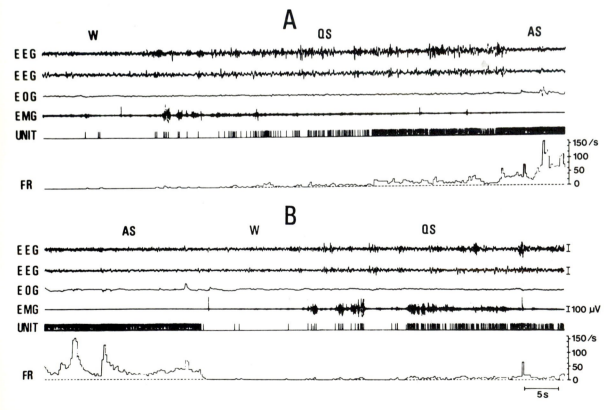

Figure 24. Discharge pattern of an extracellularly recorded medullary reticular neurons during the transition from SWS (QS) to REM sleep (AS) (A) and from REM sleep (AS) to W (B). Between A and B, records were omitted for 2 min. FR, firing rate, the number of spikes per second. Bin width 250 msec. From Chase *et al.* (1984).

sample size, and we wonder if the paucity of neurons that have been found to show this discharge signature may not reflect the participation of other neurons in REM sleep atonia. It seems entirely possible and even plausible that the neurons active in the muscle atonia of REM sleep might also be also active in the normal patterns of muscle inhibition of waking, as indeed suggested by the studies of Pompeiano (1985; this reference should also be consulted for a general review of brainstem postural control mechanisms, a subject not reviewed in this book). In this case there might not be a pure "REM-sleep-selective" pattern, a possibility noted by Chase *et al.* (1984), but the population of neurons participating in REM sleep atonia might have subsets of its members active in other states as a function of various postural adjustment mechanisms. The distinctive feature of REM sleep atonia would then lie in the simultaneous involvement of the entire population of neurons providing muscle tone suppression, a concept akin to the notion discussed in Chapter 12 that the distinctive characteristic of REM sleep in reticular formation is a population-specific activation and MP depolarization. In fact, Chase and co-workers (1981) in intracellular recordings have demonstrated the presence in REM sleep of a MP depolarization of bulbar reticular formation neurons in the same area as the extracellular recordings of the 1984 paper.

10.9.3. Role of Other Pontine Structures and the Pharmacology of REM-Sleep Muscle Atonia

With respect to the localization of descending inhibitory pathways, Mori and collaborators have found that electrical stimulation of a midline zone in the pons [from P3 to P7 and 1–2 mm below the ventricular surface, a zone straddled by the MLF in the giant-cell portion of the PRF (NRPC) and including a portion of the raphe pontis and centralis superior] produces a long-lasting suppression of postural muscle tone in both decerebrate and awake, freely moving cats (see Mori, 1987). They term this region the dorsal tegmental field (DTF). These workers believed they were activating fibers of passage, and their anatomic studies suggested that the most likely fiber pathway was that leading from the nucleus RPO (non-giant-cell field) directly to the bulbar FTG, although they could not exclude the possibility of a activation of the tegmentoreticular tract. (Ohta *et al.*, 1988). In a recent synaptic connectivity study, Takakusaki *et al.* (1988a) used spike-triggered averaging to study the relationship of extracellularly recorded discharge fluctuations of bulbar giant-cell field neurons antidromically identified as projecting in L1 spinal cord (in ventral or lateral funiculus) to the fluctuations in membrane potential of intracellularly recorded extensor and flexor motoneurons at L5–S1. The bulbar neurons so studied also were orthodromically activated by DTF stimulation at mono- or disynaptic latencies and had antidromic conduction velocities of 90 m/sec. The latency from the bulbar neuronal spike to the motoneuronal IPSP was 5 msec (3.7–8 msec range), and the segmental delay, time from the arrival of the presynaptic axonal volley to the onset of the hyperpolarizing potential, was about 1.5 msec. Since monosynaptic connections usually have synaptic delays in the range of about 0.4 msec, and disynaptic connections often have delays in the 1.5-msec time range, these workers postulated a disynaptic pathway with the inhibitory interneuron located in spinal cord. In addition, other parameters of the IPSP, such as time to peak, were not congruent with a monosynaptic projection.

This group also used carbachol (100 mM, 0.1–0.25 μl) microinjected into nucleus reticular pontis oralis (P2–P3, lateral 1–2) and found that this zone produced a very short-latency (less than 1 min) postural atonia with suppression of both flexors and extensors in acute decerebrate cats (Takakusaki *et al.*, 1988b). [It may be noted parenthetically that Yamamoto *et al.* (1988) have recently reported that carbachol injections in a similar dorsal pontine area (P1-P3; lateral 2) produce a short-latency (<5 min) induction of all REM components in intact cats.] Takakusaki *et al.* (1988b) found that these NRPO carbachol injections also induced tonic firing in bulbar FTG neurons. Electrical stimulation of the bulbar FTG (three pulses, 20–40 μA, 1 msec apart) evoked mixed PSPs in intracellularly recorded spinal α-motoneurons that became predominantly hyperpolarizing with carbachol microinjections. (cf. Chase's concept of reticular response reversal, as described above). Atropine blocked this effect, and norepinephrine (100 mM) and serotonin (50 mM) reduced the hyperpolarizing PSPs, indicating the presence of a muscarinic cholinergic–adrenergic reciprocity in this system, a finding previously reported for postural atonia systems by Pompeiano and co-workers using systemic injections (cf. review in Pompeiano, 1985, and discussion of cholinergic–monoaminergic interaction in REM sleep phenomena in Chapters 11 and 12). Electrical stimulation of medial pons (FTP and FTG) had the same effect as bulbar FTG stimulation, further suggesting the presence of pontine-to-bulbar reticular projections carrying muscle suppression information.

With respect to the pharmacology of muscle atonia, in addition to the above-cited elicitation of atonia by Mori and co-workers, it has been recognized that direct microinjection of cholinergic agonists into the dorsolateral pontine reticular formation (approximating the peri-LCα zone of Sakai) may, at times, produce muscle atonia without the other components of REM sleep (Mitler and Dement, 1974; Katayama *et al.*, 1984). Within the medial bulb, cholinergic microinjection in the caudal portion of the Magoun and Rhines muscle suppression zone (corresponding to the nucleus paramedianis) produces atonia, whereas, in contrast, non-NMDA excitatory amino acid but not cholinergic agonists were effective in the more rostral portion, corresponding to the nucleus magnocellularis (Siegel and Lai, 1988; Lai and Siegel, 1988); these same workers also reported that non-NMDA excitatory amino acids were effective in producing muscle atonia when injected into dorsolateral pons. Thus, evidence is accumulating that the muscle atonia of REM sleep may involve more than one anatomically and pharmacologically specific brainstem system.

11

Neuronal Control of the Sleep–Wake States

The first chapter of this book describes the history of much of the early lesion and stimulation work as well as the cardinal signs of sleep and the definition of behavioral state. Other chapters describe the neurophysiological and anatomic substrates of various components of EEG-synchronized sleep and REM sleep. These include the synchronized oscillations of non-REM sleep in Chapter 7, the REM-sleep components of PGO waves in Chapter 9, and the muscle atonia and rapid eye movements in Chapter 10.

In this chapter we focus on how these various components are orchestrated into the complex behavior of sleep. Chapter 7 discusses how the characteristic components of EEG-synchronized sleep occur in the absence of activating and disrupting influences from the brainstem. The first section of this chapter takes up the source of these influences in brainstem reticular neurons and the brainstem cholinergic neurons in PPT and LDT nuclei, with data from extracellular recordings of antidromically identified, thalamically projecting brainstem neurons. Our present viewpoint of EEG-synchronized sleep mechanisms is essentially a passive one; we suggest that synchronizing phenomena depend on the removal of brainstem influences. The sudden drop in both cholinergic and noncholinergic reticular input at sleep onset disfacilitates thalamocortical neurons while, at the same time, the reduction in cholinergic input facilitates the genesis of spindle oscillations in the RE thalamic nucleus. Thus, the return of brainstem cholinergic and brainstem noncholinergic activating influences with REM sleep abolishes these synchronizing events. In the next section (11.2) we address the question of the nature of neuronal population change in the reticular formation during REM sleep that leads to the production of the various REM components: intracellular recordings suggest that a common feature of REM sleep in brainstem is a REM-sleep-specific tonic membrane depolarization that lasts throughout the state. Data from extracellular recordings show the timing of the gradual onset of this influence. We suggest that sleep–wake behavioral state control may result from modulation of excitability in neuronal pools. The final section, 11.3, addresses the question of what might cause these modulations of excitability in neuronal pools. The next chapter considers REM sleep as an ultradian rhythm, with a period of about 90 min in humans and 24 min in the cat, and presents a model for its generation.

11.1. Brainstem–Thalamic Neurons Implicated in the Process of EEG Desynchronization

Studies conducted during the early 1980s investigated the waking- and sleep-related activities of rostral mesencephalic (Steriade *et al.*, 1980, 1982a) and bulbar reticular neurons (Steriade *et al.*, 1984b) with antidromically identified projections to the intralaminar and ventromedial (VM) thalamic nuclei. These thalamic targets were chosen because intralaminar and VM nuclei project over widespread cortical territories and may thus account for the diffuse cortical excitatory processes associated with EEG desynchronization. Discharges of brainstem neurons were temporally correlated to the most precocious signs of EEG desynchronization during transition from EEG-synchronized sleep to either waking or REM sleep. These data were used to evaluate the hypothesis that an increase in firing rates of brainstem neurons precedes overt signs of EEG desynchronization.

At that time, before 1985, the thalamic projections of cholinergic cell groups located at the junction between the caudal mesencephalon and the rostral pons had not yet been documented. The rationale behind searching at rostral midbrain levels for neuronal candidates involved in EEG desynchronization processes was that classical studies using stimulation and lesions pointed to the upper brainstem reticular stimulation as the critical area for inducing arousal (see Chapter 1) and that midbrain reticular neurons directly excite intralaminar thalamic cells projecting widely over the neocortex (Steriade and Glenn, 1982). There are virtually no cholinergic cells in the rostral mesencephalon, and the transmitters used by those midbrain neurons have not yet been determined. However, the established direct brainstem–thalamic excitatory actions suggest that rostral midbrain neurons probably use excitatory amino acids as neurotransmitters.

The hypothesis that bulbothalamic neurons may act synergistically with midbrain–thalamic neurons in the process of EEG desynchronization was based on the fact that electrolytic or chemical lesions of the upper brainstem reticular core failed to disrupt EEG desynchronization for long periods of time. Indeed, the excitation of midbrain perikarya by glutamate analogues induces a long-lasting (12–36 hr) EEG desynchronization associated with highly aroused behavior (Kitsikis and Steriade, 1981). At stages corresponding to the period of kainate-induced neuronal destruction, a 40–60% decrease in duration of the waking state was observed, with only phasic EEG-desynchronizing reactions, contrasting with the tonic desynchronization observed in the same animals before the kainate injection into the midbrain core (Steriade, 1983). However, this picture lasted for only 3–4 days, and both behavioral and EEG correlates of wakefulness returned to control values after 5–6 days. More recent data, using chemical lesions of upper brainstem reticular territories including cholinergic cell groups, also indicated that 10–14 days after the kainate injection, EEG desynchronization during REM sleep is not altered (Webster and Jones, 1988). These results implied an additional source of thalamocortical activation processes involved in EEG desynchronization. This source may be located in thalamically projecting neurons of the reticular formation. Since kainate-induced lesions of the pontine reticular formation do not apparently affect EEG desynchronization during REM sleep, although these lesion may have spared neurons other than the giant cells (Sastre *et al.*, 1981), the bulbar reticular formation was investigated. Fuller's data (1975) on pontine reticular neurons with thalamic projections and slow conduction velocities suggest that these neurons may also play a role in EEG desynchronization.

In fact, we do not believe that the EEG-desynchronizing neurons are confined within circumscribed regions of the brainstem reticular core, as may be the case with the mesopontine PGO-on cells (see Section 9.1). Although the role of bulbothalamic neurons involved in EEG desynchronization during REM sleep (see below, Fig 2) has not yet been tested by lesion experiments, we do not expect that such lesions would succeed in disrupting EEG desynchronization for long periods of time because, in our opinion, this process depends on activities in distributed brainstem as well as supramesencephalic networks. The desynchronization of spindle oscillations takes place in the thalamus and depends on brainstem–thalamic cholinergic neurons (see Chapter 7), whereas the disruption of slow (δ) waves is mainly a result of cholinergic actions of basal forebrain neurons on the cerebral cortex (cf. Steriade and Buzsaki, 1989). Then, any attempt at determining the efficacy of various type of lesions in disrupting EEG desynchronization should dissociate the two major rhythms of EEG synchronization.

In what follows, we briefly review data on activities of thalamically projecting neurons located in the rostral midbrain, bulbar reticular core, and cholinergic neurons of the pedunculopontine tegmental (PPT) and laterodorsal tegmental (LDT) nuclei that are temporally related to EEG desynchronization shifts on awakening and REM sleep.

11.1.1. Midbrain Reticular (Noncholinergic) Neurons

The median firing rate of midbrain reticular neurons is twice as high in waking and REM sleep (about 20/sec) as in EEG-synchronized sleep. This is valid for neurons receiving multiple converging inputs and antidromically identified as projecting to the intralaminar thalamus but is not valid for neurons with projections to the paramedian pontine reticular formation that have low firing rates (<1/sec) that do not increase on awakening (Steriade *et al.*, 1982a). Both the relatively high discharge rates of thalamically projecting midbrain reticular neurons and their extremely tonic discharge patterns during both waking and REM sleep distinguish them from paramedian pontine reticular neurons that do not seem to be related to ascending activation processes (see Section 11.2).

The role played by midbrain noncholinergic neurons in EEG desynchronization was determined by using the criterion of a statistically significant change in firing rate preceding the first change in brain electrical activity from EEG-synchronized sleep to wakefulness. Time 0 in this case is the earliest sign of decreased amplitude and increased frequency of EEG rhythms that eventually lead to generalized EEG desynchronization and overt behavioral manifestations of waking, as reflected by increased muscular tone and eye movements. In these analyses, time 0 is the onset of the transitional period between EEG-synchronized sleep and waking (see SW epoch in Fig. 1A2) that precedes by more than 15 sec the overt EEG desynchronization and motor events associated with behavioral arousal. Precursor signs of increased activity were seen in different midbrain cells 8 to 22 sec before any change in the fully synchronized EEG activity (Fig. 1B). The pooled analysis of a 25-cell group revealed that a statistically significant increase in firing rate occurs 15 sec before the end of EEG-synchronized sleep epochs that developed into waking state (Fig. 1C; Steriade *et al.*, 1982a). Similarly, midbrain reticular neurons increase firing rates in the transition from EEG-synchronized sleep to REM sleep.

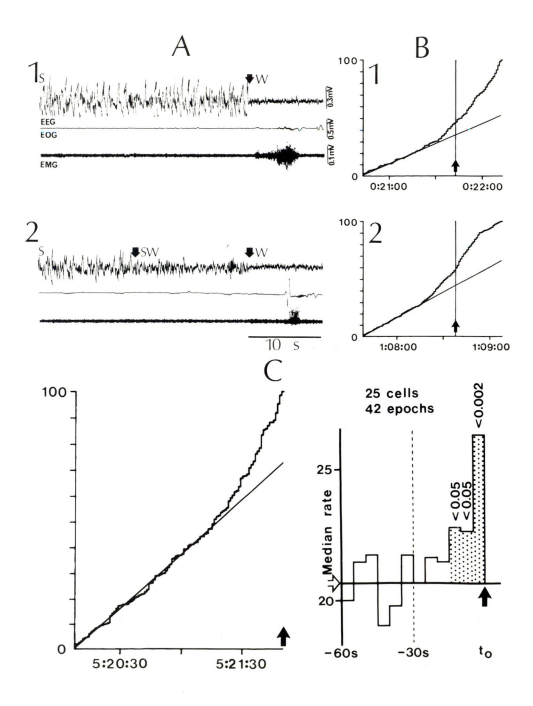

The precursor signs of decreased neuronal activity in thalamically projecting midbrain cells 1 sec before the first sequence of spindle waves during the drowsiness period were documented in Section 7.5 (see Fig. 12 of Chapter 7).

11.1.2. Bulbar Reticular (Noncholinergic) Neurons

The bulbar reticular neurons were recorded from the magno- and gigantocellular fields, and their ascending projections were antidromically identified from the midbrain reticular core and intralaminar and VM thalamic nuclei (Fig. 2A; Steriade *et al.*, 1984b). The antidromic identification from the thalamus was necessary to differentiate bulbar reticular neurons involved in EEG desynchronization from other types of medullary neurons that are related to muscular atonia (see Chapter 10). Some of the bulbothalamic neurons were phasically related to REMs and PGO waves. The focus in that study was, however, on tonically discharging neurons in order to relate their activity with the enduring event of EEG desynchronization during REM sleep.

The time 0 of EEG desynchronization associated with REM sleep follows by about 30–60 sec the onset of PGO waves during the pre-REM epoch (see Fig. 2), but in some instances the earliest sign of EEG desynchronization appears more than 2 min after the onset of PGO waves (Fig. 2B). To obtain evidence on whether the precursor signs of increased discharge rates of bulbothalamic neurons are related to the appearance of PGO waves during the fully synchronized EEG of the pre-REM epoch or if they are really related to EEG desynchronization (Fig. 2C), a group of eight cells was analyzed during at least 75 sec of EEG-synchronized sleep followed by pre-REM transitional epochs of at least 50 sec, eventually leading to REM sleep. Data showed that there was no significant difference in firing rate between the EEG-synchronized sleep and the first 30-sec period of the transitional pre-REM stage accompanied by PGO waves. Statistically significant increase in discharge frequencies began 30 sec after the onset of the pre-REM stage and continued to increase further as the earliest change from EEG synchronization to EEG desynchronization is approached (Fig. 2D; Steriade *et al.*, 1984b). These results indicate that a sample of bulbothalamic

---

Figure 1. Midbrain reticular formation (MRF) neurons with thalamic projections increase discharge rates in advance of EEG and behavioral signs of awakening from EEG-synchronized sleep in the chronically implanted cat. A: Electrographic criteria of transitional state (SW) between EEG-synchronized sleep (S) and waking (W). Abrupt (in 1) and progressive transition with an intermediate SW period (in 2). B: Percentage cumulative histogram (1-sec bins) of two MRF neurons. Abscissas, real time of recording; arrows and vertical lines, earliest signs of reduced amplitude and/or increased frequency of EEG waves (as in A, panel 2, arrow indicates time 0 of SW period). Inflection points are seen to occur 10–22 sec in advance of any change in EEG; overt signs of wakefulness (eye movements and increased muscular tone) appeared several seconds after arrows (as in A, panel 2). C: Increase in firing rate of MRF neurons before the end of S epochs developing into W. Left: Percentage cumulative histogram of neuron belonging to sample analyzed in graph depicted on right; arrows indicate first change in fully synchronized EEG waves. Right: Twenty-five cells whose global mean rate in S was at least 4/sec were analyzed during last minute of S in 42 epochs leading to SW or directly to W. Mann–Whitney test was used to compare reference rate during first 30 sec for all cells with their respective rates in the last six 5-sec bins. Note significantly increased rates in the three 5-sec bins before end of S (arrow) compared with discharge rate in the first 30 sec. Modified from Steriade *et al.* (1982a).

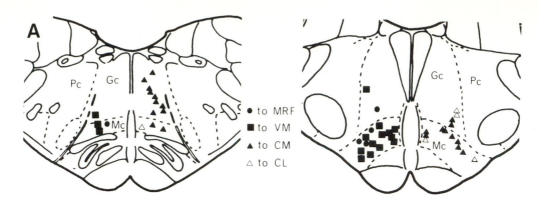

A

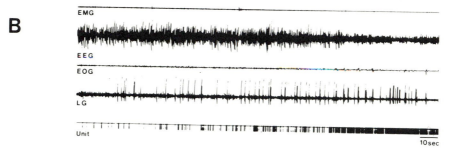

B

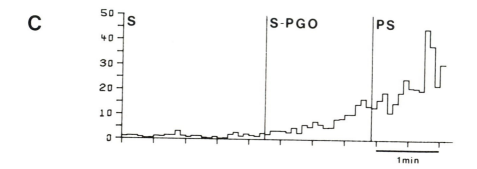

C

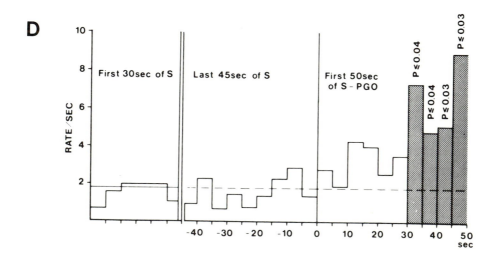

D

neurons with tonic discharge patterns significantly increase their rates of firing 20 sec in advance of EEG desynchronization with transition from EEG-synchronized sleep to REM sleep. The transmitter(s) used by these precursor neurons remain(s) to be elucidated.

11.1.3. Pedunculopontine Cholinergic Neurons

Recently, Steriade and co-workers have performed extracellular recordings in cat's PPT and LDT cholinergic nuclei at the mesopontine junction to investigate the relationship between the activity of their neurons and the tonic process of EEG desynchronization during waking and REM sleep (Datta *et al.*, 1989). The location of recorded neurons within PPT or LDT nuclei was assessed by means of lesions along microelectrode tracks combined with micrometer readings, and the sections were stained with NADPH-diaphorase histochemistry that stains cholinergic PPT and LDT neurons in the brainstem core (Fig. 3A). Of course, this method can only ascertain that the recorded cell was within a pool of cholinergic neurons. However, at the rostral PPT level (the so-called peribrachial area that, in cat, mainly extends between stereotaxic planes anterior 1 and posterior 1), where this investigation was conducted, cholinergic neurons represent about 80% of those neurons labeled by ChAT and TH immunohistochemistry (see Tables III and IV in Webster and Jones, 1988). Significant numbers of catecholaminergic neurons within the PPT nucleus appear only more caudally, at posterior planes 2 to 5 (see Fig. 1 in Section 4.1.2). Therefore, the probability that neurons located in the rostral part of the PPT nucleus are cholinergic is high. In addition, these neurons were antidromically identified as projecting to the different thalamic nuclei, mostly to LG, PUL–LP, and CL–PC intralaminar nuclei (Fig. 3B).

The majority of thalamically projecting neurons of the cholinergic PPT nucleus displayed tonic discharge patterns and increased their firing rates about 1 min before the earliest change from EEG synchronization during quiet sleep to EEG desynchronization during REM sleep (Datta *et al.*, 1989). This was shown by analyses of sequential mean frequency (SMF) in individual and in pooled PPT

Figure 2. Bulbar reticular neurons with midbrain and thalamic projections increase firing rates in advance of EEG desynchronization during REM sleep in chronically implanted cat. A: Localization of various gigantocellular (Gc), magnocellular (Mc), and parvocellular (Pv) medullary neurons projecting to midbrain reticular formation (MRF) and ventromedial (VM), centrum medianum (CM), and centrolateral (CL) thalamic nuclei, as identified by antidromic invasion. Rostrally projecting neurons are indicated on both parts of the medullary core to allow the anatomic localization of various neuronal groups (identified cells were usually found ipsilaterally to stimulating electrodes). Left section is at posterior plane 11–10, right section at posterior plane 9–8. B: Ink-written recording (EMG, cortical EEG, ocular movements (EOG), PGO waves in the LG thalamic nucleus, and discharges of a bulbothalamic cell) during transition from EEG-synchronized sleep (S) to pre-REM epoch characterized by appearance of PGO waves (S-PGO) and to paradoxical sleep (PS). Time 0 of PS (or REM sleep) is the earliest sign of EEG desynchronization. C: Sequential mean frequency (SMF), 5-sec bins, of one bulbothalamic neuron during transition from S to S-PGO and further to PS. D: Statistical evidence showing that the increased firing rate of thalamically projecting bulbar reticular neurons prior to onset of EEG desynchronization in REM sleep (during the pre-REM epoch or S-PGO) is not related to PGO waves. See details on method used in Steriade *et al.* (1984b). Modified from Steriade *et al.* (1984b).

cells (Fig. 4A,B). Since this long period of precursor changes comprises the transitional (SD = S → REM sleep) period between EEG-synchronized sleep (S) and EEG-desynchronized sleep (REM sleep), whose onset is the first PGO wave, and because many PPT cells are also PGO-on (see Chapter 9), separate SMFs were computed in which the time 0 was the onset of the transitional SD (or pre-REM) epoch. In these cases, precursor signs of increased activity were seen about

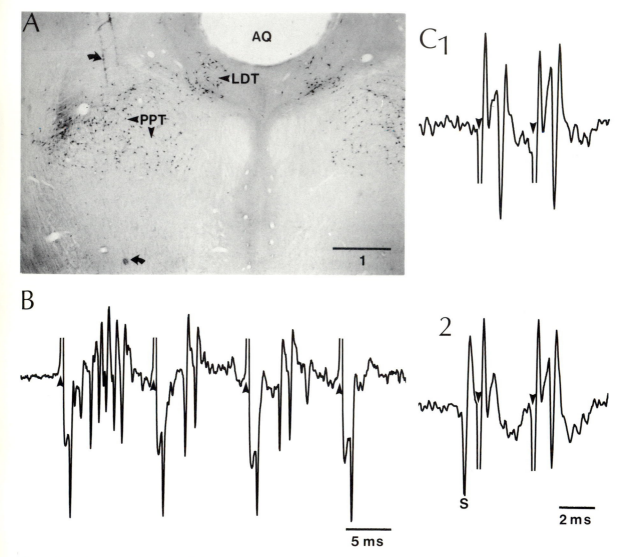

Figure 3. Cholinergic PPT and LDT brainstem nuclei and their thalamic projections as identified by cells' antidromic identification in the behaving cat. A: A frontal section stained by the NADPH–diaphorase method showing the LDT (Ch6 group) and PPT (Ch5 group) nuclei, the latter (on left part) traversed by recording microelectrodes; oblique arrow indicates the bottom lesion of a microelectrode track. AQ, aqueduct. B,C: antidromic identification of two PPT neurons from the PUL–LP thalamic complex (in B) and the LG thalamic nucleus (in C). Note fixed latency, fast-frequency following, and collision with a spontaneously occurring discharge (S in C2). The cell in B also responded orthodromically with a high-frequency burst after the antidromically elicited spike; note progressive diminution of number of spikes within the bursts at successive stimuli at 100 Hz. Unpublished data by M. Steriade, S. Datta, and D. Paré.

40 sec before the first PGO wave (Fig. 4C). These data demonstrate that neurons recorded from the cholinergic PPT nucleus, with identified thalamic projections, increase their firing rates well before the EEG desynchronization associated with REM sleep. The PPT neurons may thus be considered as the best candidates for inducing the cholinergic processes associated with EEG desynchronization, namely, direct excitation of thalamocortical cells and blockage of synchronized spindle oscillations by inhibiting RE thalamic neurons (see Chapter 7).

We discuss below the possible role of cholinergic neurons with descending projections in the induction and maintenance of REM sleep phenomena originating in pons and bulb.

11.2. Brainstem Neuronal Activity Over the Cycle of Sleep–Wake States

This section presents the brainstem neuronal activity characteristic of REM sleep. We emphasize cellular electrophysiology as offering the most definitive data about REM characteristics but include auxiliary methods as appropriate. The reason for the field's focus on the brainstem dates back to probably the most influential of the many lesion experiments, the early transection studies in the cat by Jouvet (1962). When the neuraxis was cut at the midbrain level (Fig. 5), rostral to the pons, signs of the state of REM sleep were not present rostral to the cut (with the cut between brainstem and forebrain, the pathway for all brainstem-mediated REM cortical desynchronization was absent). However, the essential signs of REM sleep were preserved in the brainstem caudal to the cut, as shown by the major REM indicator variables available for analysis in this preparation. The "pontine cat," as this preparation was called, showed periodically occurring states characterized by (1) rapid eye movements, although they were reduced in number and complexity, (2) antigravity muscle atonia, especially remarkable since it abolished the decerebrate rigidity otherwise present, and (3) spiky waves in the pontine tegmentum, the pontine component of PGO waves. The important implication of this study was that the structures caudal to the cut were necessary and sufficient for basic REM sleep phenomena, including rhythmicity. (This is not to say that more rostral structures do not enter into elaboration of REM phenomena; the phenomena in the pontine cat are simpler than those in the intact animal.) However, the presence of the major indicators of REM sleep below this transection has led to a fairly general consensus that the mechanisms for REM production are localized in the lower brainstem, although, as discussed, more precise specification of localization is still controversial (see, for example, later discussion in this chapter and the differing opinions of various workers expressed in McGinty *et al.*, 1985, and commentaries in Hobson *et al.*, 1986).

11.2.1. REM Sleep: The View from Intracellular Recordings

Our viewpoint is that intracellular recordings provide a privileged window on data relevant to the mechanisms of behavioral state control. In view of the transection evidence for the presence of the basic mechanisms of REM sleep in

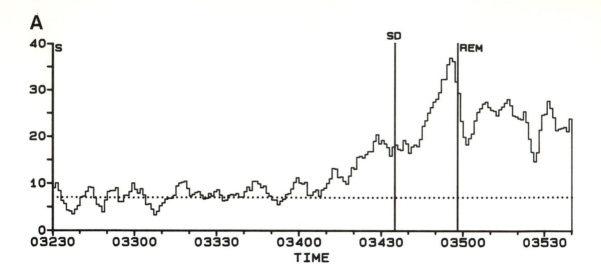

A

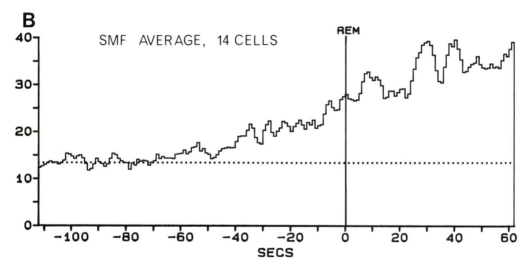

B

SMF AVERAGE, 14 CELLS

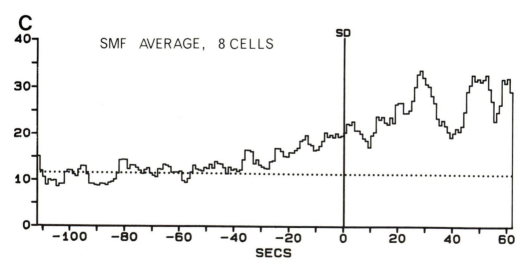

C

SMF AVERAGE, 8 CELLS

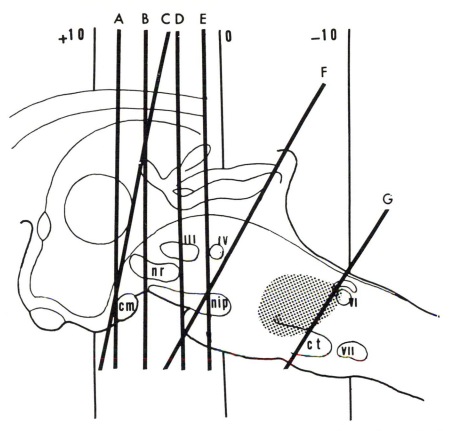

Figure 5. Neuraxis transections in the cat by Jouvet (1962). Transections A through F left the essential signs of REM sleep present caudal to the plane of the section but not rostral to it. Section G abolished the signs of REM sleep. Stippling indicates the zone where electrolytic lesions abolished REM sleep. Midline sagittal section; −10, 0, +10 are HC coordinates; Roman numerals indicate cranial nerve nuclei; red nucleus, nr; mammilary body, cm; interpeduncular nucleus, nip; trapezoid body, ct. Adapted from Jouvet (1962).

Figure 4. Pedunculopontine tegmental (PPT) neurons of cat increase firing rates in advance of EEG desynchronization during REM sleep. A: Sequential mean frequency (SMF) of a PPT neuron during transition from EEG-synchronized sleep (S) to transitional epoch (SD) from S to EEG-de-synchronized sleep (REM). Time 0 of SD (or pre-REM) epoch is the appearance of the first PGO wave. Time 0 of REM sleep is the earliest change from EEG synchronization to EEG desynchronization. Abscissa indicates real time. In this and two following panels, the spontaneous firing baseline in S is indicted by dotted line. B: An averaged SMF in a pool of 14 PPT neurons during transition from S to REM sleep. Note increased firing rates about 50 sec in advance of the first sign of EEG desynchronization. C: Since the transitional SD period comprises PGO waves, and in order to preclude that the precursor signs of increased activity in B were caused by the appearance of PGO waves, the averaged SMF in C (a pool of eight PPT neurons) shows that an increase in firing rate occurs well before (about 30 sec) the time 0 of the SD epoch. Unpublished data by M. Steriade, G. Oakson, S. Datta, and D. Paré.

brainstem, recordings in this zone may be regarded as potentially the most informative with respect to mechanism. We introduce the topic of cellular phenomena of REM sleep in the brainstem by an illustration in Fig. 6 of a prototypical continuous intracellular recording in the cat of a medial pontine reticular formation (mPRF) neuron during state passages from W to S to REM sleep and back to W. The inkwriter traces serve to highlight the indicator variables defining the various behavioral states and illustrate the temporal progression of phenomena. It can be seen that the dorsal LG–PGO waves herald the occurrence of REM sleep, whereas the occurrence of atonia, EEG desynchronization, and rapid eye movements mark the REM period proper. The time period prior to REM with PGO waves but no other signs of REM has been termed the "transition period" between slow-wave sleep and REM and is abbreviated "T" (McCarley and Hobson, 1970).

The data on the time course of membrane potential and occurrence of action potentials over the sequence of states illustrated in Fig. 6 and described below are from Ito and McCarley (1984).

1. *Synchronized sleep.* During synchronized sleep the membrane potential is polarized at about −58 mV, and there is little postsynaptic potential (PSP) activity. Little change in membrane polarization is present in quiet waking-to-synchronized sleep transitions.
2. *Pre-REM sleep changes: the transition period to REM sleep, T.* Even while the electrographic indicators are still those of synchronized sleep, the membrane potential of mPRF neurons begins to depolarize, a depolarization that progresses in the rather long, gradual approach to REM sleep. As the membrane potential depolarization progresses and the electrographic indicators of the transition period appear (onset of PGO waves), there is increased frequency and amplitude of PSPs and the onset of action potential discharge.
3. *REM sleep.* During REM sleep the membrane potential is maintained at a depolarized level, some 7–10 mV more depolarized than during quiet waking or early synchronized sleep. This state-long "tonic" depolarization is accompanied by increased frequency and amplitude of PSPs and action potential discharge. In addition to tonic depolarization there are short-duration "phasic" runs of increased PSPs and action potentials.
4. *Waking: the REM sleep–waking transition and motor activity in waking.* In the REM-sleep-to-waking state transition there is a fairly abrupt membrane repolarization of 7–10 mV, with the base-line membrane potential returning to the levels of the previous waking and early synchronized sleep periods. There is a marked reduction of PSP activity in quiet waking compared to REM sleep. Although the intracellular data discussed here were obtained in animals whose heads were atraumatically restrained to facilitate the intracellular recordings, the animals remained free to make ocular or somatomotor movements. When a somatic motor movement occurred, there was often a transient membrane depolarization and action potential activity (see Fig. 6 at the portion of the record marked Wm). After the end of the movement, the membrane potential returned to a polarized level, and action potentials ceased. In waking periods without movement there was no membrane depolarization. Other mPRF

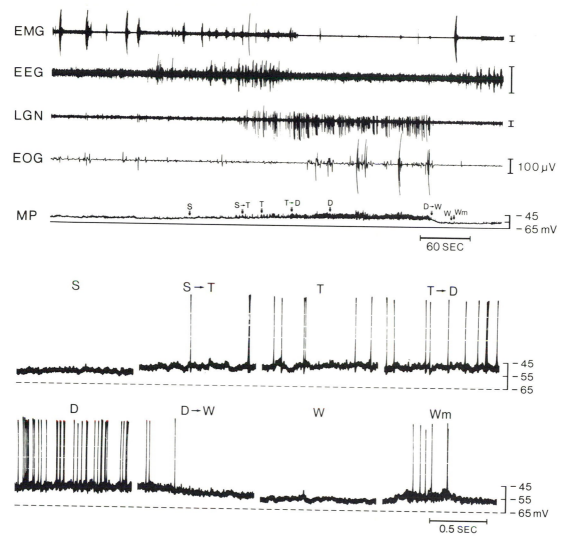

Figure 6. Changes in action potential frequency and membrane potential of an intracellularly recorded mPRF neuron in cat during changes in behavioral state. The top panel shows the inkwriter record defining state and the record of membrane potential (MP) with action potentials filtered out; the lower panel shows CRO photographs taken at the indicated points in the inkwriter record. The record begins in waking (W); note EOG activity, low-voltage fast EEG, and the EMG artifact indicating some somatic movement. In W the membrane potential was −57 mV and remained at approximately the same level with the onset of S (note EEG slow-wave activity). PSP activity in S was low. Even before the onset of the first PGO wave in the dorsal LGN record, the MP shows a gradual onset of depolarization. By the time of the first PGO wave (labeled S–T), the PSP activity is increased, and there is one action potential. With the advent of more PGO waves (segment T, transition period) and the onset of REM sleep (abbreviated as D for desynchronized sleep in this figure), there is further MP depolarization and,

pari passu, an increase in action potentials and PSPs (bottom panel, T and T–D); the increase in PSPs is visible as the thickening of the inkwriter MP trace. With the onset of full REM sleep (D) and during runs of the phasic activity of PGO waves and REMs, there are storms of depolarizing PSP activity and corresponding action potentials (segment D). The MP remains tonically depolarized at about −50 mV throughout REM sleep and shows further phasic depolarizations. With the end of REM sleep and the onset of W (D–W) there is a membrane repolarization to about the same tonic −57 mV level seen in the initial W episode. At the point marked Wm, there is a somatic movement that is accompanied by increased PSPs, a transient (phasic) membrane depolarization, and a burst of action potentials, before the MP returns to its base-line W polarization level. Abbreviations: EMG, nuchal electromyogram; EEG, sensorimotor cortex EEG; LGN, EEG record from dorsal lateral geniculate nucleus. Modified from Ito and McCarley (unpublished data).

neurons showed transient depolarizations and action potentials in waking in association with ocular movements, but a tonic membrane depolarization that persisted throughout waking was not characteristic of mPRF neurons.

To summarize: intracellular recordings show a tonic depolarization in REM sleep that is not present either in EEG-synchronized sleep or waking. In waking, transient depolarizations may occur with ocular or somatic motor movements but do not persist beyond the movement. Thus, REM sleep in the mPRF may be regarded as a state always characterized by a membrane potential depolarization, whereas in waking any depolarization is dependent on the presence of a particular behavior.

Corresponding to these changes of membrane polarization level were alterations in excitability, as measured by responses to electrical microstimulation from reticular sites in contralateral mPRF and in bulbar reticular formation (BRF; Fig. 7). Increased excitability was present in REM sleep as contrasted with EEG-synchronized sleep or waking, as measured by the effects of constant-current stimulation on monosynaptic PSP amplitude, propensity to evoke action potentials, and percentage of stimuli leading to antidromic activation.* Differences with REM sleep were most prominent in EEG-synchronized sleep (Fig. 7A) but were also present in waking (Fig. 7B) and were pervasive in the mPRF neuronal pool.

The intracellular analyses show that each behavioral state has distinctive characteristics in the mPRF neuronal pool. REM sleep is a state of heightened excitability and decreased membrane potential (e.g., depolarization) that is both extensive in the mPRF pool present in almost all (>90%) of the neurons sampled and persistent throughout the REM-sleep state. EEG-synchronized sleep is a state in which mPRF neurons show lessened excitability, increased membrane polarization, and little spontaneous EPSP activity. Waking, in contrast to REM sleep, does not have a temporally persistent heightened excitability and membrane depolarization throughout the pool. Rather, in waking, phasic membrane depolarizations appear to occur in a limited subset of the mPRF pool and in temporal association with the occurrence of specific behavioral events.

11.2.2. Sleep–Wake Behavioral State Control as Resulting from Modulation of Excitability in Neuronal Pools: Discussion of the Concept

The Sherringtonian concept of a neuronal pool with varying degrees of facilitation and suppression (Sherrington, 1906) is, we believe, a most useful concept for dealing with behavioral state alterations observable in brainstem reticular formation. The data presented suggest that one of the most salient alterations in the course of behavioral state changes is the result of different

---

*Increased antidromic activation may be present in REM sleep because of increased depolarization of the axon terminal near the stimulating electrode and/or more reliable propagation from the initial segment to the soma of the recorded neuron (see, for example, discussion in Ito and McCarley, 1987, and Glenn and Steriade, 1982).

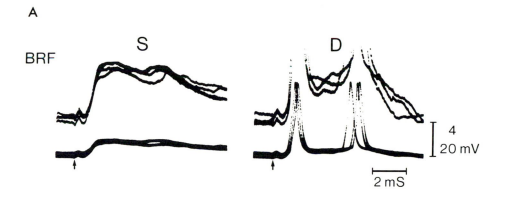

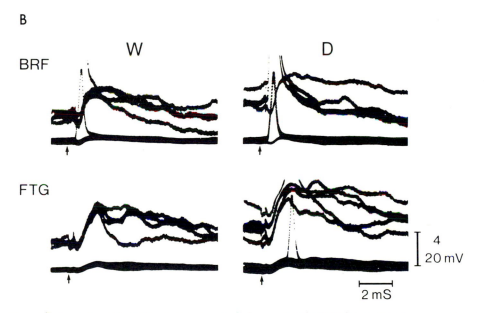

Figure 7. State-dependent excitability changes in intracellularly recorded mPRF neurons in the cat. A: Intracellular recording from an mPRF neuron showing effects of 70 μA stimulation in ipsilateral giant cell field of bulbar reticular formation (BRF) at arrow. Upper traces are high-gain A.C.-coupled (cal. 4 mV), and lower traces are low-gain D.C. (cal. 20 mV). In S, BRF stimulation evoked EPSPs with components at both monosynaptic and polysynaptic latencies but no action potentials. When the state of the animal changed to REM sleep (abbreviated as D for desynchronized sleep), stimulation at the same intensity elicited action potentials from both EPSP components. Recordings from a series of neurons during stimulation trials showed the probability of a monosynaptically elicited action potential in S was 0.13 and in REM sleep was 0.9 B: Intracellular recording of an mPRF neuron with calibration as in A. BRF stimulation of 60 μA in waking (W, upper row) produced one antidromic action potential in four trials, but in REM sleep (D), three of four trials showed antidromic invasion. Note the monosynaptic EPSP that was present when no antidromic invasion occurred. Criteria for antidromic invasion were microstimulation latency <0.6 msec with <0.1 msec variability and no preceding PSP. The lower row shows that stimulation of 75 μA in the gigantocellular tegmental field (FTG) portion of the contralateral mPRF evoked monosynaptic EPSPs with a steeper rising phase in D than in W; mean peak EPSP amplitude was also slightly (0.7 mV) higher in D than in W. One spike potential was elicited in D, but none in W. Note also that the membrane potential fluctuations caused by spontaneous PSPs were more prominent than in D. Modified from Ito and McCarley (1984).

levels of membrane polarization in different neuronal pools, which in turn lead to different levels of excitability and to different discharge pattern propensities because of the presence of voltage-sensitive membrane currents, as discussed in detail in Chapter 5. We frequently use the shorthand term of "bias" as a way of indicating alterations of excitability in neuronal pools. Figure 8 schematizes this concept of behavioral state operation by alteration of "bias" on different neuronal pools important in production of REM components. We here primarily discuss bias alterations from changes in membrane potential, since there are data available for this variable; however, we emphasize the strong possibility that the state-induced bias of neuronal pools may also utilize other mechanisms such as intracellular second messengers. Unfortunately, these other mechanisms still await experimental investigation in sleep–wake states.

All evidence from intracellular recordings points to the usefulness of this concept of behavioral state changes as operating through alterations of excitability in neuronal pools. The basic argument is straightforward: increasing the excitability of neurons in a particular brain region or nucleus will increase the probability of behaviors or physiological functions controlled or mediated by that region. Figure 8 provides an overview of the concept of behavioral state control as mediated by excitability alterations in the neuronal pools subserving

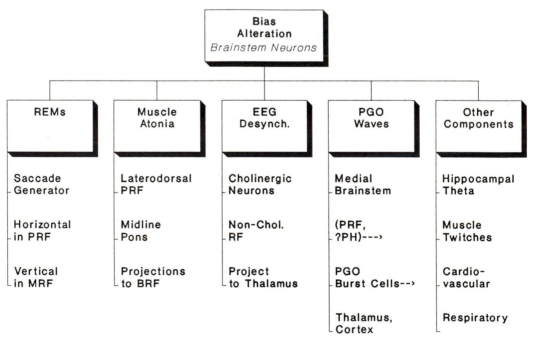

Figure 8. Schematic of REM-sleep behavioral state control by alteration of bias (excitability and other neuronal properties) within brainstem neuronal pools subserving each of the major components of the state. For example, the neuronal pool important for the REMs (the rapid eye movements) is suggested to be the brainstem saccade-generating system whose main machinery is in paramedian pontine reticular formation (Chapter 10). Although vertical saccades are fewer in REM sleep, their presence suggests similar involvement of the mesencephalic reticular formation. Information under the other system components sketches the major features of the anatomy and projections of neuronal pools important for muscle atonia, EEG desynchronization, and PGO waves, and the last part of the diagram lists other components of REM sleep.

particular components of the state. We thus see REM sleep as composed of relatively discrete "physiological modules," REM sleep components, that become active in concert because they share a common mechanism(s) of excitability modulation.

11.2.3. Sleep–Wake Behavioral State Control as Resulting from Modulation of Excitability in Neuronal Pools: Experimental Evidence

Brainstem reticular formation. Figure 9 schematizes the sleep-cycle membrane polarization levels in terms of relative levels for waking, EEG-synchronized sleep, and REM sleep for the three neuronal pools on which intracellular recordings are available.

Pontine reticular formation. We have shown that, in medial pontine reticular formation neurons, membrane depolarization and increased excitability persist throughout the state. Since, as discussed in detail in Chapters 9 and 10, much of the neuronal generating machinery for the rapid eye movements and PGO wave events lies in this zone, the increased excitability will favor the occurrence of these events. In waking, the pattern of mPRF excitability alteration revealed by the intracellular recordings is also functionally reasonable in terms of the set of the behaviors occurring in waking. In this state, discrete activation of subsets of reticular neurons with a circumscribed time duration is associated with a heightened specificity of response to particular inputs and of specificity of output (a higher signal-to-noise ratio). Were waking accompanied by the same state-long tonic increase in excitability and depolarization throughout the entire neuronal pool as found in REM sleep, behavioral responses would lose their specificity in the face of a diffuse excitation of all systems.

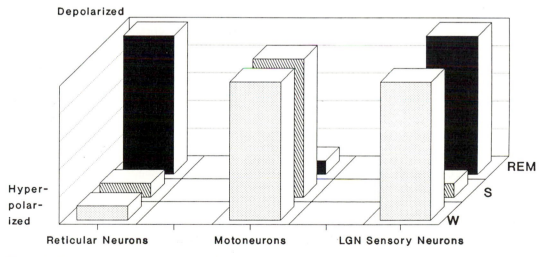

Figure 9. Sleep–wake cycle membrane polarization levels. Values are schematized as either depolarized or hyperpolarized and are relative values for waking, synchronized sleep, and REM sleep within each pool. Values represent average tonic levels and do not schematize phasic alterations; they are drawn from the neuronal populations for which intracellular data are available. (▦) Waking; (▨) synchronized sleep; (■) REM sleep.

Bulbar reticular formation neurons. Intracellular recordings of medial bulbar reticular formation neurons by Chase and collaborators (1981) indicate the presence of a REM-specific tonic membrane potential depolarization, with approximately the same level of membrane potential shift as mPRF neurons. It is of note that the membrane depolarization in BRF neurons appeared to occur later than seen in many mPRF neurons; in BRF neurons membrane depolarization occurred near the onset of muscle atonia, which, together with other data on the role of this region in atonia (Chapter 10), suggested that some of the recorded neurons may be effectors of the muscle atonia of REM sleep. State-related membrane potential changes lasted throughout the REM sleep state, thus supporting the thesis that REM sleep behavioral state changes are mediated by excitability alteration and that membrane potential alteration is one important agent of this change throughout the pontobulbar reticular pool.

Peripheral motoneurons. In both spinal α-motoneurons and trigeminal jaw-closer motoneurons there is a strong modulation of excitability during REM sleep by modulation of membrane potential. The membrane potential in these neurons is hyperpolarized during the state of REM sleep (see Fig. 9 and data from the studies of Chase and co-workers and of others cited in Chapter 10). The reduction in excitability in these motoneuronal pools is reflected in the muscle atonia of REM sleep.

Sensory system neurons. Only dorsal lateral geniculate (LG) thalamocortical neurons have been recorded intracellularly during sleep-wake states, but these data also support the thesis of behavioral state control through excitability modulation, with membrane potential alteration being an important mechanism. As schematized in Fig. 9, during EEG-synchronized sleep LG neurons are relatively hyperpolarized compared with REM sleep, and the REM sleep membrane depolarization is maintained throughout that state (Hirsch *et al.,* 1983). It is of interest that these LG neurons begin to depolarize coincident with the onset of PGO waves in the transition period from synchronized sleep to REM sleep, consistent with the notion that during REM sleep these neurons are targets of brainstem excitatory input associated with PGO waves (see Chapter 9). It is also of functional interest that, unlike some brainstem reticular neurons, the LG relay neurons are depolarized throughout waking. This is, of course, functionally reasonable since they function throughout the state of waking to transmit and modulate information from retina. In contrast, pontine reticular formation neurons do not function as a homogeneous group during waking, and thus the absence of a tonic depolarization throughout waking is also functionally reasonable.

We conclude that all available experimental evidence supports the concept that modulation of excitability is a key factor in behavioral state control and that modulation of membrane potential is an important mechanism of excitability modulation.

11.2.4. Summary of Orchestration of REM Sleep Components

In this section we indicate the evidence for localizing generation of a particular component of REM sleep to a particular set of neurons; in most cases the data have been presented in detail elsewhere in the book, and this section and

Fig. 9 can act as a summary. The order of presentation follows the left-to-right ordering of REM components in Fig. 9. Although intracellular recordings and direct monitoring of membrane potential have not been done for all sets of neurons implicated in control of REM components, the state-long persistence of changes in each component is compatible with our hypothesis of membrane potential alteration as an important mechanism of behavioral state change.

Rapid eye movements. Chapter 10 discusses the saccade generation system, most of which lies in mPRF structures. The REM sleep membrane depolarization and increased excitability bias the system toward increased saccade production during REM sleep. The presence of rapid eye movements in the REM-like states of the pontine cat indicates clearly that this component of REM sleep can be generated exclusively within the brainstem, even without the forebrain input so important in waking control.

Muscle atonia. Chapter 10 describes the extracellular recordings of dorsolateral tegmental neurons projecting to BRF; their discharge activity is highly correlated with onset and offset of REM-sleep muscle atonia, although intracellular recordings are not presently available. Chapter 10 also describes electrical and chemical stimulation evidence suggesting a possible midline component to the muscle atonia system, but there are neither extra- nor intracellular recordings of neurons in this zone relating their activity to muscle atonia. The previous chapter has also described evidence for reticulotrigeminal input important in muscle atonia.

EEG desynchronization. Section 11.1 describes data from Steriade and co-workers (1982a, 1984b, 1989a) supporting a role for cholinergic neurons in PPT and noncholinergic neurons in mesencephalic and bulbar reticular formation in mediating this component of REM sleep.

PGO waves. Chapter 9 describes intracellular data from McCarley and Ito (1983) indicating the presence of neurons in medial PRF and the tegmental reticular nucleus that discharge with long lead times before PGO waves and thus may serve to initiate the eye-movement-related PGO waves of REM sleep. Anatomic data by Higo and co-workers (1989a) indicate the presence of prepositus hypoglossi (PH) to PPT projections that may be involved in the genesis of eye-movement-triggered PGO waves, although REM-sleep recordings have not yet been done in PH. Various classes of PGO burst neurons in the PPT zone are described in Chapter 9 (Steriade *et al.*, 1989a). They represent the output pathway from brainstem to thalamus and have been recorded extracellularly in sleep (see Section 9.1) but not intracellularly.

Other components of REM sleep: θ *rhythm.* Studies by Vertes (1982, 1984) using macropotential recordings, electrical stimulation, and lesion techniques have pointed to the pontine reticular formation at more lateral sites as important for production of the hippocampal θ rhythm of REM. Unit recordings showed neurons whose onset and offset of activity were correlated with onset and offset of θ; it is of interest that this subset of neurons was tonically active in both REM sleep and waking, suggesting a state-dependent activation of this pool that may be different from the set of medial pontine reticular neurons discussed above. These neurons have not been recorded intracellularly.

Phasic muscle twitches. One of the behavioral characteristics of REM sleep is the presence of muscle twitches, especially of distal flexor muscles and, in cats, of the vibrissae and ears. These are present in the "pontine cat," and thus brainstem structures are necessary and sufficient for their occurrence. Cellular data bearing on their occurrence have been presented by Wyzinski *et al.* (1978), who recorded extracellularly from mPRF neurons antidromically identified as projecting to ventral spinal cord. These neurons showed high correlations of runs of action potentials with the presence of muscle twitches, suggesting brainstem mediation of this component of REM sleep.

Autonomic nervous system changes. The cardiovascular, respiratory, and thermoregulatory systems undergo profound alterations during slow-wave sleep and REM sleep. We shall not review here the extensive literature because a recent book has discussed this aspect of sleep physiology in some detail (Lydic and Biebuyck, 1988). We do think it useful, however, to give a brief overview of the current state of this area of physiology *vis-à-vis* brainstem control mechanisms. With respect to respiration, extracellular recording studies in cats conditioned to arrest inspiration on signal have led to the Orem's (1988) thesis that the voluntary/behavioral and the automatic/metabolic aspects of breathing are integrated at the brainstem level, and extracellular recordings indicate that some respiratory neurons have relatively "pure" respiration-related discharge activity whereas that of others is greatly influenced by behavioral state. Orem (1988) hypothesizes that non-REM sleep reflects a predominance of automatic/metabolic system control, whereas breathing during REM sleep represents a predominance of voluntary/behavioral system control (Orem, 1988). An obvious possibility is that the state-modulated respiratory neurons may have input from areas greatly affected by behavioral state changes, although the others do not. The requisite anatomic studies to test this supposition have not yet been done.

State-related changes are similarly important in the cardiovascular system. In waking there is a high degree of heart rate variability, which is transformed to a great regularity in EEG-synchronized sleep except for a nearly sinusoidal modulation from respiratory influences (sinus arrhythmia is accentuated in this state). REM sleep consistently shows much episodic variability of cardiac rate. These state-related respiratory and cardiovascular changes are sufficiently distinctive to allow machine classification of state (Harper *et al.*, 1987). As with the respiratory system, the locus of neurons accounting for the REM sleep variability has not yet been firmly identified, although influences from the brainstem parabrachial region and from the forebrain, including central nucleus of the amygdala, have been postulated (Harper *et al.*, 1988; Verrier, 1988). Parmeggiani (1985) has described the vascular-bed-specific changes in blood pressure during REM sleep. Much of the recent interest in the cardiovascular field is driven by an effort to discover associations between clinical pathology and state; in pigs, synchronized sleep, but not REM sleep, is associated with arrhythmias in ischemic heart (Skinner *et al.*, 1975), although such a clear-cut relationship between sleep stage and arrhythmias in humans is still uncertain (Verrier, 1988). Overall the investigation of cardiovascular changes during sleep is still, in general, concentrated on noncellular, "electrographic" data, and detailed central nervous system anatomic and physiological studies have just begun (McCarley, 1988).

Thermoregulation is profoundly affected during sleep, and extracellular recordings in hypothalamus suggest a decrease in thermosensitivity in synchronized sleep and an absence of thermoregulation in REM sleep, at least in cats (Parmeggiani *et al.*, 1987) and kangaroo rats (Glotzbach and Heller, 1984). Parmeggiani has summarized the behavioral-state-related changes as an absence of hypothalamic and telencephalic regulation in REM sleep and a "rhomben-cephalic" dominance of thermoregulation in this state as well as a rhomben-cephalic dominance of other physiological systems during REM sleep (Parmeggiani, 1988). As with other autonomic functions, the pathways and neurotransmitters causing these dramatic state-related alterations have not yet been defined.

11.2.5. Waking and Sleep-Related Activity of Brainstem Neurons: The Perspective from Extracellular Recordings

The previous parts of this section have detailed the dramatic alterations of membrane potential and excitability of brainstem reticular neurons that occur with REM sleep and contrasted this with the hyperpolarization of synchronized sleep and the episodic and behavior-dependent depolarizations of waking. The perspective one obtains from extracellular recordings is quite different and is useful to review, because this technique enables long-term recordings and is of historical importance for the development of concepts in the field, although the level of mechanistic insight into the nature of state-related alterations and mechanisms is necessarily less than with intracellular recordings. Extracellular unit recordings in the head-restrained cat done in the early 1970s by McCarley and Hobson (1971) and Hobson *et al.* (1974a) showed that cells in the pontine reticular formation gigantocellular field (FTG) and REM-sleep discharge rates considerably higher than those in EEG-synchronized sleep and waking. An early formulation was that this area might be a REM sleep "center." However, the work of Siegel (1979; Siegel and Tomaszewski, 1983; Siegel *et al.*, 1983) in cats and Vertes (1977, 1982) in rats showed that FTG neurons discharged in association with movements in waking in freely moving animals and that if the animals performed the movement associated with a higher discharge rate throughout the recorded waking segment, then the discharge rate in waking approximated that of REM. These studies indicated that a simple notion of the FTG as a "REM center" was not appropriate, at least in one classical definition of a center: an anatomic locus of neurons associated with one behavioral or physiological function and no other (see discussion of the center concept in Chapter 1). In fact, in extracellular recordings Siegel and Vertes did not observe any state-specific activity in any portion of the pontobulbar reticular formation; obviously these extracellular recordings could not monitor the REM-state-specific population membrane depolarization observable in intracellular recordings and described in Section 11.2.1.

Extracellular recordings are particularly valuable because they enable long-duration recordings of brainstem activity and hence a clear perspective of changes in activity profile over repeated sleep–waking cycles. Figure 10 is such an extracellular multiple-cycle recording that clearly shows the magnitude of state-related modulation of discharge activity. This neuron shows a remarkable modulation of activity. Extracellular recordings indicated that within pontine reticular formation the pattern of discharge varies from "phasic," defined by runs of clustered discharges to "tonic," with relatively little moment-to-moment discharge variation (McCarley and Hobson, 1975a); as a general rule, neurons with the most pronounced REM-sleep discharge rate increase tended to have

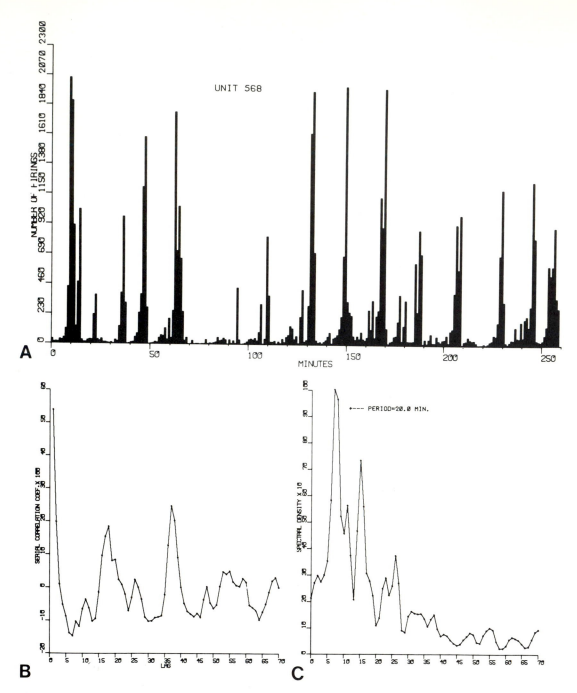

Figure 10. Extracellular recording of a pontine FTG neuron over many sleep–wake cycles in a head-restrained cat (A) and spectral analysis to show the periodicity. A: Each of the peaks of discharge activity corresponds to the occurrence of a REM-sleep episode; the use of head restraint renders waking activity minimal and further emphasizes the obligatory nature of REM sleep discharge enhancement against the behavior-dependent changes of waking. B: Au-

tocorrelogram analysis. Note periodic peaks at approximately 20-min intervals. Spectral analysis shows that maximal power is concentrated at a frequency corresponding to a period of 20 min, the period of REM sleep in this animal. The presence of substantial power on the flank of the peak is attributable to the nonsinusoidal (nonlinear) components of the activity. Adapted from McCarley (1980a).

phasic discharge patterns (clusters of discharges but without the presence of low-threshold spike "bursts" as defined in Chapter 5) and to be localized in medial pontine reticular formation (FTG), whereas those recorded more laterally were more tonic and had less change. (The neurons with discharge activity associated with muscle atonia and described in Chapter 10 were a conspicuous exception.) The neuron illustrated in Fig. 10 had a "phasic" discharge pattern.

The next section (11.3) addresses the important question of what might cause the state-related changes in pontine reticular formation neurons, but we first look at lesion data bearing on the functional role of reticular subdivisions in the production of REM-sleep components. The reader will again be reminded of our suggestion that lesions are not the most suitable technique for resolving questions of function of small groups of neurons. We list here the following potential confounds: (1) fibers of passage (electrolytic lesions may destroy fibers as well as somata), (2) imprecise boundaries (all types of lesions are not controllable with respect to extent, and the precise boundary of functional destruction/disturbance is not known), (3) ambiguity of interpretation even with complete lesions. The latter point is worthy of some elaboration. If a behavioral component vanishes, it is not known whether this implies destruction of output pathways, nonspecific interference (e.g., the animal may be rendered so ill that REM sleep will not occur), the area destroyed indeed normally mediates the behavioral component in question but other areas may be sufficient for its continued production, or the behavior, such as REM sleep, being investigated is so radically changed by the lesion that it is not clear whether or not it is present.

We have earlier discussed the Jouvet (1962) transection experiments suggesting a pontobulbar location for most of REM-sleep components. Transections at a pontomedullary level show preservation of many REM-sleep indicator variables rostral to the transection, suggesting that medullary components are not essential for REM sleep and thus pointing to the primacy of pontine and pontomesencephalic components (Siegel *et al.*, 1984, 1986; transections rostral to the 6th nucleus). Early reports by Jouvet and co-workers (Jouvet, 1962) pointed to abolishment of REM sleep by electrolytic pontine reticular (FTG) lesions. Later, kainic acid lesions of pontine FTG by two sleep research groups (Sastre *et al.*, 1981; Drucker-Colin and Pedraza, 1983) were reported to have no effects on REM sleep signs, including no effect on eye movements in waking or REM sleep, a finding in conflict with the lesion studies reported by the oculomotor researchers in the preceding chapter. Although it is difficult to reconcile these differences, absence of complete lesions of the medial pontine reticular zones important for eye movements (see Chapter 10, Fig. 2) may account for the differences; it is of interest that, although giant cells were reported as destroyed by the two sleep research groups, we now know (Chapter 4) that these giant neurons are primarily reticulospinal neurons, and the smaller neurons critical for saccade generation may have been left unlesioned. This sparing appears likely from the histological photographs presented. Lesions of the zones that may be involved in muscle atonia have been discussed in the previous chapter. It is of note that much of the early lesion work was fraught with such controversies over precise localization; as a case example of the difficulty of resolution of lesion data, the reader is referred to the detailed discussion of the precise role of various vestibular nuclei in production of the PGO wave bursts of REM sleep furnished in an annotated bibliography (Hobson and McCarley, 1974).

11.3. Questions of Causality: What Creates the Membrane Potential and Excitability Alterations of REM Sleep

In the previous section we presented the phenomenology of membrane potential changes over the sleep–wake cycle. We suggested that the components of REM sleep were elicited by an alteration of bias of the neuronal pool subserving each component. With the increased excitability associated with REM sleep, the neuronal machinery controlled by a particular neuronal pool would be set into motion. However, we have not yet addressed experimental evidence for the reasonableness of this assertion, such as presenting data indicating that experimentally induced modulation of excitability could produce the complete or partial set of REM sleep phenomena, with the partial or complete nature of production depending on which neuronal pools were activated. Nor have we yet presented either data or hypotheses relevant to how the membrane potential alterations of REM sleep are caused. We see this question as one of the most important in sleep physiology, although, at this stage of research, we must be content with presenting possible controlling factors. Three factors are discussed, and we emphasize that they are not mutually exclusive, and, indeed, there is more reason to suppose they all are important than that any one might dominate. We also add the (perhaps obvious) comment that future work will likely add to this list. At this stage of research, the potential causal factors of the reticular formation REM sleep membrane potential changes are (1) cholinergic input, (2) reticuloreticular excitatory connections, and (3) disinhibition by aminergic neurons.

11.3.1. Cholinergic Influences on REM Sleep

Chapter 4 presents anatomic evidence of cholinergic projections to mPRF from the LDT and PPT nuclei, and Chapter 6 presents *in vitro* data indicating the strong excitatory response of over 65% of mPRF neurons to carbachol, administered in micromolar concentrations. Thus, there is strong supporting evidence that acetylcholine is a physiological neurotransmitter acting on mPRF neurons. (A final but critical piece of evidence is to show that stimulation of LDT/PPT produces PSPs with the same effects and that the PSPs are blocked by antagonists in the same low concentrations as described in Chapter 6.) Given this information one might thus, on an *ad hoc* basis, choose cholinergic agonists as reasonable agents to alter the excitability of reticular neuronal pools.

In fact, the history of cholinergic injections into brainstem began in the 1960s on a much more empirical basis. Cordeau *et al.* (1963) and George *et al.* (1964) reported the induction of a REM-sleep-like state by these injections. Since then numerous published studies have reported the elicitation of some or all components of REM sleep by brainstem injections of cholinergic agonists (these include, among others: Baxter, 1969; Kostowski, 1971; Mitler and Dement, 1974; Amatruda *et al.*, 1975; Velasco *et al.*, 1979; Silberman *et al.*, 1980; van Dongen, 1980; Vivaldi *et al.*, 1980; Hobson *et al.*, 1983b; Katayama *et al.*, 1984; Baghdoyan *et al.*, 1984a,b, 1987; Shiromani and Fishbein, 1986; Shiromani and McGinty, 1986; Shiromani *et al.*, 1986).

In certain application sites in the pontine reticular formation, cholinergic agonists produce a "full" REM-sleep-like syndrome with the simultaneous presence of all major indicator variables (Fig. 11); these sites tend to be in the medial pontine reticular formation rostral to abducens and in the dorsal one-half (see also discussion of localization of cholinergic agonist effects in the final section of Chapter 10). Carbachol application at other sites, such as near the peribrachial zone and hence near PPT, may produce isolated PGO waves without other signs of REM sleep (Vivaldi *et al.*, 1980). Chapter 10 discusses how the muscle atonia of REM sleep may be produced by application of cholinergic agonists to the dorsolateral pontine reticular formation. Applications of cholinergic agonists to mesencephalic or bulbar reticular formation have not, at least in the sites so far tested, produced the full REM-sleep-like syndrome (Baghdoyan *et al.*, 1984b).

We have seen that (1) microinjection of cholinergic agonists into pontine tegmentum produces a REM-sleep-like state, (2) there are cholinergic projections from LDT and PPT to pontine reticular formation (Chapter 4), and (3) cholinergic agonists in physiological concentrations act directly on pontine reticular formation neurons to produce depolarization and increased excitability (Chapter 5).

What else must be shown before we accept a causal role? First of all, more evidence must be adduced for cholinergic projections and excitatory effects on the lateral pontine reticular formation neurons, although anecdotal anatomic evidence for projections is present (A. Mitani, R. McCarley, and S. Higo, unpublished data), and there is little reason to suspect that lateral reticular neurons will have a radically different receptor profile than medial neurons. One might also argue that the preponderance of pontobulbar reticular formation has been demonstrated to receive a cholinergic projection, thus accounting for many REM components and suggesting that, as discussed below, reticuloreticular excitatory connections might lead to a spread of excitability from medial to lateral elements, even if lateral reticular formation were not cholinergically innervated.

The main missing criterion is the *time course criterion:* cholinergic neurons projecting to PRF must be shown to increase discharge rate before the alterations in membrane potential and excitability in mPRF neurons, which occur even before the onset of PGO waves. Obviously if LDT/PPT neurons increase discharge rate after the onset of MP changes in mPRF neurons, they cannot be the cause of these changes. The data presented for thalamically projecting PPT neurons in Section 11.1 indicate a quite early pre-REM onset of discharge alterations; it will be interesting to determine the time course for PPT/LDT neurons with projections to pontine and bulbar reticular formation. Another criterion, less important, is the *selectivity of discharge* criterion: even if the discharge activity increase of LDT/PPT neurons projecting to mPRF were to precede the onset of PGO waves, thus satisfying the time course criterion, there is the possibility that the cholinergic neurons might also have a similar discharge rate during waking, a time when most mPRF neurons do not have a tonic membrane potential depolarization. The inference would then be that the cholinergic input to mPRF could not be the *exclusive* cause of the membrane potential depolarization that begins even before the onset of transition period. It might also be emphasized again that even if both the time course and selectivity criteria were satisfied, other factors still may contribute to the REM-sleep-associated changes in pontine reticular formation. We next discuss these other factors.

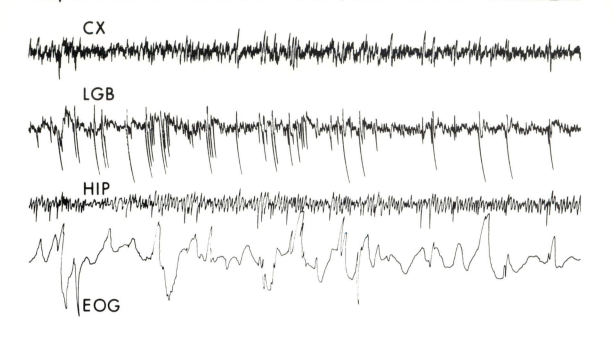

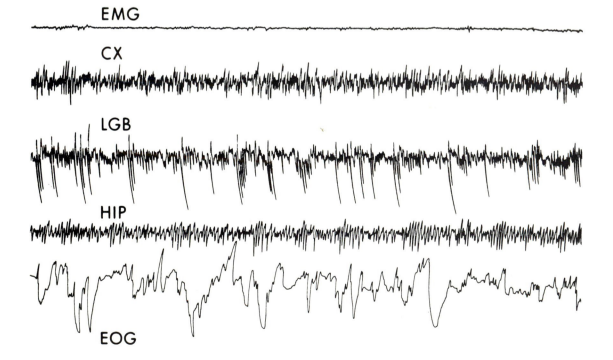

11.3.2. Reticuloreticular Excitatory Connections as Facilitating Recruitment within the Reticular Pool

Chapters 3 and 4 extensively document evidence for the presence of dense reticuloreticular excitatory connectivity. It is immediately apparent that the onset of discharge activity within this pool as REM sleep is approached would lead to the recruitment of other members through the reticuloreticular excitatory connections and that this excitatory connectivity would similarly contribute to the maintenance of REM-sleep depolarization. Stated in systems terminology, the monosynaptic excitatory connectivity in pontobulbar reticular formation may furnish the substrate for a self-augmenting positive feedback process that will result in the progressive membrane depolarization in T and will help maintain the depolarization and excitability throughout the state of REM sleep. Indeed, the data show the time course of depolarization in reticular neurons prior to REM sleep onset to be compatible with their playing this role in the process leading to initiation of this state. Figure 12 summarizes the extracellular recording data on the time course of recruitment and shows these data are matched quite nicely by an exponential curve, indicating that mutual augmentation is a good model of recruitment within the population.

11.3.3. REM-off Neurons

The neurons described in the previous section that increase discharge rate with the advent of REM are often termed "REM-on neurons." In contrast, groups of other neurons radically decrease and may nearly arrest discharge activity with the approach and onset of REM; these are often termed "REM-off" neurons. Their typical discharge activity profile is for discharge rates to be highest in waking, then decrease in synchronized sleep, and nearly cease discharging in REM sleep. REM-off neurons are distinctive both because they are in the minority in the brain and also because they are recorded in zones with neurons that use biogenic amines as neurotransmitters. The loci include a midline zone of the brainstem raphe nuclei and a more lateral bandlike zone in the rostral pons–midbrain junction that includes the nucleus locus coeruleus, a reticular zone, and the peribrachial zone, as illustrated in Fig. 13.

Raphe nuclei. Neurons with a REM-off discharge profile were first described by Harper and McGinty (1973) in the dorsal raphe nucleus, a finding confirmed by other workers (Trulson and Jacobs, 1979; Hobson *et al.*, 1983a; Lydic *et al.*, 1987a,b). Neurons with the same REM-off discharge pattern have been found in the other raphe nuclei, including nucleus linearis centralis (McCarley, 1980a; Hobson *et al.*, 1983a), centralis superior (Rasmussen *et al.*, 1984), raphe magnus (Cespuglio *et al.*, 1981; Fornal *et al.*, 1985), and raphe pallidus (Sakai *et al.*, 1983).

Figure 11. Electrographic signs of natural REM sleep and a REM-sleep-like state in the same cat induced by diffusion form a cannula filled with 4 μg carbachol in 1 μl of saline. Note the similarity of the indicator variables of EMG atonia, cortical EEG (CX) desynchronization, PGO waves in the dorsal lateral geniculate body (LGB), hippocampal θ, and the EOG record of rapid eye movements. This full REM-like syndrome, shown in the bottom panel, is typical of carbachol application to anterodorsal pons. From Vivaldi *et al.* (1980).

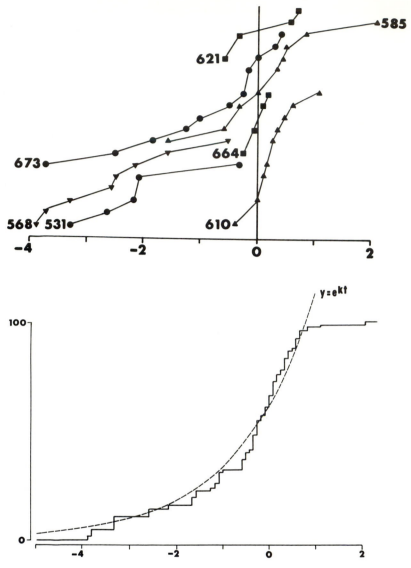

Figure 12. Time course of REM-sleep-related increase in discharge rate of brainstem reticular neurons extracellularly recorded over many sleep–wake cycles. Top panel shows the "REM sleep recruitment" time onset of five FTG neurons and two FTC neurons (531 and 673) relative to the electrographically defined time of onset of REM sleep, 0 min on the abscissa. "Recruitment" is defined as a persistent, significant discharge rate increase over the synchronized sleep baseline period ($Ps \geq 0.001$). The data are displayed as a cumulative histogram with the increment for one transition period being shown as the calibration bar. Each point for each numbered neuron represents the occurrence of one or more transition periods with the increment at this time. Thus, for example, the curve of unit 610 presents 12 transition period changes as nine points because there were three pairs of identical recruitment times. Bottom panel: Pooled cumulative histogram for the data of the top panel. Time ordinate is at top panel, and abscissa is the percentage of the pool of seven neurons showing recruitment, with the time curve for each of the neurons showing the recruitment distribution of the top panel, and with the contribution of each of the neurons weighted equally. The dotted line is a plot of $y = \exp(kt)$, the exponential growth curve. Note that the correspondence is quite close until 1 min after REM sleep onset, at which time the experimental data reach an asymptote, indicating all neurons have changed discharge rate. Modified from Hobson *et al.* (1974a).

Identification of these extracellularly recorded neurons with serotonin-containing neurons was made on the basis of recording site location in the vicinity of histochemically identified serotonin neurons and the similarity of the extracellularly recorded slow, regular discharge pattern to that of histochemically identified serotonergic neurons (see Chapters 5 and 6). Nonserotonergic neurons in the raphe system have been found to have different discharge pattern characteristics (Chapter 6). Although this extracellular identification methodology does not approach the "gold standard" of intracellular recording and labeling, the circumstantial evidence that the raphe REM-off neurons are serotonergic appears strong.

Locus coeruleus. The second major locus of REM-off neurons is the locus coeruleus, as described in cat (Chu and Bloom, 1974; Hobson *et al.*, 1973, 1975), rat (Aston-Jones and Bloom, 1981a,b), and monkey (Foote *et al.*, 1980). The argument that these extracellularly recorded discharges are from norepinephrine-containing neurons parallels that for the putative serotonergic REM-off neurons. Extracellularly recorded neurons that are putatively noradrenergic have the same slow, regular discharge as identified norepinephrine-containing neurons (see Chapter 5) and have the proper anatomic localization of recording sites, including recording sites in the compact locus coeruleus in the rat, where the norepinephrine-containing neurons are rather discretely localized. Thus, although the evidence that these REM off neurons are norepinephrine-containing is indirect and circumstantial, it nonetheless appears quite strong.

Finally, the remaining groups of REM-off neurons are principally localized to the anterior pontine tegmentum–midbrain junction either in the peribrachial zone or in a more medial extension of it (Fig. 13), recording sites that correspond to the presence of aminergic neurons scattered through this zone (see Chapters 3 and 4). The "stray" REM-off neurons in other reticular locations also correspond to dispersed adrenergic neuronal groups, although adrenergic identification in this case is much less secure. At this point we note that putatively dopaminergic neurons in substantia nigra and midbrain do not alter their discharge rate or pattern over the sleep–wake cycle (Steinfels *et al.*, 1983) and thus are unlikely to play important roles in sleep–wake cycle control.

11.3.4. REM-off Neurons and REM Sleep Control: Do REM-off Neurons Play a Permissive, Disinhibitory Role?

The intriguing reciprocity of the discharge time course of REM-off and REM-on neurons led to the initial hypothesis of interaction of these two groups, as originally proposed for the REM-off adrenergic neurons (McCarley, 1973; Hobson *et al.*, 1973, 1975; McCarley and Hobson, 1975b). The strongest kind of evidence for this interaction would be demonstration of the proper anatomic connectivity and inhibitory actions of aminergic neurotransmitter on REM effector neurons; although much is known about the connectivity that is in general consistent, we are just beginning to learn about cellular effects of aminergic transmitters in reticular formation and other sites of interest (and effects on pontine cholinergic neurons have not yet been reported), as discussed in Chapter 6. In spite of the absence of these critical data, the phenomenological and behavioral data have been sufficiently strong to lead diverse groups of

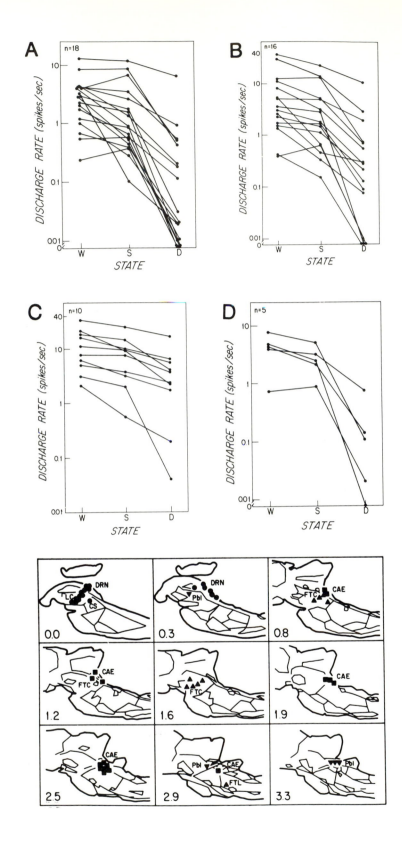

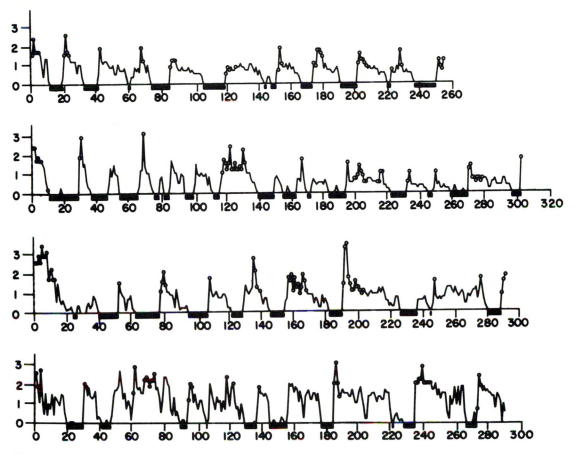

Figure 14. Long-term extracellular recording of dorsal raphe discharge over multiple sleep–wake cycles in the cat. The four sets of discharge profiles, each from the same presumptively serotonergic dorsal raphe neuron recorded on four separate days, show action potentials per second on the ordinate and time in minutes on the abscissa. Unit activity has been grouped into 1-min bins with the open circles representing samples during wakefulness and the dark bars below senting samples during wakefulness and the dark bars below

the abscissa indicating the occurrence of REM-sleep episodes. Note the consistency of the discharge profile, with highest rates in waking and lowest in REM sleep. The tendency of REM sleep to occur rhythmically is evident in these recordings, a tendency that was accentuated by recording in sessions following REM deprivation by forced locomotor activity on a slowly moving treadmill. Modified from Lydic *et al.* (1987a).

Figure 13. Top panel shows mean discharge rate by state of four groups of REM-off neurons extracellularly recorded in the cat in waking (W), synchronized sleep (S), and REM sleep (REM), and the bottom plate their anatomic location on computerized reconstructions of sagittal plates from Berman (1968). Note the near uniformity of the discharge rate profile, W > S > REM. A: The raphe group (bottom panel, circles) includes dorsal raphe, linearis centralis, and centralis superior. B: The locus coeruleus group anatomic localization is represented by the square symbols in the bottom panel. C: The reticular group (bottom panel, upright triangles). D: The peribrachial group (bottom panel, inverted triangles). Note that these three latter REM-off groups form a bandlike zone across the anterodorsal tegmentum. This particular illustrated sample of REM-off neurons, adapted from Hobson *et al.* (1983a), did not include neurons from the pontine and bulbar raphe nuclei.

investigators to propose that the REM-off neurons, as a complete or partial set, act in a permissive, disinhibitory way on some or all of the components of REM sleep. We here summarize these postulates and present the phenomenology on which they are based. Many of these theories arose in the mid 1970s, as increased technical capability led to extracellular recordings of REM-off neurons.

Raphe system REM-off neurons and PGO waves. The possibility that the dorsal raphe serotonergic neurons act to suppress PGO waves was explicitly proposed by Simon *et al.* (1973) on the basis of lesion data and the *in vivo* pharmacological experiments using reserpine, which depleted brainstem serotonin and simultaneously produced nearly continuous PGO-like waves (Brooks *et al.,* 1972). McGinty and Harper (1976), in their study of extracellularly recorded dorsal raphe REM-off neurons, also noted the inverse relationship between PGO waves and dorsal raphe unit activity. With respect to REM sleep onset, the decrease in discharge activity of presumptively serotonergic raphe neurons is remarkably consistent, as shown in Fig. 14. This time course of dorsal raphe unit activity (and other components of the sleep–wake cycle) can be averaged over multiple cycles, a procedure described in Fig. 15, so as to form a picture of the average time course. With this technique, the time course of presumptively serotonergic dorsal raphe neuronal activity over the sleep–wake cycle and its relationship to PGO waves have been described by Lydic *et al.* (1983). Figure 16, derived from this work, shows clearly the inverse relationship between PGO waves and dorsal raphe discharge. Note also the premonitory increase in dorsal raphe activity prior to the end of the REM sleep episode, a phenomenon also observed and commented on by Trulson and Jacobs (1979). Chapter 12 discusses this time course in terms of a model of REM sleep control.

On the basis of *in vivo* pharmacological experiments, Ruch-Monachon and co-workers (1976) hypothesized that serotonergic neurons inhibited PGO waves and also included adrenergic neurons as playing a suppressive role; they further suggested that cholinergic/cholinoceptive systems were actively responsible for their generation. Experiments by Cespuglio and co-workers (1979) utilized local cooling of the dorsal raphe in the unanesthetized "semichronic cat." (This preparation of spinal cord transected at T2 and deafferented above T2 showed spontaneous sleep cycles.) A cryode at +10°C furnished localized cooling without histological evidence of cellular destruction; cooling the dorsal raphe during waking produced, with a latency period of about 1 min, the onset of EEG-synchronized sleep and PGO waves (phenomena of the transition period, T, to REM sleep) in 100% of the trials, followed by full REM sleep in 35% of the trials. This sequence could be repetitively induced after a refractory period of 5 min. Cryocoagulations at the end of the experiment produced a state with cortical desynchronization and continuous PGO waves, much as in previous pure lesion experiments (Jouvet, 1969).* The cooling experiments appear to us to be one of the more convincing "lesion" studies, since the effects were both reversible and repeatable and hence less likely to be nonspecific, and the extent of temperature

---

*A historical note is useful. On the basis of systemic, *in vivo* pharmacological studies and lesion studies, Jouvet originally proposed the theory that serotonin actively promoted synchronized sleep and that norepinephrine actively promoted REM sleep, as summarized in Jouvet (1969). This theory was widely accepted until unit recordings revealed that serotonergic and noradrenergic neurons actually decreased discharge rates in synchronized and REM sleep and thus rendered it untenable.

changes could be estimated within 1–2 mm and were fairly circumscribed. These data are, of course, consistent with a suppressive, inhibitory role for the dorsal raphe nuclei in the production of the PGO waves of REM sleep and perhaps in the entire REM-sleep state.

Locus coeruleus and REM sleep phenomena: Lesion studies. Lesion studies furnish an unclear picture of the role of the LC in REM sleep. *Bilateral* electrolytic lesions of LC in cat by Jones *et al.* (1979) led these workers to conclude that the LC was

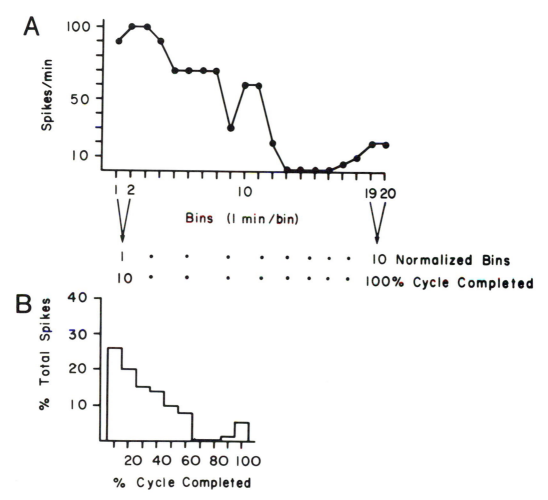

Figure 15. Illustration of the method of time normalization used for averaging neuronal activity over multiple sleep–wake cycles, using dorsal raphe neuronal activity as an example. A: The continuous time course of discharge activity of a single dorsal raphe neuron recorded over a sleep–wake cycle of 20 min duration, with the beginning of the cycle (0 min) and the end of the cycle (20 min) defined by the end of REM sleep. The computer program for time normalization converts the real-time bins into ten time-normalized bins of part B. This example shows a 2 : 1 compression for transformation of 20 real-time bins into ten normalized bins, and the same procedure is followed for other real-time sleep–wake cycle durations; e.g., a 24-min cycle would use a 2.4 : 1 compression. In B, it will be seen that the ten normalized bins are read as percentage of cycle completed and that the actual discharge rate has been converted into the percentage of total dorsal raphe spikes over the entire sleep–wake cycle that are included in each time-normalized bin. The final step is simply averaging each cycle thus time-normalized and discharge-activity-normalized to produce histograms such as seen in the next figure (Fig. 16). Modified from Lydic *et al.* (1983).

not necessary for REM sleep. In the REM-sleep-like state following the lesion there was a twofold reduction of PGO spikes, whereas the number in deep synchronized sleep increased approximately threefold, so that the total number of spikes remained approximately the same—a picture much like that following acute raphe lesions. Over time the total number of PGO spikes declined, and the percentage of REM-sleep-like state increased from about 5% to 10% compared with a control value of 15%. We use the term "REM-sleep-like" because muscle atonia was abolished and there was in fact motor activity like that described in the previous chapter for "REM sleep without atonia" following tegmental lesions; this syndrome likely resulted from spread of the lesion to the reticular area subserving atonia. Other lesion effects included loss of spontaneous micturition and defecation, a rise in mean temperature from 37.1° to 38.3°C, loss of grooming, and a loss of coordination and balance.

The picture following *unilateral* locus coeruleus lesions is quite strikingly different. Caballero and De Andres (1986) found a 50% *increase* in the percentage of REM sleep ($P < 0.001$) following unilateral electrolytic lesions of locus coeruleus in cats; cats with lesions in neighboring tegmentum and sham-operated controls showed no change. The postoperative condition of an animal with unilateral lesions was much better than after bilateral lesions; in only one unilaterally LC-lesioned animal was there urinary retention, and this was transient, and no "alteration in any other vegetative function was observed." Accordingly, Caballero and De Andres attributed the differences between their study and that

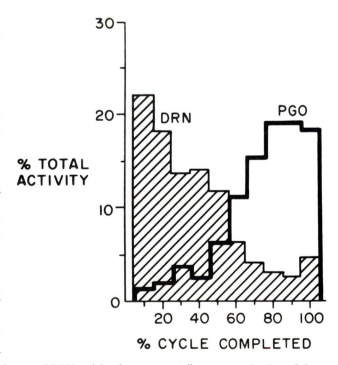

Figure 16. Simultaneously recorded time course of a single presumptively serotonergic dorsal raphe neuron (DRN) and PGO waves averaged over 11 sleep–wake cycles. The time bins on the abscissa represent the percentage (10–100%) of the sleep cycle completed, with the cycle beginning and ending at the end of REM sleep, as described in Fig. 15. The histograms show the percentage of activity in each bin relative to the total number of events; overall 10,021 DRN action potentials and 5,124 PGO waves were recorded. Note the reciprocal time course between discharge activity and PGO waves. Note also that DRN activity is lowest in the portion of the cycle with the maximal probability of REM (80–90% of cycle completed) but that there is an increase in DRN activity prior to the electrographically defined end of REM sleep, suggesting a phase advance of DRN activity that may contribute to termination of the REM-sleep episode. Chapter 12 discusses this possibility in detail. Adapted from Lydic *et al.* (1983).

of Jones *et al.* (1979) to nonspecific effects of the larger lesions that, as with almost any CNS insult, may have led to a REM sleep reduction.

Locus coeruleus cooling induces REM sleep. Cespuglio and co-workers (1982) performed unilateral and bilateral cooling of the locus coeruleus using the same methodology as described above for the dorsal raphe cooling. The effects of cooling were quite clear-cut. Three cats had five trials of bilateral cooling, and in all 15 trials there was progression to synchronized sleep (30–60 sec) and then to the transition phase with PGO waves (2–3 min), and then, in 40–50% of the trials, to full-blown REM sleep (3–4 min after cooling onset). Unilateral cooling produced exactly the same picture in 92% of the trials. In repeated cooing trials REM sleep was repetitively induced, and the percentage of REM sleep increased by 120% over control periods. Figure 17 shows that locus coeruleus cooling to +10°C induced, in sequence, synchronized sleep, then PGO waves (transition period, 2-min latency), and, finally, 2.5 min after the onset of cooling, a full-blown REM-sleep episode. Note that both phasic and tonic components of REM sleep are present: muscle atonia, cortical desynchronization, PGO waves, and rapid eye movements.

We find these cooling experiments particularly instructive both because they produce repeatable effects, implying temporary inactivation and not destruction of neuronal elements, and also because they clearly enhance REM. Nonspecific effects of destructive lesions always decrease REM, as do other CNS insults. Satinoff's comment (1988) about nonspecific effects is that "one might also say that rendering an animal unconscious by a blow to the head eliminated REM sleep. In a sense it does, but that sense is completely trivial." We agree that it is hard to draw definitive and interpretable conclusions about destructive lesions, especially those that do not enhance REM sleep. Jones, for example, concluded that her lesions showed the LC was not necessary for REM sleep in the sense of being a region actively promoting REM, as had been proposed in the early Jouvet theory. Although this interpretation appears reasonable, an important alternative interpretation is not ruled out: namely, that the LC plays a permissive, disinhibitory role but that nonspecific effects of the large lesions prevented the appearance of increased REM sleep, as we have seen did take place with both cooling and unilateral LC lesions that inactivated monoamine neurons. In summary, many nonspecific factors decrease REM, and few, if any, increase it; consequently, lesions or manipulations that increase REM are always more directly interpretable.

Site(s) of interaction of REM-off and REM-on neurons. The model of REM-sleep control presented in the next chapter discusses REM-off suppression of REM-on neurons. It must be emphasized that there are several, non-mutually-exclusive possible sites of interaction. These include direct ACh–NE interactions in the LDT and PPT. For example, there is now available preliminary evidence (M. T. Shipley, personal communication) that ChAT-labeled fibers are present in locus coeruleus, and it has long been known that the NE-containing LC neurons also stain intensely for the presence of acetylcholinesterase. Norepinephrine varicosities are present throughout the reticular formation, the LDT, and the peribrachial area that is the site of ChAT-positive neurons. Recent dopamine beta-hydroxylase (DBH) and ChAT immunohistochemical-labeling studies in the rat by Jones (1989) further indicate the contiguity of LDT and LC

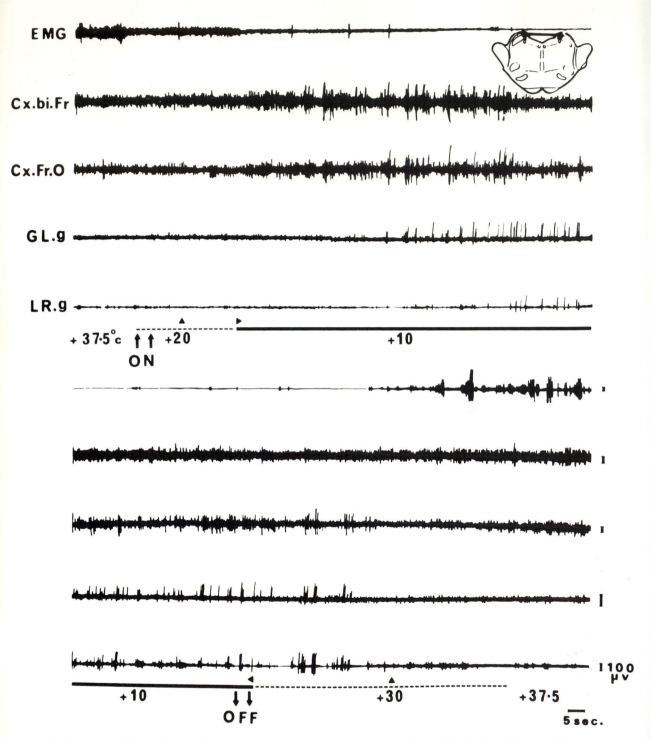

Figure 17. In the cat, bilateral localized cooling of the locus coeruleus induces cortical synchronization, then PGO waves, then both the tonic and phasic components of REM sleep. The frontal section insert is at P3 (Berman, 1968) and shows the position of the tip of the cryode in the LC zone. The dotted and solid lines indicate the time duration of cooling to +20° and then to +10°C; at +10°C, REM sleep is induced and maintained. Abbreviations: EMG, electromyogram of neck muscle; Cx.bi.Fr and Cx.Fr.O, cortical EEG from bifrontal and fronto occipital electrodes, respectively; Gl.g, record of PGO wave activity from the left (*gauche* in French) dorsal lateral geniculate nucleus; LR.g., electromyographic record of the left lateral rectus muscle, indicating the presence of leftward eye movements. From Cespuglio *et al.* (1982).

neurons and the close apposition of their axonal and dendritic processes. These findings clearly indicate the possibility of reciprocal connections between the NE- and ACh-containing neurons, including those between axons and soma/dendrites and between dendrites. Thus, adrenergic–cholinergic interactions may take place directly between these two species of neurons, and/or may take place at reticular neurons. The current evidence bearing on these possibilities is discussed in more detail in the next chapter.

12

REM Sleep as a Biological Rhythm
The Phenomenology and a Structural and Mathematical Model

12.1. Characteristics of the REM Sleep Rhythm

Biological rhythms are processes characterized by recurrence over a particular time period, with the period of recurrence often referred to as τ. The inverse of the period of a rhythm is its frequency, a measure less often used. Circadian rhythms, for example, refer to processes with a period of about a day, and ultradian rhythms are those with periods shorter than a day. REM sleep has a period of about 90 min in the adult human, about 22 min in the cat, and about 12 min in the rat. This feature of alteration of ultradian REM sleep period with body and brain size is not seen in circadian rhythms, which maintain an approximately 24-hr period across all species, regardless of size. This constancy of circadian period likely reflects function: circadian rhythms prepare behavior and physiology for events in the external world that are clocked by the circadian period of the earth's rotation, such as sunrise or sunset. Although the functions of REM sleep remain speculative, adjusting internal events to coincide with timing of external events thus seems excluded as a function. A point relating circadian rhythms and the ultradian REM sleep rhythm is that in many species, including man, the time of occurrence and other parameters of REM sleep are modulated by circadian rhythms, although the occurrence of REM sleep is not dependent on the presence of either a circadian rhythm or an intact circadian oscillator.

12.1.1. Phenomenology of the REM Sleep Rhythm

The long duration of the period of the human REM sleep cycle (90 min) and the consequent paucity of the number of consecutive cycles available for analysis, usually only three or four, and, in addition, its variability of duration makes statistical and experimental analysis of the rhythmicity difficult. Hence, study of many characteristics of REM sleep cycle is easier in animals with a more rapid rhythm and consequently more consecutive cycles available for analysis. We note that the term "REM sleep cycle" or "sleep cycle" refers to the time duration from the end of the one REM sleep period to the end of the next. Figure 1 shows the rhythmicity of REM sleep occurrence in the cat recorded in the laboratory. This figure also shows that REM sleep deprivation, produced by forced activity for 12 hr, has the effect of increasing the regularity of the REM sleep cycle and the percentage of recording time occupied by REM sleep. (Where no citation is given, the data in this section were taken from Lydic *et al.*, 1987a,b).

Examining the effects of this mild REM sleep deprivation is important in allowing us to make statements about the properties of the "REM sleep oscillator," as we refer to the system producing this ultradian rhythm. The following statements summarize the characteristics revealed by REM sleep deprivation:

1. The number of REM sleep episodes is increased by deprivation (Figure 2A,B).
2. The duration of REM-sleep episodes is only slightly, if at all, increased by REM sleep deprivation (Fig. 2C). (The duration of a REM-sleep episode is the time from onset of REM sleep to end of the same REM sleep episode and is to be contrasted with the term "REM sleep cycle" duration, the time from the end of one REM sleep episode to the end of the next.)
3. Without REM sleep deprivation the average time from end of one REM sleep episode to the end of the next is increased; more time is spent in waking and slow-wave sleep, but not in the "transition period," the pre-REM sleep time characterized by the occurrence of PGO waves. The effect of deprivation is summarized in the histograms of REM sleep cycle duration; deprivation produces a regularization of REM sleep cycle lengths to the median duration of about 22 min, whereas without deprivation there are more long REM cycles characterized by long episodes of waking and slow-wave sleep (Fig. 3).

A simple summary of these data is that the REM sleep oscillator has relatively fixed characteristics: REM sleep episode duration is relatively constant, as is the "preferred" or median REM sleep cycle length. We conclude that what varies with REM sleep deprivation is the probability of the REM sleep oscillator being turned on. When the oscillator is not "on," the animal is in waking or light slow-wave sleep (the Lydic *et al.* study did not differentiate light from deep slow-wave sleep, but other studies make it clear that light slow-wave sleep is the phase that is increased when REM sleep cycling is not present). Figure 4 emphasizes this point.

12.1.2. Mathematical Characterization of Oscillators

A mathematical characterization of these phenomena would thus seem to require a REM sleep oscillator with a variable probability of being "on" and with a limit cycle organization. By a limit cycle organization is mean that the oscillator system, once turned on, tends to follow a relatively fixed time course of change no matter what the state of the organism when the oscillator is turned on.

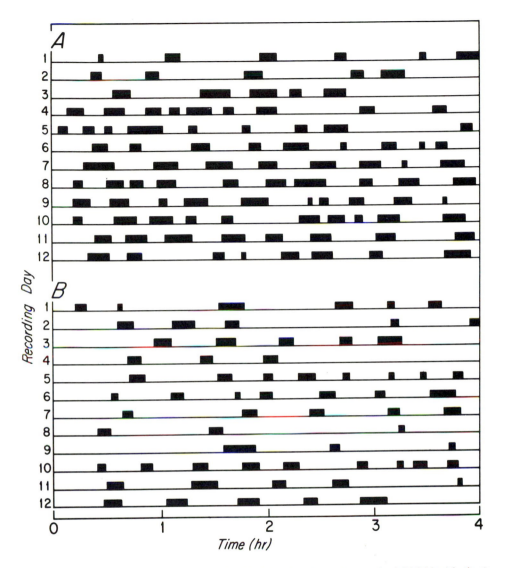

Figure 1. The occurrence of REM-sleep epochs (black bars) in the cat during the initial 4 hr (abscissa) from a randomly selected sample of 12 daily recordings, each of which followed REM-sleep deprivation by means of forced locomotor activity (A) and 12 different days of recordings that were not preceded by forced activity (B). Note the marked reduction in time to onset of the first REM-sleep epoch on each recording day (from zero on the abscissa to the first black bar) and the increased frequency of REM-sleep epochs after REM deprivation during forced activity (contrast number of black bars in A and B). This figure also illustrates the variability of REM sleep episodes, with episode-to-episode variability being less following REM-sleep deprivation by forced activity. [Duration of forced activity on a very slowly moving treadmill was 8 hr for the data in Figs. 1–4. Other studies cited in Lydic *et al.* (1987a) suggest that REM-sleep deprivation was the major cause of the REM-sleep increase; for the present purpose of illustrating how the REM-sleep control system increases the percentage of REM sleep, the possible presence of other major effects on recovery of REM is not important.] Adapted from Lydic *et al.* (1987a).

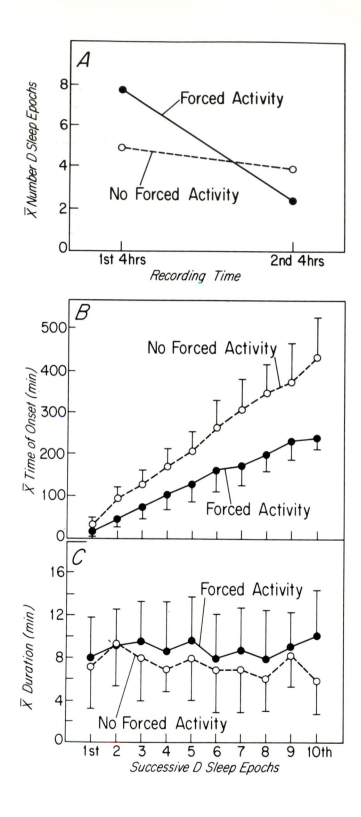

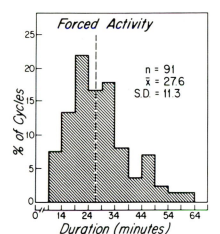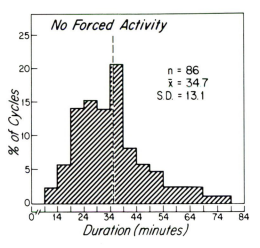

Figure 3. Frequency histograms of sleep-cycle duration in the cat following forced activity (left panel) and no forced activity (right panel). Note that forced activity had the effect of reducing the number of long-duration sleep cycles and increasing the number of shorter-duration cycles, with a stronger tendency to cluster around the modal sleep cycle duration in the cat, 22 min. *n*, number of sleep cycles (sleep cycle = time from end of one REM-sleep episode to the end of the next); $\bar{x}$, mean; S.D., standard deviation. Adapted from Lydic *et al.* (1987a).

In describing the organization of the oscillator, there are two main classes of systems to consider. The first are those depending on timing mechanisms intrinsic to individual cells, often referred to as "pacemakers." There is growing evidence that the suprachiasmatic circadian oscillator system has this kind of structure, although the pacemaker neurons themselves are sensitive to *Zeitgeber* (time-resetting) inputs from outside the suprachiasmatic nucleus and also are linked to, and perhaps modulate, each other. In contrast, there is no positive evidence that any such pacemaker neurons are responsible for the REM sleep cycle. The currently most popular class of models, and, indeed, the only class of models for the generation of the REM sleep cycle, are those depending on the interaction of neuronal populations.

To facilitate understanding of some of these concepts, this chapter first presents models of REM sleep control based on interaction of neuronal populations together with a broad sketch of the relevant neurophysiology, and a later section discusses the neurophysiological, anatomic, and pharmacological postulates of the models and links these to data presented in previous chapters. The final two sections of this chapter present details of the postulates and of construction of the models.

Figure 2. The average number (A), time of onset (B), and duration (C) of 265 REM-sleep episodes recorded following forced and no forced locomotor activity in the cat. Part A shows that forced activity doubled the number of REM-sleep episodes in the first 4 hr of the subsequent recording sessions but that this effect was not seen in the second 4 hr of recording. Part B summarizes the decreased latency to REM-sleep onset that followed forced activity. Frame C shows that forced activity produced no significant increase in the average duration of REM sleep. Thus, forced activity and REM-sleep deprivation act primarily to increase the number of REM-sleep episodes. Adapted from Lydic *et al.* (1987a).

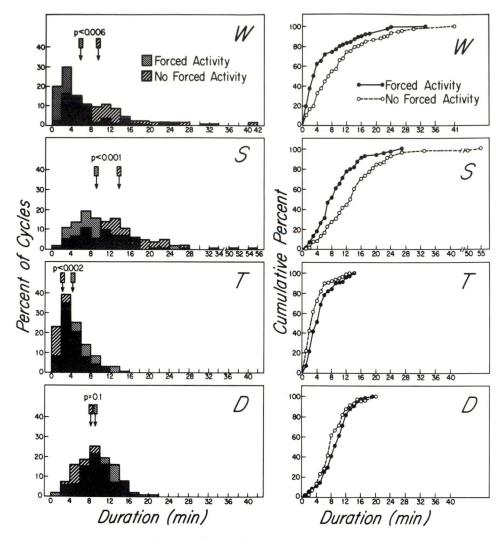

Figure 4. Histograms describing the effect of forced activity on the temporal organization of the four behavioral states comprising the sleep cycle in the cat: wakefulness (W), synchronized (S) sleep, transition (T), and REM sleep (abbreviated D for desynchronized sleep). The left panels are histograms of the durations of the individual states within each sleep cycle, and the right panels present the same data in cumulative histogram form. At a glance the panels show that forced activity decreases W and S ($P < 0.01$) by decreasing the number of long-duration episodes; note also the shift in the means. The transition period (T) duration is reduced slightly but significantly by forced activity. In contrast, REM-sleep duration (abbreviated as D) is not significantly affected. These data thus support the concept of a REM oscillator with a propensity to generate a relatively constant amount of REM sleep per sleep cycle. REM sleep percentage is increased by increasing the number of REM-sleep episodes, but the duration of the episodes is not greatly altered. A simple summary is that, following REM sleep deprivation, the REM oscillator remains "on" more of the time; with less REM sleep pressure, the oscillator is "off," and this is reflected in more waking and non-REM sleep. (Kolmogorov–Smirnow nonparametric statistical tests were used.) Adapted from Lydic *et al.* (1987a).

12.2. The Reciprocal Interaction Model and the Lotka–Volterra Equations

This mathematical model was first proposed in 1975 (McCarley and Hobson, 1975b) and used the simple Lotka–Volterra equations to describe interactions of populations of neurons postulated to be involved in REM sleep cycle production. Although this first model does not have the limit-cycle feature, the basic features of the interaction of neuronal populations and the dynamics are the same as the more recent limit-cycle REM sleep (McCarley and Massequoi, 1986a,b). We think it useful to begin with a verbal illustration of the dynamics of the simple Lotka–Volterra equations, then to present the equations, and to discuss the limit cycle model in the next section. The reader should understand that the limit-cycle model builds on the simple Lotka–Volterra equations and that the dynamics are, in general, the same.

The basic concept is of interaction of two populations of neurons. REM-on neurons (population X in Fig. 5) promote the various events of REM sleep and reciprocally interact with REM-off neurons, which are suppressive to REM sleep events. [We note that Fig 12 and Section 12.4 (below) present details of the composition of the REM-on and REM-off populations, but for this exposition the simpler structural diagram of Fig. 5 is used.)]

The REM-promoting REM-on neurons were originally identified exclusively with the medial pontine reticular formation neurons that became active long before the onset of electrographically defined REM sleep; work since then has made it clear that the neurophysiological situation is more complex and that is likely the cholinergic neurons in the laterodorsal and pedunculopontine tegmental nuclei (LDT and PPT) are critically involved (see Chapters 4, 6, and 11), as well as other reticular neurons in pons and perhaps bulb. We later discuss the current conceptualization of this very active research area but, for the present initial discussion of the dynamics of the model, suggest that the reader regard the REM-on neurons as including reticular core neurons in pons and bulb and also the LDT/PPT neurons.

The set of REM-off neurons likely includes a wide variety of aminergic neurons with the discharge activity profile of decreasing discharge activity pre-

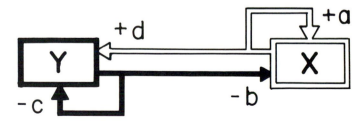

Figure 5. structural model of the X and Y population interconnections postulated by the model, with the connectivity constants corresponding to those in text equations 1 through 4. The X population is REM-promoting, excitatory, and cholinoceptive/cholinergic. The Y population is REM-suppressive, inhibitory, and uses biogenic amines as neurotransmitters. Solid lines and "−" signs indicate inhibitory connections, and open lines and "+" signs indicate excitatory connections. Adapted from McCarley and Massequoi (1986a).

ceding REM and a very low level of activity or even of silence during the REM-sleep episode. Brainstem neurons with this discharge activity profile include those utilizing norepinephrine, epinephrine, and serotonin as neurotransmitters and located in locus coeruleus, dorsal raphe, the peribrachial region, and scattered elsewhere in brainstem. Data on their possible REM-sleep-suppressive role and REM-on neuronal inhibition have been presented in Chapters 6 and 11. We emphasize that potential sites of REM-off inhibitory action on REM-on neurons are currently under intense investigation, with a consequent influx of new data and alterations of interpretations. The data currently available from the slice preparation, however, indicate that adrenergic inhibitory effects on reticular REM-on neurons are less powerful than excitatory effects (Chapter 6), and thus would support an interpretation that the adrenergic inhibitory effects may take place directly on the meso-pontine acetylcholine-containing neurons, a possibility supported by anatomical data cited in the last section of Chapter 11, and consistent with the structural model presented in Fig. 12.

12.2.1. Postulated Steps in Production of a REM Sleep Episode

To aid in intuitive understanding of the model we here summarize in words the model's postulate of steps in production of a REM-sleep episode and the repetition of this REM cycle and later introduce the mathematical equations. We point out the approximate time points of these steps by noting the percentage of cycle completed values on the time averages of neuronal activity shown in Fig. 6. (Zero indicates the beginning of a REM cycle with the end of the previous REM period, and the subsequent figures indicate the percentage of the cycle competed, with REM sleep onset occurring at about 75% of cycle completed.)

1. The slowing and near cessation of firing of REM-off neurons disinhibit the population of REM-on neurons (0–25% of cycle duration).
2. As a result of this disinhibition, the population of REM-on neurons becomes increasingly active, and this activity augments because of the excitatory interconnections in this REM-on population until the REM sleep episode is produced (25–75% of cycle duration).
3. The REM-off population becomes active as a result of excitatory input from the REM-on population (75–100% of cycle duration). When the REM-off population becomes sufficiently active, the REM episode is terminated because of the REM-off neurons' inhibition of the REM-on population.
4. The population of REM-off neurons is postulated to become less active because of inhibitory feedback, and this leads to step 1 and a resumption of the cycle.

The astute reader will also have noticed that the oscillatory system as described continues to oscillate indefinitely. Below we give a more detailed account of the model and describe the turning on and off of the oscillator through interaction with circadian and other systems.

12.2.2. Simple Lotka–Volterra Equations

The situation described verbally in the previous section and in the structural model of Fig. 5 corresponds to the structural model for the most simple of stable two-population oscillatory systems, namely, the Lotka–Volterra equations (Lotka, 1956; Volterra, 1931). These were initially used in population biology to describe the interaction of a predator population (corresponding to the REM-suppressive REM-off neurons) with a prey population (corresponding to the REM-promoting REM-on neurons).

The simple Lotka–Volterra equations are, with X representing REM-on and Y REM-off activity, and the constants corresponding to those in the structural model in Fig. 5:

$$X'(t) = aX - bXY \tag{1}$$

$$Y'(t) = -cY + dXY \tag{2}$$

These simple Lotka–Volterra (LV) equations (equations 1 and 2) yield time courses of activity that mimic the time course of REM-on neuronal discharge and

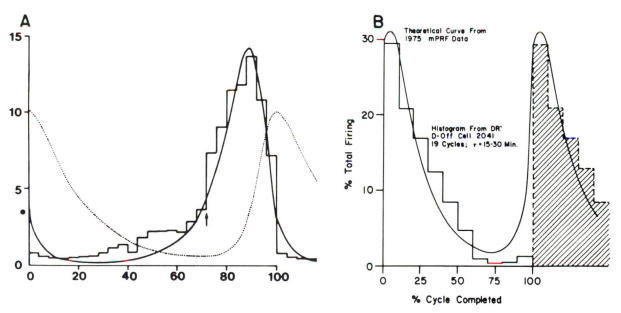

Figure 6. A: Match of the time course of averaged mPRF neuronal activity (data in bins) to time course of activity from model simulation using the simple Lotka–Volterra equations (equations 1 and 2). For model: solid line = X population; broken line = Y population. Ordinate is discharge activity in spikes per second. Point 0 on the graph represents the end of one REM episode (the start of the cycle), and 100 represents the end of the next REM episode (cycle end, 100% complete). The arrow points to the start of the bin with the most probable time of REM-sleep onset. Initial conditions and the values of model constants were set to match the observed modulation during the sleep cycle. Adapted from McCarley and Hobson (1975b). B: Theoretical curve (smooth line) for the Y population derived from data for the X population described in part A compared with averaged neuronal activity data from ten cycles of a dorsal raphe neuron (adapted from Lydic et al., 1983a; τ is sleep-cycle duration). Abscissa as in A. Averages from LC neurons showed approximately the same goodness of fit (McCarley and Hobson, 1975b). We note that the ratio of a to c reflects the fundamental nature of X–Y interaction (see text); this ratio in the new limit-cycle model presented here is approximately the same as that of the 1975 simple Lotka–Volterra model.

also of REM-off discharge, as illustrated in Fig. 6. The data fitting for the cat neuronal data to the simple Lotka–Volterra model was done by setting the strengths of the equations' constants to match the observed time course of rise of REM-on (mPRF) neuronal activity at the approach of REM sleep (see description in McCarley and Hobson, 1975b; see also Hobson *et al.*, 1975, for a discussion of the structural features of the model). We do not describe the "time domain" behavior of the system further but call attention to Fig. 7A, which describes the "phase plane" of the system and will be useful in understanding the differences between the simple LV model and the limit-cycle model. A *phase-plane graph* (refer to Fig. 7A) is constructed by plotting the level of activity of one component

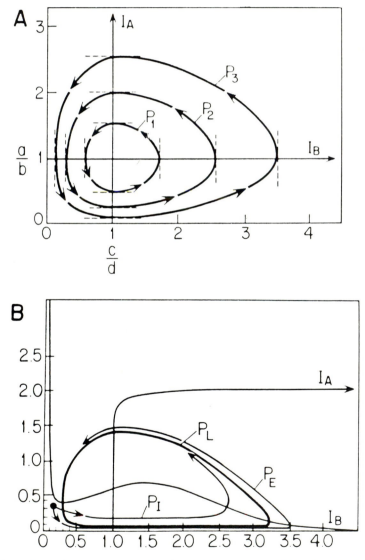

Figure 7. Schematic of phase-plane paths for simple LV system (part A) and for limit-cycle system (part B). See text for discussion. Adapted from McCarley and Massaquoi (1986a).

(*X*, REM-on discharge activity) versus the that of the other (*Y*, REM-off discharge activity) at successive points in time. In particular, the simple Lotka–Volterra solutions appear as families of simple oval orbits (paths) in the phase plane; Fig. 7 provides a schematic illustration of three such paths (P1, P2, P3), which correspond to separate solutions generated by choosing different initial conditions but having the same values for *a, b, c,* and *d*. P3 is most similar to the solution used in the 1975 model; note that it, like any stable oscillation of the *X* and *Y* population, is represented by a single closed orbit that is traversed repeatedly over time in a counterclockwise direction (note direction of arrows). All orbits have zero slope on the isocline, I_A, whereas all orbits have infinite slope on the other isocline, I_B. Section 12.6 provides more details of system behavior in terms of the phase plane.

12.2.3. Limitations of the Simple Lotka–Volterra System

The fundamental difficulty with the simple Lotka–Volterra (LV) equation system was that it displayed only neutral stability. That is, the system's long-term behavior was determined entirely by its initial conditions. This would imply that in order to generate the regular pattern of sleep cycles, the REM sleep oscillator would have to be set into motion each night with a highly reproducible precision alien to physiological systems. Furthermore, a REM sleep oscillator governed by simple LV dynamics would be unreasonably sensitive to any perturbation such as external stimuli so that even a momentary alteration of the components of the oscillator would disturb the period and other properties of REM-sleep system forever (or until specifically reset). These properties are clearly not typical of physiological oscillators; these must be able to maintain stability in the face of continuously changing internal and external influences. An additional complication of the neutral stability condition was the difficulty in modeling circadian influences, which would have necessitated postulating the existence of unreasonable phase-resetting mechanisms.

Central to the LV system's neutral stability problem was that there was no inherent limit on the frequency of neuronal discharge, and even swings to infinite frequency were possible. A reasonable first step in modeling was thus to add factors to the equation that effectively produced realistic physiological constraints on neuronal firing rates. In addition, factors were added that better described neuronal firing characteristics at low discharge rates. These changes led to a model that displayed limit-cycle stability, and the new model will be hereafter described as the limit-cycle model.

12.3. The Limit-Cycle Model

12.3.1. Summary of Changes from the Simple Lotka–Volterra Model

The limit-cycle feature of the new model results from the addition of the following postulates to the simple LV equations. (1) Constraints on maximal neuronal firing rates in both REM-on (X) and REM-off (Y) populations; further, the strength of inhibition of the REM-off population on the REM-on population is limited when the REM-on population activity is at low levels. (2) The term for growth rate of the mPRF population resulting from excitatory feedback is now a function of X level and is less for lower values of X, whereas it was constant in the simple LV model.

The other major category of change in the model is the addition of circadian modulation, a point not addressed in the original model. This feature is primarily of use for modeling human REM sleep (and that in other animals with a strong circadian REM sleep modulation); it is not utilized in the feline version because cat circadian modulation is weak, especially that observed in the usual laboratory recoding session. (Circadian REM sleep modulation in cats is relatively minimal and consists of a tendency to have more REM sleep at dawn and dusk, a "crepuscular" circadian REM sleep organization.) In the limit-cycle model for man all circadian sleep fluctuation is modeled by (1) circadian variation in the way the system begins oscillation, modeled by variation in the strength of excitatory influences on the REM-off (Y) population at sleep onset and consequent alteration of the time course of decline of this population at sleep onset—this "start-up" variation accounts for most of the observed circadian changes in REM sleep percentage—and (2) a small continuous circadian modulation (accounting for about ± 5% variation in REM parameters) that results from changing the constant d in the simple LV equations to a sinusoidally modulated circadian variable, d(circadian time phase) = d(circ). The rationale for each of these changes is discussed in detail in Section 12.7 of this chapter. The equations for the limit-cycle model, which incorporate these changes, are:

$$X'(t) = a(X)*X*S_1(X) - b(X)*X*Y \tag{3}$$

$$Y'(t) = -c*Y + d(\text{circ})*X*Y*S_2(Y) \tag{4}$$

where * is multiplication, X is REM-off neuronal activity, Y is REM-off neuronal activity, S_1 and S_2 are saturation functions constraining X and Y, a(X) is the X growth rate, smaller with smaller X, b(X) is the limitation on inhibitability of X by Y for low X values, and d(circ) = d(circadian time) is the circadian variation in amplitude of d. The graphs and discussion of the construction of S_1, S_2, a(X), b(X), and d(circ) are presented in Section 12.7 of this chapter.

12.3.2. Modeling Events at Sleep Onset, Human Sleep Patterns, and Circadian Variation

12.3.2.1. Events at the Onset of Sleep

Neuronal recordings in cats indicate that during waking the activity of the REM-off population is generally elevated ($1 \leq Y \leq 2$, cf. Fig. 3), and intracellular recordings indicate that population activity and excitability of the REM-on (X) population is low, with X typically <0.2, although, as discussed below, subsets of REM-on neurons may be phasically active during waking. Thus, in the phase-plane graph (Fig. 7B graphs the phase plane), the system points (X–Y values) cluster in the upper left-hand corner during waking (high Y values, low X values). At sleep onset there is falling Y activity and rising X activity, and thus the graph shows a downward and rightward drift and eventually begins to orbit. For the feline model without circadian variation, this time course of decline is postulated to be relatively constant, with the probability of the system being allowed to oscillate being, in part, a function of whether REM sleep deprivation had occurred previously. In a limit-cycle system all orbits, by definition, eventually converge to the limit cycle, and the graph of later cycles is insensitive to the details of the trajectory of the initial transition into sleep, providing the necessary stability in the feline cycle.

12.3.2.2. Modeling Human Sleep Patterns

However, the shape of the first cycle is critically dependent on the precise trajectory taken at sleep onset, and it is this variation that is important for modeling the human sleep pattern. Although no specific physiological mechanism has yet been clearly identified as maintaining the system in the upper left portion of the phase plane in waking, we suggest a simple, plausible explanation: that tonic excitatory input to REM-off neurons maintains the system at high Y values during waking and that one important component of the strength of this input may be circadian influences arising from hypothalamus. Computer simulations show that such an input suppresses oscillations by keeping Y high and thus X activity low. In the limit-cycle model applied to adult human sleep, the circadian waxing and waning of this input is an important factor turning the REM sleep oscillator on and off. We add that we do not wish to suggest that other physiological mechanisms having the equivalent mathematical effect are ruled out but only that this currently appears the most plausible postulate.

In summary, for the human sleep model, the difference in the time course of decline of Y (as controlled by excitation withdrawal) at sleep onset determines whether the limit cycle is entered from the interior (slow time course of decline) or from the exterior (rapid time course of decline), and thus this parameter is by far the most critical one for determining changes in REM sleep values, since it is the first REM cycle that varies the most in human sleep.

12.3.2.3. Circadian Variation in the REM Cycle

The experimentally observed circadian phase sensitivity of the initial sleep-cycle parameters (cycle period duration, REM intensity, REM latency, and REM duration) are simply modeled by varying the time course of withdrawal of excitatory influence on the Y population with circadian phase: withdrawal is more rapid near a temperature minimum and slower at a temperature maximum.

Figure 7B graphically illustrates the concept of the limit cycle and external and internal entry points. The limit cycle model solutions are families of spirals that all converge to a common, unique final oval, termed the limit cycle (P_L in the figure). This same limit cycle is approached regardless of whether the initial approach is exterior (P_E) or interior (P_I). The critical feature of this human sleep model is that an interior approach (P_I) results from a slow decline in Y and occurs near a temperature maximum (a measure of the activity of the "deep" circadian oscillator); this results in a quick-onset, short-duration, low-amplitude first REM sleep period. An exterior approach (P_E) results, in contrast, from a rapid decline in Y and occurs near a temperature minimum: this results in a slow-onset, long-duration, high-amplitude first REM sleep period. Section 12.7 describes other details of the system including the altered shape of the isoclines, I_A and I_B. Whether the approach is exterior or interior to the limit cycle depends entirely on the starting conditions and not on any alteration of a property of the oscillator.

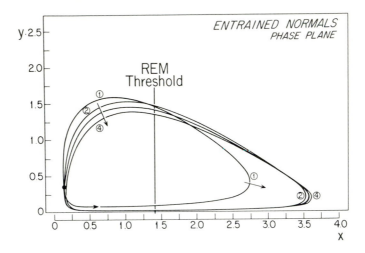

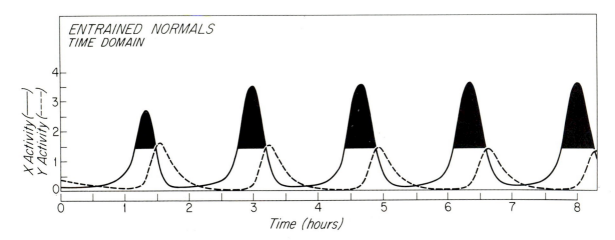

Figure 8. Model simulation of night's course of REM sleep in entrained normal humans. The top part is the phase-plane, and the bottom part the time-domain representation of this data. At bottom the solid portions of the X graph show those portions of the night with REM sleep, and the height of these peaks indicates the intensity of the REM-sleep episode. Note the short-duration, lesser-intensity first REM episode with subsequent variations being slight. The activity of the Y (REM inhibitory) population is indicated by the dotted line. In the phase-plane representation at top, each point on the graph represents the X–Y values at a particular time. The dot represents the starting point, and the interior curve 1 with the arrow shows the first REM-sleep episode values, with this curve being interior to the limit-cycle values obtained in subsequent REM cycles, labeled 2, 3, 4 in the order of their occurrence (for simplicity, sleep cycle 5 has not been graphed in the phase plane). The smaller variations in sleep cycles 2 through 4 result from circadian modulation. Adapted from McCarley and Massequoi (1986a).

In this model, when sleep is begun at the usual point on the circadian temperature cycle, soon after the occurrence of a temperature maximum, the activity trajectories illustrated in Fig. 8 for the phase plane and time domain are produced. This starting point produces an interior entry into the limit cycle and a long-latency, short-duration first REM sleep period. In contrast, when sleep is begun near a temperature minimum, there is an exterior entry into the limit cycle and a short-latency, long-duration first REM sleep period (Fig. 9).

The fit between the model and data from actual human sleep is good, both for percentage of REM sleep in thirds of the night in entrained normals (Fig. 10) and for a match between duration of successive REM sleep episodes in free-run

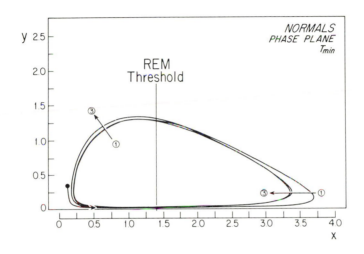

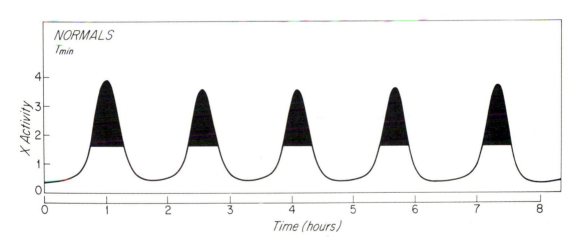

Figure 9. Phase-plane (top) and time-domain (bottom) representation of model results for sleep begun near a temperature minimum (circadian phase = 4.72 radians, 270°). Note that, in contrast to Fig. 8, the phase-plane graph shows an entry into the limit cycle from a point *exterior* to the cycle; arrows indicate the direction of change of successive phase-plane trajectories for cycles 1, 2, and 3. As can be seen, this is associated with a shorter-latency, longer-duration, and higher-intensity first REM episode than does the interior entry that occurs near a temperature maximum (cf. phase plane of Fig. 8). Adapted from McCarley and Massequoi (1986a).

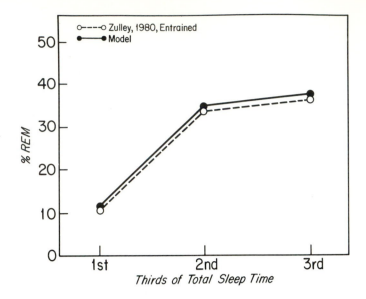

Figure 10. Empirical data (Zulley, 1979, 1980) and model indicate a low REM percentage in first third of the night and a tendency for the last third of the night to show more REM than the middle portion. Note the near-exact fit of model and data. Adapted from McCarley and Massequoi (1986a).

normal subjects when sleep is begun at a temperature minimum (Fig. 11, top) or at a temperature maximum (Fig. 11, bottom).

It perhaps does not need to be emphasized that much additional work will be needed before this model can be said to be solidly grounded on empirical data. Our reading is, however, that the currently available behavioral, pharmacological, and cellular neurophysiological data indicate the utility of such a model in terms of aiding conceptualization and for suggesting experiments. For example, the concept of interacting REM-on and REM-off populations has been used by Sakai (1985a,b; and see discussion below) and also has been useful in modeling REM sleep alterations in depression (see Chapter 13).

12.4. REM-on Neurons and Cholinergic Neurons

We next discuss several points relevant to the conceptualization of REM-on neurons, namely, LDT/PPT neurons and their input to reticular formation. As discussed in Chapter 4, advances in immunohistochemistry have made it clear that the principal sources of cholinergic neurons in brainstem are LDT and PPT and that, although pontine reticular neurons are likely cholinoceptive, few are cholinergic. Thus, the major locus of cholinergic REM-on neurons postulated by the 1975 model has been shifted to the LDT/PPT. Figure 12 illustrates our current conceptualization of the structural composition of the REM-on and REM-off neuronal populations. It will be noted that this figure includes both LDT/PPT and reticular neurons in the category of "REM-on" neurons. As is made clear below, the exact role and interrelationship of these two groups of neurons in REM are matters of current intense investigation.

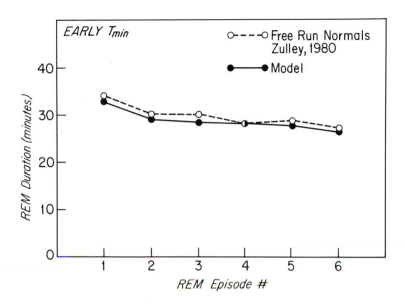

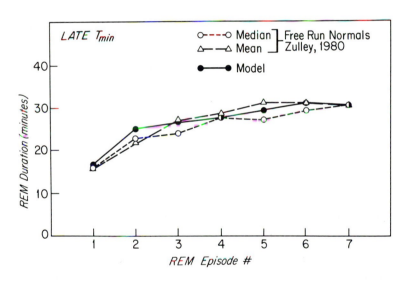

Figure 11. Top: Match of model and Zulley's data (median, open circle) for REM duration in sleep begun at temperature minimum (circadian phase = 4.72 radians) in free-run normals. Note excellent fit in general and, in particular, that the first-to-second REM-episode change is the largest, and the subsequent gradual duration decrease in both model and data REM duration. Bottom: Match of model and Zulley's data (median, circle; mean, triangle; both included because of variation in this data set) for REM duration in sleep begun near temperature maximum in free-run normals (Zulley labels these data as "late temperature minimum"). Note close approximation of model prediction; in particular, the first-to-second REM-episode increase is the largest, and there is a subsequent gradual duration increase in both model and data. Adapted from McCarley and Massequoi (1986a).

12.4.1. Reticular REM-on Neurons

As noted in the preceding chapter, from the perspective of *in vivo* intracellular recording the principal phenomenon related to the REM sleep episode is the membrane potential (MP) depolarization of virtually all members of the "medial pontine reticular pool" (Ito and McCarley, 1984; McCarley and Ito, 1985); this depolarization may also include members of the bulbar reticular formation pool (Chase *et al.*, 1981). The MP depolarization begins in many PRF neurons even before the onset of PGO waves (which occurs prior to REM sleep onset) and progresses to the 7–10 mV MP depolarization seen in REM sleep relative to slow-wave sleep. This MP depolarization is present throughout the REM sleep episode and, in the neurons thus far recorded, is followed by a repolarization on transition to the state of waking (W). During W there may be MP depolarization of specific sets of neurons in association with specific waking events—for example, eye or somatic movements—but the reticular population as a whole does not have a depolarized MP throughout W, in contrast to the situation during REM sleep. We have suggested that this reticular neuronal population MP depolarization during REM sleep (and consequent action potential production) is responsible for activation of the neuronal machinery contained within the PRF and for causing the events of REM sleep, including the rapid eye movements, the pontine component of PGO waves, the muscle twitches, and, for the dorsolateral PRF (peri-LCα), the muscle atonia. Viewed in this manner the question then becomes what processes act to produce this MP depolarization, and current data suggest that cholinergic influences on PRF may be important. Chapters 4 and 11 document the presence of reticuloreticular excitatory synapses, which may be important in the spread of this REM-sleep-associated activation.

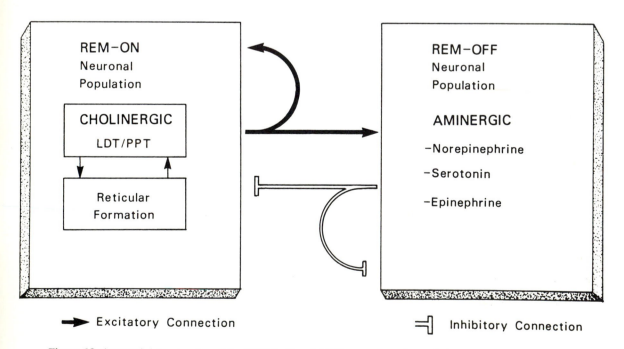

Figure 12. Anatomic/structural model of REM-off and REM-on neuronal populations and their interaction.

Figure 12 shows that we conceptualize the REM-on set of neurons as having an internal structure of excitatory interconnections between LDT/PPT and reticular formation neurons. These LDT/PPT projections to PRF, and the excitatory effects of cholinergic agonists have of course been described in Chapters 4 and 6. Figure 12 also indicates the presence of excitatory reticular projections to LDT/PPT. There is anatomic evidence for these projections (Chapter 3, Fig. 5; Paré and Steriade, 1989; S. Higo and R. McCarley, unpublished data), though it is not yet known if they are excitatory.

There appear to be two principal possible modes of action of LDT/PPT neurons on reticular neurons involving the production of a REM-sleep episode.

1. *Trigger.* If the pre-REM time of onset of LDT/PPT neuronal discharge is early enough, then they might act to "trigger" the population membrane depolarization and increased action potential discharge observable in PRF neurons prior to REM sleep. This possibility is indicated in Fig. 12 by the excitatory projection to PRF.
2. *Latch.* Even if LDT/PPT neuronal discharge begins at the same time or later than PRF neuronal discharge, the cholinergic excitatory input to PRF may act to enhance the membrane depolarization of PRF neurons. Further, as indicated in Fig. 12, it is possible that members of the LDT/PPT and reticular populations may form a mutually augmenting network during REM sleep, as indicated by the mutually excitatory projections between the two groups of neurons. We have termed this mode of interaction a "latch," since the activation of reticular neurons would be augmented and then "latched" at a high level by the interaction with LDT/PPT neurons. Note that the trigger and latch modes are not mutually exclusive.

We emphasize at the outset that we think it likely that the discharge activity of LDT/PPT neurons may not be homogeneous, that there may be several different types of cholinergic neuronal discharge patterns. Much empirical work clearly remains to be done in this area. As reviewed in Chapter 9, the present evidence is clearest for a role in PGO wave production. Studies in several laboratories have now clearly found the presence of "PGO burst neurons" in and around the brachium conjunctivum that discharge in a stereotyped way just prior to a large PGO wave in the ipsilateral LGN. These PGO burst neurons have been demonstrated to project to thalamus and are localized to "in and around the brachium conjunctivum," i.e., the zone of the PPT cholinergic neurons. Steriade *et al.* (1989a) have recorded antidromically identified LDT neurons with thalamic projections that also discharge in bursts prior to PGO waves. Chapter 9 has presented evidence that PGO waves in the dorsal part of LG nucleus are blocked by nicotinic antagonists. Thus, there is circumstantial evidence that the "PGO burst neurons" may be cholinergic neurons.* These PGO

---

*We must caution, unfortunately, that there have been no physiological recordings during sleep of identified Ch5–6 cholinergic neurons; for certainty of identification there must be a marker stain of the recorded neuron combined with a ChAT stain for double labeling. Although the reader may think the technical virtuosity demanded may render this a moot point, we believe that rapid advancement of techniques will make such double labeling commonplace.

burst neurons might, through projections to PRF as well as to thalamus, act to increase the excitability of PRF neurons. However, several factors suggest that PRF excitation from PGO burst neurons alone would not explain most of the observed PRF excitation in REM sleep. First, PRF neurons discharging in association with PGO waves (McCarley and Ito, 1983) do so with 30–300 msec lead times, much longer than the 12–15 msec of the PGO burst neurons, and thus the burst neurons could not cause the preceding activation*; secondly, the membrane potential depolarization of PRF neurons is present throughout the REM sleep period and not just during the periods where PGO waves occur.

From recordings of neurons in PPT we know that non-PGO burst neurons are also found in the area, and these increase discharge rate in anticipation of and during REM sleep (Datta *et al.*, 1989; R. McCarley, unpublished data). The data in Fig. 4 of Chapter 11 suggest an early REM-anticipatory discharge rate increase for thalamically projecting PPT neurons, but the precise timing of the onset of REM-anticipatory discharge and the waking discharge rate properties of the LDT/PPT neurons with brainstem reticular projections have not been determined. This systematic characterization is an important current task.

Evidence supporting a role of the Ch5–6 neuronal zone in production of REM sleep phenomena has recently been obtained by bilateral kainic acid lesions of this zone producing a mean reduction of 59% in the number of ChAT-positive neurons (Jones and Webster, 1988; Webster and Jones, 1988). These lesions markedly diminished LG PGO wave spike rate, which was reduced on 28 days postlesion recordings by at least 40% in all cats but one, and with a mean reduction of 73% in PGO spike rate during REM sleep. Furthermore, the overall percentage of REM sleep declined from a control mean value of 13% to 8.5% 28 days postlesion, a 35% reduction. REM sleep muscle atonia and the rapid eye movements were also reduced. Some cholinergic specificity was suggested by the fact that postlesion REM percentage and PGO spike rate correlations were highest with the number of ChAT-positive neurons destroyed; Pearson's $r = 0.69$ and -0.66, respectively, accounting for 48% and 44% of the variance. These figures were higher than the correlations with the total volume of the lesion ($r = -0.53$ and -0.32) or with the number of tyrosine-hydroxylase-positive neurons destroyed ($r = -0.18$ and -0.27). This study thus provides important suggestive evidence for a role of this region in REM sleep, and especially the role of cholinergic neurons in LG PGO wave production. Such histochemically nonspecific lesions, however, cannot offer final proof as to whether these effects are mediated through ChAT-positive or nearby non-ChAT-positive neurons. Cellular physiological studies utilizing double-labeling techniques, as described above, will likely be required for definitive conclusions.†

---

*PGO-on neurons with tonic discharges and a phasic increase in discharge rate that precedes the thalamic PGO wave by at least 150–300 msec have recently been recorded from PPT/LDT (Steriade *et al.*, 1989a; see Fig. 4 of Chapter 9). This tonic discharge pattern with a phasic increase is unlike the purely phasic pattern of the medial PRF long-lead PGO-on neurons (see Fig. 3 of Chapter 9). Recent anatomic work does indicate a projection from the zone where the PRF PGO-on neurons are recorded to the PPT (S. Higo and R. McCarley, unpublished data).

†With respect to cholinergic effects on the sleep–wake cycle, the findings in animals with heightened cholinergic activity are of interest. In rats with chronic CNS administration of scopolamine there is an increase in the number of REM-sleep bouts without marked changes in the duration of REM-sleep episodes (Shiromani and Fishbein, 1986). In a strain of rats with increased number of CNS muscarinic receptors and hypersensitivity to cholinergic agonists (Flinders sensitive line; see Over-

The set of REM-off neurons likely includes a wide variety of aminergic neurons with the discharge activity profile of decreasing discharge activity preceding REM and a very low level of activity or even of silence during the REM sleep episode. As illustrated in Fig. 12, brainstem neurons with this discharge activity profile include those utilizing norepinephrine, epinephrine, and serotonin as neurotransmitters and located in locus coeruleus, dorsal raphe, and peribrachial region, and scattered elsewhere in brainstem.* Data described in Chapter 11 have outlined the time course of discharge activity of these neurons and evidence bearing on their suppressive role in REM-sleep-related activity. The first reciprocal interaction model (McCarley and Hobson, 1975b) suggested that their inhibitory action might occur on reticular REM-on neurons. It is likely, however, that the neurophysiological situation is more complex, and that in view of the excitatory α_1 effects of NE seen on 80% of mPRF neurons that inhibitory interactions with REM on neurons should be postulated to take place directly on meso-pontine cholinergic neurons. The situation is complex, however, since, in addition to direct effects, bath-applied NE in the slice preparation also produces a barrage of synaptically mediated inhibitory PSPs, presumably from effects on glycinergic reticular neurons (see Greene *et al.*, 1989b), and this inhibitory effect, should it also occur *in vivo*, may also be important for modulation of excitability of reticular neurons in the sleep–wake cycle. Serotonin has been shown to have inhibitory effects on about half of the population of mPRF neurons (Stevens *et al.*, 1989), but the presence of excitatory effects in about an equal percentage mPRF neurons suggests that future specification of the kind of reticular neuron excited or inhibited may be an important feature for modeling.

Given the current state of rapid development of knowledge in this area, we have chosen in the sketch of the structural model in Fig. 12 to be schematic and leave open several possibilities of REM-off action on REM-on neurons. The inhibitory action of REM-off neurons on REM-on neurons may occur directly on cholinergic neurons and/or on reticular neurons. We note also that the close

---

street, 1986), Shiromani and co-workers (1988b) have also found the number of REM-sleep episodes increased without a marked change in the duration. Unfortunately from the standpoint of a test of the model, it is not known at present whether there are changes in the REM-sleep cycle duration or whether the increased number of REM sleep episodes simply represents the REM-sleep oscillator being turned "on" a higher percentage of the time. The model predicts that with an increase in model parameter *a* (i.e., increased intensity of cholinergic feedback on the REM-on population), the cycle duration should shorten. In the case of this pure alteration of *a*, the data should show, in the REM-cycle histograms, a shortened modal value during the times when the oscillator is "on," operationally defined by the times when the animal is sleeping soundly, i.e., with little or no waking, the kind of sleep present in the cat post-deprivation (Fig. 1). Unfortunately, for a simple test of the model, cholinergic alterations may also affect other interactions, such as the REM-on neurons' effect on the REM-off neurons, whose coupling strength is indicated by the *d* term in the equations. Nonetheless, our "best guess" as to the main effect of increased muscarinic sensitivity would be a shortening of the REM-sleep cycle. Other aspects of the REM-sleep cycle that might be affected are discussed in McCarley and Massaquoi (1986a,b).

*It is possible that histaminergic neurons in hypothalamus may play an analogous role, since discharge rates are maximal in waking and are greatly reduced in REM (Vanni-Mercier *et al.*, 1984); they are not included in the Fig. 12 model, since brainstem transection experiments indicate they are not necessary for REM oscillations.

anatomical apposition of GABAergic neurons with NE and cholinergic neurons (Jones, 1989) also suggests a possible role in REM-off and REM-on neuronal interaction for GABAergic neurons. With respect to the model presented here, it should be noted that in its present form the model's predictions about the REM sleep cycle are not dependent on these features of structural connectivity. The model as formulated postulates REM-off inhibition of REM-on neurons and will work just as well for connections on meso-pontine cholinergic neurons as for connections on reticular neurons, and even if an interposed GABAergic neuron provides inhibition.

In fact, as discussed in Greene and McCarley (1989), there are plausible arguments that can be marshaled for the reasonableness of cholinergic–adrenergic interaction at LC neurons in terms of the known time course of LC neuronal activity, i.e., the near silence in REM sleep and the rapid increase of activity at the end of the REM sleep period and wakefulness onset. We here briefly sketch this argument. The kinetics of the effects of cholinergic input, known to be excitatory to LC neurons (see Chapter 6), can be surmised from the known intrinsic and neurotransmitter-dependent LC currents as quantitatively described by Williams $et\ al.$ (1988a). It may be inferred that, at the hyperpolarized LC membrane potential early in the REM sleep period, acetylcholine might have relatively little depolarizing effect due to the relatively high inward rectifier conductance (G_{ir}). Williams and co-workers have described the voltage sensitivity of the G_{ir} as a sigmoid function, whose midpoint is about 90 mV. The formula for G_{ir} and further details are given in the legend for Fig. 17 of Chapter 6; for the present section the essential point is that cholinergic input will have a lesser excitatory effect at hyperpolarized membrane potentials because of the inward rectification, as has been quantitatively shown by Greene and McCarley (1989).

Still another voltage-sensitive factor influencing LC neuronal firing rates is the activation of a potassium conductance by norepinephrine α_2 receptors (G_{ne}) elicited by recurrent noradrenergic synaptic activity (Egan $et\ al.$, 1983). As was the case for G_{ir}, the voltage sensitivity of G_{ne} is described by a sigmoid function with an approximate midpoint of -50 mV (Williams $et\ al.$, 1988a; the formula for this function is given in the legend of Fig. 17, Chapter 6, where $G_{ne} = G_{ag}$). The maximal norepinephrine conductance ($maxG_{ne}$) is considerably less than $maxG_{ir}$; however, within the voltage range of -80 to -40 mV a greater fraction of G_{ne} is activated. If a $maxG_{ir}$ of 13 nS and a $maxG_{ne}$ of 1 nS is assumed (Williams $et\ al.$, 1988a), the combined conductances plotted relative to the membrane potential (see Greene and McCarley, 1989, Fig. 7B) indicate the effect a depolarizing current might exert. At a critical threshold of cholinergic input the hyperpolarizing effect of the G_{ir} and G_{ne} would be overcome. The depolarizing cholinergic effect may then be regeneratively magnified due to the voltage-sensitive deactivation of the hyperpolarizing G_{ir} and G_{ne}. A slowly increasing level of cholinergic activity would have little effect on the LC neurons until this threshold was reached. Then the LC membrane would be quickly driven to a depolarized level, with the abrupt reappearance of action potentials, as does indeed occur at the end of a REM sleep period. While this sequence of events is speculative, the availability of a quantitative model of voltage-sensitive intrinsic currents (Williams $et\ al.$, 1988a) means that the predictions could be tested with applications of acetylcholine at different membrane potentials of LC neurons.

We thus suggest the current rapid expansion of data about connectivity and neurotransmitter effects is promising for development of a future model that will be able to be more precise about the cellular basis of neuronal interactions important for control of the REM sleep cycle.

12.6. Details of Simple Lotka–Volterra Model

This section provides a more detailed account of the concepts and mathematics than in the earlier overview.

12.6.1. Significance of the Terms in the Equations

This initial formulation of the sleep cycle control model employed a simple system of first-order nonlinear differential equations known as the Lotka–Volterra system after the two mathematical biologists who first used it to model the interaction of predator and prey species. As REM-on neurons excite themselves via recurrent collaterals, they behave mathematically as an autonomous, self-replicating prey population. REM-off neurons, conversely, inhibit the growth in activity of REM-on neurons while their own activity dies off in the absence of REM-on input. Thus, they behave as a predatory population. The Lotka–Volterra system is:

$$X'(t) = aX - bXY$$

$$Y'(t) = -cY + dXY$$

where X represents the aggregate firing rate of REM-on neurons, and Y represents the aggregate firing rate of REM-off neurons.

The reciprocal interaction between the two populations is characterized by the LV system. The different terms in the system represent the contribution of each type of synapse in the model (Figs. 5 and 12) to overall system behavior.

The first term represents REM-on neurons' response to self-excitation, $X'(t) = aX$, which alone would yield unbridled exponential growth,

$$X(t) = e^{+at}$$

with growth constant a.

The second term represents REM-on neurons' response to REM-off neurons' inhibition, $Y'(t) = -(bY)X$, which alone would yield exponential decay of X activity with a rate dependent on Y activity and b:

$$X(t) = e^{-(bY)t}$$

The third terms represents REM-off neuronal response to self inhibition, $Y'(t) = -cY$, which alone would yield an exponential decay in Y activity with decay constant c:

$$Y(t) = e^{-ct}$$

The fourth term represents REM-off response to REM-on excitation, $Y'(t)$ $= (dX)Y$, which alone would yield exponential growth of REM-off activity with a growth rate dX:

$$Y(t) = e^{+(dX)t}$$

12.6.2. Phase-Plane Representation

In the phase-plane representation, any stable oscillation of X and Y populations is represented graphically as a single closed orbit that is traversed repeatedly over time in a counterclockwise direction. In particular, the simple Lotka–Volterra solutions appear as families of simple oval orbits (paths) in the phase plane; Fig. 7A provides a schematic illustration of three such paths (P_1, P_2, P_3), which correspond to separate solutions generated by choosing different initial conditions but have the same values for a, b, c, and d. P_3 is most similar to the solution used in the 1975 model.

Line I_A in Fig. 7A represents the vertically oriented isocline, the set of loci where all paths must have zero slope (hashed lines). Line I_B is the horizontally oriented isocline where all crossing paths have infinite slope. The isocline equations are: I_A, $X = c/d$; I_B, $Y = a/b$; where a, b, c, and d are the LV parameters of equations 1 and 2. Since in this figure a = b = 2c = 2d, the isoclines are located at $X = 1$ and $Y = 1$. The values c/d and a/b are termed the X and Y equilibrium values because they represent the average X and Y values over time and represent the coordinates for the system center, where no oscillation occurs.

Figure 7B and the limit-cycle system are discussed in detail below. For here we note that the limit-cycle model solutions are families of spirals that all converge to a common, unique final oval, termed the limit cycle (P_L in the figure). This same limit cycle is approached regardless of whether the initial approach is exterior (P_E) or interior (P_I); the presence of such a limiting oval graphically demonstrates the stability of the oscillatory system. Whether the approach is exterior or interior to the limit cycle depends entirely on the starting conditions and not on any alteration of a property of the oscillator.

12.7. Details of Limit-Cycle Model

This section discusses the mathematical form and the rationale for the changes in the simple LV system that lead to the limit-cycle model. We discuss the changes in approximate order of occurrence in the equations. For convenience of reference we here repeat the limit cycle model equations:

$$X'(t) = a(X)*X*S_1(X) - b(X)*X*Y \tag{3}$$

$$Y'(t) = -c*Y + d(\text{circ})*X*Y*S_2(Y) \tag{4}$$

a(X), the REM-on autoexcitation growth function, has *X* dependence and replaces the constant *a* in the simple LV system. This term makes effectiveness of REM-on-to-REM-on neuron positive feedback a function of REM-on activity level. In the limit-cycle model the term for the *X* population feedback is changed from the constant *a* in the simple LV equations into a function dependent on *X*, with a smaller growth rate at lower values of *X*. This is physiologically analogous to an assumption of a "kindling effect," since as the mean activity level grows so does the growth term, *a* (autoexcitability), with near-maximal levels of *a(X)* being reached at the threshold for REM onset (see graph in Fig. 13). Mathematically, making *a* a function of *X* in this manner destabilizes the system in the center region. In the phase-plane representation, it accounts for the system's spiraling outward toward the limit cycle when initiated in the region interior to the limit cycle (Fig. 7B, P_I).

The term *a(X)* has the form $a_{max}L(X)$, where L(*X*) is a logistic (sigmoid) function that slopes upward from 0 to 1 with peak slope occurring at $X = 0.5$ (marked by circle 1 on graph in Fig. 13) (the equation of the logistic function is given in Section 12.7.3). a_{max} is taken to be 2 such that for large *X*, $a = a_{max} = 2$, the same value used in the earlier non-limit-cycle model. Note that at REM threshold (circle 2) *a(X)* is nearly at its maximum.

This central destabilization can be heuristically understood as follows: As REM-on activity becomes suppressed by REM-off neurons, it declines to low

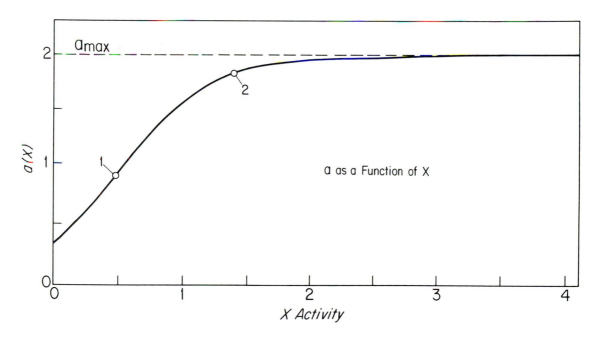

Figure 13. Shape of logistic curve describing the alteration in *a* with changes in the level of activity of the *X* population. See text for further description. Adapted from McCarley and Massequoi (1986a).

levels where it remains for a period slightly longer than that of the standard LV equations. This further removes excitation from REM-off and allows REM-off firing intensity to diminish to lower levels. This, in turn, facilitates a much more explosive growth of REM-on firing rate on the next cycle. Without this reduction in REM-on excitability at low levels and the consequent additional decrease in REM-off activity, REM-off activity would remain relatively high and constrain REM-on firing rate to progressively less rapid growth on successive cycles, and ultimately oscillations would cease entirely. In the phase-plane representation this would be seen as a progressive spiral to the center of the phase plane, to a single stable equilibrium point. Thus, reduction of the X (REM-on) firing rate growth term at low values of X is one simple mathematical postulate that leads to the repeated oscillations found physiologically.

It must be acknowledged that, at present, although there is general evidence for increased REM-on excitability and rate of REM-on membrane potential change for a given stimulus input in REM as compared with waking (Ito and McCarley, 1984), there are no specific empirical data indicating the shape of the excitability curve or suggesting the physiological mechanisms of excitability alteration. Such data and investigations of the mechanisms of such changes will likely be most readily derived from experiments on the *in vitro* brainstem, a preparation described in Chapter 5.

12.7.2. Limitations on Growth of Firing Rates: $S_1(X)$, $S_2(Y)$

An unrealistic feature of the simple LV model was the absence of limitation on neuronal firing rates; when the system was perturbed, firing rates could become arbitrarily and thus unreasonably high, even infinite. In the new model we have included constraining functions on firing rates of neurons; the shape of these constraining curves is sigmoid, in accord with data from a number of neuronal pools suggesting this to be the general form of frequency limitation (Eccles, 1964). As discussed below, physiological data dictated that the REM-off population curve has a sharper cut-off than that for the REM-on population. Below we also list the sample values for neuronal discharge activity for various components of the REM-on and REM-off populations; the values used for X and Y discharge rate activity in the graph ordinates are scaled, relative values since it would be too cumbersome to label all graphs with absolute firing rates for each of the subpopulations. We further note that, technically, the sigmoidal functions act to constrain X and Y levels by sharply attenuating the rate of neuronal firing rate growth at high firing levels of X or Y but do not directly impose a boundary on firing levels.

$S_1(X)$ is a sigmoidal saturation function (Fig. 14) that slopes from 1 to 0 as X increases, thereby effectively constraining the growth of REM-on neurons to finite levels. A logistic function is used to generate this sigmoid curve (circle in Fig. 14 indicates point of maximum slope). The particular parameters of the X population curve were selected to produce a curve consistent with extensive data indicating that the reticular population is heterogeneous with respect to both maximal firing rates and mean rates (Hobson *et al.*, 1974a; McCarley, 1980b). The slow rate of descent of the function reflects the heterogeneity of the X population; i.e., some reticular units are rate limited at relatively low rates, and others at relatively high discharge rates. It will be noted that we have placed the cut-off value close to maximal REM discharge rate values; we have done this because extracellular recordings during carbachol stimulation of reticular areas suggest very little in the way of additional increase of reticular activity under these conditions of probable near-maximal stimulation as compared with that in REM sleep. With respect to the ordinate values, X activity units should be thought of in terms of mean population discharge activity values, with each reticular group having a different absolute maximum but rescaled so that the peak rate is 3.2 and therefore the mean rate is 1.0. For the mPRF cell group, the example used in this paper, maximal values are 10.8 spikes/sec in REM, and minimal values as a population are 0.231 spikes/sec (geometric mean values). We note that the dynamics of our system of equations is not greatly altered by changes in the details of the shape of these sigmoid functions. For example, making this saturation function begin at higher values of X simply shifts the peak of REM intensity more toward the start of the REM period.

$S_2(Y)$ is sigmoidal saturation function that slopes steeply from 1 to 0 as Y increases, thereby effectively limiting the growth of REM-off discharges to finite levels. A logistic function is used to generate this sigmoid. Figure 15 indicates the point of maximum slope by a circle. The Y activity values in Fig. 15 and other figures in this paper represent scaled mean neuronal discharge rates for the entire REM-off population. For the various subgroups of REM-off neurons sample values for the mean peak rates and, in parentheses, median peak rates are: LC population, 7.9 spikes/sec (3.4); DR neurons, 3.25 spikes/sec (2.57); and peribrachial neurons, 4.4 spikes/sec (4.46) (data from Hobson *et al.*, 1983a). Because it would be cumbersome for each graph to indicate absolute maximal firing levels for each of these populations, the ordinates of the graphs are relative (scaled) firing rates, and we refer to these relative firing rates as "Y units." (We originally selected the peak Y population activity to be about 2.5 Y units such that the mean activity value would lie at $Y = 1.0$ in order to facilitate computation of parameters.)

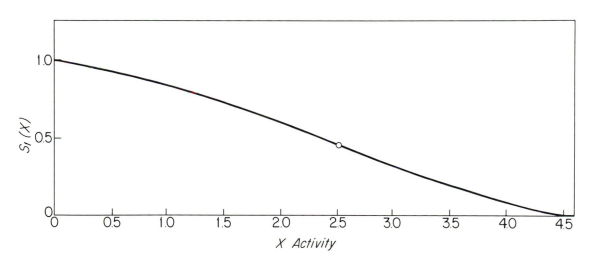

Figure 14. Shape of logistic curve indicating limitation on X population maximal firing rates; note a slower cut-off than for the Y population in Fig. 15. Adapted from McCarley and Massequoi (1986a).

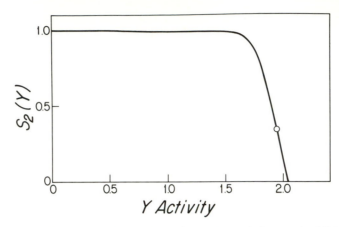

Figure 15. Shape of logistic curve indicating limitation on Y population maximal firing rates. Adapted from McCarley and Massequoi (1986a).

Extensive extracellular data have shown that the firing rate of all of these REM-off populations is severely limited at the upper end and that each population is also fairly homogeneous in terms of the firing rate of its members and the upper frequency limitation. We have accordingly used a sigmoid curve with a rapid cut-off at the upper end and a high maximum slope value of 3.

12.7.3. Use of $b(X)$ and c

$b(X)$ is the REM-on dependence on REM-off inhibitory input. Compared with the simple LV system, this is no longer a simple constant but, as in the growth function $a(X)$, depends on X, the REM-on firing level.

$$b(X) = b_{max} * \text{logistic function}(X)$$

where logistic function$(X) = 1/\{1 + \exp[-80(X - 0.11)]\}$ and $b_{max} = 2$. The logistic function has a point of maximum slope at $X = 0.11$ and is very steeply sloped so that at $X > 0.2$, this function is virtually identical to $b(X) = 2$. This function provides a limitation on inhibitability of X by Y population when X activity level is low and is significantly different from the constant b in the simple LV equations only at very low levels of X (approximately < 0.2). Its addition prevents the X population activity level from becoming zero at high and sustained levels of REM-off activity, as is postulated to occur during waking; in terms of system dynamics this alteration was empirically found to be necessary to prevent degeneration of the system to the origin. Physiologically, this corresponds to a nonzero basal level of REM-on activity that can not be suppressed by REM-off inhibition; experimental observations confirm the presence of some reticular activity throughout all behavioral states.

$$c = 1.0 \text{ (as in simple Lotka–Volterra system)}$$

12.7.4. Circadian Variation, *d*(circ), and Entry into the Limit Cycle

d(circ) is the REM-off dependence on REM-on firing rate made dependent on the phase of the circadian temperature oscillator ("circadian time," abbreviated "circ"). Circadian variation in *d* is described by the following equation:

$$d(\text{circadian time}) = d(\text{circ}) = d + A * \sin[(f*t) + p_o]$$

where d is average level, set at 0.975 in the simulations; *A* is amplitude of the oscillations, set at 0.125; p_o is the circadian phase in radians at start of simulation; *t* is the time since start of simulation; and *f* is the frequency of oscillation (period = 24 hr).

The introduction of continuous circadian variation of the parameter *d*, which describes the sensitivity of the *Y* population to activity in the *X* population, allows (1) modeling of small amounts of sleep cycle parameter variation that occur in concert with the temperature rhythm after the first sleep cycle and are especially visible in humans in extended sleep (for example, circabidean days), and (2) a more accurate modeling of the shorter latency of REM near sleep onset near temperature minima. Specifically the amplitude of *d* sinusoidally covaries with temperature; *d* is 1.1 at temperature maximum and is 0.85 at temperature minimum.

The alterations of *d*(circ) over many cycles have relatively little effect on REM parameters other than those of the first REM cycle. In humans it is the first REM cycle that is most strongly affected by circadian variation.

The experimentally observed circadian phase sensitivity of the initial sleep cycle parameters (cycle period duration, REM intensity, REM latency, and REM duration) are simply modeled by varying the time course of withdrawal of excitatory influences on the *Y* population with circadian phase: withdrawal is more rapid near a temperature minimum and slower at a temperature maximum.

Specifically, this is modeled by having a constant rate of decay of excitatory input to *Y* but having the starting strength of *Y* excitation at sleep onset vary sinusoidally and in phase with the circadian temperature oscillator (Czeisler *et al.*, 1980; Zulley *et al.*, 1981; Akerstedt and Gillberg, 1981; Endo *et al.*, 1981; Kronauer *et al.*, 1982). For sleep onset at all circadian phases the rate of decay of *Y* excitation is 0.05 units/time unit (that is, −0.05 firing rate units per 10.7 min, scaled), but the higher starting amplitude of excitation with sleep onset at $T_{\max}$ leads to a longer time course of decline in *Y* and therefore to an internal approach to the limit cycle, resulting in a longer latency, shorter duration, and smaller intensity of the first REM period. In contrast, with sleep onset near $T_{\min}$ there is a lower starting level of *Y* excitation that leads to a more rapid decline in *Y* and thus to an external approach to the limit cycle. An earlier version of this limit-cycle model was termed the "Karma model" to emphasize that the "fate" of the system depended on the way in which it was set into motion (Massaquoi and McCarley, 1982).

The sleep-onset starting level of the residual excitation was sinusoidally covaried with a maximum of 0.69 occurring at temperature maximum and a minimum of 0.09 at temperature minimum. Thereafter, the rate of linear decay was a constant 0.05 *X* units/10.7 min (scaled), with a resultant longer time course of decay near temperature maximum and a consequent interior entry into the limit cycle.

Specifically, the sleep onset level of residual excitation, *Es*, is:

$$Es = Em + A*\sin[(f*t) + p_o)]$$

where *Em* is the midpoint level of residual excitation (0.39), *A* is the amplitude of variation (0.3), *f* is the frequency of oscillation (period fixed at 24 hr), *t* is the time since start of simulation (0 at start of simulation), and p_o is the circadian phase in radians at start of simulation.

It will be noticed that this construction exactly parallels that for *d*(circ) described above. This starting level of residual excitation is then decreased linearly until it becomes zero and then remains zero throughout the simulation. Thus, until the decay of residual excitation, equation 4 becomes:

$$Y'(t) = c*Y + d(\text{circ})*(X + E)*Y*S_2$$

where *E* is the level of residual excitation (same units as *X*).

In summary, we note that it is the difference in the time course of decline of *Y* (as controlled by excitation withdrawal) at sleep onset that determines whether the limit cycle is entered from the interior (slow time course of decline) or the exterior (rapid time course of decline), and thus this parameter is by far the most critical one for determining changes in REM sleep values, since it is the first REM cycle that varies more than all others.

12.7.5. Phase-Plane Representation of Entry into the Limit Cycle

With this model the trajectory into sleep cycling is controlled by the time course of the decline in excitatory input to *Y*, the residual excitation. Slow withdrawal allows the system very slowly to begin a gentle oscillation, which increases in amplitude as the limit cycle is approached. In the phase-plane graph this corresponds to an initial trajectory that is interior to the limit cycle with a subsequent outward spiraling to reach the limit cycle (cf. Fig. 7B, path P_I, and Fig. 8). In contrast, rapid withdrawal of excitation from *Y* allows the system to accelerate into a rapid, large-amplitude oscillation that then decays slightly to the limit-cycle amplitude; this is represented in the phase-plane graph as an external approach to the limit cycle (cf. Fig. 7B, path P_E, and Fig. 9).

It is useful to use Fig. 7B to summarize some of the dynamics of the limit-cycle system. The equations governing the limit cycle isoclines are:

$$I_A, X = c/[S_2(Y)d(\text{circ})]; \text{ and } I_B, Y = a(X)S_I(X)/b(X)$$

with the terms as in equations 3 and 4. These isoclines are clearly "bent" compared with those of the simple LV system in Fig. 7A. Since all solution paths must have zero slope at the point of crossing I_A, it can be seen heuristically that if I_A is bent clockwise against the sense of path rotation, then solution paths are "forced" to curve earlier and more tightly than in the standard system. Therefore, solutions spiral inward toward the limit cycle. At larger radii from the center (>0.75 units), I_B produces the same constraining effect by being similarly bent against the direction of solution rotation. At smaller radii, however, I_B is bent counterclockwise and in the same direction as that of solution rotation. In this case solution paths near the center bend later and less tightly than in the standard system. Thus, solution paths tend to spiral outward on each revolution when initiated interior to the limit cycle. This counterclockwise bending of I_B at small radii is the graphic reflection of depressed REM-on autoexcitation at low firing rates—a property we propose is fundamental to the presence of limit-cycle behavior of the system. There are two further technical points. First, the position of I_A is shown for $d(\text{circ}) = 1$; however, since d varies with circadian phase between 0.85 and 1.1, the position of I_A will also vary with circadian phase by +0.125 abscissa units. The second point has to do with the different vertical scale factors of Fig. 12.7A and B; these do not affect system behavior or the final values of subsequently scaled neuronal discharge rates (this point is discussed in detail in McCarley and Massequoi, 1986a).

13

Brainstem Mechanisms of Dreaming and of Disorders of Sleep in Man

This chapter discusses examples of clinical disorders (Sections 13.1 and 13.2) and of the mental activity during REM sleep (dreaming, Section 13.3) that are directly related to brainstem control of behavioral state. The intent is to provide a two-way bridge between basic neuroscience investigations of brainstem function and knowledge of characteristics of human pathology and mental activity in REM sleep. We have accordingly attempted to phrase the discussion so as to be accessible to both the neuroscientist and the clinician. The cognitive phenomenology and the clinical disorders surveyed have been selected because they form excellent "case examples" of the interplay of clinical and research domains. We have further chosen the clinical pathological examples because they represent examples of the diverse roles of cholinergic and monoaminergic modulatory systems. The chapter follows the paradigm of having an "explanation" of the clinical data by models and data derived from more basic neuroscience research, and the clinical data serve as a benchmark for measuring adequacy and accuracy of the basic science explanations.

At this point it may be useful to list several useful, although perhaps obvious, conceptual guidelines.

The world of both pathological and normal human behavior, whether of dreams or psychiatric pathology, is more complex and rich than any current model or basic science data set, and consequently the clinician will always justifiably be able to point to gaps and label models as simplistic.

However, the gaps may or may not be of great importance in terms of neuroscience connectivity, since they may represent adventitious addenda to basic mechanisms that are indeed modeled correctly. Gaps can not constitute *prima facie* evidence of a fatal flaw of the model, although they clearly represent a call for more investigation, and if there are competing models, the one with more explanatory power is to be preferred.

Clinical phenomenology and diagnoses are not necessarily reflective of any fundamental principles of biological ordering. Clinical syndromes that are phenomenologically the same may have different biological causes; there may be a divergence of mechanism. Conversely, clinical syndromes that are phenomenologically quite different may be kin because they share abnormalities in the same or closely related biological systems; there may be a convergence of mechanisms. As an example of divergent mechanisms, consider the 19th-century diagnosis of "dropsy" (edema), which today we know might be the result of pathology in a number of different systems, including cardiovascular, renal, and metabolic. In contrast, some forms of the 19th-century syndromes of "apoplexy" (stroke), "acute indigestion" (myocardial infarction), and dropsy may be alike, we know today, because of the presence of abnormalities in the blood pressure regulatory system, an example of convergence of mechanisms. We have deliberately selected 19th-century medical diagnoses to emphasize the point that the behavioral sciences of neurology and psychiatry are now, in many ways, at the same point as internal medicine in the 19th century. Clinical syndromes are just now being described in terms of constituent mechanisms, and there is movement toward a more rational classification of diseases based on causal mechanisms. A final point is that different disease processes may affect the same biological system but at different sites and with different mechanisms of action. Thus, that the same system should be found to be involved in a variety of clinical diagnoses should not be surprising or discomfiting but rather act as a prod to further investigation of the sites and mechanisms affected in each disorder.

13.1. Narcolepsy: A Disorder of REM-Sleep Mechanisms

The most striking clinical disorder of REM-sleep phenomena is narcolepsy. True to its name, this disorder presents with attacks of partial or complete REM-sleep phenomena. The clinical syndrome involves several characteristic features, which are reviewed in detail in Guilleminault (1989). We group the symptom clusters into the following five classes.

(1) *Excessive daytime sleepiness* (EDS) is an uncontrollable desire to go to sleep, with the sleep episodes marked by "sleep-onset" REM-sleep episodes, i.e., REM sleep within 15 min of sleep onset. These REM episodes are often accompanied by dreamlike mentation, and the sleep episodes are typically less than 30 min in duration. We frequently refer to this sleep propensity complex as EDS.

(2) *Cataplexy* is an abrupt attack of decreased muscle tone. Mild forms may involve only a transient jaw sag or knee buckle, analogous to the normal phenomena metaphorically and physically describing bodily reaction to surprise. Indeed, in the narcoleptic, cataplexy is typically provoked by surprise or other sudden emotion such as laughter or anger. More severe cataplectic attacks may involve the entire voluntary musculature, causing a sudden, total collapse of tone with danger of bone fractures from falling. At this point the reader may be reminded of the muscle atonia system of REM sleep described in Chapter 10. There is strong evidence that the muscle atonia system, normally active only in REM sleep, becomes active at other times in the narcoleptic and is responsible for the attacks of cataplexy. For example, at the clinical level, the monosynaptic H reflex is inhibited in both REM sleep and cataplexy; there is frequently a progression of cataplexy to a full-blown state that is both electrographically identical to REM sleep and accompanied by dreamlike mentation, thus further underlining the link between cataplexy and REM-sleep phenomena. Figure 1 illustrates cataplexy in a canine model.

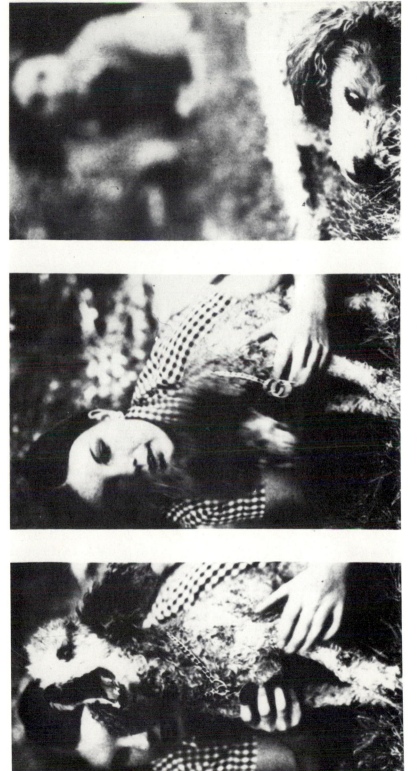

Figure 1. Cataplexy in a narcoleptic poodle being offered food. The first panel shows the excitement of the poodle over being offered food. This is followed by (second and third panels) a collapse of muscle tone and falling. (Courtesy of Dr. William Dement.)

(3) *Sleep paralysis* occurs during falling asleep or awakening. There is a paralysis of voluntary movement of limbs and of the speech and respiratory apparatus, all occurring in a state of awareness. Often the first episode of sleep paralysis is terrifying, but anxiety usually lessens if the narcoleptic is given information about the cause of these attacks and comes to realize that the episodes are brief (usually less than 10 min) and self-limiting. A useful way to conceptualize sleep paralysis is as a premature onset or delayed offset of the muscle atonia system that normally accompanies REM sleep but instead now appears with a wakinglike consciousness. Milder versions of this phenomenon are found in the sleep of normals, and informal surveys suggest that more than three-fourths of normal individuals vividly recall having forms of mild sleep paralysis (R. W. McCarley, unpublished data).

(4) *Hypnagogic hallucinations* occur at sleep onset and in a clear state of consciousness. These are typically visual, sometimes consisting of simple forms and other times of more complex imagery such as an intruder breaking into the bedroom. Auditory, somesthetic, and kinesthetic hallucinations may also be present, just as in normal dreaming; the kinesthetic hallucinations often involve sensations of floating or of being detached from the physical body. These complex hallucinations are part of the narcoleptic syndrome but may lead both the patient and the psychiatric clinician to inappropriate worry about paranoid psychoses. They are more appropriately considered breakthroughs of normal REM-sleep/dream-state phenomena, as discussed later in this chapter.

(5) *Nocturnal sleep-onset REM episodes.* The first four symptom clusters are often termed the "narcoleptic tetrad" (Daniels, 1934). With the discovery of REM sleep and its documentation with electrographic recordings, it was found that the narcoleptic clinical symptoms were associated with a nocturnal sleep-onset REM episode complete with dreaming (Yoss and Daly, 1957; Vogel, 1960). An interesting finding related to the REM sleep oscillator has been the report by Passouant and co-workers (1964) that daytime narcoleptic attacks tend to occur with the same 90-min periodicity of the human REM sleep cycle, suggesting that the REM oscillator remained turned on during the day in narcoleptics.

This above symptom constellation defines narcolepsy, with sleep paralysis and hypnogogic hallucinations occurring less frequently than EDS and cataplexy. The prevalence of narcolepsy is estimated at about 0.06%, and there is a genetic predisposition (see Guilleminault *et al.,* 1975). It has been found that most narcoleptics are positive for the human leukocyte antigen (HLA) DR2 (Juji *et al.,* 1984; Billard and Seignalet, 1985).

Canine animal models show cataplexy with emotional triggering and with a frequent progression to the full electrographic signs of REM sleep, just as in humans (Fig. 1). This disorder is heritable in Doberman pinschers and Labrador retrievers, likely by an autosomal recessive gene, and sporadic in other breeds (Foutz *et al.,* 1979).

13.1.1. Cholinergic Abnormalities in Canine Narcolepsy

The canine model (Boehme *et al.,* 1984; Baker and Dement, 1985; Kilduff *et al.,* 1986) has provided evidence for significantly increased numbers of cholinergic muscarinic receptors but no change in K_D in widespread areas of brainstem reticular formation. Reticular areas included the pontine and bulbar gigantocellular tegmental fields (FTG) that receive cholinergic projections (see Chapter 4); these zones include sites where microinjections of cholinergic agonists induce muscle atonia, with or without other REM sleep signs (see Chapter 10 and 11). Tests with pirenzepine on bulbar FTG samples suggested that an M_2 receptor type was involved. These data complemented previous pharmacological experiments of the Stanford group showing that systemic administration of muscarinic or mixed cholinergic agonists such as arecoline or physostigmine increased cataplexy, whereas nicotine and neostigmine, which does not cross the blood–brain barrier, were not effective (Baker and Dement, 1985). Cataplexy was reduced by systemic administration of the muscarinic receptor blockers atropine sulfate and scopolamine, but mecamylamine, a nicotinic blocker, and atropine methylnitrate, which does not cross the blood–brain barrier, were ineffective.

In summary, these data suggest an abnormality of muscarinic receptor number, perhaps of the M_2 type, in the brainstem reticular formation in canine narcolepsy. The data from *in vitro* pharmacological studies indicate the presence of excitatory muscarinic receptors on reticular formation neurons (Greene *et al.*, 1989a). If these receptors are present in increased number on the neurons mediating muscle atonia (and this awaits experimental demonstration), they may be responsible for the cholinergic pharmacological hypersensitivity of narcoleptic dogs. It is also possible that the observed cholinergic abnormalities play a role in the induction of spontaneous cataplectic attacks.

13.1.2. Monoamine Abnormalities in Canine Narcolepsy

In humans, drugs that increase biogenic amine concentrations have been found to be effective in treating various symptoms of narcolepsy. These include (1) the tricyclic antidepressants, which block monamine reuptake and are widely used for treating cataplexy, (2) drugs that potentiate monamine release (amphetamines and methylphenidate), widely used in treating symptoms of EDS, and (3) monamine oxidase inhibitors, used only in intractable cases because of their potential for serious side effects (Guillemenault, 1989). In both the sporadic and hereditary canine narcoleptic models (Baker and Dement, 1985), a parallelism of pharmacological effects with those seen in humans has been observed. In affected canines, tricyclic antidepressants reduced cataplexy, an effect that was partially reversed by physostigmine. Tricyclics acting primarily on norepinephrine, e.g., nisoxetine, appeared more effective than those acting on serotonin. Methylphenidate induced a short-duration reduction in cataplexy, but the side effects of monamine inhibitors made it impossible to test their effect. It was also of interest that the α_2-receptor agonist clonidine decreased cataplexy, as also has been shown in humans, but the β-adrenergic blocker propranolol did not have any effects. Recent studies suggest that low affinity α_1 receptors are involved (cf. Mingnot *et al.*, 1988); prazosin, an α_1-receptor blocker, has been found to be the most effective inducer of cataplexy in affected canines. It is of interest that atropine completely blocked the prazosin effect, implying that a cholinergic system may interact with an adrenergic system. In affected Dobermans, punch biopsies of brain assayed with HPLC showed that catecholamines (dopamine, epinephrine, norepinephrine) were elevated in a number of brainstem and forebrain regions, but serotonin and its metabolite 5-HIAA were not altered (Faull *et al.*, 1986).

These abnormalities of the catecholamine systems are not as simply interpretable as those of the cholinergic system. In general, the data of the canine model support the hypothesis of a cholinergic cataplexy-promoting system, whereas catecholamines act to suppress cataplexy (Baker and Dement, 1985), a finding that parallels aspects of REM-sleep control models (see Chapter 12). Dopamine-containing neurons do not alter discharge rate over the sleep–wake cycle (Steinfels *et al.*, 1983), and thus dopamine, unlike norepinephrine and epinephrine, had not been postulated to play a critical role in normal sleep-cycle control, although it may prove to be important in narcolepsy. Research is not far enough advanced to demonstrate the nature of the deficit in canine narcolepsy, but a neuronal membrane defect that alters acetylcholine and catecholamine release has been postulated for the hereditary form in Dobermans (Kilduff *et al.*, 1986).

13.2. Depression and Other Major Psychiatric Disorders

We here discuss those neurobiological control mechanisms likely important for both sleep and depression and thought to have important brainstem components. No attempt to cover the entire neurobiology of major mood disorders is made; this is an overly large topic for a book focused on the brainstem. However, the overlap between the mood disorders and sleep disorders is considerable and quite important, since about 90% of patients with major endogenous depressive disorders show some electrographic sleep abnormality (Kupfer, 1982; Reynolds, 1989). These abnormalities may be grouped into three categories.

(1) *REM sleep abnormalities* include *shortened "REM latency,"* a shortened interval between sleep onset and the beginning of the first REM sleep period, *increased "REM density" in the first REM sleep episode,* an increased number of rapid eye movements per unit time, and a tendency to *increased duration of the first REM-sleep episode* (Fig. 3, top, schematizes these abnormalities). REM density and REM sleep duration may also be increased in other early night REM sleep episodes in addition to the first. A number of studies suggest that these abnormalities persist beyond the stage of clinical recovery from the depressive episode. (For more details, see Gresham *et al.*, 1965; Hartmann, 1968; Kupfer and Foster, 1972; Coble *et al.*, 1976; Foster *et al.*, 1976; McPartland *et al.*, 1979.)

(2) *Synchronized sleep abnormalities* include δ-*sleep reduction.* This is a reduction in stage 3 and 4 sleep, often called δ sleep. This is especially marked in the first non-REM sleep episode (i.e., the interval between sleep onset and the first REM episode), a time when δ sleep ordinarily is at a maximum. Initial analyses also indicated reduction in power in the δ bandwidth (0.5–3.0 Hz) on frequency analysis (see Borbely *et al.*, 1984; Kupfer *et al.*, 1984).

(3) *Sleep continuity disturbances* include difficulty in falling asleep, early morning awakenings, and increased nocturnal awakenings and appear to be the least specific for depression (see reviews in Kupfer, 1982; Gillin *et al.*, 1988).

Three major theories have been advanced to account for the observed links between sleep-state disturbances and mood-state disturbances.

(1) *Monoaminergic–cholinergic alterations.* McCarley (1980a, 1982) has proposed communality of monoamine and cholinergic biological control systems to explain covarying aspects of REM sleep and mood control. This thesis grew out

of the cholinergic–adrenergic reciprocal-interaction model of sleep-cycle control described in Chapter 12 and posits at least partial parallelism with the mood regulation system, in terms of disturbances of monoaminergic control (Schildkraut and Kety, 1967), cholinergic control (reviewed in Gillin *et al.,* 1982, 1988), and cholinergic–adrenergic balance (Janowsky *et al.,* 1972).

(2) *Deficient process S.* Borbely, Daan, Beersma, and co-workers have proposed a two-process model of control of the synchronized phase of sleep (Borbely, 1982; Daan *et al.,* 1984; Beersma *et al.,* 1987). Process C (for circadian) regulates the circadian variation in sleep propensity, while process S is the momentary physiological need for sleep that is dependent on the prior history of sleep and wakefulness and is measured by the power spectrum density in the δ bandwidth. "Factor S" builds up in wakefulness and declines during sleep. A deficiency in factor S is postulated for depressives, who are hypothesized not to produce sufficient factor S to cause deep δ sleep at sleep onset (Borbely and Wirz-Justice, 1982). The postulated inhibition of REM sleep by factor S (indexed by δ sleep) means that reduced factor S (and consequently reduced δ sleep) has, as a consequence, a quicker-onset first REM-sleep period (shortened REM latency). Finally, it is postulated that the deficiency in factor S causes the shortening of sleep duration found in depressives.

(3) *Phase-advance theories of sleep disturbance in depression.* Chapter 12 has described how the latency to the first REM-sleep episode and the intensity and duration of REM-sleep episodes are under control of a circadian oscillator that also controls the temperature cycle and endocrine rhythms, such as cortisol. The phase-advance theory of depression simply states that the abnormalities of sleep and mood in depressives are a function of a phase advance in the circadian oscillator controlling both temperature and REM-sleep propensity relative to the phase of the rest–activity circadian rhythm. Thus, it is postulated, the observed pattern of REM sleep in depressives at sleep onset is like that seen near the temperature nadir of normals, which in entrained subjects occurs at about 4 a.m. (Kripke *et al.,* 1978; Wehr *et al.,* 1979). This out-of-phase relationship of the temperature–REM-sleep oscillator and the oscillator controlling the rest–activity cycle is postulated to lead to a mood disturbance.

Before reviewing the theories and relevant data, it is first important to emphasize that the separation of these theories has been done for didactic purposes and that, in fact, they are not mutually incompatible. For example, it is entirely possible that there is disturbance both in process S (synchronized sleep) and in cholinergic–adrenergic balance (controlling REM sleep). The other key point to be made is that the factors controlling circadian rhythms, REM sleep, and non-REM sleep interact, and, in fact, our review of the theories and data will emphasize interactions. We begin with a review of the monoaminergic–cholinergic disturbance theory.

13.2.1. Monoaminergic–Cholinergic Factors in Mood Disorders and Associated Sleep Abnormalities

13.2.1.1. Monoamines

The monoamine theory of depression proposes that a deficiency in monoamine activity (norepinephrine and/or serotonin systems) is responsible for the occurrence of some or all of the major depressions (Schildkraut and Kety, 1967; Maas, 1975). Almost all varieties of clinically effective tricyclic antidepressants, including those atypical ones not associated with acute blocking of monoamine reuptake such as iprindole, have been reported to change norepinephrine and serotonin receptor binding (Peroutka and Snyder, 1980; Wolfe *et al.*, 1978). Long-term administration of these agents decreases β-adrenergic and sero-tonin-2 (high affinity to [^{3}H]spiroperidol) receptors. Neuronal recordings indicate that long-term administration of tricyclic antidepressants, including the atypical ones, act on monoamine systems by increasing responsiveness to iontophoretically applied monoamines (DeMontigny and Aghajanian, 1978; Menkes and Aghajanian, 1980). A study by Blier and DeMontigny (1983) has provided some insight into the mechanisms of antidepressant action at the neuronal level; after 2 weeks of antidepressant administration, serotonergic transmission in the rat dorsal raphe–hippocampal pathway was potentiated. The initial effect of antidepressants was to cause reduced dorsal raphe firing because of depolarization blockade, with this effect vanishing over 2 weeks; it is of note that a similar lag period is present before tricyclics become clinically effective in improving human depressive symptoms. Cortes and co-workers (1988) have recently examined the binding sites in human brain of both a tricyclic antidepressant, [^{3}H]imipramine, and a nontricyclic antidepressant, [^{3}H]paroxetine, a more specific and potent serotonin uptake inhibitor. These antidepressant binding sites paralleled the serotonin system, with highest values in the midbrain raphe nuclei and ascending projections. Also of interest in view of the augmentation of REM-sleep phenomena in depression and their suppression by antidepressants was the finding of fairly dense labeling in brainstem zones related to PGO waves and eye movements (Chapter 10), namely, in the nucleus reticularis tegmenti pontis and gigantocellular portions of reticular formation (cf. Figs. 6 and 7 of Cortes *et al.*, 1988).

The implication of monoamine systems both in the regulation of mood (the monoamine theory) and in REM sleep (the reciprocal interaction theory) suggests the possibility of a link between these two systems through the monoamines. Kupfer and co-workers (1981b) have shown that one of the first indications of effectiveness of the tricyclic action on depression is the abolition of the abnormally short latency of the first REM period. In fact, almost all clinically effective antidepressants (tricyclics, monoamine oxidase inhibitors, and others) markedly suppress REM sleep and induce a characteristic REM-sleep rebound on their discontinuance* (see review by Vogel, 1989). Further supporting the

---

*The tricyclic antidepressants typically act within a few days to lengthen the abnormally short REM-sleep latency in depression; in fact, their ability to reverse the REM-sleep abnormalities of depression on an immediate basis predicts their ultimate effectiveness in reversing the lowered mood of depression (Kupfer *et al.*, 1981b). There is now growing evidence that, at the electrographic level of analysis, 5-HT$_2$ antagonists and other "new generation" compounds show different effects on sleep than previously studied tricyclics or MAO inhibitors. This is now an area of intense research, but the present diversity of data suggests that further work will be needed for precise definition of effects and mode of action. These compounds have only been studied using systemic administration (making the brain site and mode of action difficult to specify), and the *in vivo* cellular effects have not yet been examined. Ritanserin, a 5-HT$_2$ antagonist, has been reported to increase slow-wave sleep and not to suppress REM sleep in humans (Idzikowski *et al.*, 1986, 1988). In rats ritanserin has been reported to increase synchronized sleep but to suppress REM (Dugovic and Waquier, 1987); Trachsel *et al.* (1988) confirmed the REM suppression and enhancement of slow-wave activity, but

link between control mechanisms of REM sleep and depression is a study by Vogel and co-workers (1980); REM sleep deprivation, known to increase mono-amine neuronal discharge activity in animals, acts to improve depression, and with about the same efficacy as tricyclic antidepressants. REM sleep deprivation has also been shown to decrease rat cortical high-affinity binding sites for the antidepressant imipramine (Mogilnicka *et al.*, 1980), with the likely mediating event being the deprivation-induced increased firings of monoamine neurons. This monoamine communality of mood and REM control systems forms one basis of the model of REM sleep abnormalities in depression.

13.2.1.2. Cholinergic Abnormalities in the Sleep of Depressives

In addition to the monoamine abnormalities in depression, Gillin *et al.* (1982, 1988) have found that increased sensitivity to acetylcholine agonist induction of REM sleep appears to be a hallmark of many patients subject to endogenous depression (Fig. 2). These patients may have a primary cholinergic abnormality. The shorter REM latencies in rats with increased number of muscarinic receptors (Flinders sensitive line; see Overstreet, 1986) suggest the possibility of cholinergic causation of this event, although these animals also had an increased percentage of REM sleep, a finding not present in depressives (Shiromani *et al.*, 1988b). Another possibility, given the monoaminergic–cholinergic duality of control, is that the monoamine deficiency is responsible for the enhanced effectiveness of cholinergic agonists in inducing REM sleep. In general, it appears likely that various kinds of depression involve more than one causative factor and that both acetylcholine and monoamine abnormalities (in addition to other factors) could be present. Table 1 summarizes some of the evidence on parallelism of monoaminergic and cholinergic features in depression and REM-sleep control. Overall, the evidence appears stronger for a monoamine role in depression and for more parallelism between monoamine controls in depression and sleep than for cholinergic systems. Figure 3, bottom, is a qualitative sketch of how lessened monoaminergic inhibition might lead to short-latency, higher-intensity first REM-sleep episode in depressives.

The availability of quantitative predictions about the effects of monoaminergic and cholinergic factors may be of use in specifying subtypes of depression and in classifying other pathological syndromes with REM abnormalities and is discussed in the next section, as are the "phase-advance" theories of REM-sleep alterations in depression.

EEG power spectral analysis showed a bimodal distribution of low-frequency activity as contrasted with the unimodal distribution in physiological synchronized sleep. Another 5-HT_2 antagonist, seganserin, has been reported to enhance electrographically scored synchronized sleep and to suppress REM in humans; however, EEG power spectral analysis suggested that the electrographically defined synchronized sleep induced by seganserin was different from physiological synchronized sleep (Dijk and Beersma, 1988). Two other 5-HT_2 antagonists, ICI 169,369 and ICI 170,809, have been reported to suppress REM sleep but not to alter non-REM sleep in the rat (Tortella *et al.*, 1988). 5-HT_2 agonists suppress both REM and non-REM sleep (Dugovic and Waquier, 1987; Pastel, 1988). A preliminary study by Besset *et al.* (1988) indicated that toloxatone, a "new generation" MAO inhibitor, did not suppress REM sleep or cause a rebound on withdrawal.

13.2.2. Quantitative Modeling of the REM-Sleep Abnormalities in Depression

This section addresses the quantitative modeling of REM-sleep abnormalities in depression, a procedure that furnishes more precise predictions and tests than do simple qualitative assertions. This modeling uses aspects of the limit-cycle reciprocal-interaction model of sleep-cycle control presented in Chapter 12 (McCarley and Massaquoi, 1986a,b); for simplicity we hereafter refer to this model as the "limit-cycle" model. The first and most elementary question is whether a simple phase advance, as modeled by the limit-cycle model, could account for the REM-sleep abnormalities. Figure 9 of Chapter 12 shows that for sleep begun at temperature minimum, there is indeed a more intense, longer-duration REM-sleep episode that has a shorter REM latency than with sleep begun near temperature maximum, which is shown in Fig. 8 of Chapter 12.

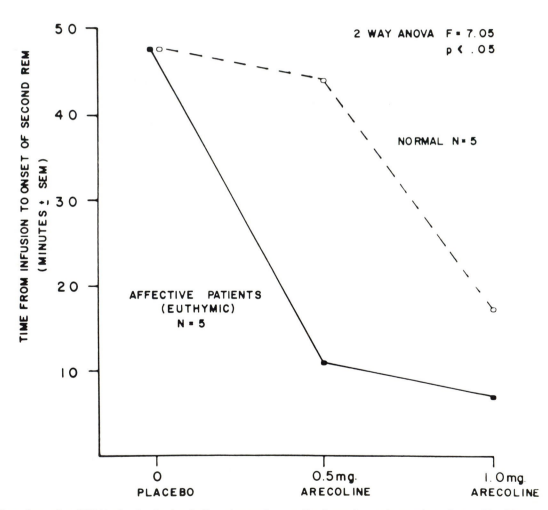

Figure 2. Dose-dependent REM induction by the cholinergic agonist arecoline has a shorter latency in patients with a history of primary depressive disorder than in normals. This phenomenon was present even though the patients were not symptomatic at time of testing. From Gillin *et al.* (1982).

Table 1. Data Bearing on Communality of Control Systems for REM Sleep and Mood

Common effect	Source of data		
	Naturalistic study	Monoamine experiments (norepinephrine, serotonin)	Cholinergic experiments
Promotion of REM sleep and depression	Endogenous depressive patients have a short-latency first REM episode with increased intensity and duration (Kupfer and Foster, 1972; McPartland et al., 1979)	Reserpine increases PGO waves in animals and produces depression; other aminergic depleting agents and aminergic blocking agents (aminergic β blockers) may produce depression as a side effect; cooling of LC and dorsal raphe in animals produces REM sleep (see McCarley, 1980a,b; Cespuglio et al., 1979, 1982).	Cholinergic agonists promote REM; endogenous depressive patients have increased sensitivity to cholinergic REM induction; cholinergic agonists mimic some depressive signs and symptoms in normal and depressive subjects and are clinically useful in acutely reducing mania (abnormally elevated mood) (Baghdoyan et al., 1985; Janowsky et al., 1972, 1980; Gillin et al., 1982, 1988; Gillin, 1989)
Suppression of REM sleep and depression	REM sleep deprivation ameliorates depression and decreases cortical imipramine binding sites (Vogel et al., 1980; Mogilnicka et al., 1980)	Tricyclic antidepressants and monoamine oxidase inhibitors decrease depressive symptoms and suppress REM-sleep phenomena; REM-sleep suppression predicts tricyclic antidepressant effectiveness (see McCarley, 1980a; Gillin, 1989; Kupfer et al., 1981b)	Anticholinergics suppress REM sleep but are not generally clinically useful as antidepressants (Gillin et al., 1982, Sitaram et al., 1982)

However, the REM latency shortening to about 45 min is not sufficient to mimic that seen in depressives, although it does match quite well the empirical findings of REM-sleep changes in normals with sleep begun at different points on the circadian oscillator. The match to empirical circadian phase data is important, since the failure to mimic could represent a problem with the limit-cycle

EEG MEASURES

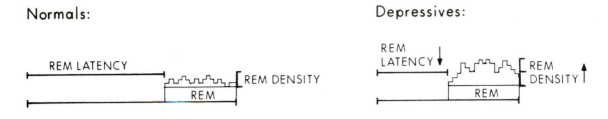

NEURONAL ACTIVITY

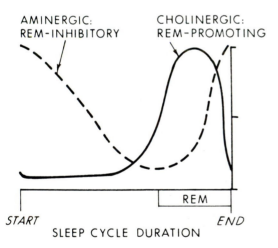
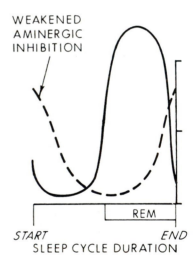

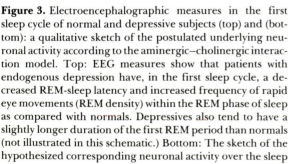

Figure 3. Electroencephalographic measures in the first sleep cycle of normal and depressive subjects (top) and (bottom): a qualitative sketch of the postulated underlying neuronal activity according to the aminergic–cholinergic interaction model. Top: EEG measures show that patients with endogenous depression have, in the first sleep cycle, a decreased REM-sleep latency and increased frequency of rapid eye movements (REM density) within the REM phase of sleep as compared with normals. Depressives also tend to have a slightly longer duration of the first REM period than normals (not illustrated in this schematic.) Bottom: The sketch of the hypothesized corresponding neuronal activity over the sleep cycle in normal subjects shows that REM sleep occurs when cholinergic and REM-promoting (REM-on) neuronal activity becomes dominant with the gradual offset of aminergic (noradrenergic, adrenergic, and serotonergic) inhibition. The hypothesized weakened aminergic inhibition in depression produces a quicker release from inhibition of the cholinergic, REM-promoting neurons and a consequently quicker onset of REM (decreased REM latency) and an increased intensity of the REM-sleep episode (increased REM density). To be compared with quantitative simulation of Fig. 4. From Mc-Carley (1982).

model and not the phase-advance theory. Additional evidence against the simple phase-advance hypothesis comes from the fact that depressives also show short REM latencies compared with normals when they nap in the daytime (Kupfer *et al.*, 1981a) and when they are awakened later in the night (Schulz and Tetzlaff, 1982); the phase-advance theory would predict a longer-duration REM latency during at least some point of the circadian cycle. Thus, both the limit-cycle model and empirical data suggest that simple phase change could not explain the REM-sleep abnormalities in depression.

Nonetheless, examination of the latency, intensity, and duration of the first REM-sleep episode when sleep is begun near a circadian temperature minimum (T_{min}) in free-running normal subjects (Fig. 9 of Chapter 12) is instructive for suggesting the kind of changes that might occur in depression. In the limit-cycle model at T_{min} there is a more rapid decline of the REM-suppressive monoamine (Y) population activity; this leads to entry into the limit cycle from the outside and hence produces a shorter-latency, larger-amplitude, and longer-duration REM episode than at points nearer circadian T_{max}.

These results suggest that the REM-sleep abnormalities in depressives might be quite simply and realistically modeled by alterations in the monoamine population activity at sleep onset (although these would need to be more pronounced that those seen with circadian modulation). A lessened monamine influence is also compatible with evidence (cited above) on monoamine alterations in depressives and the normalization of REM sleep abnormalities by antidepressants. Thus, both an initial qualitative approach (McCarley, 1980a, 1982; see Fig. 3) and subsequent quantitative modeling (Massaquoi and McCarley, 1982; McCarley and Massaquoi, 1986a,b) have worked on the postulate that the level of monoamine population activity at sleep onset is less in depressives than in normals.

The level of monoamine population activity at sleep onset, following the terminology of the previous chapter, will be described as $Y_{initial} = Y_i$. Setting the value of Y_i at 0.25 units, compared with a normal value of 0.35, produces a first REM-sleep latency of 35 min, as shown in Fig. 4. This shortened REM-sleep latency is almost exactly in accord with the mean values for depressives in the literature and also has the desirable feature of being less than most extreme values for the first REM-sleep latency in normals as tabulated by H. Schulz, J. Zulley, and G. Dirlich (unpublished data, 1984). Figure 4 further indicates that alteration of Y_i is not only able to mimic the shortened REM-sleep latency characteristic of depressives but also produces a first REM-sleep episode with a heightened amplitude (heightened REM-sleep intensity) and duration, also characteristics of the first REM-sleep episode of depressives. It is to be emphasized that the critical feature of the limit-cycle model that produces a short-latency REM-sleep episode is the rapid decline of the Y (monoamine) population activity. This change in Y_i is able to produce short REM-sleep latencies regardless of whether the simulation is begun at times near circadian T_{min} (as in the illustration in Fig. 4) or near circadian T_{max}. In both cases, subsequent REM-sleep cycles tend to converge to the limit cycle, preserving a realistic replica of sleep patterning after the initial short-latency REM-sleep episode; this important feature of the limit-cycle model was not present with the earlier simple Lotka–Volterra model (McCarley and Hobson, 1975b).

13.2.2.1. Modeling the Bimodal Distribution of REM-Sleep Latencies in Depression

The REM-sleep latency histogram from patients in at least some types of depression has been reported to show a "bimodal distribution"; there is one peak at near sleep-onset REM-sleep latency and another peak at much longer laten-

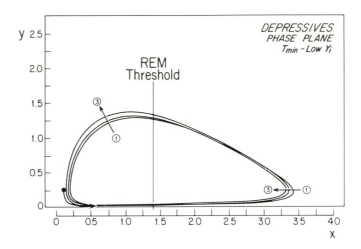

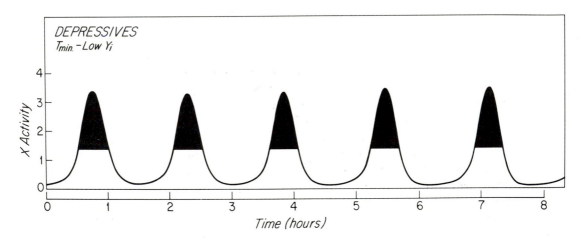

Figure 4. Quantitative simulation of REM activity of depressives by the reciprocal-interaction limit-cycle model. Time-domain (bottom) representation of REM-on neuronal activity is to be compared with Fig. 3; as in the figures of Chapter 12, X represents REM-on neuronal activity, the darkened portions of the time-domain graph represent REM-sleep episodes, and Y represents REM-off neuronal activity. The main point of this figure is that use of a lower value of $Y_{initial}$ than for the entrained normal simulation leads to a first REM episode with a shortened latency (here about 35 min), increased intensity, and longer duration compared with that of the normal first REM episode (Fig. 8 of Chapter 12). The phase-plane representation (top, part A) shows that entry into the limit cycle is external; legends and interpretation are as in Chapter 12. In this particular simulation the circadian phase used was T_{min}, but the same alterations in the first REM period were present when T_{max} was used as a circadian phase. Comparison with a simulation of T_{min} and normal Y_i (Fig. 9 of Chapter 12) shows further that a lower Y_i is required to achieve a shortened REM latency in the range of depressives. Circadian phase is as in Fig. 9 of Chapter 12 (temperature minimum, 4.72 radians), and $Y_{initial}$ is 0.25 versus the 0.35 for all simulations of normal REM in Chapter 12. See also description in text. From McCarley and Massequoi (1986a).

cies, with relatively few REM-sleep episodes in the intermediate zone (Schulz *et al.*, 1979). The limit-cycle model simulations have suggested a possible mechanism for this phenomenon. In the limit-cycle model (McCarley and Massaquoi, 1986a,b), Y (monoamine population activity) values less than approximately 0.3 were progressively less able to "hold" the X (REM-on) population at low values, i.e., 0.2 and less. If the Y values dropped below this critical zone of about 0.3 in the presleep period, there was a progressively increasing tendency for an "escape" and a gradual increase of the X (REM-on) population toward a higher value prior to onset of stage 2 sleep, which is conventionally used to define "sleep onset" and, as such, begins the graph of depressives in Fig. 4 and those of normals in Chapter 11. ["Pre-sleep," as pre-stage 2, thus includes stage 1; REM-sleep latency is measured as the time from stage 2 onset to REM-sleep onset. It will be noted that this model assumes that the initial non-REM sleep abnormalities of depression (lessened initial δ sleep) are reflections of the REM-sleep abnormalities. This "passive" model of non-REM sleep is supported by the presently available data, extensively discussed in Chapter 7 and the first section of Chapter 11 as well as briefly noted in Section 13.2.3.2 below.)

This "escape" of the X (REM-on) population activity because of the lowered Y (monoamine) population activity hastened the onset of the first REM-sleep episode. Simulations showed that the degree of shortening of REM-sleep latency as Y values decreased depended on the pre-stage-2 values of Y, which were termed Y^*. The shape of the function relating REM-sleep latency and the level of Y^* (presleep Y) was highly nonlinear, resulting in a bimodal distribution of REM-sleep latencies, as illustrated in Fig. 5, whose legend should be consulted for a more detailed description of the simulation. The very short REM-sleep latencies reflect the "escape" of the X population.

It is evident that the exact form of the REM-sleep latency distribution is contingent on the level and rate of change of Y presleep as well as the probability distribution assumed for Y^*, but McCarley and Massequoi (1986a) noted that the production of a bimodal REM-sleep latency distribution occurs under a wide variety of assumptions about the form of Y^* density and the rapidity of Y^* decline.

13.2.2.2. Earlier Quantitative Models of REM-Sleep Latency in Depression

All of the previous work has been based on the simple Lotka–Volterra (LV) model of McCarley and Hobson (1975b) (equations 1 and 2 of the previous chapter). Vogel *et al.* (1980) used cycle-to-cycle alterations of the connectivity constants a and c without explicit use of the Y population values at sleep onset. McCarley (1980a) suggested that alterations in the $Y_{initial}$ value might mimic the findings in depression, and Massaquoi and McCarley (1982) provided quantitative evidence for this in the context of the presenting the initial version of the limit-cycle model. Beersma and colleagues (1983, 1984) were the first to realize the value of a stochastic model of $Y_{initial}$ values and used this model to generate a bimodal REM-sleep latency histogram with the simple LV equations. With respect to the use of $Y_{initial}$ alteration to model the sleep of depressives, the papers of both Beersma *et al.* and Massequoi and McCarley emphasized that use of a single parameter change (Y) was to be preferred to the more elaborate suppositions about system changes used by Vogel *et al.* (1980).

However, the neutral stability of the simple LV model used by Beersma *et al.* meant that altering initial conditions created persisting alterations and consequently did not reproduce the actual data of the REM-sleep cycles. (1) In the simple LV equations with parameters used by Beersma *et al.*, lowering Y_i does shorten the REM sleep latency but unfortunately also produces a first REM-sleep episode with a less than normal intensity, not in agreement with the higher intensity found in empirical studies of depression. (2) Because of the neutral stability feature of the simple LV equations, creating a short-latency first REM-sleep episode also creates distortions of later REM/NREM sleep cycles, and the REM/NREM sleep values obtained by the Lotka–Volterra simulation do not match those observed in empirical studies. Thus, use of the limit-cycle model appears to offer marked improvements over the simple Lotka–Volterra model.

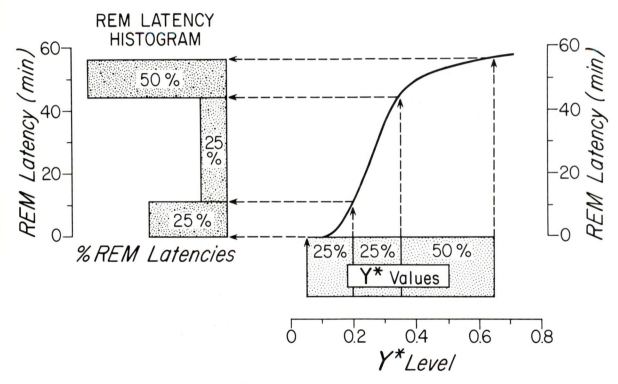

Figure 5. Reciprocal-interaction limit-cycle model simulation of bimodal REM latency distribution for depressives. Presleep variation of the value of the monoamine population activity (Y^*, abscissa) is nonlinearly related to REM latency (ordinate), producing a bimodal distribution of REM latencies because of the nonlinear, sigmoid nature of the function relating them (illustrated sigmoid function). For simplicity of computation it is assumed that the probability of a given Y^* is uniformly distributed in the range 0.05 to 0.65. The resulting map of this probability distribution onto the probability distribution of REM latencies is highly nonlinear. Note that 50% of the Y^* range is from 0.35 to 0.65 but that this range maps into a much smaller latency range, 43–56 min or 23% of latency range, producing a peak at longer REM latencies. There is a second strongly nonlinear region at the lower end, where 25% of Y^* values map into a latency range of 0–11 min (20%), producing a peak at the lower range of REM latencies. In contrast, 25% of the Y^* values map into a large middle-value REM latency range, 11–43 min (57% of entire range). Thus, a presleep stage 2 increase in X values secondary to low Y^* values produces a bimodal REM latency distribution. In this series of simulations Y^* was held constant for 30 min prior to stage 2 onset (stage 2 onset is sleep onset); in all cases other parameters, including circadian phase, were held constant at the values used in Fig. 4. From McCarley and Massequoi (1986a).

The ability of cholinergic agonists to hasten the onset of a REM-sleep episode has been mimicked by the limit-cycle model (Fig. 6), which has also produced a prediction of the normal phase-response curve to cholinergic agonists

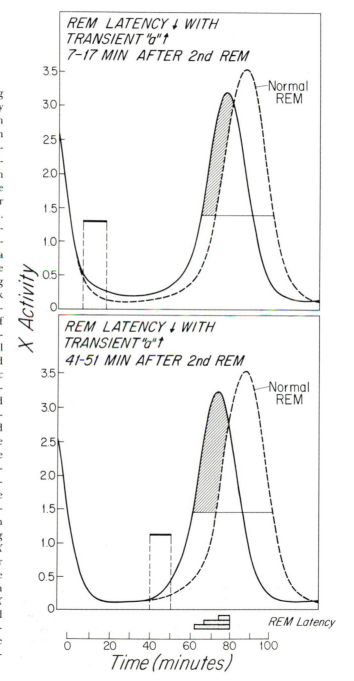

Figure 6. Examples of modeling of REM-latency shortening by experimental application of an acetylcholinesterase inhibitor. In the reciprocal-interaction limit-cycle model the parameter *a* is increased for the same duration in A and B, but the phase advance of REM (shaded area) is greater for application at the time in B. The curves model REM-on neuronal activity with REM onset defined as the point of crossing a threshold (horizontal line). In the model, *a* is the term indicating the strength of positive feedback in the excitatory, REM-on population and thus the strength of cholinergic activity. As a first approximation to the experimental conditions, simulations doubled the strength of *a* (cholinergic feedback) for 10.7 min (step function). These values produced clear-cut effects but did not severely distort the time curves and produced a phase advance of the REM episode of roughly the same order of magnitude as the single-time-point experiments of Sitaram and Gillin, whose results are illustrated in Fig. 2. These differential phase response effects can be understood as REM being much easier to induce when the *X* population is on the rising rather than in the falling phase of the sleep cycle. This has to do with both an ease of moving the *X* population into an exponential growth phase and also the absence of *Y* inhibition later in the cycle. From McCarley and Massequoi (1986a).

(Fig. 7). Patients with predisposition to affective disorder should not only have a single time-point abnormality in their response to acetylcholine agonist but should also show an abnormal phase-response curve to cholinergic agonists administered at various points in the sleep–wake cycle.

13.2.2.4. Circadian Rhythms in Depression: Decreased Amplitude Instead of a Phase Advance?

Although empirical studies cited above have failed to provide strong empirical support for a theory of phase advance in depression, more recent work has suggested that the amplitude of circadian rhythms may be reduced in endogenous depression (Schulz and Lund, 1983, 1985); Czeisler and co-workers

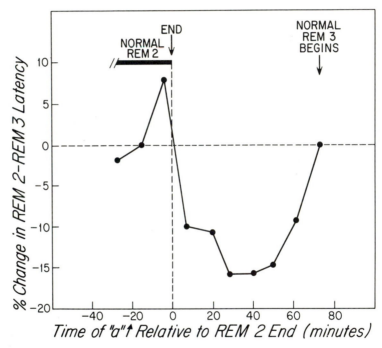

Figure 7. Predicted REM latency phase-response curve, reciprocal-interaction limit-cycle model. Each point on the curve was constructed by a simulation like the two described in Fig. 6, with *a* increased for the same 10.7-min duration but with different times of onset. Onset times of *a* increase are relative to the end of the REM period at the start of the graph, the second REM episode of the night. Negative times indicate the time before the normal (unpreturbed) end of this REM-sleep episode. Note that there is a time zone just at the end of the previous REM-sleep episode when increasing *a* prolongs the latency of the subsequent REM episode. This results from an increase in the duration of the second REM episode. The phase of the response then changes rapidly; a shortening of the REM latency of the order of 10% occurs on administrations starting after the end of the second REM episode; an increase to maximal effect (17% latency reduction) occurs with administrations about 25 to 50 min after the end of the second REM-sleep episode. Following this there is relatively less effect because the third REM sleep episode normally occurs very soon thereafter, and thus there is very little room left for shortening. This phase–response curve both is a useful test of the predictions of the model in normals and also draws attention to the fact that cholinergic system abnormalities in depressives should be marked by phase–response abnormalities as well as single-time-point abnormalities. From McCarley and Massaquoi (1986a).

(1987) have suggested that this may also hold for seasonal affective disorder. It may be useful to point out that a reduced amplitude of circadian rhythms would be highly compatible with the model just presented, since there would be a low level of monoamine activity at sleep onset, with consequent production of the abnormalities of the first REM-sleep episode.

13.2.3. Deficient Process S and Sleep Abnormalities in Depression

13.2.3.1. REM Sleep

Borbely and Wirz-Justice (1982), modifying the reciprocal-interaction model of McCarley and Hobson (1975b), have suggested that there may be a reciprocal interaction between the processes inducing REM sleep and the processes inducing non-REM sleep. Under this theory the shortened first REM latency might be a consequence of reduced "inhibition" from neurons controlling non-REM sleep. Unfortunately, this hypothesis about cellular mechanism is not supported by physiological data, since unit recordings have found no neuronal groups in the brainstem that become active in EEG-synchronized sleep, much less ones that inhibit REM-on neurons (see discussion in Chapters 1, 7, and 11). [A brainstem locus is necessary since the pontine brainstem preparation (Chapter 11, Fig. 1) indicates that the brainstem is sufficient for the rhythmic occurrence of REM sleep. REM sleep may be suppressed after synchronized sleep deprivation, but the mechanisms operative in this situation appear quite different from those producing the normal REM-sleep cycle.]

13.2.3.2. Non-REM Sleep

The hypothesis of deficient process S has stimulated considerable research and remains as a possible explanation of the disturbed synchronized sleep in depression. Reynolds *et al.* (1985), using automated scoring of δ waves, have confirmed decreased δ-wave activity prior to the first REM sleep episode in depressives as compared with normals. However, whether this δ deficiency is responsible for the short REM latency has been questioned. Schulz and Lund (1985) found no intrapatient correlation between very short REM latencies and the amount of stage 3 and 4 sleep, contrary to the deficient "process S" hypothesis, which would predict a covariation of REM latency and amount of δ sleep. Also not supporting the deficient process S—short REM latency hypothesis was a study by van den Hoofdakker and Beersma (1985): the accumulation curves of δ sleep in depressives with very short and longer REM latencies were similar, in contrast to the this theory's prediction of a covariation of REM latency and accumulation of δ sleep. These workers concluded that best explanatory model for the short REM latencies of depression abnormalities was the mathematical reciprocal interaction model (McCarley and Hobson, 1975b). Beersma and colleagues (1985) have also suggested that postulating a deficiency in process S is not necessary to account for shortening and interruption of sleep in depressives; by superimposing random noise on the circadian rhythm, they were able to stimulate both the shortening and decreased continuity of sleep in depressives. Feinberg and March (1988) argue that the apparent initial postdeprivation δ increase and exponential decline may be an artifact of not scoring a short or *forme fruste* first REM sleep episode with a consequent mistaken lumping of δ from two non-REM sleep periods. With the use of their nonlinear smoothing techniques, two discrete episodes of δ are seen at sleep onset following one night of total sleep deprivation. This area of sleep abnormalities in depression is thus one of considerable current interest and exploration.

Krueger and co-workers (1985) have isolated peptides, such as the muramyl peptides, that have the ability to induce synchronized sleep and may play a role in the increased synchronized sleep seen in infections. They have recently reviewed the role of peptides in slow wave sleep (Krueger *et al.*, 1989). It is entirely possible that similar humoral factors, although not presently identified, may play a role in natural EEG-synchronized sleep.

13.2.3.3. New Data on the Mechanism of Generation of δ Activity in Cortex

Buzsaki *et al.* (1988; also see Chapter 7) found that unilateral ibotenic acid lesions of the nucleus basalis in the rat produced an increase in δ power (1–4 Hz) on the side of the lesion. Furthermore, slow waves were present on the side of the lesion when not visible contralaterally, and when slow waves were present

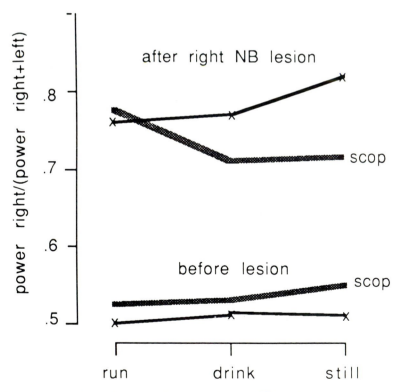

Figure 8. In the rat, unilateral lesions of the nucleus basalis (NB) produce an increase in δ power (1–4 Hz) asymmetry during different behaviors; compare bottom thin line (before lesion) with thin top line (after lesion). This asymmetry is decreased by the muscarinic antagonist scopolamine (scop) when the animal is immobile (still). From Buzsaki *et al.* (1988).

bilaterally during immobility and drowsiness, their amplitude was larger on the side of the lesion. Systemic administration of the muscarinic antagonist scopolamine decreased the δ-wave asymmetry (Fig. 8). Buzsaki *et al.* concluded that a decrease in the activity of cholinergic neurons in the nucleus basalis permitted the occurrence of δ waves in the cortex and speculated that the δ waves may represent summated long-duration after hyperpolarizations in cortical layer V pyramidal neurons. Thus, the presence of δ waves in cortex may reflect, at least partially, an absence of cholinergic input to cortex, an input that is high during REM sleep and waking (Jasper and Tessier, 1971). There is thus an important cautionary note about the use of δ power as an index of "process S." The δ power may not index "process S" (an unspecified and mechanistically undefined process related to sleep propensity) but may simply reflect an absence of REM-sleep-like and wakinglike cholinergic activity. Conversely, the decrease in δ power at sleep onset in depressives may simply reflect an increase in cholinergic activity associated with the early onset of the first REM sleep episode.

13.2.4. REM-Sleep Abnormalities in Other Psychiatric Disorders

Short REM-sleep latencies have been reported in other psychiatric disorders. These include obsessive–compulsive disorder (Rapoport *et al.*, 1981; Insel *et al.*, 1982), characterological depression (Akiskal *et al.*, 1980), and anorexia nervosa (Neil *et al.*, 1980), conditions in which antidepressants may be useful in treatment and conditions that may be related to the spectrum of affective disorders. These different clinical diagnoses may share the presence of similar biological mechanisms. The presence of shortened REM latencies in schizophrenia has been controversial. Zarcone and co-workers (1987) found no differences in REM latency between depressives and schizophrenics, with both showing a shortened REM latency compared with normals. On the other hand, Ganguli *et al.* (1987) found that schizophrenics had normal REM latencies. However, the absence of REM rebound in schizophrenics following REM deprivation, in contrast to the rebound found in normals and depressives, is a more clearly established finding (see review in Zarcone, 1989). A recent review concluded, "Given the brainstem origin of REM sleep, these REM sleep abnormalities suggest the possibility that many severe 'mental illnesses' share a common brainstem component. Whether this is cause or effect of the mental illness is unknown and remains one of the more exciting puzzles for future investigation in biological psychiatry" (Reynolds, 1989). To this we would add the important note that the communality of disturbances of sleep mechanisms may represent the operation of similar physiological mechanisms and that these mechanisms are increasingly open to elucidation by basic neuroscience research approaches.

13.3. Dreaming

Since earliest times, dreaming has attracted the interest of both mystics and naturalistic observers. Aristotle watched the pawing movements of dogs in sleep and suggested they were dreaming of the chase, thus presciently affirming both the correspondence of sleep activity in man and other animals and also the unity of mind and body in sleep. The discussion of dreams and sleep in this chapter is in this spirit of exploring links between mental activity and body (brain) activity. As for the meaning of dreams, another duality has historically been present, since dreams have often been glorified as important vehicles for messages, whether from the gods or from the unconscious, whereas, perhaps equally often, others have dismissed them as epiphenomenal gibberish. This chapter does not propose to resolve this duality of viewpoint, but it does seek to provide perspective on dreams by pointing to the clearest points of contact between mental life in sleep and the physiology of REM sleep. Although a complete historical overview of the development of mind–brain theories of dreams is beyond the scope of this chapter, we begin by examining in some detail the mind–brain theory embedded in perhaps the most celebrated theory of dreams, that of Sigmund Freud. Both the neuroscientist and the psychiatric clinician may be somewhat surprised to find neuronal circuitry furnishing a critical underpinning of psychoanalytic dream theory. This hidden neurobiology is important for understanding quirks of psychoanalytic dream theory, many of whose problems lie in its reliance on now outmoded 19th-century ideas of the brain and sleep. The final portion of this chapter outlines a modern viewpoint of the psychophysiological unity of aspects of dream form and brain state during REM sleep, the activation–synthesis hypothesis.

We first briefly review the current state of knowledge about the relationship between REM sleep and dreaming. There is an approximately 85% correspondence between the subjective experience of dreaming and the occurrence of REM sleep, a far better level of correlation than for any other complex psychophysiological relationship (see McCarley and Hobson, 1979, for a review). In fact, we suggest that even the 15% of dreaming outside of REM sleep may be related to REM-sleep phenomena, since this mental activity may occur when brain neuronal activity approximates that seen in a full-blown REM-sleep episode but has not quite reached sufficient intensity to register in the human EEG as REM sleep.* On this point, the reader may wish to examine the long pre-REM sleep time course of increasing REM-sleep-like neural activity illustrated in Chapter 11, Fig. 6.

Furthermore, data from experiments in cats discussed in Chapter 9 show that the signal-to-noise ratio (PGO-related discharge to spontaneous discharge) of lateral geniculate neurons is much higher during the period immediately preceding REM sleep (the pre-REM period or transition period) than in REM sleep proper (see Figs. 12 and 13 of Chapter 9). These data suggest that dreaming imagery related to this LG thalamic input (see later discussion) may be at least as high during this final portion of EEG-synchronized sleep as in a full-blown REM sleep episode (Steriade *et al.*, 1989c; see Section 9.2.2).

---

*The exact prominence of "dreamlike" recall in slow-wave sleep periods was at one time a subject of active debate and investigation. Although the exact percentage still remains uncertain, there is little current work. It is our opinion that imprecision of human EEG scoring relative to the underlying dream- and REM-sleep-related neuronal activity has led to the current sense of nonproductivity of work in this area and that, without refinements in human sleep recording and scoring, further work is unlikely to resolve the question. For the interested reader Herman *et al.* (1978) provide a thorough discussion and also emphasize the possible role of experimenter bias in recording non-REM sleep mentation.

Our definition of a dream is "a mental experience in sleep always characterized by hallucinoid visual imagery and usually by the experience of sensations in other sensory systems and by motor activity. The experience is delusionally accepted as real." In contrast to the vivid visual imagery and other sensory experiences in dreams, mentation during synchronized sleep is characteristically that of rambling, obsessive, and purely verbal ruminations.

13.3.1. The Neurobiologically Based Dream Theory of Sigmund Freud

The thesis of this section is that the theoretical constructs central to Freud's psychoanalytic dream theory, and indeed to psychoanalytic theory in general, were born from a marriage of the neurobiological concepts of the 1890s to the clinical phenomena observed by Freud. The theoretical model adopted by Freud may have been a reasonable one for that neurobiological era. However, it is important to appreciate that both the roots of dream theory in particular and psychoanalytic theory in general lie in now-antique biology: Freud, at the time of writing his dream theory, was working without the advantage of knowing of the existence of REM sleep and its correspondence with dreaming. Another characteristic of dreaming and REM sleep was also unknown to Freud, namely, that long-term memory storage is turned off during REM sleep and that dream recall depends on being awakened. Thus, there is a consequent need to effect a major theoretical reconstruction consonant with modern neurobiology. Otherwise, psychoanalytic theory is in danger of becoming an ineffectual and sterile hermeneutics of psychopathology. Since the first appearances of this kind of critique of psychoanalytic dream theory (see McCarley and Hobson, 1977; Sulloway, 1979, for reviews), there has been a gradual appreciation of the merits of the union of psychiatry and modern neurobiology, an effort toward which this chapter is directed.

How did Freud come to the development of psychoanalytic theory in general and dream theory in particular? Freud spent most of his early career in neurobiology (Jones, 1959; Amacher, 1965). From age 20 in 1876 to age 26 he worked at the University Physiological Institute in Vienna, doing research in histology and completing his M.D. He then did neuropathology in a hospital and in a private practice setting and was sufficiently versed in brain sciences to author an encyclopedia article on the brain (Freud, 1888) and, at age 35 in 1891, to write a book on aphasia (Freud, 1891). Even though developing interests in hypnosis and hysteria, he remained in the Viennese tradition of *Nervenartz* through the critical summer of 1895, when most of his *Project for a Scientific Psychology* (Freud, 1895) was written. It is the *Project*, as we shall refer to it, that most clearly reveals the links between psychoanalysis and the neurobiology of the 1890s.* It was this same summer that Freud tells us he developed the central

---

*It may be useful to review briefly the scientific climate of the 1890s. There are parallels between the great explosion of knowledge occurring in the field of neurobiology today and in the 1890s. In 1889 Santiago Ramon y Cajal made a victorious anabasis to Berlin where he presented to the leading scientists of the German-speaking world his dogma that the brain is composed of individual cells that are separated from each other and that the brain is not a reticulum or net as Golgi and others had believed (Ramon y Cajal, 1901–1917). Cajal's exquisite materials persuaded even the mighty

ideas of *The Interpretation of Dreams* (Freud, 1900a,b, 1887–1902), the foundation of much of psychoanalytic theory and even of many contemporary popular concepts of the meaning of dreams. These works were intertwined in temporal contiguity, in the free interchange of ideas between the *Project* and *The Interpretation of Dreams*, and by the pivotal appearance of the Irma dream in both. Freud himself remarked that the secret of dream interpretation was his after July 24, 1895, the night of the Irma dream, the first dream to be interpreted by the principles of the new psychoanalytic theory.

Freud left no doubt at what he wished to accomplish in the *Project*. "The intention is to furnish a psychology that shall be a natural science," and his mental model was formed to be consonant with, and was molded by, the neurobiology of the 1890s. We are not alone in seeing hidden neurobiology as forming the core of much of later psychoanalytic theory. Strachey, the translator and editor of the standard edition of Freud's works in English, affirms that "the *Project*, or rather its invisible ghost, haunts the whole series of Freud's theoretical writings to the very end" (Strachey, 1966), and the psychoanalytic theoretician Holt agrees that "hidden biological assumptions were retained in the construction of a psychological model" (Holt, 1965). For the reader whose introduction to Freud is through the clinically oriented papers, it is a great shock and revelation to read the *Project* since the embryos of most of Freud's major theoretical concepts are to be found here. Twenty years of concepts elaborated in clinical papers are collapsed into a few lines, and, to add to the sense of wonder, they appear in a physiological paper. For the modern neuroscientist the astonishment is of a different sort. So many of Freud's 1890 ideas about the brain are now known to be simply and fundamentally wrong. The reader acquainted with psychoanalytic theory will appreciate the irony of the disguise of hidden biological assumptions in the "manifest content" of psychoanalysis. Freud himself in his later career wanted the *Project* manuscript burned, but it was preserved and published posthumously.

Both Freud and other theorists of his day* believed in direct, simple corre-

---

Kölliker, and the Germanic establishment gave the final stamp of accord in 1891 when Waldeyer spoke favorably of the "neuron theory." The study of cells and neurons was what was new and exciting, even though knowledge of pathways and functional localization was also quite advanced and certainly beyond that of most of today's first-year medical students. Freud himself had a certain fame as the neurologist whose powers of lesion localization were so sure that a pathological report was superfluous. Compared with the neuroanatomy, the neurophysiology of the 1890s was not so far advanced, and we shall see that misconceptions in that area were to bedevil Freud's theory. At that time the precise role of electrical forces in nerve cells was unknown, although the knowledge of electrical changes associated with reflex conduction had made it apparent that electrical phenomena were important. It was Freud's misfortune to develop his theory of neuronal discharge and of the energy economy of the brain at this point of physiological uncertainty about the electrical and functional aspects of neurons.

*Biologists of that era shared a sense of excitement with other disciplines. Old dogmas were failing, new edifices were being erected—in politics, the arts, biology, and physics. In biology, vitalism was being crushed by the new armamentarium of chemistry and physics. Biologists of Freud's generation were marked by two traits. First, they were loath to be mystical in any way; hard-nosed materialism and the scientific method was their credo and their weapon against the still lingering forces of vitalism. Yet they also had an audacity, an abundance of hope and faith in the new scientific method, and the excitement of believing themselves on the verge of being scientifically able to describe that most difficult and elusive object of all, the human mind. An extremely valuable source of information about the state of physiological and anatomic knowledge in Vienna in the

spondences between brain and mental events, and thus it is not surprising to find the *Project* and *The Interpretation of Dreams* replete with examples of these simple correspondences. Our exposition summarizes the major features of Freud's neural model of the *Project* and their links with his model of the mind, i.e., psychoanalytic theory. During this discussion the reader will find it useful to refer to a sketch of Freud's model of the nervous system in the *Project* (Fig. 9) and a summary of the correspondences between his physiological and psychological models (Table 2). The major features of Freud's model follow.

(1) *The brain and mind were conceptualized as passive entities with all energy coming from outside sources.* In 1895 the histological basis of the neuron doctrine had been accepted, and there was knowledge of simple reflex activity, but unfortunately for the accuracy of Freud's neural model, the exact mode of functioning of neurons was unclear. Perhaps it was to avoid "vitalistic" notions that Freud in the *Project* conceptualized neurons as passive transmitters and reservoirs of energy derived from outside the brain, shown in Fig. 9 as originating in somatic, instinctual sources such as hunger and sex. Neurons, as passive energy reservoirs, were able to be filled or "cathected" (*Besetzung*) with greater or lesser amounts of energy, what Freud terms "nervous quantity," and passed this energy on to other neurons in graded amounts, thus functioning as power reservoirs instead of the signal transducers of modern theory. When Freud speaks of "discharge" of energy, it is analogous to the discharge of a capacitor. (It should not be surprising that Freud did not understand the true nature of neuronal function; even the existence of the membrane resting potential was unknown until 1910.)

(2) *The nervous system is a simple reflex system whose function is to discharge energy.* Building on knowledge of simple reflex experiments, Freud conceived the nervous system as acting so as to dissipate energy derived either from outside sources (usually of lesser importance, since a protective stimulus barrier, *Reizschutz*, was interposed) or from internal, instinctual drives, where no protective barrier was present.

1890s comes from a book by Sigmund Exner. Exner was a co-worker of Freud's in the day when both were neurobiologists (Amacher, 1965), and Exner went on to become the head of the department of physiology at the Royal University of Vienna. In scientific circles Exner was best known for his studies on reflexes and reflex conduction velocity and was cited both in textbooks (Horsley, 1892) and by Sherrington (1906). Yet Exner also wrote the book *A Sketch of a Physiological Explanation of Psychic Events* (1894). His book was published in 1894, just one year before the essence of Freud's theory of dreams was developed, and its title well conveys the audacity of that time, the soaring hope of a physiology of the mind. Exner explained what he wanted to do in the introduction to the book, which was, appropriately for one speaking in both physiological and psychological tongues, completed on Pentecostal Sunday. With an eye on the vitalism of the past he wrote, "A path has been broken toward [the] conviction that life processes can be explained on the basis of chemical and physical processes. . ." Looking toward the present and future and in a striking parallel to Freud's ambition, he noted that "the attempt to explain psychic events forms my assignment in life." As well as letting us see what was hoped for (the union of physiology and psychology), the book is most valuable from a documentary point of view because it allows us to scan the kind of physiological data and theory present in Vienna just before Freud's *The Interpretation of Dreams*. Exner committed himself to the neuron theory and even went so far as to postulate that inhibition was an active mechanism served by its own neural pathways (1894, p. 306; see also McCarley, 1983). This important but subtle concept of active inhibitory pathways is one that was not posited by many early neural theorists, including Freud. Exner's book may well have served as a stimulus for Freud's own attempts at a mind–body integration by combining his neurobiological training with his newly developing interest in the psyche.

(3) *Preeminence of somatic instinctual drives and conflicts associated with their discharge.* In Freud's simple reflex model conflict arose when somatic instincts raised the energy level (*Quantität nervös, Qn*) of the nervous system and this energy could not be discharged through motoric activity because of social conventions or family sanctions. This high level of energy in the psychic system (ψ in Fig. 9) was perceived as pain (unpleasure) by the conscious sensing system, and the energy (and the consequent unpleasure) remained until discharged. Of particular importance was that the "executive" aspect of the nervous system (the ego) derived its energy from internal instinctual sources and so was subject to contamination and corruption arising from the instinctual drives. A final feature of Freud's nervous system was the absence of inhibitory neurons. Perhaps because Freud conceived of neurons as transmitters and receivers of instinctual energy (something like a power network) rather than as signal transducers and transformers, he had difficulty conceiving of inhibition of neuronal activity; in

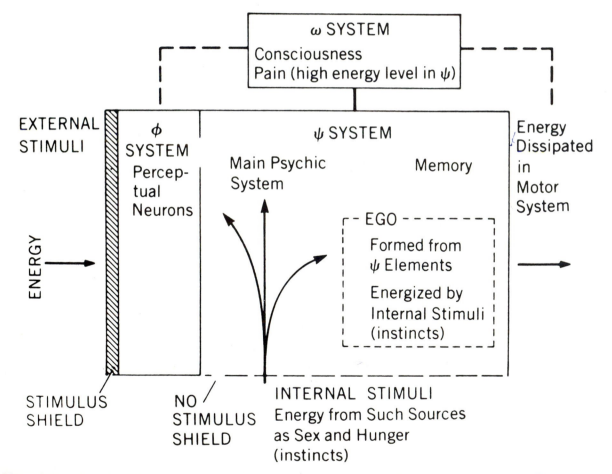

Figure 9. Freud's model of the nervous system in the *Project for a Scientific Psychology.* In Freud's model energy responsible for neural activity comes from outside the brain, especially from instincts; neurons and the brain are not autoch thonously active. The brain functions as a reflex system seeking to rid itself of excessive energy by dissipation in motoric discharge. See text for description. From McCarley and Hobson, 1977.

Table 2. Correspondences between Freud's Dream Theory and the Neuronal Model of the Project

Dream process	Neuronal process
Generator of a dream is a wish whose energy is derived from a somatic drive.	All neuronal energy comes from outside the brain, mainly from somatic sources, since these have no barrier to entry (*Reizschutz*).
Dream process is a reaction to events outside the CNS, i.e., the combination of day residue with an instinctual wish	There is no autochthonous energy source or regulatory capacities for neurons. They are the passive recipients of energy. No concept of CNS oscillators.
Regression of psychic energy after censor blocks access to consciousness.	Flow of nervous energy is reversed toward perceptual side of nervous system.
Dream work, dream hallucinations. Dream guards sleep by disguising wish.	Mechanism is overly strong cathexsis of mnemic neurons near perceptual side of nervous system. The nervous energy travels pathways toward mnemic elements associatively related to wish, and these furnish the disguised representation of the wish.
Dream forgetting is from repression.	Repression blocks access into consciousness by "inhibitory side cathexes." No concept of state-dependent absence of memory storage.

his model once instinctual energy was introduced into the brain, it remained forever until discharged. In order to divert this energy from immediate discharge Freud proposed that the ego used what he termed "inhibiting side cathexes," a process bearing no relationship to modern neurophysiological concepts of inhibition (see Fig. 10). It is of interest that the familiar psychoanalytic terms "inhibiting ego," cathexis (meaning charging of a neuron with energy), repression, ego, primary and secondary process thinking, and hallucinatory wish fulfillment are all present in the neural model of the *Project*.

13.3.1.1. Freud's Dream Model: Dream Features Result from Disguise of a Forbidden Wish

The seventh and most theoretical chapter of Freud's magnum opus, *The Interpretation of Dreams,* outlined what Freud described as a psychological model of the psychic apparatus (Fig. 11). In fact, it is virtually the same model as the brain model of the *Project* as is indicated in Table 2 and by comparison with Figure 10. The "psychological model" of Fig. 11 has the same perceptual system as the *Project,* although the symbol φ is not used. As in the *Project,* excitation from perceptual neurons flows into a main psychic system. The psychic system of *The Interpretation of Dreams* includes three subsystems: mnemic elements; the unconscious, to be thought of as those psychic elements in contact with instincts and not open to the conscious system (the unconscious elements are described in Freud's text but are not included in his sketch in Fig. 11); and, finally, the preconscious, composed of those psychic elements in close apposition to consciousness.

Freud did not include the "psychic censor" in the sketch of Fig. 11, but in his text description of psychic topography, Freud placed its elements between the

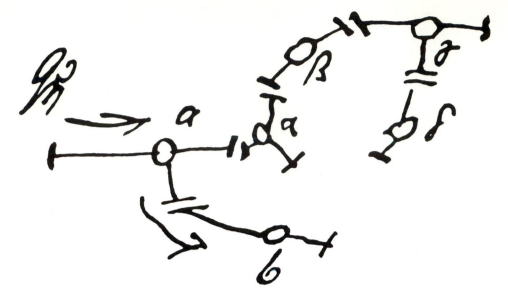

Figure 10. Freud's sketch of neurons and the flow of neural energy in the *Project* (1895). This sketch illustrates Freud's concept of diversion of neural energy through a "side-cathexis." The normal flow of energy (arrow labeled Qn in Freud's script at left) is from neuron *a* to neuron *b*. Freud postulated that a side-cathexis of neuron α would attract the Qn and divert the flow from neuron *b*. Freud believed this postsynaptic attraction of energy or side-cathexis (for which there is no experimental support) to be the neuronal mechanism underlying repression of forbidden wishes in both dreaming and waking. From Freud (1895).

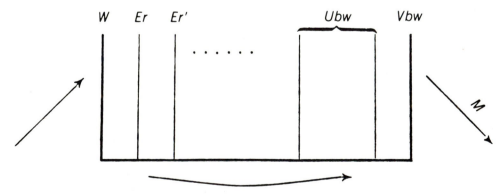

Figure 11. Freud's model of the psyche as applied to dreaming, from the seventh chapter of *The Interpretation of Dreams* (Freud, 1900a,b). W is the German abbreviation for the perceptual system (compare with φ system in Fig. 9). The constituents of the main or psychic system (not labeled as such in the original figure, but comparable to the ψ system of Fig. 9 are: *Er*, memory; *Ubw*, unconscious; and *Vbw*, preconscious. *M* indicates the motor system (as in Fig. 9). The arrows indicate the normal direction of energy flow. Although Freud did not include as much detail in this drawing, the full model outlined in his text is virtually identical to the brain model of the *Project* sketched in Fig. 9. From Freud (1900a).

unconscious and preconscious; the psychic censor acts to screen and block wishes unacceptable to consciousness. The psychic censor is conceptually derived from the set of neurons in the *Project* that were responsible for repression.

The outline of Freud's dream theory is straightforward. The ego wishes to sleep (the causal basis for this wish is not clear); it withdraws its cathexes from the motor system, resulting in sleep paralysis. The dream process begins when something in the day's experience stirs up a repressed wish in the unconscious. The "day's residue" and the repressed wish pair forces and seek to move in the usual direction of flow in Freud's model (see arrow in Fig. 11) toward the preconscious system. Entry of the undisguised wish is blocked by the censor, and there is a regressive movement of the "currents of excitation" toward the mnemic elements of the psyche, which, as in the model of the *Project,* are close to the perceptual side of the psychic apparatus. It is among the mnemic elements that the "dream's work" of condensation, displacement and symbol formation takes place; there is a disguise of the wish by the imagery of those mnemic elements with the strongest associative links to the wish. The disguised wish thus becomes acceptable to the censor and is passed into consciousness. Freud believed that the dream functioned as a guardian of sleep by preventing the intrusion of undisguised and unacceptable wishes into the conscious system, since their undisguised presence would lead to awakening.

As for dream phenomena, Freud concentrated on the symbolic grammar employed and focused his interpretive powers on unraveling the psychic meaning of symbols and the thematic material of dreams. He paid relatively little attention in *The Interpretation of Dreams* to the formal sensory, temporal, and intensity attributes of the dream but did note that the psychic or subjective intensity of a dream image reflected the underlying intensity of the wish (its charge) and the number of excitations condensed into a single symbol or wish. He suggested that the frequent subjective sense in dreams of little or no movement was related to the sensing of sleep paralysis. Most importantly, Freud asserted that the forgetting of dreams is "inexplicable unless the power of the psychic censorship is taken into account," i.e., we forget our dreams because of psychic repression. Freud saw in the forgetting of dreams the prime support for his "wish fulfillment–disguise" theory of dream generation.

Freud's psychic model for dream generation was thus quite directly derived from the physiological constructs of the *Project.* The psychic and neural agencies are virtually the same, their organizational sequence and function are the same, the direction of flow of energy is the same, and the reflex model is retained. The psychic "elements" share the properties of the *Project's* "neurons" in that "excitation" is "transmitted" according to "conductive resistance." "Association" results from "facilitating paths." Freud even talked about "currents of excitation." In short, virtually the entire neural theory of the *Project* was retained despite Freud's assertion that he was creating a psychological model.

13.3.1.2. Implications of the "Disguised Neurobiology" for Revisions of Psychoanalytic Theory

Had Freud and later workers maintained the links between psychoanalytic theory and neuroscience so boldly forged in the *Project,* then as advances in neuroscience rendered the assumptions of the *Project* invalid, revisions in the corresponding elements of psychoanalytic theory would have followed as a matter of course. It is unfortunate that this did not occur, since the split between psychoanalysis and biology would have been avoided, and there would have been a continuing reinvigoration of psychoanalytic theory. As to what changes should be made in psychoanalytic theory, we here suggest only the most salient components. One important alteration should be in the role allotted to instincts in behavior and cognitive processes. Classical psychoanalytic theory (and some interpretative practice) sees behavior and thought largely constructed from instinctual energy sources and their "derivatives," i.e., from "defenses" against the open expression and/or conscious awareness of instincts. In fact, the neurons involved in cognitive processes do not derive their "energy" from instincts but are autochthonously active, and the notion that defensive derivatives of instincts are the prime source of behavior is not supportable.

The behavioral and thought disturbances of major mental illness (such as schizophrenia, manic–depressive disorder, and autism) arise from disrupted brain processing rather than from the operation of maladaptive "primitive defenses" of psychogenic origin, as some psychoanalytic theoreticians have suggested. The notion of "sexual instinct" should be enlarged to include a neural basis for most of sexual behavior and to acknowledge that sexual instincts are much more complex than the *Project*'s simple notion of "sexual energy" seeking release. Finally, even the jewel in the crown of psychoanalytic theory, the interpretation of dreams as deriving their dreamlike characteristics as a direct consequence of the disguise of forbidden wishes (defensive derivatives), must yield to modern data. The biological state of REM sleep and its psychological counterpart of dreaming result from the rhythmic operation of a brain oscillator that internally and periodically activates brain in such a way as to produce the characteristic features of REM sleep and the distinctive formal characteristics of dreams. The forgetting of dreams is not from repression but is a state-dependent attribute of the systems involved in long-term memory storage.

13.3.2. The Form of Dreams and the Biology of Sleep

This section discusses the extent to which correspondences may be found between REM-sleep physiology and formal features of dreaming. The "activation–synthesis hypothesis" suggests that many formal features of dreaming correspond with the kind of brain activation during REM sleep (Hobson and McCarley, 1977; McCarley and Hoffman, 1981; Hobson, 1988). Inevitably in discussing mental and brain activity the question arises of how to conceptualize their relationship. As discussed in more detail elsewhere (McCarley and Hobson, 1979; McCarley, 1981, 1983), we view the proper strategy as seeking areas of contact between the conceptualizations of physiological and psychological theory, seeking possible isomorphisms between operations and objects in the two conceptual systems of mind and brain. Isomorphism literally means "of the same form," and its use is drawn from mathematics where it indicates correspondences between different algebraic systems, each composed of objects and operations on those objects. We do not assert the primacy of either mental or brain domain or that events in one domain cause events in the other, simply that they represent different conceptualizations, are isomorphic to one another. A simple example of isomorphic systems is Euclidian plane geometry, which is isomorphic with the domain of ordered pairs of numbers (Cartesian geometry). Neither system is said to "cause" the other or to be more fundamental.

The activation–synthesis model can be simply summarized. During the REM-sleep state, sensory input from the external world is restricted, but the brain is activated internally by neural activity originating in the brainstem oscillator. (It is an important parenthetical remark that this activity, unlike that of Freud's model, is "motivationally neutral," not a drive derivative but the turning on of a neural oscillator unrelated to sexual or aggressive instincts.) Both sensory and motor systems are activated, and the sensations and the feedback from neuronal command signals for muscular activity play preeminent roles in the construction of the dream experience. The generation of successive dream plots is temporally isomorphic with the successive phasic sequences of activity of brainstem neurons and the consequent activation of different motor pattern generators and sensory systems. The synthetic aspects of dream formation are the knitting together of these often disparate elements, and the resulting combinations of incongruous elements cause some of the bizarreness of the dream experience. This theory focuses on the universal, formal aspects of the dram, on the automatic generation of particular types of brain activity by the REM-sleep oscillator, and does not attempt to account for the mechanisms of synthesis other than to state that the brain seeks to knit together the internally generated stimuli in REM sleep in the same manner as it does external stimuli during waking. In the next section the correspondences between dream activity and REM-sleep physiology are discussed for various systems. Dream reports obtained from REM-sleep awakenings will illustrate the subjective experience.

13.3.2.1. Visual System: Dream Report

> Walking along, I came upon a rainbow. I don't remember if I was alone or not. But the rainbow was three dimensional and it touched earth. The rainbow was three dimensional so I took off on the rainbow just like I would a beanstalk. I continued along the steps, which I can describe to be like layer cake of different colors in the shape of steps. Little action except there were two couplets spoken. The one spoken by myself, "What am I doing down here?" And the reply, "Come back tomorrow." It's a very existential dream (McCarley and Hoffman, 1981).

Visual system activation during REM sleep is shown in depth EEG recordings in the cat by the presence of PGO waves in the pontine reticular formation near the abducens nucleus, in the dorsal lateral geniculate nucleus, and the occipital (visual) cortex. PGO waves originate in pons and project to lateral geniculate (and other thalamic nuclei) and to occipital cortex (see Chapter 9). The PGO waves herald the onset of REM sleep, occurring in the minute or so before onset of electrographically defined REM sleep (see Fig. 3 in Chapter 1). They are an excellent example of the brainstem providing nonrandom excitation of the forebrain during REM sleep. PGO waves carry information to the lateral geniculate nucleus and the visual cortex on the direction of the rapid eye movement (REM) that will begin a few milliseconds after the onset of the PGO wave.

As discussed in Chapters 9 and 11, cellular recordings have provided important information on PGO wave generation, transmission, and effects at target sites. Neuronal recordings indicate that REM-sleep PGO waves are accompanied by excitation of LGN principal cells (relay neurons), perigeniculate neurons, and neurons in occipital and association cortex (Bizzi, 1966; McCarley and Hobson, 1970; McCarley *et al.*, 1983; Steriade, 1978; Steriade *et al.*, 1989d). Furthermore, autoradiographic studies using the 2-deoxyglucose technique have demonstrated powerful increases in glucose metabolism during REM sleep in visual cortex, presumably as a consequence of intense neuronal activation (Hubel and Livingstone, 1980; Livingstone and Hubel, 1981). This input to visual system may be a substrate for dream visual experience construction. One kind of information transmitted to the visual system may be movement-related information. Because the PGO waves predict the direction of the upcoming eye movement, it has been hypothesized that they may represent a REM-sleep activation of the corollary discharge system for eye movements, whereby the rest of the brain is alerted to the impending eye movement (McCarley, 1980a; McCarley and Hobson, 1979; McCarley and Hoffman, 1981). In waking the corollary discharge system tells the rest of the brain to counteract the change in retinal input attendant on the eye movement with an equal-magnitude but directionally opposite compensation in subjective visual world. Since input from the external world is blocked in REM sleep, this corollary discharge compensation is itself perceived as movement of the visual world. This may constitute the source of (some of) the visual imagery changes of REM sleep.

The postulated sequence is:

Activation of rapid eye movement system (saccades, primarily horizontal)	→	Activation of corollary discharge system	→	Subjective perception of visual movement	→	Incorporation of visual movement into dream

That activation of the corollary discharge system without an actual eye movement or visual world alteration leads to a subjective (and illusory) sense of movement has been demonstrated in experiments in (waking) humans in whom a transient paralysis of eye movement has been induced.* Evaluations of the extensive dream set of one individual (Hobson, 1988) found evidence for many "looplike" sequences of dream gaze, corresponding to the frequent occurrence of this eye movement pattern in REM sleep (see Chapter 9).

In addition to the corollary discharge system, other visual system elements are also likely activated during REM sleep, although there are no data on the precise type of visual system neurons activated in REM sleep. Since the visual

---

*One may ask if the pre-REM sleep PGO waves, which occur without eye movement, may also represent activity in the eye-movement-related corollary discharge system. We suggest they may. Corollary discharge activity may occur in the presence of commands in the saccade-generating system for movements that do not get executed because of the as-yet-incomplete pre-REM sleep activation of oculomotor system motoneurons or other elements near the output side of the system. We note also that the mesopontine neurons that transfer PGO waves to thalamus (Chapter 9) may be excited by input other than from the saccade-related system, although input from this system appears to predominate during REM.

system is characterized by parallel processing of different aspects of visual information, such as for color, form, movement, etc., one may speculate that the systems underlying these particular aspects of information processing could be separately activated in REM sleep. The REM sleep dream introducing this section would suggest the activation of the color perception subsystem.

13.3.2.2. Activation of Other Sensory Systems in REM Sleep and Representation in Dreams: Dream Report

> I was spinning, my body was spinning around. The circus performers put the bit in their horses, and they spin around. The trapeze was spinning like that. Hands at my sides and yet there was nothing touching me. I was as nature made me, and I was revolving at 45 rpm record [speed]. Had a big hole in the center of my head. Spinning, spinning, and spinning. And at the same time, orbiting. Orbiting what, I don't know. I'd stop for a second, stop this orbit and spinning (McCarley and Hoffman, 1981).

This REM-sleep dream clearly suggests activation of the vestibular system and serves to introduce the topic of activation of other sensory systems in REM sleep and their presence in REM dream experiences. Figure 12 (from McCarley and Hoffman, 1981) tallies the percentages of dreams with the presence of various sensations as determined by explicit mention of the sensation in the dream report. The isomorphism postulate suggests that the intensity of physiological activation should parallel the order of subjective intensity as described in the figure. Although physiological data are not sufficiently complete for a complete test of this postulate, the available data show certain correspondences to be striking: all dreams are visual, and the degree and extent of REM-sleep visual system activation is indeed intense, as has been described above. Auditory system activation remains to be investigated at the cellular level, but the presence of the

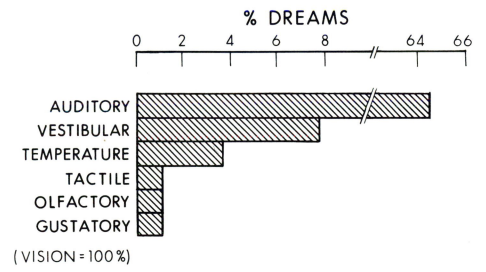

Figure 12. Frequency of sensory system reports in REM sleep dreams, scored for explicit mention of relevant sensation (96% concordance between scorers). Note that about 8% of dreams have "vestibular" sensations, defined as (1) rapid and extreme displacements of the body in space, such as spinning, sinking, going on a roller coaster or merry-go-round, and (2) floating in space, "I was just floating over the steps." From McCarley and Hoffman (1981).

phasic event of middle ear muscle activity (MEMA) suggests it is intense (Pessah and Roffwarg, 1972). It is also known that the PPT zone involved in production of LGN PGO waves also projects to the medial geniculate nucleus, and this projection may be related to auditory system activation. Of particular note in Fig. 12 is the relatively high percentage of dreams scored as having "vestibular" sensation. The vestibular system functions to sense the position of the body in space and changes in position. Consequently, in this REM-sleep dream sample, dreams were scored as having "vestibular" sensation if they included flying, floating, falling, and other rapid displacements of the body in space, such as the dream report cited above. This sensation is noteworthy because these dream experiences were not part of the everyday experience, past or present, of the student subjects whose dream reports were scored. Rather, they likely reflect the subjective aspect of physiological data from extracellular unit recordings indicating vestibular system activation during REM sleep (Bizzi *et al.*, 1964).

Finally, the absence of reports of pain in dreams in this sample was notable; other researchers also found a dearth of dream reports of pain, even in those subjects with chronic, severe pain during the day (Arkin *et al.*, 1975). This suggests that the neurophysiological systems underlying pain are not active in REM sleep, and, further, the absence of dreamed pain in those with constant daytime pain is one of the more persuasive arguments that dreams represent a separate biological state and are not merely transformations of daytime experiences.

13.3.2.3. Motor System Activity in Dreams and in REM Sleep

This topic and the correspondence of subjective and physiological aspects of motor activation are well illustrated by dream content that was accompanied by isomorphic and overt motor activity in a case of *REM-sleep behavioral disorder* (Schenck *et al.*, 1986).

> I was a halfback playing football, and after the quarterback received the ball from the center he lateraled it sideways to me and I'm supposed to go around end and cut back over tackle and—this is very vivid—as I cut back over tackle there is this big 280-pound tackle waiting, so I, according to football rules, was to give him my shoulder and bounce him out of the way. . . . [Upon abrupt awakening:] When I came to I was standing in front of our dresser and I had [gotten up out of bed and run and] knocked lamps, mirrors and everything off the dresser, hit my head against the wall and my knee against the dresser (dream report transcription by McCarley from a patient reported in Schenck *et al.*, 1986).

In the dream the dreamer fully experienced the sensation of motion while running and had very clear vision, but there was no awareness of sound until he knocked objects off the dresser and awakened to the crash. Subsequent polysomnography showed these "physically moving dreams," as the dreamer described them, occurred in REM sleep. Figure 13 shows the polygraphic record of another case of REM-sleep behavioral disorder.

The important principles underlying both normal and abnormal REM sleep and dreaming as illustrated by this and other cases (Salva and Guilleminault, 1986) of REM-sleep behavioral disorder can be summarized as follows:

1. The motor system is activated during REM sleep, and commands for complex behaviors are given that are isomorphic with the dream experience.

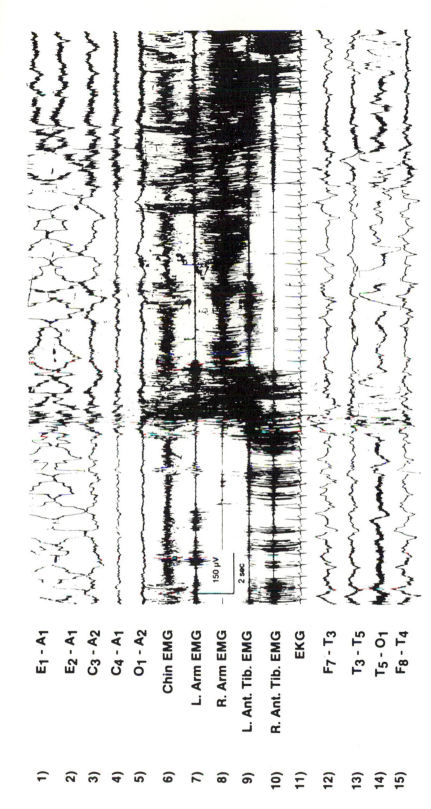

Figure 13. Polygraphic record of a patient with REM-sleep behavior disorder and movements during REM sleep. Polygraphic record is of REM sleep; note the presence of out-of-phase high-amplitude activity in EOG channels (1–2) indicating conjugate rapid eye movements and the presence of a low-voltage fast (activated) EEG (3–5, 12–15). The EKG (11) shows a constant rate of 65 beats/min, consistent with REM sleep and highly inconsistent with a normal arousal and waking. Chin EMG tone (6) is augmented with phasic increases, while arms (7–8) and legs (9–10) show aperiodic bursts of intense EMG activity that accompanied the overt behaviors noted by the technician. This sequence ends with a spontaneous awakening (note end of conjugate EOG activity in last 5 sec of record). The patient reported a dream of running down a hill in Duluth, MN, taking shortcuts through backyards, and in an abrupt scene shift, suddenly finding himself on a barge that is rocking back and forth. He feels haunted and desperately reaches about to hold onto anything he can grasp to prevent the barge's rocking making him fall into the cargo hold, which is full of skeletons. He awakens at this point in the dream. Videotape of behavior while in REM sleep showed arm movements consistent with this last dream scene. Modified from Mahowald and Schenck (1989).

2. Ordinarily the commands for motor activity are not executed because of a powerful inhibition of the motoneurons directly innervating musculature. However, in this pathological syndrome, this inhibition has been destroyed, much as was done in experimental lesions in animals in Jouvet's and Morrison's laboratories (Jouvet and Delorme, 1965; Sastre and Jouvet, 1979; Jouvet, 1979; Morrison, 1979; Hendricks *et al.*, 1982; see muscle atonia system discussion in Chapter 10).

We now discuss these issues in more detail. First of all, the case reported here and the other described provide strong support for the postulate of isomorphism between subjective dream experience and REM-sleep physiology: the dreamed motor activity directly paralleled the commands for motor activity, which were executed in this pathological case. The second point has to do with how the motor system is activated in REM sleep; extracellular recordings have shown that both motor cortex and subcortical, including brainstem, motor areas are activated during REM sleep (see reviews in McCarley and Hobson, 1979; Steriade and Hobson, 1976; Hobson and Steriade, 1986). This case suggests that the motor system activation in REM sleep is comprised of commands for organized, coherent motor acts, as during waking, rather than, for example, a jumble of commands with consequent random excitation of antagonistic muscles.

The third point has to do with the mode of origination of subjective motor experience in dreams; the above data suggest that the commands for muscle activity are incorporated into the dreams; that is, the "acts are dreamed out" rather than the "dream is acted out." Basically this argument rests on the fact that brainstem-commanded motor activity (eye movements, MEMA, somatic muscle twitches) is present during REM sleep in animals even when the forebrain is totally absent; since forebrain is necessary for conscious experience (including dream experience), one must conclude that REM-sleep phenomena in brainstem intrinsically involve motor system activation. Physiological studies have shown that many of the "routine" motor acts, such as walking and running, involve the activation of lower centers, which then direct the coordinated sequence of muscle activity necessary for the performance of the motor act (for a recent review, see Cohen *et al.*, 1988). For example, there is a brainstem "stepping generator" whose activation, even by electrical stimulation, leads to stepping and whose more intense activation leads to running. It is hypothesized that REM-sleep activation of these centers for repetitive, stereotyped motor acts leads to the corresponding presence of the corresponding subjective experience in dreams. This subjective experience may enter by action of the "corollary" discharge system: as with the oculomotor system, when somatomotor activity is commanded, in addition to the neuronal discharge acting to effect the motor act, there is a "corollary" discharge that acts to inform the rest of the brain of the upcoming movement, so that the brain will interpret the movement as "self-initiated" and not externally imposed. This corollary discharge is of equal magnitude but opposite in direction so that it will "cancel" the perception of the self-initiated movement.

As proposed by McCarley and Hobson (1979), the hypothesis is that motor system activation in REM sleep leads to corollary discharge, which is subjectively perceived as movement in the absence of the execution of movement as in REM sleep (or in the absence of sensory feedback from the movement in the case of

REM sleep without atonia, sensory input is curtailed in REM sleep). This subjective perception is then incorporated into the dream experience.

This sequence may be summarized:

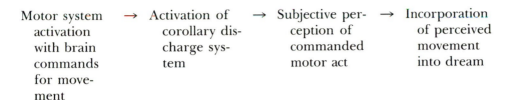

Motor system activation with brain commands for movement → Activation of corollary discharge system → Subjective perception of commanded motor act → Incorporation of perceived movement into dream

The hypothesis of isomorphism would predict, given the high level of motor system activation, that there would also be an equally high level of dreamed motor activity. Figure 14 (from McCarley and Hoffman, 1981) shows that indeed there is a very high percentage of dreams with motor activity; lower extremity movement was tallied because it was a variable with high scoring reliability. Overall, 37% of all dream verbs were those expressing lower extremity movement.

In closing this section we wish to emphasize how closely the human syndrome of "REM-sleep behavior disorder" (see discussion in Mahowald and Schenck, 1989) resembles that of "REM sleep without atonia" in cats, and indeed the knowledge of the animal syndrome led to understanding of the human symptoms and to a prediction of the type of lesion that would be found (McCarley, 1989). Of course, final demonstration of the similarity of these syndromes awaits demonstration that the human lesion sites overlap those of the experimental

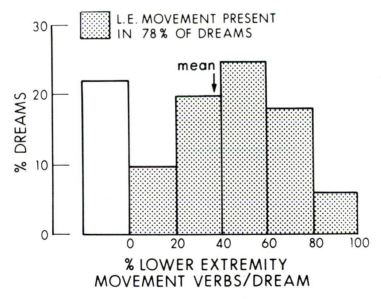

Figure 14. REM-sleep dreams with reports of lower extremity motor activity. Lower extremity motor activity is common in dream reports, being present in 78.8% of all dreams, and with 36.8 of all dream report verbs being verbs that express lower extremity movement. From McCarley and Hoffman (1981).

animals. Morrison (1979) has presented evidence that, in animals, experimental lesions in some locations along the tegmentoreticular pathway not only disrupt the atonia of REM sleep but may also favor increased motor activity in waking and, for some lesion locations, may promote aggressive behavior in waking. Neither of these phenomena has been present in waking in the human cases thus far described, but an increase in aggression in dreams of some patients may be present (see Mahowald and Schenck, 1989).

13.3.2.4. Dream Bizarreness

Dream bizarreness is a distinctive formal property of dreams; in dreams impossible events may occur—the dreamer flies or talks with persons dead or fictional, and in the scenery rocks may float on water. Added to this unusual set of dramatis personae and scenery of dreams is a striking fluidity; there are frequent and sudden transformations of persons and even of the entire dream world, a kind of bizarreness described as "scene shifts" (McCarley and Hoffman, 1981). Judged by the presence of bizarreness in the categories of inanimate environment, animate characters, and transformations, such as scene shifts, about two-thirds of dreams contain at least one bizarre element, with scene shifts being the most frequent and present in 37% of REM-sleep dreams (McCarley and Hoffman, 1981). The brief dream summary in the caption of Fig. 13 contains a scene shift, as does the following dream report, which combines the bizarre with the banal activity of walking (cf. previous section):

> The first part of the dream: I was an investigator policeman, and we were looking for vampires . . . so the very first place I walk into was a john, must have been some public building. I walk in and there is a man on the wall with a stick going up through his chin. I turned around and walked out the door and turned around and said to whoever I was with, "Who's been in here?" So I walked back in again and he was definitely dead. Then I heard something in one of the stalls, the toilet stalls. So I walk around, but just as I was getting ready to look down through the top of it, this lady bites this man in the neck. They both drop dead right there. Blood flowing freely. . . Then the dream changed sort of. I was walking along some street. . . There were four little people yelling out, each was trying to decide which one sounded the most serious. Which to help first. Then the one up in the fourth room started climbing out the window. Then the dream changed. I was a door-to-door salesman of some books or something . . . this car pulls up and started following me along the street and I thought to myself, "They're trying to sell books too." I'm doing all the work peddling doors while they just drive along and make a sale (McCarley and Hoffman, 1981).

In contrast to the psychoanalytic suggestion that dream bizarreness is inserted to disguise forbidden wishes, the activation–synthesis hypothesis suggests that bizarreness occurs as a concomitant of the physiology of the REM state. In this state there is a different mode of brain activation—internal instead of external, as in waking—and there is simultaneous activation of many brain sensory and motor systems not ordinarily activated together in waking; both often occur with an extremely high degree of intensity. The synthesis of these brain events may proceed as in waking, but bizarreness may result from the attempt to knit together the often contradictory and incongruent elements. Dream scene shifts may be a concomitant of the runs of phasic activity that characterize REM sleep; each sequence of phasic activity may activate different motor and sensory elements, which are interpreted as a scene shift.

In this section emphasis has been placed on the nonforebrain elements of dream generation, since the prime "dream generator" is the REM-sleep oscillator, and the essential elements of REM sleep are present without the forebrain. Nonetheless, there is no question that forebrain activity may contribute to dream formation both in the interpretation of brainstem signals and in adding to the complexity of REM-sleep activity, although there are currently no data to indicate the relative strength of this contribution.

In this regard, a comment on meaning in dreams may be useful. The activation–synthesis theory suggests that there is no intrinsic meaning to dreams. That is to say, the REM-sleep brain activation does not arise from forbidden wishes or from motivationally linked sources.* However, as in interpreting a Rorschach card, meaning may be *attributed* to a dream, since all stimuli, internally or externally generated, may be seen as meaningful in the context of individual experience. In the *attributed* meaning, motivationally relevant themes may arise. Starving men dream of food, but in an undisguised way. Similarly, sexual wishes are presented without disguise, although these and other dream elements are couched in the language of the dream, which is visual, plastic, sensory, action-rich, not verbal, obsessive, and abstract. In psychotherapy the dream is an ally, not because it disguises but because it expresses.

---

*It is probable that systems relevant to memory and drive are also directly activated by the brainstem oscillator, and, isomorphically, dream elements associated with this direct activation are likely present. However, at present, little is known about the relevant neurophysiology: this subject remains a topic for future work.

References

Adams, D. J., Smith, S. J., and Thompson, S. H., 1980, Ionic currents in molluscan soma, *Annu. Rev. Neurosci.* **3**:141–167.

Adams, D. J., Constanti, A., Brown, D. A., and Clark, R. B., 1982, Intracellular Ca^{2+} activates a fast voltage-sensitive K^+ current in vertebrate sympathetic neurones, *Nature* **296**:746–749.

Adams, R. W., Lambert, G. A., and Lance, J. W., 1988, Brainstem facilitation of electrically evoked visual response in the cat. Source, pathway and role of nicotinic receptors, *Electroencephalogr. Clin. Neurophysiol.* **69**:45–54.

Adrian, E. D., 1936, The spread of activity in the cerebral cortex, *J. Physiol. (Lond.)* **88**:127–161.

Aghajanian, G. K., 1981, The modulatory role of serotonin of multiple receptors in brain, in: *Serotonin Neurotransmission and Behavior* (B. L. Jacobs and A. Gelperin, eds.), MIT Press, Cambridge, pp. 156–185.

Aghajanian, G. K., 1985, Modulation of a transient outward current in serotonergic neurones by alpha 1 adrenoceptors, *Nature* **315**:501–503.

Aghajanian, G. K., and Lakoski, J. M., 1984, Hyperpolarization of serotonergic neurons by serotonin and LSD: Studies in brain slices showing increased K^+ conductance, *Brain Res.* **305**:1818–185.

Aghajanian, G. K., and VanderMaelen, C. P., 1982a, Intracellular recordings from serotonergic dorsal raphe neurons: Pacemaker potentials and the effect of LSD, *Brain Res.* **238**:463–469.

Aghajanian, G. K., and VanderMaelen, C. P., 1982b, Intracellular identification of central noradrenergic and serotonergic neurons by a new double labeling procedure, *J. Neurosci.* **2**:1786–1792.

Aghajanian, G. K., and Wang, E. Y., 1977, Habenular and other midbrain raphe afferents demonstrated by a modified retrograde tracing technique, *Brain Res.* **122**:229–242.

Aghajanian, G. K., Cedarbaum, J. M., and Wang, R. Y., 1977, Evidence for norepinephrine mediated collateral inhibition of locus coeruleus neurons, *Brain Res.* **136**:570–577.

Aghajanian, G. K., Wang, R. Y., and Baraban, J., 1978, Serotonergic and nonserotonergic neurons of the dorsal raphe: Reciprocal changes in firing induced by peripheral nerve stimulation, *Brain Res.* **153**:169–175.

Ahlsén, G., 1984, Brain stem neurones with differential projection to functional subregions of the dorsal lateral geniculate complex in the cat, *Neuroscience* **12**:817–838.

Ahlsén, G., Lindström, S., and Lo, F. S., 1984, Inhibition from the brain stem of inhibitory interneurones in the cat's dorsal lateral geniculate nucleus, *J. Physiol. (Lond.)* **347**:593–609.

Akerstedt, T., and Gillberg, M., 1981, The circadian variation of experimentally displaced sleep, *Sleep* **4**:159–169.

Akiskal, H. S., Rosenthal, T. L., Haykal, R. F., Lemmi, H., Rosenthal, R. H., and Scott-Strauss, A., 1980, Characterological depressions. Clinical and sleep EEG findings separating "subaffective dysthymias" from "character spectrum disorders," *Arch. Gen. Psychiatry* **37**:777–783.

Albanese, A., and Butcher, L. L., 1980, Acetylcholinesterase and catecholamine distribution in the locus coeruleus of the rat, *Brain Res. Bull.* **5**:127–124.

Albe-Fessard, D., Levante, A., and Lamour, Y., 1974, Origin of spinothalamic and spinoreticular pathways in cats and monkeys, in: *Advances in Neurology*, Vol. 4 (J. J. Bonica, ed.), Raven Press, New York, pp. 157–166.

Alley, K., Baker, R., and Simpson, J. I., 1975, Afferents to the vestibulocerebellum and the origin of the visual climbing fibers in the rabbit, *Brain Res.* **98**:582–589.

Alonso, A., and Garcia-Ausst, E., 1987a, Neuronal sources of theta rhythm in the entorhinal cortex of the rat. I. Laminar distribution of theta field potentials, *Exp. Brain Res.* **67**:493–501.

Alonso, A., and Garcia-Ausst, E., 1987b, Neuronal sources of theta rhythm in the entorhinal cortex of the rat. II. Phase relations between unit discharges and theta field potentials, *Exp. Brain Res.* **67**:502–509.

Alonso, A., and Llinás, R., 1988, Voltage-dependent calcium conductances and mammillary body neurons autorhythmicity: An *in vitro* study, *Soc. Neurosci. Abstr.* **14**:900.

Amacher, P., 1965, *Freud's Neurological Education and Its Influence on Psychoanalytic Theory, Psychological Issues*, Monograph 16, International Universities Press, New York.

Amatruda, T. T., Black, D. A., McKenna, R. M., McCarley, R. W., and Hobson, J. A., 1975, Sleep cycle control and cholinergic mechanisms: Differential effects of carbachol injections at pontine brain stem sites, *Brain Res.* **98**:501–515.

Andersen, P., and Andersson, S. A., 1968, *Physiological Basis of Alpha Rhythm*, Appleton-Century-Crofts, New York.

Andersen, P., and Curtis, D. R., 1964a, The excitation of thalamic neurones by acetylcholine, *Acta Physiol. Scand.* **61**:85–99.

Andersen, P., and Curtis, D. R., 1964b, The pharmacology of the synaptic and acetylcholine-induced excitation of ventrobasal thalamic neurones, *Acta Physiol. Scand.* **61**:100–120.

Andersen, P., and Eccles, J. C., 1962, Inhibitory phasing of neuronal discharges, *Nature* **196**:645–647.

Andersen, P., and Sears, T. A., 1964, The role of inhibition in the phasing of spontaneous thalamo-cortical discharges, *J. Physiol. (Lond.)* **173**:459–480.

Andrade, R., Malenka, R. C., and Nicoll, R. A., 1986, A G binding protein couples serotonin and GABA$_B$ receptors to the same channels in hippocampus, *Science* **243**:1261–1265.

Andrezik, J. A., Chan-Palay, V., and Palay, S., 1981a, The nucleus paragigantocellularis lateralis in the rat. Conformation and cytology, *Anat. Embryol.* **161**:355–371.

Andrezik, J. A., Chan-Palay, V., and Palay, S., 1981b, The nucleus paragigantocellularis lateralis in the rat. Demonstration of afferents by the retrograde transport of horseradish peroxidase, *Anat. Embryol.* **161**:373–390.

Araki, M., McGeer, P. L., and McGeer, E. G., 1984, Presumptive γ-aminobutyric acid pathways from the midbrain to the superior colliculus studied by a combined horseradish peroxidase–γ-aminobutyric acid transaminase pharmacohistochemical method, *Neuroscience* **13**:433–439.

Arkin, A. M., Sanders, K. I., Ellman, S. J., Antrobus, J. S., Farber, J., and Nelson, W. T., 1975, The rarity of pain sensation in sleep mentation reports, *Sleep Res.* **4**:179.

Armstrong, D. M., Saper, C. B., Levey, A. I., Wainer, B. H., and Terry, R. D., 1983, Distribution of cholinergic neurons in rat brain demonstrated by the immunocytochemical localization of choline acetyltransferase, *J. Comp. Neurol.* **216**:53–68.

Arsenault, M. Y., Parent, A., Séguéla, P., and Descarries, L., 1988, Distribution and morphological characteristics of dopamine-immunoreactive neurons in the midbrain of the squirrel monkey (*Saimiri sciureus*), *J. Comp. Neurol.* **267**:489–506.

Arthur, D. L., and Starr, A., 1984, Task-relevant late positivity component of the auditory event-related potential in monkeys resembles P300 in humans, *Science* **223**:186–188.

Artola, A., and Singer, W., 1987, Long-term potentiation and NMDA receptors in rate visual cortex, *Science* **330**:649–662.

Asanuma, C., 1989, Basal forebrain projections to the reticular thalamic nucleus in rat, *Proc. Natl. Acad. Sci. U.S.A.* **86**:4746–4750.

Ascher, P., and Nowak, L., 1987, Electrophysiological studies of NMDA receptors, *Trends Neurosci.* **10**:284–287.

Aserinsky, E., and Kleitman, N., 1953, Regularly occurring periods of eye motility, and concomitant phenomena during sleep, *Science* **118**:273–274.

Aserinsky, E., Lynch, J. A., Mack, M. E., Tzankoff, S. P., and Hurn, E., 1985, Comparison of eye motion in wakefulness and REM sleep, *Psychophysiology* **22**:1–10.

Aston-Jones, G., and Bloom, F. E., 1981a, Activity of norepinephrine-containing locus coeruleus neurons in behaving rats anticipates fluctuations in the sleep–waking cycle, *J. Neurosci.* **1**:876–886.

Aston-Jones, G., and Bloom, F. E., 1981b, Norepinephrine-containing locus coeruleus neurons in behaving rat exhibit pronounced responses to non-noxious environmental stimuli, *J. Neurosci.* **1**:887–900.

Aston-Jones, G., Segal, M., and Bloom, F. E., 1980, Brain aminergic axons exhibit marked variability in conduction velocity, *Brain Res.* **195:**215–222.

Aston-Jones, G., Shaver, R., and Dinan, T., 1984, Cortically projecting nucleus basalis neurons in rat are physiologically heterogeneous, *Neurosci. Lett.* **46:**19–24.

Aston-Jones, G., Foote, S. L., and Segal, M., 1985, Impulse conduction properties of noradrenergic locus coeruleus axons projecting to monkey cerebrocortex, *Neuroscience* **15:**765–777.

Aston-Jones, G., Ennis, M., Pieribone, V. A., Nickell, W. T., and Shipley, M. T., 1986, The brain nucleus locus coeruleus: Restricted afferent control of a broad efferent network, *Science* **234:**734–737.

Avoli, M., 1986, Inhibitory potentials in neurons of the deep layers of the *in vitro* neocortical slice, *Brain Res.* **370:**165–170.

Baghdoyan, H. A., Monaco, A. P., Rodrigo-Angulo, M. L., Assens, F., McCarley, R. W., and Hobson, J. A., 1984a, Microinjection of neostigmine into the pontine reticular formation enhances desynchronized sleep signs, *J. Pharmacol. Exp. Ther.* **231:**173–180.

Baghdoyan, H. A., Rodrigo-Angulo, M. L., McCarley, R. W., and Hobson, J. A., 1984b, Site-specific enhancement and suppression of desynchronized sleep signs following cholinergic stimulation of three brainstem regions, *Brain Res.* **306:**39–52.

Baghdoyan, H. A., McCarley, R. W., and Hobson, J. A., 1985, Cholinergic manipulation of brainstem reticular systems: Effects on desynchronized sleep generation, in: *Sleep: Neurotransmitters and Neuromodulators* (A. Waquier, J. Monti, J. P. Gaillard, and M. Radulovacki, eds.), Raven Press, New York, pp. 15–27.

Baghdoyan, H. A., Rodrigo-Angulo, M. L., McCarley, R. W., and Hobson, J. A., 1987, A neuroanatomical gradient in the pontine tegmentum for the cholinoceptive induction of desynchronized sleep signs, *Brain Res.* **414:**245–261.

Bagnoli, P., Beaudet, A., Stella, M., and Cuénod, M., 1981, Selective retrograde labeling of cholinergic neurons with (^{3}H)choline, *J. Neurosci.* **1:**691–695.

Baker, R., and McCrea, R., 1979, The parabducens nucleus, in: *Integration in the Nervous System* (H. Asanuma and V.J. Wilson, eds.), Igaku-Shoin, New York, pp. 97–121.

Baker, T. L., and Dement, W. C., 1985, Canine narcolepsy–cataplexy syndrome: Evidence for an inherited monoaminergic–cholinergic imbalance, in: *Brain Mechanisms of Sleep* (D. McGinty, R. Drucker-Colin, A. Morrison, and P. L. Parmeggiani, eds.), Raven Press, New York, pp. 63–80.

Ball, G. J., Gloor, P., and Schaul, N., 1977, The cortical electromicrophysiology of pathological delta waves in the electroencephalogram of cats, *Electroencephalogr. Clin. Neurophysiol.* **43:**346–361.

Baraban, J. H., and Aghajanian, G. K., 1981, Noradrenergic innervation of serotonergic neurons in the dorsal raphe: Demonstration by electron microscopic autoradiography, *Brain Res.* **204:**1–11.

Barrett, E. F., and Barrett, J. N., 1976, Separation of two voltage-sensitive potassium currents, and demonstration of a tetrodotoxin-resistant calcium current in frog motoneurons, *J. Physiol. (Lond.)* **255:**737–774.

Bartee, T. C., Lebow, I. L., and Reed, I. S., 1962, *Theory and Design of Digital Machines*, McGraw-Hill, New York.

Basbaum, A. I., Clanton, C. H., and Fields, H. L., 1978, Three bulbospinal pathways from the rostral medulla of the cat: An autoradiographic study of pain modulating systems, *J. Comp. Neurol.* **178:**209–224.

Batini, C., Moruzzi, G., Palestini, M., Rossi, G. F., and Zanchetti, A., 1958, Persistent patterns of wakefulness in the pretrigeminal midpontine preparation, *Science* **128:**30–32.

Batsel, H. L., 1960, Electroencephalographic synchronization and desynchronization in the chronic "cerveau isolé" of the dog, *Electroencephalogr. Clin. Neurophysiol.* **12:**421–430.

Baughman, R. W., and Gilbert, C. D., 1980, Aspartate and glutamate as possible neurotransmitters of cells in layer 6 of the visual cortex, *Nature* **287:**848–849.

Baughman, R. W., and Gilbert, C. D., 1981, Aspartate and glutamate as possible neurotransmitters in the visual cortex, *J. Neurosci.* **1:**427–439.

Baxter, B. L., 1969, Induction of both emotional behavior and a novel form of REM sleep by chemical stimulation applied to cat mesencephalon, *Exp. Neurol.* **23:**220–229.

Beaudet, A., and Descarries, L., 1978, The monoamine innervation of rat cerebral cortex: Synaptic and nonsynaptic axon terminals, *Neuroscience* **3:**851–860.

Beaudet, A., and Descarries, L., 1984, Fine structure of monoamine axon terminals in cerebral cortex, in: *Monoamine Innervation of Cerebral Cortex* (L. Descarries, T. Reader, and H. H. Jasper, eds.), Alan R. Liss, New York, pp. 77–93.

Beck, S. G., Clarke, W. P., and Goldfarb, J., 1985, Spiperone differentiates multiple 5-hydroxytryptamine responses in rat hippocampal slices *in vitro*, *Eur. J. Pharmacol.* **116:**195–197.

Beckstead, R. M., 1983, Long collateral branches of substantia nigra pars reticulata axons to thalamus, superior colliculus and reticular formation in monkey and cat. Multiple retrograde neuronal labeling with fluorescent dyes, *Neuroscience* **10**:767–779.

Beckstead, R. M., and Frankfurter, A., 1982, The distribution and some morphological features of substantia nigra neurons that project to the thalamus, superior colliculus and pedunculopontine nucleus in the monkey, *Neuroscience* **10**:2377–2388.

Beckstead, R. M., Edwards, S. B., and Frankfurter, A., 1981, A comparison of the intranigral distribution of nigrotectal neurons labeled with horseradish peroxidase in the monkey, cat, and rat, *J. Neurosci.* **1**:121–125.

Beersma, D. G. M., van den Hoofdakker, R. H., Daan, S., and van Berkestijn, J. W. B. M., 1983, REM sleep and depression, in: *Sleep 1982 (Abstracts of the 6th European Congress on Sleep Research, Zurich 1982)*, S. Karger, Basel, pp. 349–351.

Beersma, D. G. M., Daan, S., and van den Hoofdakker, R. H., 1984, Distribution of REM latencies and other sleep phenomena in depression as explained by a single ultradian rhythm disturbance, *Sleep* **7**:126–136.

Beersma, D. G. M., Daan, S., and van den Hoofdakker, R. H., 1985, The timing of sleep depression: Theoretical considerations, *Psychiatr. Res.* **16**:253–262.

Beersma, D. G. M., Daan, S., and Dijk, D. J., 1987, Sleep intensity and timing—a model for their circadian control, in: *Lectures on Mathematics in the Life Sciences*, Vol. 19, *Some Mathematical Questions in Biology: Circadian Rhythms* (G. A. Carpenter, ed.), The American Mathematical Society, Providence, RI, pp. 39–61.

Belin, M. F., Aguera, M., Tappaz, M., McRae-Dequeurce, A., Bobillier, P., and Pujol, J. F., 1979, GABA-accumulating neurons in the nucleus raphe dorsalis and periaqueductal gray in the rat: A biochemical and radioautographic study, *Brain Res.* **170**:279–297.

Benardo, L. S., and Prince, D. A., 1982a, Cholinergic pharmacology of mammalian hippocampal pyramidal cells, *Neuroscience* **7**:1703–1712.

Benardo, L. S., and Prince, D. A., 1982b, Cholinergic excitation of mammalian hippocampal pyramidal cells, *Brain Res.* **249**:315–331.

Ben-Ari, Y., Dingledine, R., Kanazawa, I., and Kelly, J. S., 1976, Inhibitory effects of acetylcholine on neurones in the feline nucleus reticularis thalami, *J. Physiol. (Lond.)* **261**:647–671.

Ben-Ari, Y., Krnjevic, K., Reinhardt, W., and Ropert, N., 1981, Intracellular observations on the disinhibitory action of acetylcholine in the hippocampus, *Neuroscience* **6**:2475–2484.

Bender, M. B., Shanzer, S., and Wagman, I. H., 1964, On the physiologic decussation concerned with head turning, *Confin. Neurol.* **24**:169–181.

Bentivoglio, M., Macchi, G., and Albanese, A., 1981, The cortical projections of the thalamic intralaminar nuclei, as studied in cat and rat with the multiple fluorescent retrograde tracing technique, *Neurosci. Lett.* **26**:5–10.

Berger, H., 1930, Uber das Elektroenkephalogram des Menschen. Zweite Mitteilung, *J. Psychol. Neurol.* **40**:160–179.

Berger, H., 1933, Uber das Elektrenkephalogram des Menschen. Sechste Mitteilung, *Arch. Psychiatr. Nervenkr.* **99**:555–574.

Berlucchi, G. Maffei, L., Moruzzi, G., and Strata, P., 1964, EEG and behavioral effects elicited by cooling of medulla and pons, *Arch. Ital. Biol.* **102**:372–392.

Berman, A. L., 1968, *The Brain Stem of the Cat*, University of Wisconsin Press, Madison.

Berry, D. J., Ohara, P. T., Jeffery, G., and Lieberman, A. R., 1986, Are there connections between the thalamic reticular nucleus and the brainstem reticular formation?, *J. Comp. Neurol.* **243**:347–362.

Besset, A., Billiard, M., Brissaud, L., and Touchon, J., 1988, Effects of toloxatone on sleep architecture, *Abstr. Eur. Sleep Res. Soc.* **205**.

Billard, J., and Seignalet, J., 1985, Extraordinary association between HLA-DR2 and narcolepsy, *Lancet* **2**:226–227.

Bizzi, E., 1966, Discharge patterns of single geniculate neurons during the rapid eye movements of sleep, *J. Neurophysiol.* **29**:1087–1095.

Bizzi, E., Pompeiano, O., and Somogyi, I., 1964, Spontaneous activity of single vestibular neurons of unrestrained cats during sleep and wakefulness, *Arch. Ital. Biol.* **104**:425–458.

Bjorklund, A., and Hökfelt, T., eds., 1985, *Handbook of Chemical Neuroanatomy*, Vol. 4, *GABA and Neuropeptides in the CNS*, Elsevier, Amsterdam.

Bjorklund, A., and Lindvall, O., 1984, Dopamine-containing systems in the CNS, in: *Handbook of Chemical Neuroanatomy*, Vol. II: *Classical Transmitters in the CNS*, Part I (A. Bjorklund and T. Hökfelt, eds.), Elsevier, Amsterdam, pp. 55–122.

Bjorklund, A., and Lindvall, O., 1986, Catecholaminergic brain stem regulatory systems, in: *Handbook of Physiology*, Section 1, Vol. IV: *Intrinsic Regulatory Systems of the Brain* (V. B. Mountcastle and F. E. Bloom, eds.), American Physiological Society, Bethesda, pp. 155–235.

Blake, J. F., Brown, M. W., and Collingridge, G. L., 1988, CNQX blocks amino acid depolarizations and synaptic components mediated by non-NMDA receptors in rat hippocampal slices, *Neurosci. Lett.* **55**:89–94.

Blier, P., and De Montigny, C., 1983, Electrophysiological investigations on the effect of repeated zimelidine administration on serotonergic neurotransmission in the rat, *J. Neurosci.* **3**:1270–1278.

Bloom, F., 1978, Central noradrenergic systems: Physiology and pharmacology, in: *Psychopharmacology: Generation of Progress* (M. A. Lipton, A. Di Mascio, and K. S. Killam, eds.), Raven Press, New York, pp. 131–141.

Bloom, F. E., Battenberg, E., Rossier, J., Ling, N., and Guillemin, R., 1978, Neurons containing beta-endorphin in rat brain exist separately from those containing enkephalin: Immunocytochemical studies, *Proc. Natl. Acad. Sci. U.S.A.* **75**:1591–1595.

Bobillier, P., Sequin, S., Petitjean, F., Salvert, D., Touret, M., and Jouvet, M., 1976, The raphe nuclei of cat brain stem: A topographical atlas of their efferent projections as revealed by autoradiography, *Brain Res.* **113**:449–486.

Boehme, R. H., Baker, T. L., Mefford, I. N., Barchas, J. D., Dement, W. C., and Ciaranello, R. D., 1984, Narcolepsy: Cholinergic receptor changes in an animal model, *Life Sci.* **34**:1824–1828.

Bon, L., Corazza, R., and Inchingolo, P., 1980, Eye movements during the waking sleep cycle of the *encephale isolé* semichronic cat preparation, *Electroencephalogr. Clin. Neurophysiol.* **48**:327–340.

Borbely, A. A., 1982, A two process model of sleep regulation, *Hum. Neurobiol.* **1**:195–204.

Borbely, A. A., and Wirz-Justice, A., 1982, Sleep, sleep deprivation and depression—a hypothesis derived from a model of sleep regulation, *Hum. Neurobiol.* **1**:205–210.

Borbely, A. A., Tobler, I., Loepfe, M., Kupfer, D. J., Ulrich, R. F., Grochocinski, V., Doman, J., and Matthews, G., 1984, All-night spectral analysis of the sleep EEG in untreated depressives and normal controls, *Psychiatr. Res.* **12**:27–33.

Borst, J. G. G., Leung, L. W. S., and MacFabe, D. F., 1987, Electrical activity of the cingulate cortex. II. Cholinergic modulation, *Brain Res.* **407**:81–93.

Bouyer, J. J., Montaron, M. F., Rougeul-Buser, A., and Buser, P., 1980, A thalamocortical rhythmic system accompanying high vigilance levels in the cat, in: *Rhythmic EEG Activities and Cortical Functioning* (G. Pfurtscheller, P. Buser, F. H. Lopes da Silva, and H. Petsche, eds.), Elsevier/North Holland, Amsterdam, pp. 63–77.

Bouyer, J. J., Montaron, M. F., and Rougeul, A., 1981, Fast fronto-parietal rhythms during combined focused attentive behaviour and immobility in cat: Cortical and thalamic localizations, *Electroencephalogr. Clin. Neurophysiol.* **51**:244–252.

Bouyer, J. J., Montaron, M. F., Vahnée, J. M., Albert, J. M., and Rougeul, A., 1987, Anatomical localization of cortical beta rhythms in cat, *Neuroscience* **22**:863–869.

Bowery, N. G., Hudson, A. L., and Price, G. W., 1987, GABA$_A$ and GABA$_B$ receptor site distribution in the rat central nervous system, *Neuroscience* **20**:365–383.

Bowsher, D., and Westman, J., 1970, The gigantocellular reticular region and its spinal afferents: A light and electron microscopic study in the cat, *J. Anat. (Lond.)* **106**:23–36.

Boylan, M. K., Fisher, R. S., Hull, C. D., Buchwald, N. A., and Levine, M. S., 1986, Axonal branching of basal forebrain projections to the neocortex: A double-labeling study in the cat, *Brain Res.* **375**:176–181.

Bradshaw, C. M., Sheridan, R. D., and Szabadi, E., 1987, Involvement of M_1-muscarinic receptors in the excitation of neocortical neurones by acetylcholine, *Neuroscience* **26**:1195–1200.

Brashear, H. R., Zaborski, L., and Heimer, L., 1986, Distribution of GABAergic and cholinergic neurons in the rat diagonal band, *Neuroscience* **17**:439–451.

Breitwiesser, G. E., and Szabo, G., 1985, Uncoupling of cardiac muscarinic and beta-adrenergic receptors from ion channels by a guanine nucleotide analogue, *Nature* **317**:538–540.

Bremer, F., 1935, Cerveau "isolé" et physiologie du sommeil, *C.R. Soc. Biol. (Paris)* **118**:1235–1241.

Bremer, F., 1937, L'activité cérébrale au cours du sommeil et de la narcose. Contribution a l'étude du mécanisme du sommeil, *Bull. Acad. R. Med. Belg.* **4**:68–86.

Bremer, F., 1938, L'activité électrique de l'écorce cérébrale et le probleme physiologique du sommeil, *Boll. Soc. Ital. Biol. Sper.* **13**:271–290.

Bremer, F. G. N., 1975, The isolated brain and its aftermath, in: *The Neurosciences: Paths of Discovery* (F. G. Worden, J. P. Swazey, and G. Adelman, eds.), The MIT Press, Cambridge, MA and London, pp. 267–274.

Bremer, F., and Stoupel, N., 1959, Facilitation et inhibition des potentiels évoqués corticaux dans l'éveil cérébral, *Arch. Int. Physiol.* **67:**240–275.

Bremer, F., and Terzuolo, C., 1954, Contribution a l'étude des mecanismes physiologiques du maintien de l'activité vigile du cerveau. Intéraction de la formation reticulée et de l'ecorcé cerebrale dans le processus de l'eveil, *Arch. Int. Physiol.* **62:**157–178.

Brezina, V., Eckert, R., and Erxleben, C., 1987, Modulation of potassium conductances by an endogenous neuropeptide in neurones of *Aplysia californica, J. Physiol. (Lond.)* **382:**267–290.

Bridges, R. J., Stevens, D. R., Kahle, J. S., Nunn, P. B., Kadri, M., and Cotman, C. W., 1989, Structure–function studies on *N*-oxalyl-diamino-dicarboxylic acids and excitatory amino acid receptors: Evidence that beta-L-ODAP is a selective non-NMDA agonist, *J. Neurosci.* **9:**2073–2079.

Brodal, A., 1957, *The Reticular Formation of the Brain Stem: Anatomical Aspects and Functional Correlations,* Oliver & Boyd, Edinburgh.

Brooks, D. C., and Gershon, M. D., 1971, Eye movement potentials in the oculomotor and visual systems in the cat: A comparison of reserpine induced waves with those present during wakefulness and rapid eye movement sleep, *Brain Res.* **27:**223–239.

Brooks, D. C., Gershon, M. D., and Simon, R. P., 1972, Brain stem serotonin depletion and ponto-geniculo-occipital wave activity in the cat treated with reserpine, *Neuropharmacology* **11:**511–520.

Brown, D. A., and Adams, P. R., 1980, Muscarinic suppression of a novel voltage-sensitive K current in a vertebrate neurone, *Nature* **283:**673–676.

Brownstein, M., 1975, Biogenic amine content of the hypothalamic nuclei, in: *Anatomical Neuroendocrinology* (W. E. Stumpf and L. D. Grant, eds.), S. Karger, Basel, pp. 393–396.

Burlhis, T. M., and Aghajanian, G. K., 1987, Pacemaker potentials of serotonergic dorsal raphe neurons: Contribution of a low-threshold Ca^{2+} conductance, *Synapse* **1:**582–588.

Buser, P., Richard, D., and Lescop, J., 1969, Contrôle, par le cortex sensorimoteur, de la réactivité des cellules réticulaires mésencephaliques chez le chat, *Exp. Brain Res.* **9:**83–95.

Butcher, L. L., Talbot, K., and Bilezikjian, L., 1975, Acetylcholinesterase neurons in dopamine-containing regions of the brain, *J. Neural. Transm.* **37:**127–153.

Büttner, J. A., and Henn, V., 1976, An autoradiographic study of the pathways from the pontine reticular formation involved in horizontal eye movements, *Brain Res.* **108:**155–164.

Büttner, U., and Henn, V., 1977, Vertical eye movement related unit activity in the rostral mesencephalic reticular formation of the alert monkey, *Brain Res.* **130:**239–152.

Büttner, U., Hepp, K., and Henn, V., 1977, Neurons in the rostral mesencephalic and paramedian pontine reticular formation generating fast eye movements, in: *Controls of Gaze by Brain Stem Neurons* (R. Baker and A. Berthoz, eds.), Elseiver/North-Holland, New York, pp. 309–318.

Büttner-Ennever, J. A., 1977, Pathways from the pontine reticular formation to structures controlling horizontal and vertical eye movements in the monkey, in: *Control of Gaze by Brain Stem Neurons* (R. Baker and A. Berthoz, eds.), Elsevier/North-Holland, New York, pp. 89–98.

Büttner-Ennever, J. A., and Büttner, U., 1978, A cell group associated with vertical eye movements in the rostral mesencephalic reticular formation of the monkey, *Brain Res.* **151:**31–47.

Büttner-Ennever, J. A., Cohen, B., Pause, M., and Fries, W., 1988, Raphe nucleus of the pons containing omnipause neurons of the oculomotor system in the monkey, and its homologue in man, *J. Comp. Neurol.* **267:**307–321.

Buzsaki, G., Leung, L. W. S., and Vanderwolf, C. H., 1983, Cellular bases of hippocampal EEG in the behaving rat, *Brain Res. Rev.* **6:**139–171.

Buzsaki, G., Bickford, R. G., Ponomareff, G., Thal L. J., Mandel, R., and Gage, F. H., 1988, Nucleus basalis and thalamic control of neocortical activity in the freely moving rat, *J. Neurosci.* **8:** 4007–4026.

Caballero, A., and De Andres, I., 1986, Unilateral lesions in locus coeruleus area enhance paradoxical sleep, *Electroencephalogr. Clin. Neurophysiol.* **64:**339–346.

Cairns, H., Oldfield, R. C., Pennybacker, J. B., and Whitteridge, D., 1941, Akinetic mutism with an epidermoid cyst of the 3rd ventricle, *Brain* **64:**273–290.

Calvet, J., Calvet, M. C., and Scherrer, J., 1964, Etude stratigraphique corticale de l'activité EEG spontanée, *Electroencephalogr. Clin. Neurophysiol.* **17:**109–125.

Calvo, J. M., Badillo, S., Morales-Ramirez, M., and Palacios-Salas, P., 1987, The role of the temporal lobe amygdala in ponto-geniculo-occipital activity and sleep organization in cats, *Brain Res.* **403:**22–30.

Cannon, S. C., and Robinson, D. A., 1987, Loss of the neural integrator of the oculomotor system from brain stem lesions in monkey, *J. Neurophysiol.* **57:**1383–1409.

Carbone, E., and Lux, H. D., 1984, A low voltage-activated, fully inactivating Ca channel in verte-brate sensory neurones, *Nature* **310**:501–502.

Carli, G., Diete-Spiff, K., and Pompeiano, O., 1967, Presynaptic and postsynaptic inhibition of somatic afferent volleys through the cuneate nucleus during sleep, *Arch. Ital. Biol.* **105**:52–82.

Carstens, E., and Trevino, D. L., 1978, Laminar origins of spinothalamic projections in the cat as determined by the retrograde transport of horseradish peroxidase, *J. Comp. Neurol.* **182**:151–166.

Carter, D. A., and Fibiger, H. C., 1977, Ascending projections of presumed dopamine-containing neurons in the ventral tegmentum of the rat as demonstrated by horseradish peroxidase, *Neuroscience* **2**:569–576.

Castaigne, P., Buge, A., Escourolle, R., and Masson, M., 1962, Ramollissement pedonculaire median, tegmento-thalamique avec ophtalmoplegie et hypersomnie, *Rev. Neurol. (Paris)* **106**:357–367.

Catsman-Berrevoets, C. E., and Kuypers, H. G. J. M., 1975, Pericruciate cortical neurons projecting to brain stem reticular formation, dorsal column nuclei and spinal cord in the cat, *Neurosci. Lett.* **1**:257–262.

Catsman-Berrevoets, C. E., and Kuypers, H. G. J. M., 1981, A search for corticospinal collaterals to the thalamus and mesencephalon by means of multiple retrograde fluorescent tracers in cat and rat, *Brain Res.* **218**:15–33.

Cauller, L. J., and Kulics, A. T., 1988, A comparison of awake and sleeping cortical states by analysis of the somatosensory-evoked response of postcentral area 1 in rhesus monkey, *Exp. Brain Res.* **72**:584–592.

Cechetto, D. F., Standaert, D. G., and Saper, C. B., 1985, Spinal and trigeminal dorsal horn projections to the parabrachial nucleus in the rat, *J. Comp. Neurol.* **240**:153–160.

Cederbaum, J. M., and Aghajanian, G. K., 1976, Noradrenergic neurons of the locus coeruleus: Inhibition by epinephrine and activation by the alpha-antagonist piperoxane, *Brain Res.* **112**:413–419.

Cederbaum, J. M., and Aghajanian, G. K., 1978, Afferent projections to the rat locus coeruleus as determined by a retrograde tracing technique, *J. Comp. Neurol.* **178**:1–16.

Celesia, G. G., and Jasper, H. H., 1966, Acetylcholine released from cerebral cortex in relation to state of activation, *Neurology (Minneap.)* **16**:1053–1064.

Cespuglio, R., Gomez, M. E., Walker, E., and Jouvet, M., 1979, Effets du refroidissement et de la stimulation des noyaux du systeme du raphe sur les etats de vigilance chez le chat, *Electroencephalogr. Clin. Neurophysiol.* **47**:289–308.

Cespuglio, R., Faradji, H., Gomez, M. E., and Jouvet, M., 1981, Single unit recordings in the nuclei raphe dorsalis and magnus during the sleep–waking cycle of semi-chronic prepared cats, *Neurosci. Lett.* **24**:133–138.

Cespuglio, R., Gomez, M. E., Faradji, H., and Jouvet, M., 1982, Alterations in the sleep-waking cycle induced by cooling of the locus coeruleus area, *Electroencephalogr. Clin. Neurophysiol.* **54**:570–578.

Champagnat, J., Jacquin, T., and Richter, D. W., 1986, Voltage-dependent currents in neurones of the nuclei of the solitary tract of rat brainstem slices, *Pflugers Arch.* **406**:372–379.

Chandler, S. H., Chase, M. H., and Nakamura, Y., 1980, Intracellular analysis of synaptic mechanisms controlling trigeminal motoneurons activity during sleep and wakefulness, *J. Neurophysiol.* **44**:359–371.

Chase, M. H., and Morales, F. R., 1983, Subthreshold excitatory activity and motoneuron discharge during REM periods of active sleep, *Science* **221**:1195–1198.

Chase, M. H., and Morales, F. R., 1985, Postsynaptic modulation of spinal cord motoneuron membrane potential during sleep, in: *Brain Mechanisms of Sleep* (D. J. McGinty, A. Morrison, R. Drucker-Colin, and P. L. Parmeggiani, eds.), Raven Press, New York, pp. 45–61.

Chase, M. H., Chandler, S. H., and Nakamura, Y., 1980, Intracellular determination of membrane potential of trigeminal motoneurons during sleep and wakefulness, *J. Neurophysiol.* **44**:349–358.

Chase, M. H., Enomoto, S., Murakami, R., Nakamura, Y., and Taira, M., 1981, Intracellular potential of medullary reticular neurons during sleep and wakefulness, *Exp. Neurol.* **71**:226–233.

Chase, M. H., Enomoto, S., Hiraba, K., Katoh, M., Nakamura, Y., Sahara, Y., and Tiara, M., 1984, Role of medullary reticular neurons in the inhibition of trigeminal motoneurons during active sleep, *Exp. Neurol.* **84**:364–373.

Chase, M. H., Morales, F. R., Boxer, P. A., Fung, S. J., and Soja, P. J., 1986, Effect of stimulation of

442

REFERENCES

the nucleus reticularis gigantocellularis on the membrane potential of cat lumbar motoneurons during sleep and wakefulness, *Brain Res.* **386**:237–244.

Chase, M. H., Soja, P. J., and Morales, F. R., 1989, Evidence that glycine mediates the postsynaptic potentials that inhibit lumbar motoneurons during the atonia of active sleep, *J. Neurosci.* (in press).

Chéron, G., Godaux, E., Laune, J. M., and VanDerkelen, B., 1986a, Lesions in the cat prepositus: Effects on the vestibulo-ocular reflex and saccades, *J. Physiol. (Lond.)* **372**:75–94.

Chéron, G., Gillis, P., and Godaux, E., 1986b, Lesions in the cat prepositus complex: Effects on the optokinetic system, *J. Physiol. (Lond.)* **372**:95–111.

Chevalier, G., Deniau, J. M., Thierry, A. M., and Féger, J., 1981a, The nigro-tectal pathway. An electrophysiological reinvestigation in the rat, *Brain Res.* **213**:253–263.

Chevalier, G., Thierry, A. M., Shibazaki, T., and Féger, J., 1981b, Evidence for a GABAergic inhibitory nigrotectal pathway in the rat, *Neurosci. Lett.* **21**:67–70.

Chi, C. C., and Flynn, J. P., 1971, Neuroanatomic projections related to biting attack elicited from hypothalamus in cats, *Brain Res.* **35**:49–66.

Childs, J. A., and Gale, K., 1983, Neurochemical evidence for a nigrotegmental GABAergic projection, *Brain Res.* **258**:109–114.

Chu, N. S., and Bloom, R. E., 1974, Activity patterns of catecholamine-containing neurons in the dorsolateral tegmentum of unrestrained cats, *J. Neurobiol.* **5**:527–544.

Claes, E., 1939, Contribution à l'étude physiologique de la fonction visuelle. I. Analyse oscillographique de l'activité spontanée et sensoriella de l'aire visuelle corticale chez le chat non anesthesié, *Arch. Int. Physiol.* **48**:181–237.

Clarke, P. B. S., Schwartz, R. D., Paul, S. M., Pert, C. B., and Pert, A., 1985, Nicotinic binding in rat brain: Autoradiographic comparison of (^{3}H)acetylcholine, (^{3}H)nicotine, and ($_{125}$I)-α-bungarotoxin, *J. Neurosci.* **5**:1307–1315.

Coben, L. A., Danziger, W. L., and Berg, L., 1983, Frequency analysis of the resting awake EEG in mild senile dementia of Alzheimer type, *Electroenceph. Clin. Neurophysiol.* **55**:372–380.

Coble, P., Foster, F. G., and Kupfer, D. J., 1976, Electroencephalographic sleep diagnosis of primary depression, *Arch. Gen. Psychiatry* **33**:1124–1127.

Coenen, A. M. L., and Vendrik, A. J. H., 1972, Determination of the transfer ratio of cat's geniculate neurons through quasi-intracellular recordings and the relation with the level of alertness, *Exp. Brain Res.* **14**:227–242.

Cohen, A. H., Rossignol, S., and Grillner, S., eds., 1988, *Neural Control of Rhythmic Movements in Vertebrates,* John Wiley & Sons, New York.

Cole, A. E., and Nicoll, R. A., 1983, Acetylcholine mediates a slow synaptic potential in hippocampal pyramidal cells, *Science* **221**:1299–1301.

Collier, B., and Mitchell, J. F., 1967, The central release of acetylcholine during consciousness and after brain lesions, *J. Physiol. (Lond.)* **188**:83–98.

Collingridge, G. L., and Bliss, T. V. P., 1987, NMDA receptors—their role in long-term potentiation, *Trends Neurosci.* **10**:288–293.

Conner, J. A., and Stevens, C. F., 1971, Voltage clamp studies of a transient outward membrane current in gastropod neural somata, *J. Physiol. (Lond.)* **213**:21–30.

Consolazione, A., Priestley, J. V., and Cuello, A. C., 1984, Serotonin-containing projections to the thalamus in the rat revealed by a horseradish peroxidase and peroxidase antiperoxidase double-staining technique, *Brain Res.* **322**:233–243.

Cordeau, J. P., Moreau, A., Beaulnes, A., and Laurin, C., 1963, EEG and behavioral changes following microinjections of acetylcholine and adrenaline in the brain stem of cats, *Arch. Ital. Biol.* **101**:30–47.

Cortes, R., Soriano, E., Pazos, A., Probst, A., and Palacios, J. M., 1988, Autoradiography of antidepressant binding sites in the human brain: Localization using [^{3}H]imipramine and [^{3}H]paroxetine, *Neuroscience* **27**:473–496.

Cotman, C. W., Flatman, J. A., Ganong, A. H., and Perkins, M. N., 1986, Effects of excitatory amino acid antagonists on evoked and spontaneous excitatory potentials in guinea-pig hippocampus, *J. Physiol. (Lond.)* **378**:403–415.

Cotman, C. W., Monaghan, D. T., Ottersen, O. P., and Storm-Mathisen, J., 1987, Anatomical organization of excitatory amino acid receptors and their pathways, *Trends Neurosci.* **10**:273–280.

Cowan, W. M., Gottlieb, D. I., Hendrickson, A. E., Price, J. L., and Woolsey, T. A., 1972, The autoradiographic demonstration of axonal connections in the central nervous system, *Brain Res.* **37**:21–51.

Cowan, W. M., Woolsey, T. A., Wann, D. F., and Dierker, M. L., 1975, The computer analysis of Golgi-impregnated neurons, in: *Golgi Centennial Symposium* (M. Santini, ed.), Raven Press, New York, pp. 81–85.

Crawford, J. M., and Curtis, D. R., 1966, Pharmacological studies on feline Betz cells, *J. Physiol. (Lond.)* **186:**121–138.

Crepel, F., Debono, M., and Flores, R., 1987, Alpha-adrenergic inhibition of rat cerebellar purkinje cells *in vitro:* A voltage-clamp study, *J. Physiol. (Lond.)* **383:**487–498.

Creutzfeldt, O. D., Watanabe, S., and Lux, H. D., 1966, Relations between EEG phenomena and potentials of single cells. I. Evoked responses after thalamic and epicortical stimulation, *Electroencephalogr. Clin. Neurophysiol.* **20:**1–18.

Creutzfeldt, O., Grunewald, G., Simonova, O., and Schmiz, H., 1969, Changes of the basic rhythms of the EEG during the performance of mental and visuomotor tasks, in: *Attention in Neurophysiology* (C. R. Evans and T. B. Mulholland, eds.), Butterworths, London, pp. 148–168.

Cropper, E. C., Eisenman, J. S., and Azmitia, E. C., 1985, An immunocytochemical study of the serotonergic innervation of the thalamus of the rat, *J. Comp. Neurol.* **234:**38–50.

Crosby, E., Humphrey, T., and Lauer, E., 1962, *Correlative Anatomy of the Nervous System*, Macmillan, New York.

Crunelli, V., and Segal, M., 1985, An electrophysiological study of neurones in the rat median raphe and their projections to septum and hippocampus, *Neuroscience* **15:**47–60.

Crunelli, V., Leresche, N., and Pirchio, M., 1985, Non-NMDA receptors mediate the optic nerve input to the rat LGN *in vitro, J. Physiol. (Lond.)* **360:**40P.

Crunelli, V., Kelly, J. S., Leresche, N., and Pirchio, M., 1987a, The ventral and dorsal lateral geniculate nucleus of the rat: Intracellular recordings *in vitro, J. Physiol. (Lond.)* **384:**587–601.

Crunelli, V., Kelly, J. S., Leresche, N., and Pirchio, M., 1987b, On the excitatory postsynaptic potential evoked by stimulation of the optic tract in the rat lateral geniculate nucleus, *J. Physiol. (Lond.)* **384:**603–618.

Crunelli, V., Leresche, N., and Parnavelas, J. G., 1987c, Membrane properties of morphologically identified X and Y cells in the lateral geniculate nucleus of the rat *in vitro, J. Physiol. (Lond.)* **390:**243–256.

Crunelli, V., Haby, M., Jassik-Gerschenfeld, D., Leresche, N., and Pirchio, M., 1988, Cl⁻ and K⁺ dependent inhibitory postsynaptic potentials evoked by interneurones in the rat lateral geniculate nucleus, *J. Physiol. (Lond.)* **399:**153–176.

Crutcher, M. D., Branch, M. H., DeLong, M. R., and Georgopoulos, A. P., 1980, Activity of zona incerta neurons in the behaving primate, *Soc. Neurosci. Abstr.* **6:**676.

Cuénod, M., Bagnoli, P., Beaudet, A., Rustioni, A., Wiklund, L., and Streit, P., 1982, Transmitter-specific retrograde labeling of neurons, in: *Cytochemical Methods in Neuroanatomy* (V. Chan-Palay and S. Palay, eds.), Alan R. Liss, New York, pp. 17–43.

Cull-Candy, S. G., and Usowicz, M. M., 1987, Multiple-conductance channels activated by excitatory amino acids in cerebellar neurons, *Nature* **325:**525–528.

Cunningham, E. T., and LeVay, S., 1986, Laminar and synaptic organization of the projection from the thalamic nucleus centralis to primary visual cortex in the cat, *J. Comp. Neurol.* **254:**65–77.

Curtis, D. R., and Eccles, R. M., 1958, The excitation of Renshaw cells by pharmacological agents applied electrophoretically, *J. Physiol. (Lond.)* **141:**435–445.

Curtis, D. R., and Ryall, R. W., 1966a, The excitation of Renshaw cells by cholinomimetics, *Exp. Brain Res.* **2:**49–65.

Curtis, D. R., and Ryall, R. W., 1966b, The acetylcholine receptors of Renshaw cells, *Exp. Brain Res.* **2:**66–80.

Czeisler, C. A., Zimmerman, J. C., Ronda, J. M., Moore-Ede, M. C., and Weitzman, E. D., 1980, Timing of REM sleep is coupled to the circadian rhythm of body temperature in man, *Sleep* **2:**329–346.

Czeisler, C. A., Kronauer, R. E., Mooney, J. J., Anderson, J. L., and Allan, J. S., 1987, Biologic rhythm disorders, depression, and phototherapy, *Psychiatr. Clin. North Am.* **10:**687–709.

Daan, S., Beersma, D. G. M., and Borbely, A. A., 1984, Timing of human sleep: Recovery process gated by a circadian pacemaker, *Am. J. Physiol.* **246**(15)**:**R161–178.

Dahlström, A., and Fuxe, K., 1964, Evidence for the existence of monoamine-containing neurones in the central nervous system. I. Demonstration of monoamines in the cell bodies of brain stem neurones, *Acta Physiol. Scand. [Suppl.]* **232:**1–55.

Daniels, L., 1934, Narcolepsy, *Medicine* **13:**1–122.

Datta, S., Paré, D., Oakson, G., and Steriade, M., 1989, Thalamic-projecting neurons in brainstem cholinergic nuclei increase their firing rates one minute in advance of EEG desynchronization associated with REM-sleep, *Soc. Neurosci. Abstr.* **15:**452.

Delagrange, P., Tadjer, D., Rougeul, A., and Buser, P., 1987, Activité unitaire de neurones du noyau ventral postérieur du thalamus pour divers degrés de vigilance chez le chat normal, *C.R. Acad. Sci. (Paris)* **305:**149–155.

Delgado-Garcia, J. M., del Pozo, F., and Baker, R., 1988a, Behavior of neurons in the abducens nucleus of the alert cat—I. Motoneurons, *Neuroscience* **17:**929–952.

Delgado-Garcia, J. M., del Pozo, F., and Baker, R., 1988b, Behavior of neurons in the abducens nucleus of the alert cat—II. Internuclear neurons, *Neuroscience* **17:**953–973.

DeLima, A. D., and Singer, W., 1987, The brainstem projection to the lateral geniculate nucleus in the cat: Identification of cholinergic and monoaminergic elements, *J. Comp. Neurol.* **259:**92–121.

DeLima, A. D., Montero, V. M., and Singer, W., 1985, The cholinergic innervation of the visual thalamus: An EM immunocytochemical study, *Exp. Brain Res.* **59:**206–212.

Dell, P. C., 1958, Some basic mechanisms of the translation of bodily needs into behaviour, in: *Neurological Basis of Behaviour* (G. E. W. Wolstenholme and C. M. O'Connor, eds.), Churchill, London, pp. 187–203.

Dement, W. C., 1958, The occurrence of low voltage, fast, electroencephalogram patterns during behavioral sleep in the cat, *Electroencephalogr. Clin. Neurophysiol.* **10:**291–296.

Dement, W. C., and Kleitman, N., 1957, The relation of eye movements during sleep to dream activity: An objective method for the study of dreaming, *J. Exp. Psychol.* **53:**339–346.

Dement, W. C., Ferguson, J., Cohen, H., and Barchas, J., 1969, Non-chemical methods and data using a biochemical model: The REM quanta, in: *Psychochemical Research in Man—Methods, Strategy and Theory* (A. Mandell and M. P. Mandell, eds.), Academic Press, New York, pp. 275–325.

DeMontigny, C., and Aghajanian, G. K., 1978, Tricyclic antidepressants: Long-term treatment increases responsivity of rat forebrain neurons to serotonin, *Science* **202:**1303–1306.

Descarries, L., Watkins, K. C., and Lapierre, Y., 1977, Noradrenergic axon terminals in the cerebral cortex of rat. III. Topometric ultrastructural analysis, *Brain Res.* **133:**197–222.

Descarries, L., Berthelot, F., Garcia, S., and Beaudet, A., 1986, Dopaminergic projection from nucleus raphe dorsalis to neostriatum in the rat, *J. Comp. Neurol.* **249:**511–520.

Deschênes, M., and Steriade, M., 1988, The neuronal mechanism of thalamic PGO waves, in: *Cellular Thalamic Mechanisms* (M. Bentivoglio, G. Macchi, and R. Spreafico, eds.), Elsevier, Amsterdam, pp. 197–206.

Deschênes, M., Roy, J. P., and Steriade, M., 1982, Thalamic bursting mechanism: A slow inward current revealed by membrane hyperpolarization, *Brain Res.* **239:**289–293.

Deschênes, M., Paradis, M., Roy, J. P., and Steriade, M., 1984, Electrophysiology of neurons of lateral thalamic nuclei in cat: Resting properties and burst discharges, *J. Neurophysiol.* **51:**1196–1219.

Desmedt, J. E., 1981, Scalp-recorded cerebral event-related potentials in man as point of entry into the analysis of cognitive processing, in: *The Organization of the Cerebral Cortex* (F. O. Schmitt, F. G. Worden, G. Adelman, and S. G. Dennis, eds.), MIT Press, Cambridge, MA, London, pp. 441–473.

Desmedt, J. E., and Bourguet, M., 1985, Color imaging of parietal and frontal somatosensory potential fields evoked by stimulation of median or posterior tibial nerve in man, *Electroencephalogr. Clin. Neurophysiol.* **62:**1–17.

Desmedt, J. E., Brunko, E., and Debecker, J., 1980, Maturation and sleep correlates of the somatosensory evoked potential, in: *Clinical Uses of Cerebral, Brainstem and Spinal Somatosensory Evoked Potentials* (J. E. Desmedt, ed.), S. Karger, Basel, pp. 146–161.

Desmedt, J. E., Huy, N. T., and Bourguet, M., 1983, The cognitive P40, N60 and P100 components of somatosensory evoked potentials and the earliest electrical signs of sensory processing in man, *Electroencephalogr. Clin. Neurophysiol.* **56:**272–282.

Detari, L., Juhasz, G., and Kukorelli, T., 1987, Neuronal firing in the pallidal region: Firing patterns during sleep–wakefulness cycle in cats, *Electroencephalogr. Clin. Neurophysiol.* **67:**159–166.

Deutch, A. V., Kalivas, P. W., Goldstein, M., and Roth, R. M., 1986, Interconnections of the mesencephalic dopamine cell groups, *Soc. Neurosci. Abstr.* **12:**875.

Dijk, D. J., and Beersma, D. G. M., 1988, Effects of seganserin, a $5\text{-}HT_2$ receptor antagonist, on human SWS and EEG power spectra, *Abstr. Eur. Sleep Res. Soc.* p. 250.

Dingledine, R., 1983, N-Methyl aspartate activates voltage-dependent calcium conductance in rat hippocampal pyramidal cells, *J. Physiol. (Lond.)* **343:**385–405.

Dingledine, R., and Kelly, J. S., 1977, Brain stem stimulation and the acetylcholine-evoked inhibition of neurones in the feline nucleus reticularis thalami, *J. Physiol. (Lond.)* **271:**135–154.

Divac, I., 1975, Magnocellular nuclei of the basal forebrain project to neocortex, brain stem, and olfactory bulb. Review of some functional correlates, *Brain Res.* **93:**385–398.

Dodd, J., Dingledine, R., and Kelly, J. S., 1981, The excitatory action of acetylcholine on hippocampal neurones of the guinea pig and rat maintained *in vitro*, *Brain Res.* **207:**109–127.

Domich, L., Oakson, G., and Steriade, M., 1986, Thalamic burst patterns in the naturally sleeping cat: A comparison between cortically-projecting and reticularis neurones, *J. Physiol. (Lond.)* **379:**429–450.

Donoghue, J. P., and Carroll, K. L., 1987, Cholinergic modulation of sensory responses in rat primary somatic sensory cortex, *Brain Res.* **408:**367–371.

Donoghue, J. P., and Ebner, F. F., 1981, The laminar distribution and ultrastructure of fibers projecting from three thalamic nuclei to the somatic sensory–motor cortex of the opossum, *J. Comp. Neurol.* **198:**389–420.

Drew, T., Dubuc, R., and Rossignol, S., 1986, Discharge patterns of reticulospinal and other reticular neurons in chronic unrestrained cats walking on a treadmill, *J. Neurophysiol.* **55:**375–401.

Drucker-Colin, R., and Pedraza, J. G. B., 1983, Kainic acid lesions of gigantocellular tegmental field (FTG) neurons do not abolish REM sleep, *Brain Res.* **272:**387–391.

Drummond, A. H., Benson, J. A., and Levitan, I. B., 1980, Serotonin-induced hyperpolarization of an identified *Aplysia* neuron is mediated by cyclic AMP, *Proc. Natl. Acad. Sci. U.S.A.* **77:**5013–5017.

Duggan, A. W., and Hall, J. G., 1975, Inhibition of thalamic neurones by acetylcholine, *Brain Res.* **100:**445–449.

Dugovic, C., and Waquier, A., 1987, 5-HT_2 receptors could be primarily involved in the regulation of slow-wave sleep in the rat, *Eur. J. Pharmacol.* **137:**145–146.

Dunlap, K., and Fischbach, G. D., 1981, Neurotransmitters decrease the calcium conductance activated by depolarization of embryonic chick sensory neurones, *J. Physiol. (Lond.)* **317:**519–535.

Eccles, J. C., 1964, *The Physiology of Synapses*, Academic Press, New York.

Eccles, J. C., Nicoll, R. A., Taborikova, H., and Wiley, T. J., 1975, Medial reticular neurons projecting rostrally, *J. Neurophysiol.* **38:**531–538.

Eccles, J. C., Nicoll, R. A., Schwarz, D. W. F., Taborikova, H., and Willey, T. J., 1976, Topographic studies on medial reticular nucleus, *J. Neurophysiol.* **38:**109–118.

Eckenstein, F., Barde, Y. A., and Thoenen, H., 1981, Production of specific antibodies to choline acetyltransferase purified from pig brain, *Neuroscience* **6:**993–1000.

Economo, C. von, 1929, Schlaftheorie, *Ergeb. Physiol.* **28:**312–339.

Edstrom, J. P., and Phillis, J. W., 1980, A cholinergic projection from the globus pallidus to cerebral cortex, *Brain Res.* **189:**524–529.

Edwards, D. L., Johnston, K. M., Poletti, C. E., and Foote, W. E., 1987, Morphology of pontomedullary raphe and reticular neurons in the brainstem of the cat: An intracellular HRP study, *J. Comp. Neurol.* **256:**257–273.

Edwards, S. B., 1975, Autoradiographic studies of the projections of the midbrain reticular formation: Descending projections of nucleus cuneiformis, *J. Comp. Neurol.* **161:**341–358.

Edwards, S. B., 1980, The deep cell layers of the superior colliculus: Their reticular characteristics and structural organization, in: *The Reticular Formation Revisited* (J. A. Hobson and M. A. B. Brazior, eds.), Raven Press, New York, pp. 193–209.

Edwards, S. B., and DeOlmos, J. S., 1976, Autoradiographic studies of the projections of the midbrain reticular formation: Ascending projections of nucleus cuneiformis, *J. Comp. Neurol.* **165:**417–432.

Egan, T. M., and North, R. A., 1985, Acetylcholine acts on M_2-muscarinic receptors to excite rat locus coeruleus neurons, *Br. J. Pharmacol.* **85:**733–735.

Egan, T. M., and North, R. A., 1986a, Acetylcholine hyperpolarizes central neurones by acting on a muscarinic receptor subtype, *Nature* **319:**405–407.

Egan, T. M., and North, R. A., 1986b, Actions of acetylcholine and nicotine on rat locus coeruleus neurons *in vitro*, *Neuroscience* **19:**565–571.

Egan, T. M., Henderson, G., North, R. A., and Williams, J. T., 1983, Noradrenaline-mediated synaptic inhibition in rat locus coeruleus neurones, *J. Physiol. (Lond.)* **345:**477–488.

Ehlers, C., Hendricksen, S. J., Wang, M., Rivier, J., Vale, W., and Bloom, F. E., 1983, Corticotropin releasing factor produces increases in brain excitability and convulsive seizures in rats, *Brain Res.* **278:**332–336.

Elliott, H. C., 1969, *Textbook of Neuroanatomy*, Lippincott, Philadelphia.

Emerson, R. G., Sgro, J. A., Pedley, T. A., and Hauser, A., 1988, State-dependent changes in the N20 component of the median nerve somatosensory evoked potential, *Neurology (N.Y.)* **38**:64–67.

Endo, K., Araki, T., and Ito, K., 1977, Short latency EPSPs and incrementing PSPs of pyramidal tract cells evoked by stimulation of the nucleus centralis lateralis of the thalamus, *Brain Res.* **132**:541–546.

Endo, S., Kobayashi, T., Yamamoto, T., Fukuda, H., Sasaki, M., and Ohta, T., 1981, Persistence of the circadian rhythm of REM sleep: A variety of experimental manipulations of the sleep–wake cycle, *Sleep* **4**:319–328.

Ennis, M., and Aston-Jones, G., 1988, Activation of locus coeruleus from nucleus paragigantocellularis: A new excitatory amino acid pathway in brain, *J. Neurosci.* **8**:3644–3657.

Evarts, E. V., and Tanji, J., 1976, Reflex and intended responses in motor cortex pyramidal tract neurons of monkey, *J. Neurophysiol.* **39**:1069–1080.

Evarts, E. V., Shinoda, Y., and Wise, S. P., 1984, *Neurophysiological Approaches to Higher Brain Functions*, John Wiley & Sons, New York.

Evinger, G., Kaneko, C. R. S., and Fuchs, A., 1982, Activity of omnipause neurons in alert cats during saccadic eye movements and visual stimuli, *J. Neurophysiol.* **47**:827–844.

Exner, S., 1894, *Entwurf zu einer Physiologichen Erklarung der Psychischen Ercheinungen*, Deuticke, Vienna.

Eysel, U. T., Pape, H. C., and van Schayck, R., 1986, Excitatory and differential disinhibitory actions of acetylcholine in the lateral geniculate nucleus of the cat, *J. Physiol. (Lond.)* **370**:233–254.

Facon, E., Steriade, M., and Wertheim, N., 1958, Hypersomnie prolongée engendrée par des lésions bilatérales du système activateur médial. Le syndrome thrombotique de la bifurcation du tronc basilaire, *Rev. Neurol. (Paris)* **98**:117–133.

Fadiga, E., and Pupilli, G. C., 1964, Teleceptive components of the cerebellar function, *Physiol. Rev.* **44**:432–486.

Fallon, J. H., 1981, Collateralization of monoamine neurons: Mesotelencephalic dopamine projections to caudate, septum, and frontal cortex, *J. Neurosci.* **1**:1361–1368.

Fatt, P., and Ginsborg, B. L., 1958, The ionic requirements for the production of action potentials in crustacean muscle fibres, *J. Physiol. (Lond.)* **142**:516–543.

Faull, K. F., Zeller-DeAmicis, L. C., Radde, L., Bowersox, S. S., Baker, T. L., Kilduff, T. S., and Dement, W. C., 1986, Biogenic amine concentrations in the brains of normal and narcoleptic canines: Current status, *Sleep* **9**:107–110.

Feinberg, I., and March, J. D., 1988, Cyclic delta peaks during sleep: Result of a pulsatile endocrine process? *Arch. Gen. Psychiatry* **45**:1141–1142.

Ferster, D., and Lindström, S., 1986, Augmenting responses evoked in area 17 of the cat by intracortical axon collaterals by cortico-geniculate cells, *J. Physiol. (Lond.)* **367**:217–232.

Fibiger, H. C., 1982, The organization and some projections of cholinergic neurons of the mammalian forebrain, *Brain Res. Rev.* **4**:327–388.

Filion, M., Lamarre, Y., and Cordeau, J. P., 1971, Neuronal discharges of the ventrolateral nucleus of the thalamus during sleep and wakefulness, *Exp. Brain Res.* **12**:499–508.

Finlayson, P. G., and Marshall, K. C., 1986, Locus coeruleus neurons in culture have a developmentally transient alpha-1-adrenergic response, *Dev. Brain Res.* **25**:292–295.

Flatman, J. A., Schwindt, P. C., Crill, W. E., and Stafstrom, C. E., 1983, Multiple actions of N-methyl-D-aspartate on cat neocortical neurons *in vitro*, *Brain Res.* **266**:169–173.

Foehring, R. C., Schwindt, P. C., and Crill, W. E., 1989, Norepinephrine selectively reduces slow Ca^{2+} and Na^+-mediated K^+ currents in cat neocortical neurons, *J. Neurophysiol.* **61**:245–256.

Foote, S. L., Aston-Jones, G., and Bloom, F. E., 1980, Impulse activity of locus coeruleus neurons in awake rats and monkeys is a function of sensory stimulation and arousal, *Proc. Natl. Acad. Sci. U.S.A.* **77**:3033–3037.

Foote, S. L., Bloom, F. E., and Aston-Jones, G., 1983, Nucleus locus ceruleus: New evidence of anatomical and physiological specificity, *Physiol. Rev.* **63**:844–914.

Fornal, C., Auerbach, S., and Jacobs, B. L., 1985, Activity of serotonin containing neurons in nucleus raphe magnus in freely moving cats, *Exp. Neurol.* **88**:590–608.

Forscher, P., and Oxford, G. S., 1985, Modulation of calcium channels by norepinephrine in internally dialyzed avian sensory neurons, *J. Gen. Physiol.* **85**:743–764.

Foster, F. G., Kupfer, D. J., Coble, P., and McPartland, R. J., 1976, Rapid eye movement sleep density, *Arch. Gen. Psychiatry* **33**:1119–1123.

Foster, J. A., 1980, Intracortical origin of recruiting responses in the cat cortex, *Electroencephalogr. Clin. Neurophysiol.* **48:**639–653.

Foutz, A. S., Mitler, M. M., Cavalli-Sforza, L. L., and Dement, W. C., 1979, Genetic factors in canine narcolepsy, *Sleep* **1:**413–422.

Francesconi, W., Müller, C. M., and Singer, W., 1988, Cholinergic mechanisms in the reticular control of transmission in the cat lateral geniculate nucleus, *J. Neurophysiol.* **59:**1690–1718.

Freedman, J. E., and Aghajanian, G. K., 1987, Role of phosphoinositide metabolites in the prolongation of afterhyperpolarizations by alpha 1-adrenoceptors in rat dorsal raphe neurons, *J. Neurosci.* **7:**3897–3906.

Freud, S., 1888, Gehirn, in: *Handwoerterbuch der Gesamten Medizin,* F. Enke, Stuttgart.

Freud, S., 1891, *Zur Auffassung der Aphasien,* Deuticke, Vienna.

Freud, S., 1895, Project for a scientific psychology, in: *Complete Psychological Works,* standard ed., Vol. 1 (translated and edited by J. Strachey), Hogarth Press, London, pp. 294–397.

Freud, S., 1900a, Die Traumdeutung, in: *Gesammelte Schriften,* Vol. II, Internationaler Psychoanalytischer Verlag, Vienna, reprinted 1925.

Freud, S., 1900b, The interpretation of dreams, in: *Complete Psychological Works,* standard ed., Vols. 4 and 5 (translated and edited by J. Strachey), Hogarth Press, London, reprinted 1966.

Freud, S., 1887–1902, *The Origins of Psychoanalysis: Letters to Wilhelm Fliess, Drafts and Notes: 1887–1902,* Basic Books, New York, reprinted 1954.

Freund, T. J., Powell, J. F., and Smith, A. D., 1984, Tyrosine hydroxylase-immunoreactive boutons in synaptic contact with identified striatonigral neurons, with particular reference to dendritic spines, *Neuroscience* **13:**1189–1215.

Friedman, L., and Jones, B. E., 1984, Study of sleep–wakefulness by computer graphics and cluster analysis before and after lesions of the pontine tegmentum in the cat, *Electroencephalogr. Clin. Neurophysiol.* **57:**43–56.

Fuchs, A. F., and Ron, S., 1968, An analysis of rapid eye movements of sleep in the monkey, *Electroencephalogr. Clin. Neurophysiol.* **25:**244–251.

Fuchs, A. F., Kaneko, C. R. S., and Scuddar, C. A., 1985, Brainstem control of saccadic eye movements, *Annu. Rev. Neurosci.* **8:**307–337.

Fujita, Y., and Sato, T., 1964, Intracellular records from hippocampal pyramidal cells in rabbits during theta rhythm activity, *J. Neurophysiol.* **27:**1011–1025.

Fukuda, A., Minami, T., Nabekura, J., and Oomura, Y., 1987, The effects of noradrenaline on neurones in the rat dorsal motor nucleus of the vagus, *in vitro, J. Physiol. (Lond.)* **393:**213–231.

Fuller, J. H., 1975, Brain stem reticular units: Some properties of the course and origin of the ascending trajectory, *Brain Res.* **83:**349–367.

Fulwiler, C. E., and Saper, C. B., 1984, Subnuclear organization of the efferent connections of the parabrachial nucleus in the rat, *Brain Res. Rev.* **7:**229–259.

Fung, S. J., Boxer, P. A., Morales, F. R., and Chase, M. H., 1982, Hyperpolarizing membrane responses induced in lumbar motoneurons during active sleep, *Brain Res.* **248:**267–273.

Gacek, R. R., 1979, Location of abducens afferent neurons in the cat, *Exp. Neurol.* **64:**342–353.

Galambos, R., and Hillyard, S. A., 1981, Electrophysiological approaches to human cognitive processing, *Neurosci. Res. Prog. Bull.* **20:**141–265.

Galvan, M., and Adams, P. R., 1982, Control of calcium current in rat sympathetic neurons by norepinephrine, *Brain Res.* **244:**135–144.

Ganguli, R., Reynolds, C. F., and Kupfer, D. J., 1987, EEG sleep in young, never medicated, schizophrenic patients: A comparison with delusional and nondelusional depressives and with healthy controls, *Arch. Gen. Psychiatry* **44:**36–45.

Gastaut, H., 1952, Etude electrographique de la reactivité des rhythmes rolandiques, *Rev. Neurol. (Paris)* **87:**176–182.

Gaudin-Chazal, G., Daszuta, A., Faudon, M., and Ternaux, J. P., 1979, 5-HT concentration in cat's brain, *Brain Res.* **160:**281–293.

Geffard, M., Buijs, R. M., Séguéla, P., Pool, C. W., and Le Moal, M., 1984, First demonstration of highly specific and sensitive antibodies against dopamine, *Brain Res.* **294:**161–165.

Geffard, M., Patel, S., Dulluc, J., and Rock, A. M., 1986, Specific detection of noradrenaline in the rat brain using antibodies, *Brain Res.* **363:**395–400.

George, R., Haslett, W. L., and Jenden, D. J., 1964, A cholinergic mechanism in the brainstem reticular formation: Induction of paradoxical sleep, *Int. J. Neuropharmacol.* **3:**541–552.

Gerber, U., Greene, R. W., and McCarley, R. W., 1989a, Repetitive firing properties of medial pontine reticular formation neurones of the rat recorded *in vitro, J. Physiol. (Lond.)* **410:**533–560.

Gerber, U., Green, R. W., and McCarley, R. W., 1989b, Muscarinic receptors modulate neuronal membrane properties in medial pontine reticular formation, *Sleep Res.* **18**:10.

Gerfen, C. R., and Sawchenko, P. E., 1984, An anterograde neuroanatomical tracing method that shows the detailed morphology of neurons, their axons and terminals: Immunohistochemical localization of an axonally transported plant lectin, *Phaseolus vulgaris* leucoagglutinin (PHA-L), *Brain Res.* **290**:219–238.

Gerschenfeld, H. M., and Paupardin-Tritsch, D., 1974, Ionic mechanisms and receptor properties underlying the responses of molluscan neurones to 5-hydroxytryptamine, *J. Physiol. (Lond.)* **243**:427–456.

Giesler, G. J., Jr., Menetrey, D., and Basbaum, A. I., 1979, Differential origin of spinothalamic tract projections to medial and lateral thalamus in the rat, *J. Comp. Neurol.* **184**:107–126.

Giesler, G. J., Jr., Yezierski, R. P., Gerhart, K. D., and Willis, W. D., 1981, Spinothalamic tract neurons that project to medial and/or lateral thalamic nuclei: Evidence for a physiologially novel population of spinal cord neurons, *J. Neurophysiol.* **46**:1285–1308.

Gillin, J. C., 1989, Sleep and affective disorders: theoretical perspectives, in: *Principles and Practice of Sleep Medicine* (M. H. Kryger, T. Roth, and W. C. Dement, eds.), Saunders, Philadelphia, pp. 420–422.

Gillin, J. C., Sitaram, N., and Mendelson, W. B., 1982, Acetylcholine, sleep and depression, *Hum. Neurobiol.* **1**:211–219.

Gillin, J. C., Mendelson, W. B., and Kupfer, D. J., 1988, The sleep disturbances of depression: Clues to pathophysiology with special reference to the circadian rapid eye movement rhythm, in: *Biological Rhythms and Mental Disorders* (D. J. Kupfer, T. H. Monk, and J. D. Barchas, eds.), Guilford, New York, pp. 27–54.

Glaser, E. M., and van der Loos, H., 1965, A semi-automatic computer-microscope for the analysis of neuronal morphology, *IEEE Trans. Biomed. Eng.* **12**:22–31.

Glenn, L. L., and Dement, W. C., 1981, Membrane potential, synaptic activity and excitability of hindlimb motoneurons during wakefulness and sleep, *J. Neurophysiol.* **46**:839–854.

Glenn, L. L., and Steriade, M., 1982, Discharge rate and excitability of cortically projecting intra-laminar thalamic neurons during waking and sleep states, *J. Neurosci.* **2**:1387–1404.

Glenn, L. L., Hada, J., Roy, J. P., Deschenes, M., and Steriade, M., 1982, Anterograde tracer and field potential analysis of the neocortical layer I projection from nucleus ventralis medialis of the thalamus in cat, *Neuroscience* **7**:1861–1877.

Gloor, P., and Fariello, R. G., 1988, Generalized epilepsy: Some of its cellular mechanisms differ from those of focal epilepsy, *Trends Neurosci.* **11**:63–68.

Glotzbach, S. F., and Heller, H. C., 1984, Changes in the thermal characteristics of hypothalamic neurons during sleep and wakefulness, *Brain Res.* **309**:17–26.

Godfraind, J. M., 1978, Acetylcholine and somatically evoked inhibition on perigeniculate neurons in the cat, *J. Pharmacol.* **63**:295–302.

Godfraind, J. M., and Meulders, M., 1969, Effets de la stimulation sensorielle somatique sur les champs visuels des neurones de la région genouillée chez le chat anesthésié au chloralose, *Exp. Brain Res.* **9**:183–200.

Goebel, H. H., Komatsuzaki, A., Bender, M. B., and Cohen, B., 1971, Lesions of the pontine tegmentum and conjugate gaze paralysis, *Arch. Neurol.* **24**:431–440.

Gogolak, G., Stumpf, C. H., Petsche, H., and Sterc, F., 1968, The firing patterns of septal neurons and the form of hippocampal theta wave, *Brain Res.* **7**:201–207.

Gonzalez-Lima, F., and Scheich, H., 1985, Ascending reticular activating system in the rat: A 2-deoxyglucose study, *Brain Res.* **344**:70–88.

Goodwin, G. M., and Green, A. R., 1985, A behavioural and biochemical study in mice and rats of putative selective agonists and antagonists for 5-HT1 and 5-HT2 receptors, *Br. J. Pharmacol.* **84**:743–753.

Gorman, A. L. F., Hermann, A., and Thomas, M. V., 1982, Ionic requirements for membrane oscillations and their dependence on the calcium concentration in a molluscan pacemaker neurone, *J. Physiol. (Lond.)* **327**:185–217.

Grantyn, A., and Berthoz, A., 1987, Reticulo-spinal neurons participating in the control of synergic eye and head movements during orienting in the cat. I. Behavioral properties, *Exp. Brain Res.* **66**:339–354.

Grantyn, A., and Grantyn, R., 1976, Synaptic actions of tectofugal pathways on abducens motoneurons in the cat, *Brain Res.* **105**:269–285.

Grantyn, A., and Grantyn, R., 1982, Axonal patterns and sites of termination of cat superior colliculus neurons projecting in the tecto-bulbo-spinal tract, *Exp. Brain Res.* **46:**243–256.

Grantyn, R., and Grantyn, A., 1978, Morphological and electrophysiological properties of cat abducens motoneurons, *Exp. Brain Res.* **31:**249–279.

Grantyn, R., Baker, R., and Grantyn, A., 1980, Morphological and physiological identification of excitatory pontine reticular neurons projecting to the cat abducens nucleus and spinal cord, *Brain Res.* **198:**221–228.

Grantyn, R., Jacques, V. O., and Berthoz, A., 1987, Reticulo-spinal neurons participating in the control of synergic eye and head movements during orienting in the cat. II. Morphological properties as revealed by intra-axonal injections of horseradish peroxidase, *Exp. Brain Res.* **66:**355–377.

Grantyn, A., Hardy, O., and Berthoz, A., 1988, Activity and ponto-bulbar connectivity of reticulospinal neurons subserving visually triggered eye and head movements, *Soc. Neurosci. Abstr.* **14:**956.

Gray, B. G., and Dostrovsky, J. O., 1985, Inhibition of feline spinal cord dorsal horn neurons following electrical stimulation of nucleus paragigantocellularis lateralis. A comparison with nucleus raphe magnus, *Brain Res.* **348:**261–273.

Gray, C. M., Konig, P., Engel, A., and Singer, W., 1988, Spatio-temporal distribution of stimulus-specific oscillations in the cat visual cortex. I. Local interactions, *Soc. Neurosci. Abstr.* **14:**899.

Gray, R., and Johnston, D., 1987, Noradrenaline and beta-adrenoceptor agonists increase activity of voltage-dependent calcium channels in hippocampal neurons, *Nature* **327:**620–622.

Graybiel, A. M., 1977a, Direct and indirect preoculomotor pathways of the brainstem: An autoradiographic study of the pontine reticular formation in the cat, *J. Comp. Neurol.* **175:** 37–78.

Graybiel, A. M., 1977b, Organization of oculomotor pathways in the cat and rhesus monkey, in: *Control of Gaze by Brain Stem Neurons,* (R. Baker and A. Berthoz, eds.), Elsevier/North-Holland, New York, pp. 79–88.

Graybiel, A. M., 1978a, Organization of the nigrotectal connection: An experimental tracer study in the cat, *Brain Res.* **143:**339–348.

Graybiel, A. M., 1978b, A stellite system of the superior colliculus: The parabigeminal nucleus and its projections to the superficial collicular layers, *Brain Res.* **145:**365–374.

Graybiel, A. M., and Elde, R. P., 1983, Somatostatin-like immunoreactivity characterizes neurons of the nucleus reticularis thalami in the cat and monkey, *J. Neurosci.* **3:**1308–1321.

Greene, R. W., and Carpenter, D. O., 1985, Actions of neurotransmitters on pontine medial reticular formation neurons of the cat, *J. Neurophysiol.* **54:**520–531.

Greene, R. W., and McCarley, R. W., 1989, Cholinergic neurotransmission in the brainstem: Implications for behavioral state control, in: *Brain Cholinergic Systems* (M. Steriade and D. Biesold, eds.), Oxford University Press, Oxford, New York (in press).

Greene, R. W., Haas, H. L., and McCarley, R. W., 1986, A low threshold calcium spike mediates firing pattern alterations in pontine reticular neurons, *Science* **234:**738–740.

Greene, R. W., Gerber, U., and McCarley, R. W., 1989a, Cholinergic activation of medial pontine reticular formation neurons *in vitro, Brain Res.* **476:**154–159.

Greene, R. W., Gerber, U., Haas, H. L., and McCarley, R. W., 1989b, Noradrenergic actions on neurons of the medial pontine reticular formation *in vitro, Sleep Res.* **18:**11.

Gresham, S. C., Agnew, H. W., and Williams, R. L., 1965, The sleep of depressed patients, *Arch. Gen. Psychiatry* **13:**503.

Griffith, W. H., 1988, Membrane properties of cell types within guinea pig basal forebrain nuclei *in vitro, J. Neurophysiol.* **59:**1590–1612.

Grofova, I., Ottersen, O. P., and Rinvik, E., 1978, Mesencephalic and diencephalic afferents to the superior colliculus and periaqueductal gray substance demonstrated by retrograde axonal transport of horseradish peroxidase in the cat, *Brain Res.* **146:**205–220.

Grzanna, R., and Molliver, M. E., 1980, The locus coeruleus in the rat: An immunocytochemical delineation, *Neuroscience* **5:**21–40.

Gücer, G., 1979, The effect of sleep upon the transmission of afferent activity in the somatic afferent system, *Exp. Brain Res.* **34:**287–298.

Guilleminault, C., 1989, Narcolepsy syndrome, in: *Principles and Practices of Sleep Medicine* (M. H. Kryger, T. Roth, and W. C. Dement, eds.), Saunders, New York, pp. 338–347.

Guilleminault, C., Dement, W. C., and Passouant, P., eds., 1975, *Narcolepsy,* Spectrum, New York.

Guillery, R. W., 1966, A study of Golgi preparations from the dorsal lateral geniculate neurons of the cat, *J. Comp. Neurol.* **128:**21–50.

Gunning, R., 1987, Increased numbers of ion channels promoted by an intracellular second messenger, *Science* **235:**80–82.

Gustafsson, B., Galvan, M., Grafe, P., and Wigstrom, H., 1982, A transient outward current in a mammalian central neurone blocked by 4-aminopyridine, *Nature* **299:**252–254.

Guyenet, P. G., and Brown, D. L., 1986, Nucleus paragigantocellularis lateralis and lumbar sympathetic discharge in the rat, *Am. J. Physiol.* **250:**R1081–R1094.

Guyenet, P. G., and Young, B. S., 1987, Projections of nucleus paragigantocellularis lateralis to locus coeruleus and other structures in rat, *Brain Res.* **406:**171–184.

Haas, H. L., 1982, Cholinergic disinhibition in hippocampal slices of the rat, *Brain Res.* **233:**200–204.

Haas, H. L., and Greene, R. W., 1986, Effects of histamine on hippocampal pyramidal cells of the rat *in vitro*, *Exp. Brain Res.* **62:**123–130.

Haas, H. L., and Rose, G. M., 1987, Noradrenaline blocks potassium conductance in rat dentate granule cells *in vitro*, *Neurosci. Lett.* **78:**171–174.

Haas, H. L., Schaerer, B., and Vosmansky, M., 1979, A simple perfusion chamber for the study of nervous tissue slices *in vitro*, *J. Neurosci. Meth.* **1:**323–325.

Hagiwara, S., and Takahashi, K., 1974, The anomalous rectification and cation selectivity of the membrane of a starfish egg cell, *J. Membr. Biol.* **18:**61–80.

Halgren, E., Walter, R. D., Cherlow, D. G., and Crandal, P. H., 1978, Mental phenomena evoked by electrical stimulation of the human hippocampal formation and amygdala, *Brain* **101:**83–117.

Hallanger, A. E., Levey, A. I., Lee, H. J., Rye, D. B., and Wainer, B. H., 1987, The origins of cholinergic and other subcortical afferents to the thalamus in the rat, *J. Comp. Neurol.* **262:**105–124.

Halliwell, J. V., and Adams, P. R., 1982, Voltage-clamp analysis of muscarinic excitation in hippocampal neurons, *Brain Res.* **250:**71–92.

Hammer, R. P., Jr., Lindsay, R. D., and Scheibel, A. B., 1981, Development of the brain stem reticular core: An assessment of dendritic state and configuration in the perinatal rat, *Dev. Brain Res.* **7:**179–190.

Harper, R. M., Schechtman, V. L., and Kluge, K. A., 1987, Machine classification of infant sleep state using cardiorespiratory measures, *Electroencephalogr. Clin. Neurophysiol.* **67:**379–387.

Harper, R. M., Frysinger, R. C., Zhang, J., Trelease, R. B., and Terreberry, R. R., 1988, Cardiac and respiratory interactions maintaining homeostasis during sleep, in: *Clinical Physiology of Sleep*, (R. Lydic and J. F. Biebuyck, eds.), American Physiological Society, Bethesda, pp. 67–78.

Harris, E. W., Ganong, A. H., Monaghan, D. T., Watkins, J. C., and Cotman, C. W., 1986, Action of 3-((+/−)-2-carboxypiperaxin-4-yl)-propyl-1-phosphonic acid (CPP): A new and highly potent antagonist of N-methyl-D-aspartate receptors in the hippocampus, *Brain Res.* **382:**174–177.

Harris, R. M., 1987, Axon collaterals in the thalamic reticular nucleus from thalamocortical neurons of the rat ventrobasal thalamus, *J. Comp. Neurol.* **258:**397–406.

Harting, J. K., 1977, Descending pathways from the superior colliculus: An autoradiographic analysis in the rhesus monkey (*Macaca mulatta*), *J. Comp. Neurol.* **173:**583–612.

Hartmann, E., 1968, Longitudinal studies of sleep and dreams in manic–depressed patients, *Arch. Gen. Psychiatry* **19:**312–329.

Hartzell, H. C., Kuffler, S. W., Stickgold, R., and Yoshikami, D., 1977, Synaptic excitation and inhibition resulting from direct action of acetylcholine on two types of chemoreceptors on individual amphibian parasympathetic neurones, *J. Physiol. (Lond.)* **271:**817–846.

Head, H., 1923, The conception of nervous and mental energy. II. "Vigilance": A physiological state of the nervous system, *Br. J. Psychol.* **14:**126–147.

Hebb, D. O., 1972, *Textbook of Physiology*, Saunders, Philadelphia.

Hendricks, J. C., Morrison, A. R., and Mann, G. L., 1982, Different behaviors during paradoxical sleep without atonia depend on pontine lesion site, *Brain Res.* **239:**81–105.

Henn, V., and Cohen, B., 1976, Coding of information about rapid eye movements in the pontine reticular formation of alert monkeys, *Brain Res.* **108:**307–325.

Henn, V., Baloh, R. W., and Hepp, K., 1984a, The sleep–wake transition in the oculomotor system, *Exp. Brain Res.* **54:**166–176.

Henn, V., Lang, W., Hepp, K., and Reisine, H., 1984b, Experimental gaze palsies in monkeys and their relation to human pathology, *Brain* **107:**619–636.

Hepp, K., and Henn, V., 1983, Neurodynamics of the oculomotor system: Space–time recording and a nonequilibrium phase transition, in: *Springer Series in Synergetics* (E. Basar, H. Flohr, and H. Haken, eds.), Springer, Berlin, Heidelberg, New York, pp. 139–154.

Herkenham, M., 1979, The afferent and efferent connections of the ventromedial thalamic nucleus in the rat, *J. Comp. Neurol.* **183:**487–518.

Herkenham, M., 1987, Mismatches between neurotransmitter and receptor localizations in brain: Observations and implications, *Neuroscience* **23:**1–38.

Herman, J. H., Ellman, S. J., and Roffwarg, H. P., 1978, The problem of NREM dream recall re-examined, in: *The Mind in Sleep: Psychology and Psychophysiology* (A. M. Arkin, J. S. Antrobus, and S. J. Ellman, eds.), Lawrence Erlbaum, Hillsdale, NJ, pp. 59–92.

Herman, J. H., Barker, D. R., and Roffwarg, H. P., 1983, Similarity of eye movement characteristics in REM sleep and the awake state, *Psychophysiology* **20:**537–543.

Hermann, A., and Gorman, A. L. F., 1981, Effects of tetraethylammonium on potassium currents in a molluscan neuron, *J. Gen. Physiol.* **78:**87–110.

Herrling, P. L., 1985, Pharmacology of the corticoaudate excitatory postsynaptic potential in the cat: Evidence for its mediation by quisqualte- or kainate-receptors, *Neuroscience* **14:**417–426.

Highstein, S. M., Karabelas, A., Baker, R., and McCrea, R. A., 1982, Comparison of the morphology of physiologically identified abducens motor and internuclear neurons in the cat: A light micro-scopic study employing the intracellular injection of horseradish peroxidase, *J. Comp. Neurol.* **208:**369–381.

Higo, S., Ito, K., Fuchs, D., and McCarley, R. W., 1989, Pontine and bulbar afferents to the per-ibrachial PGO burst cell zone in the cat, *Sleep Res.* **18:**20.

Higo, S., Ito, K., Fuchs, D., and McCarley, R. W., 1989a, Pontine and bulbar afferents to the peribrachial PGO burst cell zone in the cat, *Sleep Res.* **18:**28.

Higo, S., Ito, K., Fuchs, D., Rye, D., Wainer, B., and McCarley, R. W., 1989b, Topography of pedunculopontine tegmental nucleus (PPT) interconnections with the lateral geniculate nucleus (LGN) and n. prepositus hypoglossi (PH) in the cat, *Soc. Neurosci. Abstr.* **15:**(in press).

Hikosaka, O., and Wurtz, R. H., 1983a, Visual and oculomotor functions of monkey substantia nigra pars reticulata. I. Relation of visual and auditory responses to saccades, *J. Neurophysiol.* **49:**1230–1253.

Hikosaka, O, and Wurtz, R. H., 1983b, Visual and oculomotor functions of monkey substantia nigra pars reticulate. IV. Relation of substantia nigra to superior colliculus, *J. Neurophysiol.* **49:**1285–1301.

Hikosaka, O., and Wurtz, R. H., 1985a, Modification of saccadic eye movements by GABA-related substances. I. Effect of muscimol and bicuculline in monkey superior colliculus, *J. Neurophysiol.* **53:**266–291.

Hikosaka, O., and Wurtz, R. H., 1985b, Modification of saccadic eye movements by GABA-related substances. II. Effects of muscimol in monkey sustantia nigra pars reticulata, *J. Neurophysiol.* **53:**292–308.

Hikosaka, O., Igusa, Y., Nakao, S., and Shimazu, H., 1978, Direct inhibitory synaptic linkage of pontomedullary reticular burst neurons with abducens motoneurons in the cat, *Exp. Brain Res.* **33:**337–352.

Hille, B., 1984, *Ionic Channels of Excitable Membranes,* Sinauer Associates, Sunderland, MA.

Hillyard, S. A., and Picton, T. W., 1987, Electrophysiology of cognition, in: *Handbook of Physiology,* Section 1, Vol. V, part 2 (V. B. Mountcastle and F. Plum, eds.), American Physiological Society, Bethesda, pp. 519–584.

Hirsch, J. C., and Burnod, Y., 1987, A synaptically evoked hyperpolarization in the rat dorsolateral geniculate neurons *in vitro, Neuroscience* **23:**457–468.

Hirsch, J. C., Fourment, A., and Marc, M. E., 1983, Sleep-related variations of membrane potential in the lateral geniculate body relay neurons of the cat, *Brain Res.* **259:**308–312.

Hobson, J. A., 1988, *The Dreaming Brain,* Basic Books, New York.

Hobson, J. A., and McCarley, R. W., 1974, *Neuronal Activity in Sleep: An Annotated Bibliography,* Brain Information Service, Los Angeles.

Hobson, J. A., and McCarley, R. W., 1977, The brain as a dream state generator: An activation–synthesis hypothesis of the dream process, *Am. J. Psychiatry* **134:**1335–1348.

Hobson, J. A., and Steriade, M., 1986, Neuronal basis of behavioral state control, in: *Handbook of Physiology,* Section 1, Vol. IV (V. B. Mountcastle and F. E. Bloom, eds.), American Physiological Society, Bethesda, pp. 701–823.

Hobson, J. A., McCarley, R. W., Wyzinski, P. A., and Pivik, R. T., 1973, Reciprocal firing by two neuronal groups during the sleep cycle, *Soc. Neurosci. Abstr.* **3:**373.

Hobson, J. A., McCarley, R. W., Freedman, R., and Pivik, R. T., 1974, Time course of discharge rate changes by cat pontine brainstem neurons during the sleep cycle, *J. Neurophysiol.* **37:**1297–1309.

Hobson, J. A., McCarley, R. W., Pivik, R. T., and Freedman, R., 1974a, Selective firing by cat pontine brain stem neurons in desynchronized sleep, *J. Neurophysiol.* **37:**497–511.

Hobson, J. A., McCarley, R. W., Freedman, R., and Pivik, R. T., 1974b, Time course of discharge rate changes by cat pontine brainstem neurons during the sleep cycle, *J. Neurophysiol.* **37:**1297–1309.

Hobson, J. A., McCarley, R. W., and Wyzinski, P. W., 1975, Sleep cycle oscillation: Reciprocal discharge by two brain stem neuronal groups, *Science* **189:**55–58.

Hobson, J. A., McCarley, R. W., and Nelson, J. P., 1983a, Location and spike-train characteristics of cells in anterodorsal pons having selective decreases in firing rate during desynchronized sleep, *J. Neurophysiol.* **50:**770–783.

Hobson, J. A., Goldberg, M., Vivaldi, E., and Riew, D., 1983b, Enhancement of desynchronized sleep signs after pontine microinjection of the muscarinic agonist bethanechol, *Brain Res.* **275:**127–136.

Hobson, J. A., Lydic, R., and Baghdoyan, H. A., 1986, Evolving concepts of sleep cycle generation: From brain centers to neuronal populations, *Behav. Brain Sci.* **9:**371–448.

Hökfelt, T., 1987, Neuronal communication through multiple coexisting messengers, in: *Synaptic Function* (G. M. Edelman, W. E. Gall, and W. M. Cowan, eds.), John Wiley & Sons, New York, pp. 179–211.

Hökfelt, T., Johansson, O., and Goldstein, M., 1984, Central catecholamine neurons as revealed by immunohistochemistry with special reference to adrenaline neurons, in: *Handbook of Chemical Neuroanatomy*, Vol. 2, *Classical Transmitters in the CNS*, Elsevier, Amsterdam, pp. 156–276.

Holets, V. R., Hökfelt, T., Rokaeus, A., Terenius, L., and Goldstein, M., 1988, Locus coeruleus neurons in the rat containing neuropeptide Y, tyrosine hydroxylase or galanin and their efferent projections to the spinal cord, cerebral cortex and hypothalamus, *Neuroscience* **24:**893–906.

Holmes, C. J., Webster, H. H., Zikman, S., and Jones, B. E., 1988, Quisqualic acid lesions of the ventromedial medullary reticular formation: Effects upon sleep–wakefulness states, *Soc. Neurosci. Abstr.* **14:**1308.

Holsheimer, J., 1982, Generation of theta activity (RSA) in the cingulate cortex of the rat, *Exp. Brain Res.* **47:**309–312.

Holstege, G., 1987, Some anatomical observations on the projections from the hypothalamus to brainstem and spinal cord: An HRP and autoradiographic tracing study in the cat, *J. Comp. Neurol.* **260:**98–126.

Holstege, G., and Kuypers, H. G. J. M., 1982, The anatomy of brain stem pathway to the spinalcord in cat. A labeled amino acid tracing study, *Prog. Brain Res.* **57:**145–175.

Holstege, J. C., and Kuypers, H. G. J. M., 1987, Brainstem projections to spinal motoneurons: An update, *Neuroscience* **23:**809–821.

Holstage, G., and Kuypers, H. G. J. M., 1988, Brainstem projections to lumbar motoneurons in rat—I. An ultrastructural study using autoradiography and the combination of autoradiography and horseradish peroxidase histochemistry, *Neuroscience* **21:**345–365.

Holt, R., 1965, A review of some of Freud's biological assumptions and their influence on his theories, in: *Psychoanalysis and Current Biological Thought* (N. Greenfield and W. Lewis, eds.), University of Wisconsin Press, Madison, pp. 93–124.

Honore, T., Davies, S. D., Drejer, J., Fletcher, E. J., Jacobsen, P., Lodge, D., and Nielsen, 1987, Potent competitive antagonism at non-NMDA receptors by FG9041 and FG9065, *Soc. Neurosci. Abstr.* **13:**383.

Hopkins, D. A., and Holstege, G., 1978, Amygdaloid projections to the mesencephalon, pons and medulla oblongata in the cat, *Exp. Brain Res.* **32:**529–547.

Horsley, V., 1892, *The Structure and Functions of the Brain and Spinal Cord*, Blakiston, Philadelphia.

Hotson, J. R., and Prince, D. A., 1980, A calcium-activated hyperpolarization follows repetitive firing in hippocampal neurons, *J. Neurophysiol.* **43:**409–419.

Houser, C. R., Vaughn, J. E., Barber, R. P., and Roberts, E., 1980, GABA neurons are the major cell type of the nucleus reticularis thalami, *Brain Res.* **200:**341–354.

Houser, C. R., Crawford, G. D., Salvaterra, P. M., and Vaughn, J. E., 1985, Immunocytochemical localization of choline acetyltransferase in rat cerebral cortex: A study of cholinergic neurons and synapses, *J. Comp. Neurol.* **234:**17–34.

Howe, R. C., and Sterman, M. B., 1972, Cortical–subcortical EEG correlates of suppressed motor behavior during sleep and waking in the cat, *Electroencephalogr. Clin. Neurophysiol.* **32**:681–695.

Hreib, K. K., Rosene, D. L., and Moss, M. B., 1985, Basal forebrain efferents to the medial dorsal thalamic nucleus in the rhesus monkey, *Soc. Neurosci. Abstr.* **11**:1226.

Hu, B., Bouhassira, D., Steriade, M., and Deschênes, M., 1988, The blockage of ponto–geniculo–occipital waves in the cat lateral geniculate nucleus by nicotinic antagonists, *Brain Res.* **473**:394–397.

Hu, B., Steriade, M., and Deschênes, M., 1989a, The effects of brainstem peribrachial stimulation on reticular thalamic neurons: The blockage of spindle waves, *Neuroscience* **31**:1–12.

Hu, B., Steriade, M., and Deschênes, M., 1989b, The effects of brainstem peribrachial stimulation on neurons of the lateral geniculate nucleus, *Neuroscience* **31**:13–24.

Hu, B., Steriade, M., and Deschênes, M., 1989c, The cellular mechanism of thalamic ponto–geniculo–occipital (PGO) waves, *Neuroscience* **31**:25–35.

Hubel, D. H., 1960, Single unit activity in lateral geniculate body and optic tract of unrestrained cats, *J. Physiol. (Lond.)* **150**:91–104.

Hubel, D. H., and Livingstone, M. S., 1980, A comparison between sleeping and waking spontaneous and visually evoked activity in cat striate cortex examined by single cell recording and 2-deoxyglucose autoradiography, *Soc. Neurosci. Abstr.* **6**:314.

Hughes, H. C., and Mullikin, W. H., 1984, Brainstem afferents to the lateral geniculate nucleus of the cat, *Exp. Brain Res.* **54**:253–258.

Hunt, S. P., Henke, H., Kunzle, H., Reubi, J. C., Schenker, T., Streit, P., Felix, D., and Cuénod, M., 1976, Biochemical neuroanatomy of the pigeon optic tectum, in: *Afferent and Intrinsic Organization of Laminated Structures in the Brain* (O. Creutzfeldt, ed.), Springer, New York, pp. 521–525.

Hyde, J. E., and Eason, R. G., 1959, Characteristics of ocular movements evoked by stimulation of brain stem of cat, *J. Neurophysiol.* **22**:666–678.

Ibuka, N., Inouye, S. T., and Kawamura, H., 1977, Analysis of sleep–wakefulness rhythms in male rats after suprachiasmatic nucleus lesions and ocular enucleations, *Brain Res.* **122**:33–47.

Idzikowski, C., Mills, F. J., and Glennard, R., 1986, 5-Hydroxytryptamine-2 antagonist increases human slow wave sleep, *Brain Res.* **378**:164–168.

Idzikowski, C., Burton, S. W., and James, R., 1988, The effects on sleep of 1 mg ritanserin given for four weeks, *Abstr. Eur. Sleep Res. Soc.* 199.

Igusa, Y., Sasaki, S., and Shimazu, H., 1980, Excitatory premotor burst neurons in the cat pontine reticular formation related to the quick phase of vestibular nystagmus, *Brain Res.* **182**:451–456.

Inouye, S. T., and Kawamura, H., 1979, Persistence of circadian rhythmicity in a mammalian hypothalamic "island" containing the suprachiasmatic nucleus, *Proc. Natl. Acad. Sci. U.S.A.* **76**:5962–5966.

Insel, T. R., Gillin, J. C., Moore, A., Mendelson, W. B., Loewenstein, R. J., and Murphy, D. L., 1982, The sleep of patients with obsessive–compulsive disorder, *Arch. Gen. Psychiatry* **39**:1372–1377.

Isaacson, L. G., and Tanaka, D., Jr., 1986, Cholinergic and non-cholinergic projections from the canine pontomesencephalic tegmentum (Ch5 area) to the caudal intralaminar thalamic nuclei, *Exp. Brain Res.* **62**:179–188.

Ito, K., and McCarley, R. W., 1984, Alterations in membrane potential and excitability of cat medial pontine reticular formation neurons during naturally occurring sleep–wake states, *Brain Res.* **292**:169–175.

Ito, K., and McCarley, R. W., 1987, Physiological studies of brainstem reticular connectivity. I. Responses of mPRF neurons to stimulation of bulbar reticular formation, *Brain Res.* **409**:97–110.

Ito, M., Udo, M., and Mano, N., 1970, Long inhibitory and excitatory pathways converging onto cat reticular and Deiters' neurons and their relevance to reticulofugal axons, *J. Neurophysiol.* **33**:210–226.

Iwamura, Y., Tanaka, M., Sakamoto, M., and Hikosaka, O., 1985, Vertical neuronal arrays in the postcentral gyrus signaling active touch: A receptive field study in the conscious monkey, *Exp. Brain Res.* **58**:412–420.

Jackson, A., and Crossman, A. R., 1981, Basal ganglia and other afferent projections to the peribrachial region in the rat: A study using retrograde and anterograde transport of horseradish peroxidase, *Neuroscience* **6**:1537–1549.

Jahnsen, H., and Llinás, R., 1984a, Electrophysiological properties of guinea-pig thalamic neurones: An *in vitro* study, *J. Physiol. (Lond.)* **349**:205–226.

Jahnsen, H., and Llinás, R., 1984b, Ionic basis for the electroresponsiveness and oscillatory properties of guinea-pig thalamic neurones *in vitro, J. Physiol. (Lond.)* **349:**227–247.

Jahr, C. E., and Stevens, C. F., 1987, Glutamate activates multiple single channel conductances in hippocampal neurons, *Nature* **325:**522–525.

Janowsky, D. S., El-Yousef, M. K., and Davis, J. M., 1972, A cholinergic–adrenergic hypothesis of mania and depression, *Lancet* **2:**632–635.

Janowsky, D. S., Risch, C., Parker, D., Huey, L., and Judd, L., 1980, Increased vulnerability to cholinergic stimulation in affective disorder patients, *Psychopharmacol. Bull.* **16:**29–31.

Jasper, H. H., 1958, Recent advances in our understanding of ascending activities of the reticular system, in: *Reticular Formation of the Brain* (H. H. Jasper, L. D. Proctor, R. S. Knighton, W. C. Noshay, and R. T. Costello, eds.), Little, Brown, Boston, Toronto, pp. 319–331.

Jasper, H. H., and Tessier, J., 1971, Acetylcholine liberation from cerebral cortex during paradoxical (REM) sleep, *Science* **172:**601–602.

Jeannerod, M., Mouret, J., and Jouvet, M., 1965, Etude de la motricité oculaire au cours de la phase paradoxale du sommeil chez le chat, *Electroencephalogr. Clin. Neurophysiol.* **18:**554–566.

Jibiki, I., Avoli, M., Gloor, P., Giaretta, D., and McLachlan, R. S., 1986, Thalamocortical and intra-thalamic interactions during slow repetitive stimulation of n. centralis lateralis, *Exp. Brain Res.* **61:**245–257.

Johnson, J. W., and Ascher, P., 1987, Glycine potentiates the NMDA response in cultured mouse brain neurons, *Nature* **325:**529–531.

Jones, B. E., 1989, The relationship among acetylcholine, norepinephrine and GABA neurons within the pons of the rat, *Anat. Record* **223:**57a.

Jones, B. E., and Beaudet, A., 1987a, Distribution of acetylcholine and catecholamine neurons in the cat brain stem studied by choline acetyltransferase and tyrosin hydroxylase immunohistochemistry, *J. Comp. Neurol.* **261:**15–32.

Jones, B. E., and Beaudet, A., 1987b, Retrograde labeling of neurons in the brain stem following injections of (^{3}H)choline into the forebrain of the rat, *Exp. Brain Res.* **65:**437–448.

Jones, B. E., and Moore, R. Y., 1977, Ascending projections of the locus coeruleus in the rat. II. Autoradiographic study, *Brain Res.* **127:**23–53.

Jones, B. E., and Webster, H. H., 1988, Neurotoxic lesions of the dorsolateral pontomesencephalic tegmentum–cholinergic cell area in the cat. I. Effects upon the cholinergic innervation of the brain, *Brain Res.* **451:**13–32.

Jones, B. E., and Yang, T. Z., 1985, The efferent projections from the reticular formation and the locus coeruleus studied by anterograde and retrograde axonal transport in the rat, *J. Comp. Neurol.* **242:**56–92.

Jones, B. E., Harper, S. T., and Halaris, A. E., 1977, Effects of locus coeruleus lesions upon cerebral monoamine content, sleep–wakefulness states and the response to amphetamine in the cat, *Brain Res.* **124:**473–496.

Jones, E., 1959, *The Life and Work of Sigmund Freud,* Vols. 1–3, Basic Books, New York.

Jones, E. G., 1985, *The Thalamus,* Plenum Press, New York.

Jones, E. G., Burton, H., Saper, C. B., and Swanson, L. W., 1976, Midbrain, diencephalic and cortical relationships of the basal nucleus of Meynert and associated structures in primates, *J. Comp. Neurol.* **167:**385–420.

Jones, L. S., Gauger, L. L., and Davis, J. N., 1985a, Anatomy of brain alpha 1-adrenergic receptors: *In vitro* autoradiography with [^{125}]-HEAT, *J. Comp. Neurol.* **231:**190–208.

Jones, L. S., Gauger, L. L., Davis, J. N., Slotkin, T. A., and Bartolome, J. V., 1985b, Postnatal development of brain alpha 1 adrenergic receptors: *In vitro* autoradiography with [^{125}]HEAT in normal rats and rats treated with alpha-difluoromethylornithine, a specific, irreversible inhibitor of ornithine decarboxylase, *Neuroscience* **15:**1195–1202.

Jouvet, M., 1962, Recherches sur les structures nerveuses et les mécanismes responsables des différentes phases du sommeil physiologique, *Arch. Ital. Biol.* **100:**125–206.

Jouvet, M., 1965a, Behavioral and EEG effects of paradoxical sleep deprivation in the cat, in: *Proceedings XXIII International Congress of Physiological Sciences: Lectures and Symposia,* Excerpta Medica Foundation, Amsterdam, pp. 344–353.

Jouvet, M., ed., 1965b, Discussion générale, in: *Neurophysiologie des Etats de Sommeil,* Editions du Centre National de la Recherche Scientifique, Paris, pp. 613–650.

Jouvet, M., 1967, Neurophysiology of the states of sleep, *Physiol. Rev.* **47:**117–177.

Jouvet, M., 1969, Biogenic amines and the states of sleep, *Science* **163:**32–41.

Jouvet, M., 1972, The role of monoamine and acetylcholine-containing neurons in the regulation of the sleep–waking cycle, *Ergebn. Physiol.* **64:**166–307.

Jouvet, M., 1979, What does a cat dream about? *Trends Neurosci.* **2:**15–16.

Jouvet, M., and Delorme, J. F., 1965, Locus coeruleus et sommeil paradoxal, *C.R. Soc. Biol. (Paris)* **159:**895–899.

Jouvet, M., and Michel, F., 1959, Corrélations electromyographiques du sommeil chez le chat décortiqué et mésencephalique chronique, *C.R. Soc. Biol. (Paris)* **153:**422–425.

Jouvet, M., Michel, F., and Courjon, J., 1959, Sur un stade d'activité électrique cérébrale rapide au cours du sommeil physiologique, *C.R. Soc. Biol. (Paris)* **153:**1024–1028.

Jouvet, M., Mounier, D., and Astic, L., 1968, Etude de l'évolution du sommeil du raton au cours du premier mois post natal, *C.R. Soc. Biol. (Paris)* **162:**119–123.

Juji, T., Satake, M., Honda, Y., and Doi. Y., 1984, HLA antigens in Japanese patients with narcolepsy—all the patients were DR2 positive, *Tissue Antigens* **24:**316–319.

Kalia, M., and Fuxe, K., 1985, Rat medulla oblongata. I. Cytoarchitechtonic considerations, *J. Comp. Neurol.* **233:**285–307.

Kanamori, N., Sakai, K., and Jouvet, M., 1980, Neuronal activity specific to paradoxical sleep in the ventromedial medullary reticular formation of unrestrained cats, *Brain Res.* **189:**251–255.

Kaneko, C. R. S., and Fuchs, A. F., 1981, Inhibitory burst neurons in alert trained cats: Comparison with excitatory burst neurons and functional implications, in: *Progress in Oculomotor Research* (A. F. Fuchs and W. Becker, eds.), Elsevier/North-Holland, New York, pp. 63–70.

Kaneko, C. R. S., Evinger, C., and Fuchs, A. F., 1981, Role of cat pontine burst neurons in generation of saccadic eye movement, *J. Neurophysiol.* **46:**387–408.

Karabelas, A. B., and Purpura, D. P., 1980, Evidence for autapses in the substantia nigra, *Brain Res.* **200:**467–473.

Katayama, Y., DeWitt, D. S., Becker, D. P., and Hayes, R. L., 1984, Behavioral evidence for a cholinoceptive pontine inhibitory area: Descending control of spinal motor output and sensory input, *Brain Res.* **296:**241–262.

Katz, B., 1949, Les constantes électriques de la membrane du muscle, *Arch. Sci. Physiol.* **3:**285.

Kayama, Y., Negi, T., Sugitani, M., and Iwama, K., 1982, Effects of locus coeruleus stimulation on neuronal activities of dorsal lateral geniculate nucleus and perigeniculate reticular nucleus of the rat, *Neuroscience* **7:**655–666.

Kayama, Y., Sumitomo, I., and Ogawa, T., 1986a, Does the ascending cholinergic projection inhibit or excite neurons in the rat thalamic reticular nucleus? *J. Neurophysiol.* **56:**1310–1320.

Kayama, Y., Takagi, M., and Ogawa, T., 1986b, Cholinergic influence of the laterodorsal tegmental nucleus on neuronal activity in the rat lateral geniculate nucleus, *J. Neurophysiol.* **56:**1297–1309.

Kellaway, P., 1985, Sleep and epilipsy, *Epilepsia* **26**(Suppl. 1):15–30.

Keller, E. L., 1974, Participation of medial pontine reticular formation in eye movement generation in monkey, *J. Neurophysiol.* **37:**316–332.

Keller, E. L., 1980, Oculomotor specificity within subdivisions of the brain stem reticular formation, in: *The Reticular Formation Revisited* (J. A. Hobson and M. A. B. Brazier, eds.), Raven Press, New York, pp. 227–280.

Kelly, J. P., and Van Essen, D. C., 1974, Cell structure and function in the visual cortex of the cat, *J. Physiol. (Lond.)* **328:**515–547.

Kelly, J. S., Godfraind, J. M., and Maruyama, S., 1979, The presence and nature of inhibition in small slices of the dorsal lateral geniculate nucleus of rat and cat incubated *in vitro, Brain Res.* **168:**388–392.

Kemp, J. A., Roberts, H. C., and Sillito, A. M., 1982, Further studies on the action of 5-hydroxytryptamine in the dorsal lateral geniculate nucleus of the rat, *Brain Res.* **246:**334–337.

Kennedy, C., 1983, Changes in glucose utilization in relation to activity in the central nervous system, in: *Basic Mechanisms of Neural Hyperexcitability* (H. H. Jasper and N. M. van Gelder, eds.), Alan R. Liss, New York, pp. 399–421.

Khachaturian H., Lewis, M. E., and Watson, S. J., 1983, Enkephalin systems in diencephalon and brainstem of the rat, *J. Comp. Neurol.* **220:**310–273.

Kievit, J., and Kuypers, H. G. J. M., 1972, Fastigial cerebellar projections to the ventrolateral nucleus of the thalamus and the organization of the descending pathways, in: *Corticothalamic Projections and Sensorimotor Activities* (T. Frigyesi, E. Rinvik, and M. D. Yahr, eds.), Raven Press, New York, pp. 91–111.

Kilduff, T. S., Bowersox, S. S., Kaitin, K. I., Baker, T. L., Ciaranello, R. D., and Dement, W. C., 1986, Muscarinic cholinergic receptors and the canine model of narcolepsy, *Sleep* **9**:102–106.

Kimura, H., McGeer, P. L., Peng, J. H., and McGeer, E. G., 1981, The central cholinergic system studied by choline acetyltransferase immunohistochemistry in the cat, *J. Comp. Neurol.* **200**:151–201.

King, W. M., and Fuchs, A. F., 1979, Reticular control of vertical saccadic eye movements by mesencephalic burst neurons, *J. Neurophysiol.* **42**:861–876.

Kita, H., and Katai, S. T., 1986, Electrophysiology of rat thalamocortical relay neurons: An *in vitvro* intracellular recording and labeling study, *Brain Res.* **371**:80–89.

Kitsikis, A., and Steriade, M., 1981, Immediate behavioral effects of kainic acid injections into the midbrain reticular core, *Behav. Brain Res.* **3**:361–380.

Kitt, C. A., Mitchell, S. J., DeLong, M. R., Wainer, B. H., and Price, D. L., 1987, Fiber pathways of basal forebrain cholinergic neurons in monkeys, *Brain Res.* **406**:192–206.

Klee, A., 1961, Akinetic mutism: Review of the literature and report of a case, *J. Nerv. Ment. Dis.* **133**:536–553.

Kleitman, N., 1929, Sleep, *Physiol. Rev.* **9**:624–665.

Kleitman, N., 1963, *Sleep and Wakefulness,* Chicago University Press, Chicago.

Konopacki, J., MacIver, M. B., Bland, B. H., and Roth, S. H., 1987, Carbachol-induced EEG "theta" activity in hippocampal brain slices, *Brain Res.* **405**:196–198.

Kosaka, T., Kosaka, K., Hataguchi, Y., Nagatsu, I., Wu, J. Y., Ottersen, O. P., Storm-Mattisen, J., and Hama, K., 1987, Catecholaminergic neurons containing GABA-like and/or glutamic acid decarboxylase-like immunoreactivities in various brain regions of the rat, *Exp. Brain Res.* **66**:191–210.

Kostowski, W., 1971, Effects of some cholinergic and anticholinergic drugs injected intracerebrally to the midline pontine area, *Neuropharmacology* **10**:595–605.

Kreindler, A., and Steriade, M., 1964, EEG patterns of arousal and sleep induced by stimulating various amygdaloid levels in the cat, *Arch. Ital. Biol.* **102**:576–586.

Kripke, D. F., Mullaney, D. J., Atkinson, M., and Wolf, S., 1978, Circadian rhythm disorders in manic–depressives, *Biol. Psychiatry* **13**:335–351.

Kristensson, K., and Olsson, Y., 1971, Retrograde axonal transport of protein, *Brain Res.* **29**:363–365.

Krnjević, K., 1974, Chemical nature of synaptic transmission in vertebrates, *Physiol. Rev.* **54**:418–540.

Krnjević, K., and Phillis, J. W., 1963a, Acetylcholine-sensitive cells in the cerebral cortex, *J. Physiol. (Lond.)* **166**:296–327.

Krnjević, K., and Phillis, J. W., 1963b, Pharmacological properties of acetylcholine-sensitive cells in the cerebral cortex, *J. Physiol. (Lond.)* **166**:328–350.

Krnjević, K., and Ropert, N., 1981, Septo-hippocampal pathway modulates hippocampal activity by a cholinergic mechanism, *Can. J. Physiol. Pharmacol.* **59**:911–914.

Krnjević, K., Pumain, R., and Renaud, L., 1971, The mechanism of excitation by acetylcholine in the cerebral cortex, *J. Physiol. (Lond.)* **215**:247–268.

Krnjević, K., Puil, E., and Werman, R., 1976, Is cyclic guanosine monophosphate the internal "second messenger" for cholinergic actions on central neurons?, *Can. J. Physiol. Pharmacol.* **54**:172–176.

Kronauer, R. E., Czeisler, C. A., Pilato, S. F., Moore-Ede, M. C., and Weitzman, E. D., 1982, Mathematical model of the human circadian system with two interacting oscillators, *Am. J. Physiol.* **242**(11):R3–R17.

Krueger, J., Walter, J., and Levin, C., 1985, Factor S and related somnogens: An immune theory for slow-wave sleep, in: *Brain Mechanisms of Sleep* (D. McGinty, R. Drucker-Colin, A. Morrison, and P. L. Parmeggiani, eds.), Raven Press, New York, pp. 253–275.

Krueger, J. M., Obal, Jr., F., Opp, M., Johansen, L., Cady, A. B., and Toth, L., 1989, Immune response modifiers and sleep, in: *Interactions between Neuroendocrine and Immune Systems* (K. Masek and G. Nistico, eds.), Pythagora Press, Rome (in press).

Kucera, P., and Favrod, P., 1979, Suprachiasmatic nucleus projection to mesencephalic central gray in the woodmouse (*Apodemus sylvaticus L.*), *Neuroscience* **4**:1705–1715.

Kulics, A. T., 1982, Cortical neural evoked correlates of somatosensory stimulus detection in the rhesus monkey, *Electroencephalogr. Clin. Neurophysiol.* **53**:78–93.

Kulics, A. T., Lineberry, C. G., and Roppolo, J. R., 1977, Neurophysiological correlates of cutaneous discrimination performance in rhesus monkey, *Brain Res.* **136**:360–365.

Kupfer, D. J., 1982, EEG sleep as biological markers in depression, in: *Biological Markers in Psychiatry and Neurology* (E. Usdin and I. Hanin, eds.), Pergamon Press, New York, pp. 387–396.

Kupfer, D. J., and Foster, F. G., 1972, Interval between onset of sleep and rapid eye movement as an indicator of depression, *Lancet* **2**:684–686.

Kupfer, D. J., Gillin, J. C., Coble, P. A., Spiker, D. G., Shaw, D. H., and Holtzer, B., 1981a, REM sleep, naps, and depression, *Psychiatry Res.* **5**:195–203.

Kupfer, D. J., Spiker, D. G., Coble, P. A., Neil, J. F., Ulrich, R., and Shaw, D. H., 1981b, Sleep and treatment prediction in endogeneous depression, *Am. J. Psychiatry* **138**:429–434.

Kupfer, D. J., Ulrich, R. F., Coble, P. A., Jarrett, D. B., Grochocinski, V., Doman, J., Matthews, G., and Borbely, A. A., 1984, Application of automated REM and slow wave sleep analysis: II. Testing the assumptions of the two-process model of sleep regulation in normal and depressed subjects, *Psychiatry Res.* **13**:335–343.

Kuypers, H. G. J. M., 1958, Cortico-bulbar connexions to the pons and lower brain stem in man. An anatomical study, *Brain* **81**:364–388.

Kuypers, H. G. J. M., Bentivoglio, M., Catsman-Berrevoets, C. E., and Bharos, A. T., 1980, Double retrograde neuronal labeling through divergent axon collaterals, using two fluorescent tracers with the same excitation wave length which label different features of the cell, *Exp. Brain Res.* **40**:383–392.

Lai, Y. Y., and Siegel, J. M., 1988, Medullary regions mediating atonia, *J. Neurosci.* **8**:4790–4796.

Lamour, Y., Dutar, P., and Jobert, A., 1982, Excitatory effect of acetylcholine on different types of neurons in the first somatosensory neocortex of the rat: Laminar distribution and pharmacological characteristics, *Neuroscience* **7**:1483–1494.

Lamour, Y., Dutar, P., and Jobert, A., 1983, A comparative study of two populations of acetylcholine sensitive neurons in rat somatosensory cortex, *Brain Res.* **289**:157–167.

Lamour, Y., Dutar, P., and Jobert, A., 1984, Septo-hippocampal and other medial septum–diagonal band neurons: Electrophysiological and pharmacological properties, *Brain Res.* **309**:227–239.

Lancaster, B., and Nicoll, R. A., 1987, Properties of two calcium-activated hyperpolarizations in rat hippocampal neurones, *J. Physiol. (Lond.)* **389**:187–203.

Lang, W. Henn, V., and Hepp, K., 1982, Gaze palsies after selective pontine lesions in monkeys, in: *Physiological and Pathological Aspects of Eye Movements* (A. Roucoux and M. Crommelinck, eds.), Junk, The Hague, pp. 209–218.

Lang, W. Lang, M., Kornhuber, A., Deeke, L., and Kornhuber, H. H., 1983, Human cerebral potentials and visuomotor learning, *Pflugers Arch.* **399**:342–344.

Langer, T., Fuchs, A. F., Scudder, C. A., and Chubb, M. C., 1985, Afferents to the flocculus of the cerebellum in the rhesus macaque as revealed by retrograde transport of horseradish peroxidase, *J. Comp. Neurol.* **235**:1–25.

Langer, T., Kaneko, C. R. S., Scudder, C. A., and Fuchs, A. F., 1986, Afferents to the abducens nucleus in the monkey and the cat, *J. Comp. Neurol.* **245**:379–400.

Lasek, R., Joseph, B. S., and Whitlock, D. G., 1968, Evaluation of a radioautographic neuroanatomical tracing method, *Brain Res.* **8**:319–336.

LaVail, J. H., and LaVail, M. M., 1972, Retrograde axonal transport in the central nervous system, *Science* **176**:1416–1417.

Leichnetz, G., Smith, D. J., and Spencer, R. F., 1984, Cortical projections to the paramedian tegmental and basila pons in the monkey, *J. Comp. Neurol.* **228**:388–408.

Leichnetz, G. R., Gonzalo-Ruiz, A., DeSalles, A. A. F., and Hayes, R. L., 1987, The origin of brainstem afferents of the paramedian pontine reticular formation in the cat, *Brain Res.* **422**:389–397.

Leonard, C. S., and Llinás, R., 1987, Low threshold calcium conductance in parabrachial reticular neurons studied *in vitro* and its blockade by octanol, *Soc. Neurosci. Abstr.* **13**:1012.

Leonard, C. S., and Llinás, R., 1988, Electrophysiology of thalamic-projecting cholinergic brainstem neurons and their inhibition by acetylcholine, *Soc. Neurosci. Abstr.* **14**:297.

Leonard, C. S., and Llinás, R., 1989, *In vitro* study of pedunculopontine neurons and ACh actions, in: *Brain Cholinergic Systems* (M. Steriade and D. Biesold, eds.), Oxford University Press, Oxford, New York (in press).

Leontovitch, T. A., and Zhukova, G. P., 1963, The specificity of the neuronal structure and topography of the reticular formation in the brain and spinal cord of carnivora, *J. Comp. Neurol.* **121**:347–389.

Leung, L. W. S., and Borst, J. G. G., 1987, Electrical activity of the cingulate cortex. I. Generating mechanisms and relations to behavior, *Brain Res.* **407**:68–80.

Levey, A. I., Armstrong, D. M., Atweh, S. F., Terry, R. D., and Wainer, B. H., 1983a, Monoclonal antibodies to choline acetyltransferase: Production, specificity, and immunohistochemistry, *J. Neurosci.* **3:**1–9.

Levey, A. I., Wainer, B. H., Mufson, E. J., and Mesulam, M. M., 1983b, Co-localization of acetylcholinesterase and choline acetyltransferase in the rat cerebrum, *Neuroscience* **9:**9–22.

Levey, A. I., Hallanger, A. E., and Wainer, B. H., 1987a, Choline acetyltransferase-immunoreactivity in the rat thalamus, *J. Comp. Neurol.* **257:**317–332.

Levey, A. I., Hallanger, A. E., and Wainer, B. H., 1987b, Cholinergic nucleus basalis neurons may influence the cortex via the thalamus, *Neurosci. Lett.* **74:**7–13.

Levitt, P., and Moore, R. Y., 1978, Noradrenaline neuron innervation of the neocortex in the rat, *Brain Res.* **139:**219–231.

Levitt, P., and Moore, R. Y., 1979, Origin and organization of brainstem catecholamine innervation in the rat, *J. Comp. Neurol.* **186:**505–528.

Lhermitte, F., Gautier, J. C., Marteau, R., and Chain, F., 1963, Troubles de la conscience et mutisme akinetique, *Rev. Neurol. (Paris)* **109:**115–131.

Lidov, H. G. W., Grzanna, R., and Molliver, M. E., 1980, The serotonin innervation of the cerebral cortex in the rat—an immunohistochemical analysis, *Neuroscience* **5:**207–227.

Lin, J.-S., Luppi, P.-H., Salvert, D., Sakai, K., and Jouvet, M., 1986, Neurones immunoreactifs a l'histamine dans l'hypothalamus chez le chat, *C.R. Acad. Sci. (Paris)* **303:**371–376.

Lindsley, D. B., Bowden, J. W., and Magoun, H. W., 1949, Effect upon the EEG of acute injury to the brain stem activating system, *Electroencephalogr. Clin. Neurophysiol.* **1:**475–486.

Lindsley, D. B., Schreiner, L. H., Knowles, W. B., and Magoun, H. W., 1950, Behavioral and EEG changes following chronic brain stem lesions in the cat, *Electroencephalogr. Clin. Neurophysiol.* **2:**483–498.

Lindvall, O., and Bjorklund, A., 1974, The organization of the ascending catecholamine neuron systems in the rat brain as revealed by the glyoxylic acid fluorescence method, *Acta Physiol. Scand. [Suppl.]* **412:**1–48.

Lindvall, O., Bjorklund, A., Nobin, A., and Stenevi, U., 1974, The adrenergic innervation of the rat thalamus as revealed by the glyoxylic acid fluorescence method, *J. Comp. Neurol.* **154:**317–348.

Lindvall, O., Bjorklund, A., and Divac, I., 1978, Organization of catecholamine neurons projecting to the frontal cortex in the rat, *Brain Res.* **142:**1–24.

Livingstone, M. S., and Hubel, D. H., 1981, Effects of sleep and arousal on the processing of visual information in the cat, *Nature* **291:**554–561.

Ljungdahl, A., Hokfelt, T., and Nilsson, G., 1978, Distribution of substance P-like immunoreactivity in the central nervous system of the rat. I. Cell bodies and terminals, *Neuroscience* **3:**861–943.

Llinás, R. R., 1988, The intrinsic electrophysiological properties of mammalian neurons: Insights into central nervous system function, *Science* **242:**1654–1664.

Llinás, R., and Hillman, D. E., 1975, A multipurpose tridimensional reconstruction computer system for neuroanatomy, in: *Golgi Centennial Symposium* (M. Santini, ed.), Raven Press, New York, pp. 71–79.

Llinás, R., and Jahnsen, H., 1982, Electrophysiology of mammalian thalamic neurones *in vitro,* *Nature* **297:**406–408.

Llinás, R., and Muhlethaler, M., 1988, An electrophysiological study of the *in vitro,* perfused brain stem–cerebellum of adult guinea-pig, *J. Physiol. (Lond.)* **404:**215–240.

Llinás, R., and Sugimori, M., 1980, Electrophysiological properties of *in vitro* Purkinje cell dendrites in mammalian cerebellar slices, *J. Physiol. (Lond.)* **305:**171–195.

Llinás, R., and Yarom, Y., 1981, Electrophysiology of mammalian inferior olivary neurones *in vitro,* *J. Physiol. (Lond.)* **315:**549–567.

Llinás, R., and Yarom, Y., 1986, Specific blockage of the low threshold calcium channel by high molecular weight alcohols, *Soc. Neurosci. Abstr.* **12:**174.

Llinás, R., Paré, D., Deschênes, M., and Steriade, M., 1987, Differences between thalamo-cortical spindling and PGO generation demonstrated by low-threshold Ca blockage by octanol, *Soc. Neurosci. Abstr.* **13:**1012.

Lopes da Silva, F., 1987, Dynamics of EEGs as signals of neuronal populations: Models and theoretical considerations, in: *Electroencephalography* (E. Niedermeyer and F. Lopes da Silva, eds.), Schwartzenberg, Baltimore, Munich, pp. 15–28.

Lopes da Silva, F. H., Vos, J. E., Mooibroek, J., and van Rotterdam, A., 1980, Partial coherence analysis of thalamic and cortical alpha rhythms in dog. A contribution towards a general model of the cortical organization of rhythmic activity, in: *Rhythmic EEG Activities and Cortical Function-*

ing (G. Pfurtscheller, P. Buser, and F. H. Lopes da Silva, eds.), Elsevier/North-Holland, Amsterdam, pp. 33–59.

Lotka, A., 1956, *Elements of Physical Biology*, Dover Press, New York.

Lucki, I., Nobler, M. S., and Frazer, A., 1984, Differential actions of serotonin antagonists on two behavioral models of serotonin receptor activation in the rat, *J. Pharmacol. Exp. Ther.* **228:**133–139.

Luschei, E. S., and Fuchs, A. F., 1972, Activity of brain stem neurons during eye movements of alert monkeys, *J. Neurophysiol.* **35:**445–461.

Lydic, R., and Biebuyck, J. F., eds., 1988, *Clinical Physiology of Sleep*, American Physiological Society, Bethesda.

Lydic, R., McCarley, R. W., and Hobson, J. A., 1983, The time-course of dorsal raphe discharge, PGO waves, and muscle tone averaged across multiple sleep cycles, *Brain Res.* **274:**365–370.

Lydic, R., McCarley, R. W., and Hobson, J. A., 1987a, Serotonin neurons and sleep: I. Long term recordings of dorsal raphe discharge frequency and PGO waves, *Arch. Ital. Biol.* **125:**317–343.

Lydic, R., McCarley, R. W., and Hobson, J. A., 1987b, Serotonin neurons and sleep: II. Time course of dorsal raphe discharge, PGO waves, and behavioral states, *Arch. Ital. Biol.* **126:**1–28.

Maas, J. W., 1975, Biogenic amines and depression: Biochemical and pharmacological separation of two types of depression, *Arch. Gen. Psychiatry* **32:**1357–1361.

Macchi, G., Bentivoglio, M., Molinari, M., and Minciacchi, D., 1984, The thalamo-caudate versus thalamo-cortical projections as studied in the cat with fluorescent retrograde double labeling, *Exp. Brain Res.* **54:**225–239.

MacDermott, A. B., Mayer, M. L., Westbrook, G. L., Smith, S. J., and Barker, J. L., 1986, NMDA-receptor activation increases cytoplasmic calcium concentration in cultured spinal cord neurones, *Nature* **321:**519–522.

MacDonald, J. F., and Wojtowicz, J. M., 1980, Two conductance mechanisms activated by applications of L-glutamatic, L-aspartic, DL-homocysteic, N-methyl-D-aspartic, and DL-kainic acids to cultured mammalian central neurones, *Can. J. Physiol. Pharmacol.* **58:**1393–1397.

Maciewicz, R. J., Eagen, K., Kaneko, C. R. S., and Highstein, S. M., 1977, Vestibular and medullary brain stem afferents to the abducens nucleus in the cat, *Brain Res.* **123:**229–240.

MacLeod, N. K., and James, T. A., 1984, Regulation of cerebello-cortical transmission in the rat ventromedial thalamic nucleus, *Exp. Brain Res.* **55:**535–552.

MacLeod, N. K., James, T. A., and Starr, M. S., 1984, Muscarinic action of acetylcholine in the rat ventromedial thalamic nucleus, *Exp. Brain Res.* **55:**553–561.

Madison, D. V., and Nicoll, R. A., 1984, Control of the repetitive discharge of rat CA1 pyramidal pyramidal neurones *in vitro*, *J. Physiol. (Lond.)* **354:**319–331.

Madison, D. V., and Nicoll, R. A., 1986a, Actions of noradrenaline recorded intracellularly in rat hippocampal CA1 neurones, *in vitro*, *J. Physiol. (Lond.)* **372:**221–244.

Madison, D. V., and Nicoll, R., 1986b, Cyclic adenosine 3′,5′-monophosphate mediates Beta-receptor actions of noradrenaline in rat hippocampal pyramidal cells, *J. Physiol. (Lond.)* **372:**245–259.

Madison, D. V., and Nicoll, R. A., 1988, Norepinephrine decreases synaptic inhibition in the rat hippocampus, *Brain Res.* **442:**131–138.

Madison, D. V., Lancaster, B., and Nicoll, R. A., 1987, Voltage clamp analysis of cholinergic action in the hippocampus, *J. Neurosci.* **7:**733–741.

Maekawa, K., and Purpura, D. P., 1967a, Properties of spontaneous and evoked synaptic activities of thalamic ventrobasal neurons, *J. Neurophysiol.* **30:**360–381.

Maekawa, K., and Purpura, D. P., 1967b, Intracellular study of lemniscal and nonspecific synaptic interactions in thalamic ventrobasal neurons, *Brain Res.* **4:**308–323.

Maffei, L., Moruzzi, G., and Rizzolatti, G., 1965a, Geniculate unit responses to sine-wave photic stimulation during wakefulness and sleep, *Science* **149:**563–564.

Maffei, L., Moruzzi, G., and Rizzolatti, G., 1965b, Influence of sleep and wakefulness on the response of lateral geniculate units to sinewave photic stimulation, *Arch. Ital. Biol.* **103:**596–608.

Maffei, L., Moruzzi, G., and Rizzolatti, G., 1965c, Effects of synchronized sleep on the response of lateral geniculate units to flashes of light, *Arch. Ital. Biol.* **103:**609–622.

Magni, F., and Willis, W. D., 1963, Identification of reticular formation neurons by intracellular recording, *Arch. Ital. Biol.* **101:**681–702.

Magni, F., Moruzzi, G., Rossi, G. F., and Zanchetti, A., 1959, EEG arousal following inactivation of the lower brain stem by selective injection of barbiturate into the vertebral circulation, *Arch. Ital. Biol.* **97:**33–46.

Magoun, H. W., 1975, The role of research institutes in the advancement of neuroscience: Ranson's institute of neurology, 1928–1942, in: *The Neurosciences: Paths of Discovery* (F. G. Worden, J. P. Swazey, and G. Adelman, eds.), The MIT Press, Cambridge, MA, London, pp. 515–527.

Magoun, H. W., and Rhines, R., 1946, An inhibitory mechanism in the bulbar reticular formation, *J. Neurophysiol.* **9:**119–152.

Mahowald, M. W., and Schenck, C. H., 1989, REM sleep behavior disorder, in: *Principles and Practices of Sleep Medicine* (M. H. Kryger, T. Roth, and W. C. Dement, eds.), Saunders, New York, pp. 389–401.

Malenka, R. C., Madison, D. V., Perkel, D. J., and Nicoll, R. A., 1986, Actions of norepinephrine and carbachol on granule cells of the dentate gyrus *in vitro*, *Soc. Neurosci. Abstr.* **12:**729.

Mancia, M., Mariotti, M., and Spreafico, R., 1974, Caudo-rostral brainstem reciprocal influences in the cat, *Brain Res.* **80:**41–51.

Mannen, H., 1975, Morphological analysis of an individual neuron with Golgi's method, 1975, in: *Golgi Centennial Symposium* (M. Santini, ed.), Raven Press, New York, pp. 61–70.

Marchetti, C., Carbone, E., and Lux, H. D., 1986, Effects of dopamine and noradrenaline on Ca channels of cultured sensory and sympathetic neurons of chick, *Pflugers Arch.* **406:**104–111.

Mariotti, M., Soja, P. J., Morales, F. R., and Chase, M. H., 1986, The spontaneous IPSPs which bombard trigeminal motoneurons during active sleep appear to be generated at somatic and proximal dendritic loci, *Abstr. Soc. Neurosci.* **12:**250.

Marks, G. A., and Roffwarg, H. P., 1987, The role of acetylcholine in the control of state-related activity of thalamic relay cells, *Sleep Res.* **16:**20.

Marshall, K. C., and McLennan, H., 1972, The synaptic activation of neurones of the feline ventrolateral thalamic nucleus: Possible cholinergic mechanisms, *Exp. Brain Res.* **15:**472–483.

Marshall, K. C., and Murray, J. S., 1980, Cholinergic facilitation of thalamic relay transmission in the cat, *Exp. Neurol.* **69:**318–333.

Martin, G. F., and Waltzer R. P., 1984a, A double-labelling study of reticular collaterals to the spinal cord and cerebellum of the North American opossum, *Neurosci. Lett.* **47:**185–191.

Martin, G. F., and Waltzer, R. P., 1984b, A study of overlap and collateralization of bulbar reticular and raphe neurons which project to the spinal cord and diencephalon of the North American opossum, *Brain Behav. Evol.* **24:**109–123.

Martin, G. F., Humbertson, A. O., Laxson, C. L., Panneton, W. M., and Tschismadia, I., 1979, Spinal projections from the mesencephalic and pontine reticular formation in the North American opossum: A study using axonal transport techniques, *J. Comp. Neurol.* **187:**373–400.

Martin, L. J., Koliatsos, V. E., Nauta, H. J. W., DeLong, M. R., and Price, D. L., 1987, Substantia innominata and pedunculopontine tegmental nucleus in the rat: Evidence for predominantly noncholinergic reciprocal innervation, *Soc. Neurosci. Abstr.* **13:**1567.

Mash, D. C., and Potter, L. T., 1986, Autoradiographic localization of M_1 and M_2 muscarine receptors in the rat brain, *Neuroscience* **19:**551–564.

Massaquoi, S. G., and McCarley, R. W., 1982, Extension of the reciprocal interaction sleep stage control model: A "Karma" control model, *Sleep Res.* **11:**216.

Mathiesen, J. S., and Blackstad, T. W., 1964, Cholinesterase in the hippocampal region. Distribution and relation to architectonics and afferent systems, *Acta Anat.* **56:**216–253.

Mauguière, F., and Courjon, J., 1983, The origins of short-latency somatosensory evoked potentials in humans, *Ann. Neurol.* **9:**607–611.

Maunz, R. A., Pitts, N. G., and Peterson, B. W., 1978, Cat spinoreticular neurons: Locations, responses and changes in responses during repetitive stimulation, *Brain Res.* **148:**365–379.

May, P. J., and Hall, W. C., 1986, The sources of the nigrotectal pathway, *Neuroscience* **19:**159–180.

Mayer, M. L., and Westbrook, G. L., 1983, A voltage-clamp analysis of inward (anomalous) rectification in mouse spinal sensory ganglion neurons, *J. Physiol. (Lond.)* **340:**19–45.

Mayer, M. L., and Westbrook, G. L., 1987, The physiology of excitatory amino acids in the vertebrate central nervous system, *Progr. Neurobiol.* **28:**197–276.

Mayer, M. L., Westbrook, G. L., and Guthrie, P. B., 1984, Voltage-dependent block by Mg^{2+} of NMDA responses in spinal cord neurones, *Nature* **309:**261–263.

Mays, L. E., and Sparks, D. L., 1980, Dissociation of visual and saccade-related responses in superior colliculus neurons, *J. Neurophysiol.* **43:**207–233.

McCance, I., Phillis, J. W., and Westerman, R. A., 1968a, Acetylcholine-sensitivity of thalamic neurones: Its relationship to synaptic transmission, *Br. J. Pharmacol. Chemother.* **32:**635–651.

McCance, I., Phillis, J. W., Tebecis, A. K., and Westerman, R. A., 1968b, The pharmacology of acetylcholine-excitation of thalamic neurones, *Br. J. Pharmacol. Chemother.* **32:**652–662.

McCarley, R. W., 1973, A model for the periodicity of brain stem neuronal discharges during the sleep cycle, *Sleep Res.* **2**:30.

McCarley, R. W., 1980a, Reciprocal discharge of reticular and non-reticular brainstem neurons and a model for state-dependent changes in neuronal activity, in: *The Brainstem Core: Sensorimotor Integration and Behavioral State Control* (J. A. Hobson and A. B. Schiebel, eds.), *Neurosci. Res. Prog. Bull.* **18**:101–112.

McCarley, R. W., 1980b, Mechanisms and models of behavioral state control, in: *The Reticular Formation Revisited* (J. A. Hobson and M. A. B. Brazier, eds.), Raven Press, New York, pp. 375–403.

McCarley, R. W., 1981, Mind-body isomorphisms and the study of dreams, in: *Advances in Sleep Research,* Vol. IV (W. Fishbein, ed.), Spectrum Publications, New York.

McCarley, R. W., 1982, REM sleep and depression: Common neurobiological control mechanisms, *Am. J. Psychiatry* **139**:565–570.

McCarley, R. W., 1983, REM dreams, REM sleep, and their isomorphisms, in: *Sleep Disorders: Basic and Clinical Research* (M. Chase and E. D. Weitzman, eds.), Spectrum Publications, New York, pp. 363–392.

McCarley, R. W., 1988, Foreward, in: *Clinical Physiology of Sleep* (R. Lydic and J. F. Biebuyck, eds.), American Physiological Society, Bethesda, pp. v–ix.

McCarley, R. W., 1989, The biology of dreaming sleep, in: *Principles and Practices of Sleep Medicine* (M. H. Kryger, T. Roth, and W. C. Dement, eds.), Saunders, New York, pp. 173–183.

McCarley, R. W., and Hobson, J. A., 1970, Cortical unit activity in desynchronized sleep, *Science* **167**:901–903.

McCarley, R. W., and Hobson, J. A., 1971, Single neuron activity in cat gigantocellular tegmental field: Selectivity of discharge in desynchronized sleep, *Science* **174**:1250–1252.

McCarley, R. W., and Hobson, J. A., 1975a, Discharge patterns of cat pontine brain stem neurons during desynchronized sleep, *J. Neurophysiol.* **38**:751–766.

McCarley, R. W., and Hobson, J. A., 1975b, Neuronal excitability modulation over the sleep cycle: A structural and mathematical model, *Science* **189**:58–60.

McCarley, R. W., and Hobson, J. A., 1977, The neurobiological origins of psychoanalytic dream theory, *Am. J. Psychiatry* **134**:1211–1221.

McCarley, R. W., and Hobson, J. A., 1979, The form of dreams and the biology of sleep, in: *Handbook of Dreams: Research, Theory, and Applications* (B. Wolman, ed.), Van Nostrand Reinhold, New York, pp. 76–130.

McCarley, R. W., and Hoffman, E. A., 1981, REM sleep dreams and the activation–synthesis hypothesis, *Am. J. Psychiatry* **138**:904–912.

McCarley, R. W., and Ito, K., 1983, Intracellular evidence linking medial pontine reticular formation neurons to PGO generation, *Brain Res.* **280**:343–348.

McCarley, R. W., and Ito, K., 1985, Desynchronized sleep-specific changes in membrane potential and excitability in medial pontine reticular formation neurons: Implications for concepts and mechanisms of behavioral state control, in: *Brain Mechanisms of Sleep* (D. McGinty, R. Drucker-Colin, A. Morrison, and P. L. Parmeggiani, eds.), Raven Press, New York, pp. 63–80.

McCarley, R. W., and Massaquoi, S. G., 1986a, A limit cycle mathematical model of the REM sleep oscillator system, *Am. J. Physiol.* **251**:R1011–R1029.

McCarley, R. W., and Massaquoi, S. G., 1986b, Further discussion of a model of the REM sleep oscillator, *Am. J. Physiol.* **251**:R1033–R1036.

McCarley, R. W., Nelson, J. P., and Hobson, J. A., 1978, Ponto-geniculo-occipital (PGO) burst neurons: Correlative evidence for neuronal generators of PGO waves, *Science* **201**:269–272.

McCarley, R. W., Benoit, O., and Barrionuevo, G., 1983, Lateral geniculate nucleus unitary discharge in sleep and waking: State and rate specific aspects, *J. Neurophysiol.* **50**:798–818.

McCarley, R. W., Ito, K., and Rodrigo-Angulo, M. L., 1987, Physiological studies of brainstem reticular connectivity. II. Responses of mPRF neurons to stimulation of mesencephalic and contralateral pontine reticular formation, *Brain Res.* **409**:111–127.

McCormick, D. A., 1989a, Cellular mechanisms of cholinergic control of neocortical and thalamic neuronal excitability, in: *Brain Cholinergic Systems* (M. Steriade and D. Biesold, eds.), Oxford University Press, Oxford (in press).

McCormick, D. A., 1989b, Cholinergic and noradrenergic modulation of thalamocortical processing, *Trends Neurosci.* **12**:215–221.

McCormick, D. A., and Pape, H. C., 1988, Acetylcholine inhibits identified interneurones in the cat lateral geniculate nucleus, *Nature* **334**:246–248.

REFERENCES

McCormick, D. A., and Prince, D. A., 1985, Two types of muscarinic response to acetylcholine in mammalian cortical neurons, *Proc. Natl. Acad. Sci. U.S.A.* **82:**6344–6348.

McCormick, D. A., and Prince, D. A., 1986a, Mechanisms of action of acetylcholine in the guinea pig cerebral cortex, *in vitro, J. Physiol. (Lond.)* **375:**169–194.

McCormick, D. A., and Prince, D. A., 1986b, ACh induces burst firing in thalamic reticular neurones by activating a K conductance, *Nature* **319:**402–405.

McCormick, D. A., and Prince, D. A., 1987a, Actions of acetylcholine in the guinea-pig and cat medial and lateral geniculate nuclei, *in vitro, J. Physiol. (Lond.)* **392:**147–165.

McCormick, D. A., and Prince, D. A., 1987b, Acetylcholine causes rapid nicotinic excitation in the medial habenular nucleus of guinea pig, *in vitro, J. Neurosci.* **7:**742–752.

McCormick, D. A., and Prince, D. A., 1987c, Neurotransmitter modulation of thalamic neuronal firing pattern, *J. Mind Behav.* **8:**573–590.

McCormick, D. A., and Prince, D. A., 1987d, Actions of acetylcholine in the guinea-pig and cat medial and lateral geniculate nuclei, *in vitro, J. Physiol. (Lond.)* **392:**147–165.

McCormick, D. A., and Prince, D. A., 1988, Noradrenergic modulation of firing pattern in guinea pig and cat thalamic neurons *in vitro, J. Neurophysiol.* **59:**978–996.

McCormick, D. A., Connors, B. W., Lighthall, J. W., and Prince, D. A., 1985, Comparative electrophysiology of pyramidal and sparsely spiny stellate neurons of the neocortex, *J. Neurophysiol.* **54:**782–806.

McGinty, D. J., and Harper, R. M., 1976, Dorsal raphe neurons: Depression of firing during sleep in cats, *Brain Res.* **101:**569–575.

McGinty, D. J., and Sterman, M. B., 1968, Sleep suppression after basal forebrain lesions in the cat, *Science* **160:**1253–1255.

McGinty, D., Drucker-Colin, R., Morrison, A., and Parmeggiani, P. L., eds., 1985, *Brain Mechanisms of Sleep*, Raven Press, New York.

McHaffie, J. G., and Stein, B. E., 1982, Eye movements evoked by electrical stimulation in the superior colliculus of rats and hamsters, *Brain Res.* **247:**243–253.

McLennan, H., 1983, Receptors for the excitatory amino acids in the mammalian central nervous system, *Prog. Neurobiol.* **20:**251–271.

McLennan, H., and Hicks, T. P., 1978, Pharmacological characterization of the excitatory cholinergic receptors of rat central neurons, *Neuropharmacology* **17:**329–334.

McPartland, R. J., Kupfer, D. J., Coble, P., Shaw, D. H., and Spiker, D. G., 1979, An automated analysis of REM sleep in primary depression, *Biol. Psychiatry* **14:**767–776.

Melker, R. J., and Purpura, D. P., 1972, Maturational features of neurons and synaptic relations in raphe and reticular nuclei of neonatal kittens, *Anat. Rec.* **172:**366–367.

Menetrey, D., Chaouch, A., and Besson, J. M., 1980, Location and properties of dorsal horn neurons at origin of spinoreticular tract in lumbar enlargement of the rat, *J. Neurophysiol.* **44:**862–877.

Menkes, D. B., and Aghajanian, G. K., 1980, Chronic antidepressant treatment enhances alpha-adrenergic responses in brain: A microiontophoretic study, *Soc. Neurosci. Abstr.* **6:**860.

Mesulam, M. M., 1978, Tetramethyl benzidine for horseradish peroxidase neurohistochemistry: A non-carcinogenic blue reaction-product with superior sensitivity for visualizing neural afferents and efferents, *J. Histochem. Cytochem.* **26:**106–117.

Mesulam, M. M., 1982, Principles of horseradish peroxidase neurohistochemistry and their applications for tracing neural pathways—axonal transport, enzyme histochemistry and light microscopic analysis, in: *Tracing Neural Connections with Horseradish Peroxidase* (M. M. Mesulam, ed.), John Wiley & Sons, New York, pp. 1–151.

Mesulam, M. M., and Mufson, E. J., 1980, The rapid anterograde transport of horseradish peroxidase, *Neuroscience* **5:**1277–1286.

Mesulam, M. M., and Rosene, D. L., 1979, Sensitivity in horseradish peroxidase neurohistochemistry: A comparative and quantitative analysis of nine methods, *J. Histochem. Cytochem.* **27:**763–773.

Mesulam, M. M., Mufson, E. J., Wainer, B. H., and Levey, A. I., 1983, Central cholinergic pathways in the rat: An overview based on an alternative nomenclature (Ch1–Ch6), *Neuroscience* **10:**1185–1201.

Mesulam, M. M., Mufson, E. J., Levey, A. I., and Wainer, B. H., 1984, Atlas of cholinergic neurons in the forebrain and upper brainstem of the macaque based on monoclonal choline acetyltransferase immunohistochemistry and acetyl-cholinesterase histochemistry, *Neuroscience* **12:**669–686.

Metherate, R., Tremblay, N., and Dykes, R. W., 1987, Acetylcholine permits long-term enhancement of neuronal responsiveness in cat primary somatosensory cortex, *Neuroscience* **22:**75–81.

Metherate, R., Tremblay, N., and Dykes, R. W., 1988a, The effects of acetylcholine on response properties of cat somatosensory cortical neurons, *J. Neurophysiol.* **59**:1231–1252.

Metherate, R., Tremblay, N., and Dykes, R. W., 1988b, Transient and prolonged effects of acetylcholine on responsiveness of cat somatosensory cortical neurons, *J. Neurophysiol.* **59**:1253–1276.

Meulders, M., and Godfraind, J. M., 1969, Influence de l'éveil d'origine réticulaire sur l'étendue des champs visuels des neurones de la région genouillée chez le chat avec cerveau intact ou avec cerveau isolé, *Exp. Brain Res.* **9**:201–220.

Meynert, T., 1872, Vom Gehirn der Saugetiere, in: *Handbuch der Lehre von den Geweben des Menschen und Tiere,* Vol. 2 (S. Stricker, ed.), Engelmann, Leipzig, pp. 694–808.

Mignot, E., Guilleminault, C., Bowersox, S., Rapport, A., and Dement, W. C., 1988, Role of central alpha-1 adrenoceptors in canine narcolepsy, *J. Clin. Investig.* **82**:885–894.

Milner, T. A., and Pickel, V. M., 1986, Ultrastructural localization and afferent sources of substance P in the rat parabrachial region, *Neuroscience* **17**:687–707.

Minciacchi, D., Bentivoglio, M., Molinari, M., Kultas-Ilinski, K., Ilinski, I. A., and Macchi, G., 1986, Multiple cortical targets of one thalamic nucleus: The projections of the ventral medial nucleus in the cat studied with retrograde tracers, *J. Comp. Neurol.* **252**:106–129.

Mitani, A., Ito, K., Mitani, Y., and McCarley, R. W., 1988a, Descending projections from the gigantocellular tegmental field in the cat: Origins of the descending pathways and their funicular trajectories, *J. Comp. Neurol.* **268**:546–566.

Mitani, A., Ito, K., Mitani, Y., and McCarley, R. W., 1988b, Morphological and electrophysiological identification of gigantocellular tegmental field neurons. I. Pons, *J. Comp. Neurol.* **268**:527–545.

Mitani, A., Ito, K., Mitani, Y., and McCarley, R. W., 1988c, Morphological and electrophysiological identification of gigantocellular tegmental field neurons with descending projections in the cat. II. Bulb, *J. Comp. Neurol.* **274**:371–386.

Mitani, A., Ito, K., Hallanger, A. H., Wainer, B. H., Kataoka, K., and McCarley, R. W., 1988d, Cholinergic projections from the laterodorsal and pedunculopontine tegmental nuclei to the pontine gigantocellular tegmental field in the cat, *Brain Res.* **451**:397–402.

Mitler, M. M., and Dement, W. C., 1974, Cataplectic-like behavior in cats after microinjections of carbachol in pontine reticular formation, *Brain Res.***68**:335–343.

Mize, R. R., and Payne, M. P., 1987, The innervation density of serotonergic (5-HT) fibers varies in different subdivisions of the rat lateral geniculate nucleus complex, *Neurosci. Lett.* **82**:133–139.

Mizuno, N., Clemente, C. D., and Sauerland, E. K., 1969, Fiber projections from rostral basal forebrain structures in the cat, *Exp. Neurol.* **25**:22–237.

Mogilnicka, E., Arbilla, S., and Depoortere, H., 1980, Rapid-eye-movement sleep deprivation decreases the density of ^{3}H-dihydroalprenolol and ^{3}H-imipramine binding sites in the rat cerebral cortex, *Eur. J. Pharmacol.* **65**:289–299.

Molinari, M., Hendry, S. H. C., and Jones, E. G., 1987, Distributions of certain neuropeptides in the primate thalamus, *Brain Res.* **426**:270–289.

Montaron, M. F., Bouyer, J. J., Rougeul, A., and Buser, P., 1982, Ventral mesencephalic tegmentum (VMT) controls electrocortical beta rhythms and associated attentive behavior in the cat, *Behav. Brain Res.* **6**:129–145.

Moon-Edley, S., and Graybiel, A. M., 1983, The afferent and efferent connections of the feline nucleus tegmenti pedunculopontinus, pars compacta, *J. Comp. Neurol.* **217**:187–215.

Moore, R. Y., and Bloom, F. E., 1978, Central catecholamine systems: Anatomy and physiology of the dopamine system, *Annu. Rev. Neurosci.* **1**:29–69.

Moore, S. D., Madamba, S. G., Joels, M., and Siggins, G. R., 1988, Somatostatin augments the M-current in hippocampal neurons, *Science* **239**:278–280.

Morales, F. R., and Chase, M. H., 1978, Intracellular recording of lumbar motoneuron membrane potential during sleep and wakefulness, *Exp. Neurol.* **62**:821–827.

Morales, F. R., and Chase, M. H., 1981, Postsynaptic control of lumbar motoneuron excitability during active sleep in the chronic cat, *Brain Res.* **225**:279–295.

Morales, F. R., Boxer, P., and Chase, M. H., 1987a, Behavioral state-specific postsynaptic potentials impinge on cat lumbar motoneurons during active sleep, *Exp. Neurol.* **98**:418–435.

Morales, F. R., Engelhardt, J. K., Soja, P. J., Pereda, A. E., and Chase, M. H., 1987b, Motoneuron properties during motor inhibition produced by microinjection of carbachol into the pontine reticular formation of the decerebrate cat, *J. Neurophysiol.* **57**: 1118–1129.

Mori, S., 1987, Integration of posture and locomotion in acute decerebrate cats and in awake, freely moving cats, *Prog. Neurobiol.* **28**:161–196.

Morin, D., and Steriade, M., 1981, Development from primary to augmenting responses in primary somatosensory cortex, *Brain Res.* **205:**49–66.

Morison, R. S., and Bassett, D. L., 1945, Electrical activity of the thalamus and basal ganglia in decorticated cats, *J. Neurophysiol.* **8:**309–314.

Morison, R. S., and Dempsey, E. W., 1942, A study of thalamo-cortical relations, *Am. J. Physiol.* **135:**281–292.

Morrell, J. I., Greensberger, L. M., and Pfaff, D. W., 1981, Hypothalamic, other diencephalic and telencephalic neurons that project to the dorsal midbrain, *J. Comp. Neurol.* **201:**589–620.

Morrison, A. R., 1979, Brain-stem regulation of behavior during sleep and wakefulness, in: *Progress in Psychobiology and Physiological Psychology*, Vol. 8 (J. M. Sprague and A. N. Epstein, eds.), Academic Press, New York, pp. 91–131.

Morrison, J. H., and Foote, S. L., 1986, Noradrenergic and serotonergic innervation of cortical, thalamic, and tectal visual structures in Old and New World monkeys, *J. Comp. Neurol.* **243:**117–138.

Morrison, J. H., Molliver, M. E., Grzanna, M. E., and Coyle, J. T., 1981, The intracortical trajectory of the coeruleo-cortical projection in the rat: A tangentially organized cortical afferent, *Neuroscience* **6:**139–158.

Morrison, J. H., Foote, S. L., O'Connor, D., and Bloom, F. E., 1982, Laminar, tangential and regional organization of the noradrenergic innervation of monkey cortex: Dopamine-β-hydroxylase immunohistochemistry, *Brain Res. Bull.* **9:**309–319.

Moruzzi, G., 1963, Active processes in the brain stem during sleep, *Harvey Lect.* **58:**233–297.

Moruzzi, G., 1964, The historical development of the deafferentation hypothesis of sleep, *Proc. Am. Phil. Soc.* **108:**19–28.

Moruzzi, G., 1969, Sleep and instinctive behavior, *Arch. Ital. Biol.* **107:**175–216.

Moruzzi, G., 1972, The sleep-waking cycle, *Ergeb. Physiol.* **64:**1–165.

Moruzzi, G., and Magoun, H. W., 1949, Brain stem reticular formation and activation of the EEG, *Electroencephalogr. Clin. Neurophysiol.* **1:**455–473.

Moschovakis, A. K., Karabelas, A. B., and Highstein, S. M., 1988a, Structure–function relationships in the primate superior colliculus. I. Morphological classification of efferent neurons, *J. Neurophysiol.* **60:**232–262.

Moschovakis, A. K., Karabelas, A. B., and Highstein, S. M., 1988b, Structure–function relationships in the primate superior colliculus. II. Morphological identity of presaccadic neurons, *J. Neurophysiol.* **60:**232–262.

Mosko, S. B., and Jacobs, B. L., 1976, Recording of dorsal raphe unit activity *in vitro, Neurosci. Lett.* **2:**195–200.

Mosko, S., Lynch, G., and Cotman, C. W., 1973, The distribution of septal projections to the hippocampus of the rat, *J. Comp. Neurol.* **152:**163–174.

Mosko, S., Haubrich, D., and Jacobs, B. L., 1977, Serotonergic afferents to the dorsal raphe nucleus: Evidence from HRP and synaptosomal uptake studies, *Brain Res.* **119:**269–290.

Mountcastle, V. B., Andersen, R. A., and Motter, B. C., 1981, The influence of attentive fixation upon the excitability of the light-sensitive neurons of the posterior parietal cortex, *J. Neurosci.* **1:**1218–1235.

Mountcastle, V. B., Motter, B. C., Steinmetz, M. A., and Duffy, C. J., 1984, Looking and seeing: The visual functions of the parietal lobe, in: *Dynamic Aspects of Neocortical Function* (G. M. Edelman, W. E. Gall, and W. M. Cowan, eds.), Wiley-Interscience, New York, pp. 159–193.

Mufson, E. J., Martin, T. L., Mash, D. C., Wainer, B. H., and Mesulam, M. M., 1986, Cholinergic projections from the parabigeminal nucleus (Ch8) to the superior colliculus in the mouse: A combined analysis of horseradish peroxidase transport and choline acetyltransferase immunohistochemistry, *Brain Res.* **370:**144–148.

Mulle, C., Steriade, M., and Deschênes, M., 1985, The effects of QX314 on thalamic neurons, *Brain Res.* **333:**350–354.

Mulle, C., Madariaga, A., and Deschênes, M., 1986, Morphology and electrophysiological properties of reticularis thalamic neurons in cat: *In vivo* study of a thalamic pacemaker, *J. Neurosci.* **6:**2134–2145.

Nagai, T., Satoh, K., Imamoto, K., and Maeda, T., 1981, Divergent projections of catecholamine neurons of the locus coeruleus as revealed by fluorescent retrograde double labeling technique, *Neurosci. Lett.* **23:**117–123.

Nagai, T., McGeer, P. L., and McGeer, E. G., 1983, Distribution of GABA-T-intensive neurons in the rat forebrain and midbrain, *J. Comp. Neurol.* **218:**220–238.

Nakamura, H., and Kawamura, S., 1988, The ventral lateral geniculate nucleus in the cat: Thalamic and commissural connections revealed by the use of WGA-HRP transport, *J. Comp. Neurol.* **277:**509–528.

Nakamura, Y., Takatori, S., Nozaki, S., and Kikuchi, M., 1975, Monosynaptic reciprocal control of trigeminal motoneurons from the medial bulbar reticular formation, *Brain Res.* **89;**144–148.

Nakao, S., and Shiraishi, Y., 1983, Excitatory and inhibitory synaptic inputs from the medial mesodiencephalic junction to vertical eye movement-related montoneurons in the cat oculomotor nucleus, *Neurosci. Lett.* **42:**125–130.

Nakazato, T., 1987, Locus coeruleus neurons projecting to the forebrain and the spinal cord in the cat, *Neuroscience* **23:**529–538.

Nauta, W. J. H., 1946, Hypothalamic regulation of sleep in rats, *J. Neurophysiol.* **9:**285–316.

Nauta, W. J. H., 1958, Hippocampal projections and related neural pathways to the midbrain in the cat, *Brain Res.* **81:**319–340.

Nauta, W. J. H., and Kuypers, H. G. J. M., 1958, Some ascending pathways in the brain stem reticular formation, in: *Reticular Formation of the Brain* (H. H. Jasper, L. D. Proctor, R. S. Knighton, W. C. Noshay, and R. T. Costello, eds.), Little, Brown, Boston, pp. 3–30.

Neher, E., 1971, Two fast transient current components during voltage clamp on snail neurons, *J. Gen. Physiol.* **58:**36–53.

Neil, J. F., Merikanges, J. R., Foster, F. G., Merikanges, K. R., Spiker, D. G., and Kupfer, D. J., 1980, Waking and all-night sleep EEGs in anorexia nervosa, *Clin. Electroencephalogr.* **11:**9–15.

Nelson, J. P., McCarley, R. W., and Hobson, J. A., 1983, REM sleep burst neurons, PGO waves, and eye movement information, *J. Neurophysiol.* **50:**784–797.

Netick, A., Orem, J., and Dement, W. C., 1977, Neuronal activity specific to REM sleep and its relationship to breathing, *Brain Res.* **120:**197–207.

Neville, H. J., and Foote, S. L., 1984, Auditory event-related potentials in the squirrel monkey: Parallels to human late wave responses, *Brain Res.* **298:**107–116.

Newberry, N. R., and Nicoll, R. A., 1984, A bicuculline-resistant inhibitory postsynaptic potential in rat hippocampal pyramidal cells *in vitro, J. Physiol. (Lond.)* **348:**239–254.

Newman, D. B., 1985a, Distinguishing rat brainstem reticulospinal nuclei by their morphology. I. Medullay nuclei, *J. Hirnforsch.* **26:**187–226.

Newman, D. B., 1985b, Distinguishing rat brainstem reticulospinal nuclei by their neuronal morphology. II. Pontine and mesencephalic nuclei, *J. Hirnforsch.* **26:**385–418.

Newman, D. B., and Liu, R. P. C., 1987, Nuclear origins of brainstem reticulocortical systems in the rat, *Am. J. Anat.* **178:**279–299.

Noble, D., 1985, Ionic mechanisms in rhythmic firing of heart and nerve, *Trends Neurosci.* **89:**499–504.

Noda, T., and Oka, H., 1984, Nigral inputs to the pedunculopontine region: Intracellular analysis, *Brain Res.* **322:**223–227.

Noma, A., and Trautwein, W., 1978, Relaxation of the acetylcholine-induced potassium current in the rabbit sinoatrial node cell, *Pflugers Arch.* **377:**193–200.

North, R. A., 1986a, Mechanisms of autonomic integration, in: *Handbook of Physiology,* Section 1, Vol. IV (V. B. Mountcastle and F. E. Bloom, eds.), American Physiological Society, Bethesda, pp. 115–153.

North, R. A., 1986b, Receptors on individual neurones, *Neuroscience* **17:**899–907.

North, R. A., and Williams, J. T., 1985, On the potassium conductance increased by opioids in rat locus coeruleus neurones, *J. Physiol. (Lond.)* **364:**265–280.

North, R. A., and Yoshimura, M., 1984, The actions of noradrenaline on neurones of the rat substantia gelatinosa *in vitro, J. Physiol. (Lond.)* **349:**43–55.

North, R. A., Williams, J. T., Surprenant, A., and Christie, M. J., 1987, Mu and delta receptors both belong to a family of receptors which couple to a potassium conductance, *Proc. Natl. Acad. Sci. U.S.A.* **84:**5487–5491.

Nowak, L., Bregestovski, P., Ascher, P., Herbet, A., and Prochiantz, A., 1984, Magnesium gates glutamate-activated channels in mouse central neurones, *Nature* **307:**462–465.

Nowycky, M. C., Fox, A. P., and Tsien, R. W., 1985, Three types of neuronal calcium channel with different calcium agonist sensitivity, *Nature* **316:**440–446.

Oades, R. D., and Halliday, G. M., 1987, Ventral tegmental (A10) system: Neurobiology. I. Anatomy and connectivity, *Brain Res. Rev.* **12:**117–165.

Oakson, G., and Steriade, M., 1982, Slow rhythmic rate fluctuations of cat midbrain reticular neurons in synchronized sleep, *Brain Res.* **247:**277–288.

Oakson, G., and Steriade, M., 1983, Slow rhythmic oscillations of EEG slow-wave amplitudes and their relations to midbrain reticular discharge, *Brain Res.* **269:**386–390.

Oertel, W. H., Graybiel, A. M., Mugnaini, E., Elde, R. P., Schmechel, D. E., and Kopin, I. J., 1983, Coexistence of glutamic acid decarboxylase- and somatostatin-like immunoreactivity in neurons of the feline nucleus reticularis thalami, *J. Neurosci.* **3:**1322–1332.

Ohta, Y., Mori, S., and Kimua, H., 1988, Neuronal structures of the brainstem participating in postural suppression in cats, *Neurosci. Res.* **5:**181–202.

Oka, H., Ito, J., and Kawamura, M., 1982, Identification of thalamo-cortical neurons responsible for cortical recruiting and spindling activities in cats, *Neurosci. Lett.* **33:**13–18.

Olivier, A., Parent, A., and Poirier, L., 1970, Identification of the thalamic nuclei on the basis of their cholinesterase content in the monkey, *J. Anat. (Lond.)* **106:**37–50.

Olpe, H. R., 1981, The cortical projection of the dorsal raphe nucleus: Some electrophysiological and pharmacological properties, *Brain Res.* **216:**61–71.

Olschowska, J. A., Molliver, M. E., Grzanna, R., Rice, F. L., and Coyle, J. T., 1981, Ultrastructural demonstration of noradrenergic synapses in the rat central nervous system by dopamine-β-hydroxylase immunocytochemistry, *J. Histochem. Cytochem.* **29:**271–280.

Olszewski, J., and Baxter, D., 1954, *Cytoarchitecture of the Human Brain Stem,* S. Karger, Basel.

Onteniente, B., Geffard, M., and Calas, A., 1984, Ultrastructural immunocytochemical study of the dopaminergic innervation of the rat lateral septum with anti-dopamine antibodies, *Neuroscience* **13:**385–393.

Onteniente, B., Geffard, M., Campistron, G., and Calas, A., 1987, An ultrastructural study of GABA-immunoreactive neurons and terminals in the septum of the rat, *J. Neurosci.* **7:**48–54.

Orem, J., 1988, Neural basis of behavioral and state-dependent control of breathing, in: R. Lydic and J. F. Biebuyck, eds., *Clinical Physiology of Sleep,* American Physiological Society, Bethesda, pp. 79–96.

Osmanovic, S. S., and Shefner, S. A., 1987, Anomalous rectification in rat locus coeruleus neurons, *Brain Res.* **417:**161–166.

Ottersen, O. P., Fisher, B. O., and Storm-Mathisen, J., 1983, Retrograde transport of D-^{3}H-aspartate in thalamocortical neurones, *Neurosci. Lett.* **42:**19–24.

Overstreet, D. H., 1986, Selective breeding for increased cholinergic function: Development of a new animal model of depression, *Biol. Psychiatry* **221:**49–58.

Panneton, W. M., and Burton, H., 1985, Projections from the paratrigeminal nucleus and the medullary and spinal horns to the peribrachial area in the cat, *Neuroscience* **3:**779–797.

Pape, H. C., and Eysel, U. T., 1987, Modulatory action of the reticular transmitters norepinephrine and 5-hydroxytryptamine (serotonin) in the cat's visual thalamus, *Soc. Neurosci. Abstr.* **13:**86.

Pape, H. C., and Eysel, U. T., 1988, Cholinergic excitation and inhibition in the visual thalamus of the cat—Influences of cortical inactivation and barbiturate anaesthesia, *Brain Res.* **440:**79–86.

Paré, D., Steriade, M., Deschênes, M., and Oakson, G., 1987, Physiological characteristics of anterior thalamic nuclei, a group devoid of inputs from reticular thalamic nucleus, *J. Neurophysiol.* **57:**1669–1685.

Paré, D., Smith, Y., Parent, A., and Steriade, M., 1988, Projections of upper brainstem cholinergic and non-cholinergic neurons of cat to intralaminar and reticular thalamic nuclei, *Neuroscience* **25:**69–88.

Paré, D., Steriade, M., Deschênes, M., and Bouhassira, D., 1989, Prolonged enhancement in synaptic responsiveness of anterior thalamic neurons by stimulating a brainstem cholinergic nucleus, *J. Neurosci.* (in press).

Paré, D., Smith, Y., Parent, A., and Steriade, M., 1989b, Neuronal activity of posterior hypothalamic neurons with identified projections to the brainstem peribrachial area of the cat, *Neurosci. Lett.* (in press).

Parent, A., 1984, Comparative anatomy of monoaminergic systems, in: *Handbook of Chemical Neuroanatomy,* Vol. 2 (A. Bjorklund, T. Hökfelt, and M. Kuhar, eds.), Elsevier, Amsterdam, pp. 409–439.

Parent, A., and Steriade, M., 1981, Afferents from the periaqueductal gray, medial hypothalamus and medial thalamus to the midbrain reticular core, *Brain Res. Bull.* **7:**411–418.

Parent, A., and Steriade, M., 1984, Midbrain tegmental projections of nucleus reticularis thalami of cat and monkey: A retrograde transport and antidromic identification study, *J. Comp. Neurol.* **229:**548–558.

Parent, A., Descarries, L., and Beaudet, A., 1981, Organization of ascending serotonin systems in the adult rat brain. A radioautographic study after intraventricular administration of (^{3}H)5-hydroxytryptamine, *Neuroscience* **6:**115–138.

Parent, A., Mackey, A., and DeBellefeuille, L., 1983, The subcortical afferents to caudate nucleus and putamen in primate: A fluorescent retrograde double labeling study, *Neuroscience* **10:**1137–1150.

Parent, A., Paré, D., Smith, Y., and Steriade, M., 1988, Basal forebrain cholinergic and non-cholinergic projections to the thalamus and brainstem in cats and monkeys, *J. Comp. Neurol.* **277:**281–301.

Park, M. R., 1987, Intracellular horseradish peroxidase labeling of rapidly firing dorsal raphe projection neurons, *Brain Res.* **402:**117–130.

Parmeggiani, P. L., 1985, Homeostatic regulation during sleep: Facts and hypotheses, in: *Brain Mechanisms of Sleep* (D. McGinty, R. Drucker-Colin, A. Morrison, and P. L. Parmeggiani, eds.), Raven Press, New York, pp. 385–397.

Parmeggiani, P. L., 1988, Thermoregulation during sleep from the viewpoint of homeostasis, in: *Clinical Physiology of Sleep,* (R. Lydic and J. F. Biebuyck, eds.), American Physiological Society, Bethesda, pp. 159–169.

Parmeggiani, P. L., Cevolani, D., Azzaroni, A., and Ferrari, G., 1987, Thermosensitivity of anterior hypothalamic–preoptic neurons during the waking–sleeping cycle: A study in brain functional states, *Brain Res.* **415:**79–89.

Passouant, P., Schwab, R. S., Cadilhac, J., and Baldy-Moulinier, M., 1964, Narcolepsie–cataplexie. Etude du sommeil de nuit et du sommeil de jour, *Rev. Neurol. (Paris)* **3:**415–426.

Pastel, R. H., 1988, The effects of DOI, a selective 5 HT-2 agonist, on sleep in the rat, *Abstr. Eur. Sleep Res. Soc.* 202.

Paupardin-Tritsch, D., Hammond, C., and Gerschenfeld, H. M., 1986, Serotonin and cyclic GMP both induce an increase of the calcium current in the same identified molluscan neurons, *J. Neurosci.* **6:**2715–2723.

Pavlov, I. P., 1928, *Lectures on Conditioned Reflexes* (H. W. Gantt, trans.), International, New York.

Pazos, A., and Palacios, J. M., 1985, Quantitative autoradiographic mapping of serotonin receptors in the rat brain. I. Serotonin-1-receptors, *Brain Res.* **346:**205–230.

Pazos, A., Cortes, R., and Palacios, J. M., 1985, Quantitative autoradiographic mapping of serotonin receptors in the rat brain. II. Serotonin-2 receptors, *Brain Res.* **346:**231–249.

Pedigo, N. W., Yamamura, H. I., and Nelson, D. L., 1981, Discrimination of multiple [^{3}H]5-hydroxytryptamine binding sites by the neuroleptic spiperone in rat brain, *J. Neurochem.* **36:**220.

Pellmar, T. C., and Carpenter, D. O., 1980, Serotonin induces a voltage-sensitive calcium current in neurons of *Aplysia californica, J. Neurophysiol.* **44:**423–439.

Perkins, M. N., and Stone, T. W., 1982, An iontophoretic investigation of the actions of convulsant kynurenines and their interaction with the endogenous excitant quinolinic acid, *Brain Res.* **247:**184–187.

Peroutka, S. J., and Snyder, S. H., 1980, Long-term antidepressant treatment decreases spiroperidol-labeled serotonin receptor binding, *Science* **210:**88–90.

Peroutka, S. J., Lebovitz, R. M., and Snyder, S. H., 1981, Two distinct central serotonin receptors with different physiological functions, *Science* **212:**827–829.

Pessah, M. A., and Roffwarg, H. P., 1972, Spontaneous middle ear muscle activity in man: A rapid eye movement sleep phenomenon, *Science* **178:**773–776.

Peters, S., Koh, J., and Choi, D. W., 1987, Zinc selectivity blocks the action of N-methyl-D-aspartate on cortical neurons, *Science* **236:**589–593.

Peterson, B. W., 1977, Identification of reticulospinal projections that may participate in gaze control, in: *Control of Gaze by Brainstem Neurons* (R. Baker and A. Berthoz, eds.), Elsevier, New York, pp. 243–152.

Peterson, B. W., Franck, J. I., Pitts, N. G., and Daunton, N. G., 1976, Changes in responses of medial pontomedullary reticular neurons during repetitive cutaneous, vestibular, cortical, and tectal stimulation, *J. Neurophysiol.* **39:**564–581.

Petrovicky, P., 1980, *Reticular Formation and its Raphe System,* Acta Universitatis Carolinae Medica, Prague.

Petsche, H., Gogolak, G., and van Zwieten, P. A., 1965, Rhythmicity of septal cell discharges at various levels of reticular excitation, *Electroencephalogr. Clin. Neurophysiol.* **19:**25–33.

Petsche, H., Pockberger, H., and Rappelsberger, P., 1984, On the search for the sources of the electroencephalogram, *Neuroscience* **11**:1–27.

Pfaffinger, P. J., Martin, J. M., Hunter, D. D., Nathanson, N. M., and Hille, B., 1985, GTP-binding proteins couple cardiac muscarinic receptors to a K channel, *Nature* **317**:536–540.

Phillipson, O. T., 1979, Afferent projections to the ventral tegmental area of Tsai and interfascicular nucleus: A horseradish peroxidase study in the rat, *J. Comp. Neurol.* **187**:117–144.

Phillis, J. W., 1970, *The Pharmacology of Synapses*, Pergamon, Oxford.

Phillis, J. W., 1971, The pharmacology of thalamic and geniculate neurons, *Int. Rev. Neurobiol.* **14**:1–48.

Phillis, J. W., and Tebecis, A. K., 1967, The responses of thalamic neurones to iontophoretically applied monoamines, *J. Physiol. (Lond.)* **192**:715–745.

Pickel, V. M., Segal, M., and Bloom, F. E., 1974, A radioautographic study of the efferent pathways of the nucleus locus coeruleus, *J. Comp. Neurol.* **155**:15–42.

Pickel, V. M., Joh, T. H., and Reis, D. J., 1977, A serotonergic innervation of noradrenergic neurons in nucleus locus coeruleus: Demonstration by immunocytochemical localization of the transmitter specific enzymes tyrosine and tryptophan hydroxylase, *Brain Res.* **131**:197–214.

Pickel, V. M., Joh, T. H., Reis, D. J., Leeman, S. E., and Miller, R. J., 1979, Electron microscopic localization of substance P and enkephalin in axon terminals related to dendrites of catecholaminergic neurons, *Brain Res.* **160**:387–400.

Picton, T. W., Woods, D. L., Baribeau-Braun, J., and Healy, T. M. G., 1977, Evoked potential audiometry, *J. Otolaryngol.* **6**:90–119.

Picton, T. W., Campbell, K. B., Baribeau-Braun, J., and Proulx, G. B., 1978, The neurophysiology of humkan attention: A tutorial view, in: *Attention and Performance* (J. Requin, ed.), Hillsdale, NJ, pp. 429–467.

Pineda, J. A., Foote, S. L., Neville, H. J., and Holmes, T. C., 1988, Endogenous event-related potentials in monkey, in: The role of task relevance, stimulus probability, and behavioral response, *Electroencephalogr. Clin. Neurophysiol.* **70**:155–171.

Pivik, R. T., McCarley, R. W., and Hobson, J. A., 1976, Eye movement-associated discharge in brain stem neurons during desynchronized sleep, *Brain Res.* **121**:59–76.

Pollock, J. D., Bernier, L., and Camardo, J. S., 1985, Serotonin and cyclic adenosine 3′:5′-monophosphate modulate the potassium current in tail sensory neurons in the pleural ganglion of *Aplysia*, *J. Neurosci.* **5**:1862–1871.

Pompeiano, O., 1967a, The neurophysiological mechanisms of the postural and motor events during desynchronized sleep, *Proc. Assoc. Res. Nerv. Ment. Dis.* **45**:351–423.

Pompeiano, O., 1967b, Sensory inhibition during motor activity in sleep, in: *Neurophysiological Basis of Normal and Abnormal Motor Activities* (M. D. Yahr and D. P. Purpura, eds.), Raven Press, New York, pp. 323–375.

Pompeiano, O., 1973, Reticular formation, in: *Handbook of Sensory Physiology, Somatosensory System*, Vol. II (A. Iggo, ed.), Springer, Berlin, pp. 381–488.

Pompeiano, O., 1976, Mechanisms responsible for spinal inhibition during desynchronized sleep: Experimental study, in: *Advances in Sleep Research*, Vol. 3, *Narcolepsy* (C. Guilleminault, W. C. Dement, and P. Passouant, eds.), Spectrum, New York, pp. 411–449.

Pompeiano, O., 1985, Cholinergic mechanisms involved in the gain regulation of postural reflexes, in: *Sleep: Neurotransmitters and Neuromodulators* (A. Wauquier, J. M. Gaillard, J. M. Monti, and M. Radulovacki, eds.), Raven Press, New York, pp. 165–184.

Pompeiano, O., and Valentinuzzi, M., 1976, A mathematical model for the mechanism of rapid eye movements induced by an anticholinesterase in the decerebrate cat, *Arch. Ital. Biol.* **114**:103–154.

Price, J. L., and Amaral, D. G., 1981, An autoradiographic study of the projections of the central nucleus of the monkey amygdala, *J. Neurosci.* **1**:1242–1259.

Price, J. L., and Stern, R., 1983, Individual cells in the nucleus basalis–diagonal band complex have restricted axonal projections to the cerebral cortex in the rat, *Brain Res.* **269**:352–356.

Puizillout, J. J., and Ternaux, J. P., 1974, Origine pyramidale des variations phasiques bulbaires observées lors de l'endormement, *Brain Res.* **66**:85–102.

Purpura, D. P., Shofer, R. J., and Musgrave, F. S., 1964, Cortical intracellular potentials during augmenting and recruiting responses. II. Patterns of synaptic activities in pyramidal and non-pyramidal tract neurons, *J. Neurophysiol.* **27**:133–151.

Purpura, D. P., McMurtry, J. G., and Maekawa, K., 1966, Synaptic events in ventrolateral thalamic neurons during suppression of recruiting responses by brain stem reticular stimulation, *Brain Res.* **1**:63–76.

Ramon-Moliner, E., 1975, Specialized and generalized dendritic patterns, in: *Golgi Centennial Symposium* (M. Santini, ed.), Raven Press, New York, pp. 87–100.

Ramon-Moliner, E., and Nauta, W. J. H., 1966, The isodendritic core of the brain stem, *J. Comp. Neurol.* **126:**311–336.

Ramon y Cajal, S., 1901–1917, Recuerdos De Mi Vida, (translated as *Recollections of My Life* by E. H. Cragie with the assistance of J. Cano, 1966) MIT Press, Cambridge, MA.

Ranson, S. W., 1939, Somnolence caused by hypothalamic lesions in the monkey, *Arch. Neurol. Psychiatry* **41:**1–23.

Ranson, S. W., and Clark, S. L., 1953, *The Anatomy of the Nervous System,* ninth ed., W. B. Saunders, Philadelphia, London.

Rapoport, J., Elkins, R., Langer, D. H., Sceery, W., Buchsbaum, M. S., Gillin, J. C., Murphy, D. L., Zahn, T. P., Lake, R., Ludlow, C., and Medelson, W. B., 1981, Childhood obsessive–compulsive disorder, *Am. J. Psychiatry* **138:**1545–1554.

Rasler, F. E., 1984, Behavioral and electrophysiological manifestations of bombesin: Excessive grooming and elimination of sleep, *Brain Res.* **321:**187–198.

Rasmussen, K., Heym, J., and Jacobs, B. L., 1984, Activity of serotonin containing neurons in nucleus centralis superior of freely moving cats, *Exp. Neurol.* **83:**302–317.

Ray, J. P., and Price, J. L., 1987, Possible interdigitation of basal forebrain afferents in the mediodorsal thalamic nucleus of the rat, *Soc. Neurosci. Abstr.* **13:**445.

Ray, W. J., and Cole, H. W., 1985, EEG alpha activity reflects attentional demands and beta activity reflects emotional and cognitive processes, *Science* **228:**750–752.

Raybourn, M. S., and Keller, E. L., 1977, Colliculoreticular organization in primate oculomotor system, *J. Neurophysiol.* **40:**861–878.

Reader, T. A., 1978, Effects of dopamine, noradrenaline and serotonin in visual cortex of cat, *Experientia* **34:**1568–1588.

Reader, T. A., Masse, P., and Champlain, J., 1979, The intracortical distribution of norepinephrine, dopamine and serotonin in the cerebral cortex of the cat, *Brain Res.* **177:**499–513.

Reynolds, C. F. III, 1989, Sleep in affective disorders, in: *Principles and Practices of Sleep Medicine* (M. H. Kryger, T. Roth, and W. C. Dement, eds.), Saunders, New York, pp. 413–415.

Reynolds, C. F. III, Kupfer, D. J., Taska, L. S., Hoch, C. C., Sewich, D. E., and Grochocinski, V. J., 1985, Slow wave sleep in elderly depressed, demented, and healthy subjects, *Sleep* **8:**155–159.

Richardson, B. P., and Engel, G., 1986, The pharmacology and function of 5-HT$_3$ receptors, *Trends Neurosci.* **9:**424–428.

Rinvik, E., Grofova, I., and Ottersen, O. P., 1976, Demonstration of nigrotectal and nigroreticular projections in the cat by axonal transport of proteins, *Brain Res.* **112:**388–394.

Rivner, M., and Sutin, J., 1981, Locus coeruleus modulation of the motor thalamus: Inhibition in nuclei ventralis lateralis and ventralis anterior, *Exp. Neurol.* **73:**651–673.

Robertson, R. T., and Feiner, A. R., 1982, Diencephalic projections from the pontine reticular formation: Autoradiographic studies in the cat, *Brain Res.* **239:**3–16.

Robinson, D. A., 1975, Oculomotor control signals, in: *Basic Mechanisms of Ocular Motility and Their Clinical Implications* (G. Lennerstrand and P. Bach-y-Rita, eds.), Pergamon, Oxford, pp. 337–374.

Robinson, D. A., and Zee, D. S., 1981, Theoretical considerations of the function and circuitry of various rapid eye movements in: *Progress in Oculomotor Research* (A. F. Fuchs and W. Becker, eds.), Elsevier/North-Holland, New York, pp. 3–9.

Roffwarg, H. P., Dement, W. C., Muzio, J. N., and Fisher, C., 1962, Dream imagery: Relationship to rapid eye movements of sleep, *Arch. Gen. Psychiatry* **7:**235–258.

Rogawski, M. A., and Aghajanian, G. K., 1980a, Activation of lateral geniculate neurons by norepinephrine: Mediation by an α-adrenergic receptor, *Brain Res.* **182:**345–359.

Rogawski, M. A., and Aghajanian, G. K., 1980b, Norepinephrine and serotonin: Opposite effects on the activity of lateral geniculate neurons evoked by optic pathway stimulation, *Exp. Neurol.* **69:**678–694.

Rogawski, M. A., and Aghajanian, G. K., 1982, Activation of lateral geniculate neurons by locus coeruleus or dorsal noradrenergic bundle stimulation: Selective blockade by the alpha$_1$-adrenoreceptor antagonist prozosin, *Brain Res.* **250:**31–39.

Rogers, A. W., 1979, *Techniques of Autoradiography,* Elsevier/North-Holland, Amsterdam.

Roldan, M., and Reinoso-Suarez, F., 1981, Cerebellar projections to the superior colliculus in the cat, *J. Neurosci.* **1:**827–834.

Rolls, E. T., Murzi, E., Yaxley, S., Thorpe, S. J., and Simpson, S. J., 1986, Sensory-specific satiety:

Food-specific reduction in responsiveness of ventral forebrain neurons after feeding in the monkey, *Brain Res.* **368**:79–86.

Room, P., Postema, F., and Korf, J., 1981, Divergent axon collaterals of rat locus coeruleus neurons: Demonstration by a fluorescent double labeling technique, *Brain Res.* **221**:219–230.

Ropert, N., and Steriade, M., 1981, Input–output organization of the midbrain reticular core, *J. Neurophysiol.* **46**:17–31.

Rosen, R., 1970, *Dynamical System Theory in Biology,* Vol. 1: *Stability Theory and Its Applications,* John Wiley & Sons, New York.

Ross, C. A., Ruggiero, D. A., Reis, and Reis, D. J., 1985, Projections from the nucleus tractus solitarii to the rostral ventrolateral medulla, *J. Comp. Neurol.* **242**:511–534.

Rossi, G. F., and Brodal, A., 1956, Corticofugal fibres to the brain stem reticular formation: An experimental study in the cat, *J. Anat. (Lond.)* **90**:42–62.

Roth, S. R., Sterman, M. B., and Clemente, C. D., 1967, Comparison of EEG correlates of reinforcement, internal inhibition and sleep, *Electroencephalogr. Clin. Neurophysiol.* **23**:509–520.

Rougeul, A., Bouyer, J. J., Dedet, L., and Debray, O., 1979, Fast somatoparietal rhythms during combined focal attention and immobility in baboon and squirrel monkey, *Electroencephalogr. Clin. Neurophysiol.* **46**:310–319.

Rougeul-Buser, A., Bouyer, J. J., Montaron, M. F., and Buser, P., 1983, Patterns of activities in the ventrobasal thalamus and somatic cortex SI during behavioral immobility in the awake cat: Focal waking rhythms, *Exp. Brain Res. (Suppl.)* **7**:69–87.

Rowntree, C. J., and Bland, B. H., 1986, An analysis of cholinoceptive neurons in the hippocampal formation by direct microinfusion, *Brain Res.* **362**:98–113.

Roy, J. P., Clercq, M., Steriade, M., and Deschênes, M., 1984, Electrophysiology of neurons of the lateral thalamic nuclei in cat: Mechanisms of long-lasting hyperpolarizations, *J. Neurophysiol.* **51**:1220–1235.

Ruch-Monachon, M. A., Jalfre, M., and Haefeley, W., 1976, Drugs and PGO waves in the lateral geniculate body of the curarized rat. I–V, *Arch. Int. Pharmacodyn. Ther.* **219**:251–346.

Ruggiero, D. A., Ross, C. A., Anwar, M., Park, D. H., Joh, T. H., and Reis, D. J., 1985, Distribution of neurons containing phenylethanolamine N-methyltransferase in medulla and hypothalamus of rat, *J. Comp. Neurol.* **239**:127–154.

Russchen, F. T., Amaral, D. G., and Price, J. L., 1985, The afferent connections of the substantia innominata in the monkey, *Macaca fascicularis, J. Comp. Neurol.* **242**:1–27.

Russell, G. V., 1955, The nucleus locus coeruleus (*dorsolateralis tegmenti*), *Tex. Rep. Biol. Med.* **13**:939–988.

Rustioni, A., Schmechel, D. E., Spreafico, R., Cheema, S., and Cuénod, M., 1983, Excitatory and inhibitory amino acid putative neurotransmitters in the ventralis posterior complex: An autoradiographic and immunocytochemical study in rats and cats, in: *Somatosensory Integration in the Thalamus* (G. Macchi, A. Rustioni, and R. Spreafico, eds.), Elsevier, Amsterdam, pp. 365–383.

Rye, D. B., Wainer, B. H., Mesulam, M. M., Mufson, E. J., and Saper, C. B., 1984, Cortical projections arising from the basal forebrain: A study of cholinergic and noncholinergic components employing combined retrograde tracing and immunohistochemical localization of choline acetyltransferase, *Neuroscience* **13**:627–643.

Rye, D. B., Saper, C. B., Lee, H. J., and Wainer, B. H., 1987, Pedunculopontine tegmental nucleus of the rat: Cytoachitecture, cytochemistry, and some extrapyramidal connections of the mesopontine tegmentum, *J. Comp. Neurol.* **259**:483–528.

Rye, D. B., Lee, H. J., Saper, C. B., and Wainer, B. H., 1988, Medullary and spinal efferents of the pedunculopontine tegmental nucleus and adjacent mesopontine tegmentum in the rat, *J. Comp. Neurol.* **269**:315–341.

Sakaguchi, T., and Nakamura, S., 1987, The mode of projections of single locus coeruleus neurons to the cerebral cortex in rats, *Neuroscience* **20**:221–230.

Sakai, K., 1980, Some anatomical and physiological properties of ponto-mesencephalic tegmental neurons with special reference to the PGO waves and postural atonia during paradoxical sleep in the cat, in: *The Reticular Formation Revisited* (J. A. Hobson and M. A. B. Brazier, eds.), Raven Press, New York, pp. 427–447.

Sakai, K., 1985a, Anatomical and physiological basis of paradoxical sleep, in: *Brain Mechanisms of Sleep* (D. J. McGinty, A. Morrison, R. Drucker-Colin, and P. L. Parmeggiani, eds.), Raven Press, New York, pp. 111–137.

Sakai, K., 1985b, Neurons responsible for paradoxical sleep, in: *Sleep: Neurotransmitters and Neuromodulators* (A. Wauquier, J. M. Gaillard, J. M. Monti, and M. Radulovacki, eds.), Raven Press, New York, pp. 29–42.

Sakai, K., 1986, Central mechanisms of paradoxical sleep, *Brain Dev.* **8**:402–407.

Sakai, K., and Jouvet, M., 1980, Brainstem PGO-on cells projecting directly to the cat lateral geniculate nucleus, *Brain Res.* **194**:500–505.

Sakai, K., Salvert, D., Touret, M., and Jouvet, M., 1977a, Afferent connections of the nucleus raphe dorsalis in the cat as visualized by the horseradish peroxidase technique, *Brain Res.* **137**:11–35.

Sakai, K., Touret, M., Salvert, D., Leger, L., and Jouvet, M., 1977b, Afferent projections to the cat locus coeruleus as visualized by the horseradish peroxidase technique, *Brain Res.* **119**:21–41.

Sakai, K., Sastre, J. P., Salvert, D., Touret, M., and Jouvet, M., 1979, Tegmentoreticular projections with special reference to the muscular atonia during paradoxical sleep in the cat: An HRP study, *Brain Res.* **176**:233–254.

Sakai, K., Sastre, J., Kanamori, N., and Jouvet, M., 1981, State specific neurons in the pontomedullary reticular formation with special reference to the postural atonia during paradoxical sleep in the cat, in: *Brain Mechanisms of Perceptual Awareness and Purposeful Behavior* (C. Ajmone-Marsan and O. Pompeiano, eds.), Raven Press, New York, pp. 405–429.

Sakai, K., Vanni-Mercier, G., and Jouvet, M., 1983, Evidence for the presence of PS-off neurons in the ventromedial oblongata of freely moving cats, *Exp. Brain Res.* **49**:311–314.

Sakakura, H., 1968, Spontaneous and evoked unitary activities of cat lateral geniculate neurons in sleep and wakefulness, *Jpn. J. Physiol.* **18**:23–42.

Sakmann, B., Noma, A., and Trautwein, W., 1983, Acetylcholine activation of single muscarinic K$^+$ channels in isolated pacemaker cells of the mammalian heart, *Nature* **303**:250–253.

Sallanon, M., Denoyer, M., Kitahama, K., Aubert, C., Gay, N., and Jouvet, M., 1989, Long-lasting insomnia induced by preoptic neuron lesions and its transient reversal by muscimol injection into the posterior hypothalamus in the cat, *Neuroscience* (in press).

Salva, M. A. Q., and Guilleminault, C., 1986, Olivopontocerebellar degeneration, abnormal sleep, and REM sleep without atonia, *Neurology* **36**:576–577.

Saper, C. B., 1984, Organization of cerebral cortical afferent systems in the rat. I. Magnocellular basal nucleus, *J. Comp. Neurol.* **222**:313–342.

Saper, C. B., and Loewy, A. D., 1982, Projections of the pedunculopontine tegmental nucleus in the rat: Evidence for additional extrapyramidal circuitry, *Brain Res.* **252**:367–372.

Saper, C. B., Standaert, D. G., Currie, M. G., Schwartz, D., Geller, D. M., and Needleman, P., 1985, Atriopeptin-immunoreactive neurons in the brain: Presence in cardiovascular regulatory areas, *Science* **227**:1047–1049.

Sasaki, K., Staunton, H. P., and Dieckman, G., 1970, Characteristic features of augmenting and recruiting responses in the cerebral cortex, *Exp. Neurol.* **26**:369–392.

Sasaki, K., Matsuda, Y., Oka, H., and Mizuno, N., 1975, Thalamo-cortical projections for recruiting responses and spindling-like responses in the parietal cortex, *Exp. Brain Res.* **22**:87–96.

Sasaki, S., and Shimazu, H., 1981, Reticulovestibular organization participating in generation of horizontal fast eye movement, *Ann. N.Y. Acad. Sci.* **374**:130–143.

Sastre, J. P., and Jouvet, M., 1979, Le comportement onirique du chat, *Physiol. Behav.* **22**:979–989.

Sastre, J. P., Sakai, K., and Jouvet, M., 1981, Are the gigantocellular tegmental field neurons responsible for paradoxical sleep? *Brain Res.* **229**:147–161.

Satinoff, E., 1988, Thermal influences on REM sleep, in: *Clinical Physiology of Sleep,* (R. Lydic and J. F. Biebuyck, eds.), American Physiological Society, Bethesda, pp. 135–144.

Satoh, K., and Fibiger, H. C., 1986, Cholinergic neurons of the laterodorsal tegmental nucleus: Efferent and afferent connections, *J. Comp. Neurol.* **253**:277–302.

Satoh, M., Akaike, A., Nakazawa, T., and Takagi, H., 1980, Evidence for involvement of separate mechanisms in the projection of analgesia by electrical stimulation of the nucleus reticularis paragigantocellularis and nucleus raphe mangnus in the rat, *Brain Res.* **194**:525–529.

Scarnati, E., Proia, A., Di Loreto, S., and Pacitti, C., 1987, The reciprocal electrophysiological influence between the nucleus tegmenti pedunculopontinus and the substantia nigra in normal and decorticated rats, *Brain Res.* **423**:116–124.

Scheibel, M. E., and Scheibel, A. B., 1958, Structural substrates for integrative patterns in the brain stem reticular core, in: *Reticular Formation of the Brain* (H. H. Jasper, L. D. Proctor, R. S. Knighton, W. C. Noshay, and R. T. Costello, eds.), Little, Brown, Boston, pp. 31–55.

Scheibel, M. E., and Scheibel, A. B., 1965, Periodic sensory nonresponsiveness in reticular neurons, *Arch. Ital. Biol.* **103**:300–316.

Scheibel, M. E., and Scheibel, A. B., 1975, Dendrites as neuronal couplers: The dendrite bundle, in: *Golgi Centennial Symposium* (M. Santini, ed.), Raven Press, New York, pp. 347–354.

Scheibel, M. E., Scheibel, A. B., Moruzzi, G., and Mollica, A., 1955, Convergence and interaction of afferent impulses on single units of reticular formation, *J. Neurophysiol.* **18**:309–331.

Schenck, C. H., Bundlie, S. R., Ettinger, M. G., and Mahowald, M. W., 1986, Chronic behavioral disorders of human REM sleep: A new category of parasomnia, *Sleep* **9**:293–308.

Schildkraut, J. J., and Kety, S. S., 1967, Biogenic amines and emotion, *Science* **156**:21–30.

Schiller, P., and Stryker, M., 1972, Single-unit recording and stimulation in superior colliculus of the alert rhesus monkey, *J. Neurophysiol.* **35**:915–924.

Schlag, J., and Waszak, M., 1971, Electrophysiological properties of units in the thalamic reticular complex, *Exp. Neurol.* **32**:79–97.

Schulman-Galambos, C., and Galambos, R., 1979, Brainstem evoked response audiometry in newborn hearing screening, *Arch. Otolaryngol.* **105**:86–90.

Schulz, H., and Lund, R., 1983, Sleep onset REM periods are associated with circadian parameters of body temperature. A study in depressed patients and normal controls, *Biol. Psychiatry* **18**:1411–1426.

Schulz, H., and Lund, R., 1985, On the origin of early REM episodes in the sleep of depressed patients: A comparison of three hypotheses, *Psychiatry Res.* **16**:65–77.

Schulz, H., and Tetzlaff, W., 1982, Distribution of REM latencies after sleep interruption in depressive patients and control subjects, *Biol. Psychiatry* **18**:1411–1426.

Schulz, H., Lund, R., Cording, C., and Dirlich, G., 1979, Bimodal distribution of REM sleep latencies in depression, *Biol. Psychiatry* **14**:595–600.

Schwartz, J. C., Pollard, H., and Quach, T. T., 1980, Histamine as a neurotransmitter in mammalian brain: Neurochemical evidence, *J. Neurochem.* **35**:26–33.

Schwartzkroin, P. A., and Stafstrom, C. E., 1980, Effects of EGTA on the calcium-activated afterhyperpolarization in hippocampal CA3 pyramidal cells, *Science* **210**:1125–1126.

Schwindt, P. C., Spain, W. J., Foehring, R. C., Stafstrom, C. E., Chubb, M. C., and Crill, W. E., 1988, Multiple potassium conductances and their functions in neurons from cat sensorimotor cortex *in vitro*, *J. Neurophysiol.* **59**:424.

Scudder, C. A., 1988, A new local feedback model of the saccadic burst generator, *J. Neurophysiol.* **59**:1455–1475.

Scudder, C. A., Langer, T. P., and Fuchs, A. F., 1982, Probable inhibitory burst neurons in the monkey, *Soc. Neurosci. Abstr.* **8**:157.

Scudder, C. A., Fuchs, A. F., and Langer, T. P., 1988, Characteristics and functional identification of saccadic inhibitory burst neurons in the alert monkey, *J. Neurophysiol.* **59**:1430–1454.

Segal, M., 1980, The action of serotonin in the rat hippocampal slice preparation, *J. Physiol. (Lond.)* **303**:423–439.

Segal, M., and Landis, S., 1974, Afferents to the hippocampus of the rat studied with the method of retrograde transport of horseradish peroxidase, *Brain Res.* **78**:1–15.

Segraves, M. A., and Goldberg, M. E., 1987, Functional properties of corticotectal neurons in the monkey's frontal eye field, *J. Neurophysiol.* **58**:1387–1419.

Séguéla, P., Watkins, K. C., and Descarries, L., 1988, Ultrastructural features of dopamine axon terminals in the anteromedial and the suprarhinal cortex of adult rat, *Brain Res.* **442**:11–22.

Semba, K., Reiner, P. B., McGeer, E. G., and Fibiger, H. C., 1988, Brainstem afferents to the magnocellular basal forebrain studied by axonal transport, immunohistochemistry and electrophysiology in the rat, *J. Comp. Neurol.* **267**:433–453.

Serafin, M., and Muhlethaler, M., 1988, Spindle activity in the thalamus *in vitro*, *Soc. Neurosci. Abstr.* **14**:1024.

Shammah-Lagnado, S. J., Negrao, N., and Ricardo, J. A., 1985, Afferent connections of the zona incerta: A horseradish peroxidase study in the rat, *Neuroscience* **15**:109–134.

Shammah-Lagnado, S. J., Negrao, N., Silva, B. A., and Ricardo, J. A., 1987, Afferent connections of the nuclei reticularis pontis oralis and caudalis: A horseradish peroxidase study in the rat, *Neuroscience* **20**:961–989.

Sherrington, C. S., 1906, *Integrative Action of the Nervous System*, Yale University Press, New Haven.

Shiromani, P. J., and Fishbein, W., 1986, Continuous pontine cholinergic microinfusion via minipump induces sustained alterations in rapid eye movement (REM) sleep, *Pharmacol. Biochem. Behav.* **25**:1253–1261.

Shiromani, P. J., and McGinty, D. J., 1986, Pontine neuronal response to local cholinergic infusion: Relation to REM sleep, *Brain Res.* **386**:20–31.

Shiromani, P. J., Siegel, J. M., Tomaszewski, K. S., and McGinty, D. J., 1986, Alterations in blood pressure and REM sleep after pontine carbachol microinfusion, *Exp. Neurol.* **91**:285–292.

Shiromani, P. J., Armstrong, D. M., and Gillin, J. C., 1988a, Cholinergic neurons from the dorsalateral pons project to the medial pons: A WGA–HRP and choline acetyltransferase immunohistochemical study, *Neurosci. Lett.* **95**:19–23.

Shiromani, P. J., Overstreet, D., Levy, D., Goodrich, C. A., Campbell, S. S., and Gillin, J. C., 1988b, Increased REM sleep in rats selectively bred for cholinergic hyperactivity, *Neuropsychopharmacology* **1**:129–133.

Shute, C. C. D., and Lewis, P. R., 1967a, The ascending cholinergic reticular system: Neocortical olfactory and subcortical projections, *Brain* **90**:497–520.

Shute, C. C. D., and Lewis, P. R., 1967b, The cholinergic limbic system: Projections to hippocampal formation, medial cortex, nuclei of the ascending cholinergic reticular system, and the subfornical organ and supra-optic crest, *Brain* **90**:521–540.

Siegel, J. M., 1979, Behavioral functions of the reticular formation, *Brain Res. Rev.* **1**:69–105.

Siegel, J. M., and Lai, Y. Y., 1988, Receptors mediating suppression of muscle tone produced by glutamate in dorsolateral pons and medial medulla, *Soc. Neurosci. Abstr.* **14**:1309.

Siegel, J. M., and Tomaszewski, K. S., 1983, Behavioral organization of reticular formation studies in the unrestrained cat. I. Cells related to axial, limb, eye and other movements, *J. Neurophysiol.* **50**:696–716.

Siegel, J. M., Tomaszewski, K. S., and Wheeler, R. L., 1983, Behavioral organization of reticular formation: Studies in the unrestrained cat. II. Cells related to facial movements, *J. Neurophysiol.* **50**:717–723.

Siegel, J. M., Nienhuis, R., and Tomaszewski, K. S., 1984, REM sleep signs rostral to chronic transections at the pontomedullary junction, *Neurosci. Lett.* **45**:241–246.

Siegel, J. M., Tomaszewski, K. S., and Nienhuis, R., 1986, Behavioral states in the chronic medullary and midpontine cat, *Electroencep. Clin. Neurophysiol.* **63**:274–288.

Siegelbaum, S. A., Camardo, J. S., and Kandel, E. R., 1982, Serotonin and cyclic AMP close single potassium channels in *Aplysia* sensory neurones, *Nature* **299**:413–417.

Siggins, G. R., and Gruol, D. L., 1986, Mechanisms of transmitter action in the vertebrate central nervous system, in: *Handbook of Physiology*, Section 1, Vol. IV (V. B. Mountcastle, and F. E. Bloom, eds.), American Physiological Society, Bethesda, pp. 1–114.

Siggins, G. R., Champagnat, J., Jacquin, T., and Denavit-Saubie, M., 1987, Somatostatin depresses neuronal excitability in the solitary tract complex (STC) via hyperpolarization and augmentation of the M-current, *Soc. Neurosci. Abstr.* **13**:1443.

Silberman, E. K., Vivaldi, E., Garfield, J., McCarley, R. W., and Hobson, J. A., 1980, Carbachol triggering of desynchronized sleep phenomena: Enhancement via small volume infusions, *Brain Res.* **191**:215–224.

Sillito, A. M., 1987, Synaptic processes and neurotransmitters operating in the central visual system: A system approach, in: *Synaptic Function* (G. M. Edelman, W. E. Gall, and W. M. Cowan, eds.), John Wiley & Sons, New York, pp. 329–371.

Sillito, A. M., and Kemp, J. A., 1983, Cholinergic modulation of the functional organization of the cat visual cortex, *Brain Res.* **289**:143–155.

Sillito, A. M., Kemp, J. A., and Berardi, N., 1983, The cholinergic influence on the function of the cat dorsal lateral geniculate nucleus (dLGN), *Brain Res.* **280**:299–307.

Simon, R. P., Gershon, M. P., and Brooks, D. C., 1973, The role of the raphe nuclei in the regulation of ponto-geniculo-occipital wave activity, *Brain Res.* **58**:313–330.

Singer, W., 1973, The effects of mesencephalic reticular stimulation on intracellular potentials of cat lateral geniculate neurons, *Brain Res.* **61**:35–54.

Singer, W., 1977, Control of thalamic transmission by corticofugal and ascending reticular pathways in the visual system, *Physiol. Rev.* **57**:386–420.

Singer, W., 1979, Central-core control of visual cortex functions, in: *The Neurosciences: Fourth Study Program* (F. O. Schmitt and F. G. Worden, eds.), MIT Press, Cambridge, pp. 1093–1110.

Singer, W., Gray, C. M., Engel, A., and Konig, P., 1988, Spatio-temporal distribution of stimulus-specific oscillations in the cat visual cortex. II. Global interactions, *Soc. Neurosci. Abstr.* **14**:899.

Sirkin, D. W., Schallert, T., and Teitelbaum, P., 1980, Involvement of the pontine reticular formation in head movements and labyrinthine righting in the rat, *Exp. Neurol.* **69**:435–457.

Sitaram, N., Nurnberger, J. I., Jr., Gershon, E. S., and Gillin, J. C., 1982, Cholinergic regulation of mood and REM sleep: Potential model and marker of vulnerability to affective disorder, *Am. J. Psychiatry* **139**:571–576.

Skinner, J. E., Mohn, D. N., and Kellaway, P., 1975, Sleep-stage regulation of ventricular arrhythmias in the unanesthetized pig, *Circ. Res.* **37**:342–349.

Smith, S. J., and Thompson, S. H., 1987, Slow membrane currents in bursting pace-maker neurones of *Tritonia*, *J. Physiol. (Lond.)* **382**:425–448.

Smith, T. G., Barker, J. L., and Gainer, H., 1975, Requirements for bursting pacemaker potential in molluscan neurones, *Nature* **253**:450–452.

Smith, Y., Parent, A., Séguéla, P., and Descarries, L., 1987, Distribution of GABA-immunoreactive neurons in the basal ganglia of the squirrel monkey, *J. Comp. Neurol.* **259:**50–64.

Smith, Y., Paré, D., Deschênes, M., Parent, A., and Steriade, M., 1988, Cholinergic and non-cholinergic projections from the upper brainstem core to the visual thalamus in the cat, *Exp. Brain Res.* **70:**166–180.

Sofroniew, M. V., Priestley, J. V., Consolazione, A., Eckenstein, F., and Cuello, A. C., 1985, Cholinergic projections from the midbrain and pons to the thalamus in rat, identified by combined retrograde tracing and choline acetyltransferase immunohistochemistry, *Brain Res.* **329:**213–223.

Soja, P., Finch, D. M., and Chase, M. H., 1987a, Effect of inhibitory amino acid antagonists on masseteric reflex suppression during active sleep, *Exp. Neurol.* **96:**178–193.

Soja, P. J., Morales, F. R., Baranyi, A., and Chase, M. H., 1987b, The effect of inhibitory amino acid antagonists on IPSPs induced in lumbar motoneurons upon stimulation of the nucleus reticularis gigantocellularis during active sleep, *Brain Res.* **423:**353–358.

Soja, P. J., Lopez, F., Morales, F. R., and Chase, M. H., 1988, Depolarizing synaptic events influencing cat lumbar motoneurons during rapid eye movement episodes of active sleep are blocked by kynurenic acid, *Soc. Neurosci. Abstr.* **14:**941.

Soltesz, I., Haby, M., Leresche, N., and Crunelli, V., 1988, The GABA$_B$ antagonist phaclofen inhibits the late potassium-dependent IPSP in cat and rat thalamic and hippocampal neurones, *Brain Res.* **448:**351–354.

Somogyi, P., 1978, The study of Golgi stained cells and of experimental degeneration under the electron microscope: A direct method for the identification in the visual cortex of three successive links in a neuron chain, *Neuroscience* **3:**167–180.

Somogyi, P., Hodgson, A. J., and Smith, A. D., 1979, An approach to tracing neuron networks in the cerebral cortex and basal ganglia. Combination of Golgi staining, retrograde transport of horseradish peroxidase and anterograde degeneration of synaptic boutons in the same material, *Neuroscience* **4:**1805–1852.

Somogyi, P., Freund, T. F., Wu, J. Y., and Smith, A. D., 1983, The section–Golgi impregnation procedure. 2. Immunocytochemical demonstration of glutamate decarboxylase in Golgi-impregnated neurons and in their afferent synaptic boutons in the visual cortex of the cat, *Neuroscience* **9:**475–490.

Soury, J., 1899, *Le Système Nerveux Central. Histoire Critique des Theories et des Doctrines*, Vol. 2, Carré et Naud, Paris.

Sparks, D. L., and Mays, L. E., 1983, Spatial localization of saccade targets. I. Compensation for stimulation-induced pertubations in eye position, *J. Neurophysiol.* **49:**45–63.

Sparks, D. L., Mays, L. E., and Porter, J. D., 1987, Eye movements induced by pontine stimulation: Interaction with visually triggered saccades, *J. Neurophysiol.* **58:**300–318.

Spencer, W. A., and Brookhart, J. M., 1961a, Electrical patterns of augmenting and recruiting waves in the depths of the sensorimotor cortex of cat, *J. Neurophysiol.* **24:**26–49.

Spencer, W. A., and Brookhart, J. M., 1961b, A study of spontaneous spindle waves in sensorimotor cortex of cat, *J. Neurophysiol.* **24:**50–65.

Standaert, D. G., Saper, C. B., Rye, D. B., and Wainer, B. H., 1986, Colocalization of atriopeptin-like immunoreactivity with choline acetyltransferase and substance P-like immunoreactivity in the pedunculopontine and laterodorsal tegmental nuclei in the rat, *Brain Res.* **382:**163–168.

Stanfield, P. R., 1983, Tetraethylammonium ions and the potassium permeability of excitable cells, *Rev. Physiol. Biochem. Pharmacol.* **97:**167.

Stanton, G. B., and Greene, R. W., 1981, Brain stem afferents to the periabducens reticular formation (PARF) in the cat, *Exp. Brain Res.* **44:**419–426.

Stanton, G. B., Goldberg, M. E., and Bruce, C. J., 1988, Frontal eye field efferents in the macaque monkey. II. Topography of terminal field in midbrain and pons, *J. Comp. Neurol.* **271:**493–506.

Steinbush, H. W. M., 1981, Distribution of serotonin-immunoreactivity in the central nervous system of the rat, *Neuroscience* **6:**557–618.

Steinbusch, H. W. M., and Nieuwehuys, R., 1983, The raphe nuclei of the rat brainstem: A cytoarchitectonic and immunohistochemical study, in: *Chemical Neuroanatomy* (P. C. Emson, ed.), Raven Press, New York, pp. 131–207.

Steinbusch, H. W. M., van der Kooy, D., Verhofstad, A. A. J., and Pellegrino, A., 1980, Serotonergic and non-serotonergic projections from the nucleus raphe dorsalis to the caudate–putamen complex in the rat, studied by a combined immunofluorescence and fluorescent retrograde axonal labeling technique, *Neurosci. Lett.* **19:**137–142.

Steinfels, G. F., Heym, J., Strecker, R. E., and Jacobs, B. L., 1983, Behavioral correlates of dopaminergic unit activity in freely moving cats, *Brain Res.* **258**:217–228.

Stephan, F. K., Berkley, K. J., and Moss, R. L., 1981, Efferent connections of the rat suprachiasmatic nucleus, *Neuroscience* **6**:2625–2641.

Steriade, M., 1969, *Physiologie des Voies et des Centres Visuels,* Masson, Paris.

Steriade, M., 1970, Ascending control of thalamic and cortical responsiveness, *Int. Rev. Neurobiol.* **12**:87–144.

Steriade, M., 1974, Interneuronal epileptic discharges related to spike-and-wave cortical seizures in behaving monkeys, *Electroencephalogr. Clin. Neurophysiol.* **37**:247–263.

Steriade, M., 1978, Cortical long-axoned cells and putative interneurons during the sleep–waking cycle, *Behav. Brain Sci.* **3**:465–514.

Steriade, M., 1980, State-dependent changes in the activity of rostral reticular and thalamocortical elements, *Neurosci. Res. Prog. Bull.* **18**:83–91.

Steriade, M., 1981, Mechanisms underlying cortical activation: Neuronal organization and properties of the midbrain reticular core and intralaminar thalamic nuclei, in: *Brain Mechanisms and Perceptual Awareness* (O. Pompeiano and C. Ajmone-Marsan, eds.), Raven Press, New York, pp. 327–377.

Steriade, M., 1983, Cellular mechanisms of wakefulness and slow-wave sleep, in: *Sleep Mechanisms and Functions in Humans and Animals. An Evolutionary Perspective* (A. Mayes, ed.), Van Nostrand-Reinhold, Wokingham, UK, pp. 161–216.

Steriade, M., 1984, The excitatory–inhibitory response sequence of thalamic and neocortical cells: State-related changes and regulatory systems, in: *Dynamic Aspects of Neocortical Function* (G. M. Edelman, W. E. Gall, and W. M. Cowan, eds.), John Wiley & Sons, New York, pp. 107–157.

Steriade, M., 1989, Spindling, incremental thalamocortical responses and spike–wave epilepsy, in: *Generalized Epilepsy* (M. Avoli, P. Gloor, G. Kostopoulos, and R. Naquet, eds.), Birkhauser, Boston (in press).

Steriade, M., and Buzsaki, G., 1989, Parallel activation of thalamic and cortical neurons by brainstem and basal forebrain cholinergic systems, in: *Brain Cholinergic Systems* (M. Steriade and D. Biesold, eds.), Oxford University Press, Oxford, New York (in press).

Steriade, M., and Demetrescu, M., 1960, Unspecific systems of inhibition and facilitation of potentials evoked by intermittent light, *J. Neurophysiol.* **23**:602–617.

Steriade, M., and Deschênes, M., 1974, Inhibitory processes and interneuronal apparatus in motor cortex during sleep and waking. II. Recurrent and afferent inhibition of pyramidal tract neurons, *J. Neurophysiol.* **37**:1093–1113.

Steriade, M., and Deschênes, M., 1984, The thalamus as a neuronal oscillator, *Brain Res. Rev.* **8**:1–63.

Steriade, M., and Deschênes, M., 1988, Intrathalamic and brainstem–thalamic networks involved in resting and alert states, in: *Cellular Thalamic Mechanism* (M. Bentivoglio and R. Spreafico, eds.), Elsevier, Amsterdam, pp. 37–62.

Steriade, M., and Glenn, L. L., 1982, Neocortical and caudate projections of intralaminar thalamic neurons and their synaptic excitation from the midbrain reticular core, *J. Neurophysiol.* **48**:352–371.

Steriade, M., and Hobson, J. A., 1976, Neuronal activity during the sleep–waking cycle, *Prog. Neurobiol.* **6**:155–376.

Steriade, M., and Llinás, R., 1988, The functional states of the thalamus and the associated neuronal interplay, *Physiol. Rev.* **68**:649–742.

Steriade, M., and Morin, D., 1981, Reticular influences on primary and augmenting responses in the somatosensory cortex, *Brain Res.* **205**:67–80.

Steriade, M., and Paré, D., 1989, Brainstem genesis and thalamic transfer of internal signals during dreaming sleep: Cellular data and hypotheses, in: *Basic Mechanisms of Sleep* (J. Montplaisir and R. Godbout, eds.), Oxford University Press, New York (in press).

Steriade, M., and Stoupel, N., 1960, Contribution à l'étude des relations entre l'aire auditive du cervelet et l'écorce cérébrale chez le chat, *Electroencephalogr. Clin. Neurophysiol.* **12**:119–136.

Steriade, M., and Yossif, G., 1974, Spike-and-wave afterdischarges in cortical somatosensory neurons of cat, *Electroencephalogr. Clin. Neurophysiol.* **37**:633–648.

Steriade, M., Botez, M. I., and Petrovici, I., 1961, On certain dissociations of consciousness levels within the syndrome of akinetic mutism, *Psychiatr. Neurol. (Basel)* **141**:38–58.

Steriade, M., Iosif, G., and Apostol, V., 1969, Responsiveness of thalamic and cortical motor relays during arousal and various stages of sleep, *J. Neurophysiol.* **32**:251–265.

Steriade, M., Apostol, V., and Oakson, G., 1971, Control of unitary activities in cerebellothalamic pathways during wakefulness and synchronized sleep, *J. Neurophysiol.* **34**:384–413.

Steriade, M., Deschênes, M., and Oakson, G., 1974a, Inhibitory processes and interneuronal apparatus in motor cortex during sleep and waking. I. Background firing and responsiveness of pyramidal tract neurons and interneurons, *J. Neurophysiol.* **37**:1065–1092.

Steriade, M., Deschênes, M., Wyzinski, P., and Hallé, J. Y., 1974b, Input–output organization of the motor cortex during sleep and waking, in: *Basic Sleep Mechanisms* (O. Petre-Quadens and J. Schlag, eds.), Academic Press, New York, pp. 144–200.

Steriade, M., Oakson, G., and Diallo, A., 1976, Cortically elicited spike–wave afterdischarges in thalamic neurons, *Electroencephalogr. Clin. Neurophysiol.* **41**:641–644.

Steriade, M., Diallo, A., Oakson, G., and White-Guay, B., 1977a, Some synaptic inputs and ascending projections of lateralis posterior thalamic neurons, *Brain Res.* **131**:39–53.

Steriade, M., Oakson, G., and Diallo, A., 1977b, Reticular influences on lateralis posterior thalamic neurons, *Brain Res.* **131**:55–71.

Steriade, M., Kitsikis, A., and Oakson, G., 1978, Thalamic inputs and subcortical targets of cortical neurons in areas 5 and 7 of cat, *Exp. Neurol.* **60**:420–442.

Steriade, M., Ropert, N., Kitsikis, A., and Oakson, G., 1980, Ascending activating neuronal networks in midbrain reticular core and related rostral systems, in: *The Reticular Formation Revisited* (J. A. Hobson and M. A. B. Brazier, eds.), Raven Press, New York, pp. 125–167.

Steriade, M., Oakson, G., and Ropert, N., 1982a, Firing rates and patterns of midbrain reticular neurons during steady and transitional states of the sleep–waking cycle, *Exp. Brain Res.* **46**:37–51.

Steriade, M., Parent, A., Ropert, N., and Kitsikis, A., 1982b, Zona incerta and lateral hypothalamic afferents to the midbrain reticular core of the cat—an HRP and electrophysiological study, *Brain Res.* **238**:13–28.

Steriade, M., Parent, A., and Hada, J., 1984a, Thalamic projections of nucleus reticularis thalami of cat: A study using retrograde transport of horseradish peroxidase and double fluorescent tracers, *J. Comp. Neurol.* **229**:531–547.

Steriade, M., Sakai, K., and Jouvet, M., 1984b, Bulbothalamic neurons related to thalamocortical activation processes during paradoxical sleep, *Exp. Brain Res.* **54**:463–475.

Steriade, M., Deschênes, M., Domich, L., and Mulle, C., 1985, Abolition of spindle oscillations in thalamic neurons disconnected from nucleus reticularis thalami, *J. Neurophysiol.* **54**:1473–1497.

Steriade, M., Domich, L., and Oakson, G., 1986, Reticularis thalami neurons revisited: Activity changes during shifts in states of vigilance, *J. Neurosci.* **6**:68–81.

Steriade, M., Domich, L., Oakson, G., and Deschênes, M., 1987a, The deafferented reticular thalamic nucleus generates spindle rhythmicity, *J. Neurophysiol.* **57**:260–273.

Steriade, M., Parent, A., Paré, D., and Smith, Y., 1987b, Cholinergic and noncholinergic neurons of cat basal forebrain project to reticular and mediodorsal thalamic nuclei, *Brain Res.* **408**:372–376.

Steriade, M., Paré, D., Parent, A., and Smith, Y., 1988, Projections of cholinergic and non-cholinergic neurons of the brainstem core to relay and associational thalamic nuclei in the cat and macaque monkey, *Neuroscience* **25**:47–67.

Steriade, M., Datta, S., Paré, D., Deschênes, M., and Oakson, G., 1989a, Different classes of PGO-on neurons in pedunculopontine and laterodorsal tegmental brainstem cholinergic nuclei, *Soc. Neurosci. Abstr.* **15**:452.

Steriade, M., Jones, E. G., and Llinás, R. R., 1989b, *Thalamic Oscillations and Signalling*, Wiley-Interscience, New York.

Steriade, M., Paré, D., Bouhassira, D., Deschênes, M., and Oakson, G., 1989c, Phasic activation of lateral geniculate and perigeniculate thalamic neurons during sleep with ponto-geniculo-occipital waves, *J. Neurosci.* **9**:2215–2229.

Steriade, M., Paré, D., Hu, B., and Deschênes, M., 1989d, The visual thalamocortical system and modulation thereof by the brainstem core, in: *Progress in Sensory Physiology,* Vol. 10 (D. Ottosen, ed.), Springer, Berlin, Heidelberg, New York, pp. 1–121.

Sterman, M. B., and Clemente, C. D., 1962, Forebrain inhibitory mechanisms: Sleep patterns induced by basal forebrain stimulation in the behaving cat, *Exp. Neurol.* **6**:103–117.

Sterman, M. B., and Wyrwicka, W., 1967, EEG correlates of sleep: Evidence for separate forebrain substrates, *Brain Res.* **6**:143–163.

Stevens, D. R., Greene, R. W., and McCarley, R. W., 1989, Excitatory and inhibitory actions of serotonin on medial pontine reticular formation neurons mediated by opposing actions on potassium conductance(s), *Sleep Res.* **18**:23.

Stichel, C. C., and Singer, W., 1985, Organization and morphological characteristics of choline acetyltransferase-containing fibers in the visual thalamus and striate cortex of the cat, *Neurosci. Lett.* **53**:155–160.

Stone, T. W., and Taylor, D. A., 1977, Microiontophoretic studies of the effects of cyclic nucleotides on excitability of neurones in the rat cerebral cortex, *J. Physiol. (Lond.)* **266**:523–543.

Stone, T. W., Taylor, D. A., and Bloom, F. E., 1975, Cyclic AMP and cyclic GMP may mediate opposite neuronal responses in the rat cerebral cortex, *Science* **187**:845–847.

Storm, J. F., 1987, Action potential repolarization and a fast afterhyperpolarization in rat hippocampal pyramidal cells, *J. Physiol. (Lond.)* **385**:733–759.

Strachey, J., 1966, Editor's introduction to project for a scientific psychology, in: *Complete Psychological Works*, Vol. 1, (translated and edited by J. Strachey), Hogarth Press, London, pp. 283–293.

Strassman, A., Highstein, S. M., and McCrea, R. A., 1986, Anatomy and physiology of saccadic burst neurons in the alert squirrel monkey. II. Inhibitory burst neurons, *J. Comp. Neurol.* **249**:358–380.

Streit, P., 1980, Selective retrograde labeling indicating the transmitter of neuronal pathways, *J. Comp. Neurol.* **191**:429–463.

Sugimoto, T., and Hattori, T., 1984, Organizational and efferent projections of nucleus tegmenti pedunculopontinus pars compacta with special reference to its cholinergic aspects, *Neuroscience* **11**:931–946.

Sulloway, F. J., 1979, *Freud, Biologist of the Mind*, Basic Books, New York.

Sutton, R. E., Koob, G. F., Le Moal, M., Rivier, J., and Vale, W., 1982, Corticotropin releasing factor produces behavioral activation in rats, *Nature* **297**:31–33.

Svensson, T. H., and Engberg, G., 1980, Effect of nicotine on single cell activity in the noradrenergic nucleus locus coeruleus, *Acta. Physiol. Scand. [Suppl.]* **479**:31–34.

Swadlow, H. A., and Weyand, T. G., 1987, Corticogeniculate neurons, corticotectal neurons, and suspected interneurons in visual cortex of awake rabbits: Receptive-field properties, axonal properties, and effects of EEG arousal, *J. Neurophysiol.* **57**:977–1001.

Swanson, L. W., 1976, The locus coeruleus: A cytoarchitectonic Golgi and immunohistochemical study in the albino rat, *Brain Res.* **110**:39–56.

Swanson, L. W., 1977, Immunohistochemical evidence for a neurophysin-containing autonomic pathway in the paraventricular nucleus of the hypothalamus, *Brain Res.* **128**:346–353.

Swanson, L. W., and Hartman, B. K., 1975, The central adrenergic system. An immunofluorescence study of the location of cell bodies and their efferent connections in the rat utilizing dopamine-β-hydroxylase as a marker, *J. Comp. Neurol.* **163**:467–506.

Swanson, L. W., Mogenson, G. J., Gerfen, C. R., and Robinson, P., 1984, Evidence for a projection from the lateral preoptic area and substantia innominata to the "mesencephalic locomotor region" in the rat, *Brain Res.* **295**:161–178.

Swanson, L. W., Mogenson, G. J., Simerly, R. B., and Wu, M., 1987, Anatomical and electrophysiological evidence for a projection from the medial preoptic area to the "mesencephalic and subthalamic locomotor regions" in the rat, *Brain Res.* **405**:108–122.

Szerb, J. C., 1967, Cortical acetylcholine release and electroencephalographic arousal, *J. Physiol. (Lond.)* **192**:329–345.

Szymusiak, R., and McGinty, D., 1986, Sleep-related neuronal discharge in the basal forebrain of cats, *Brain Res.* **370**:82–92.

Taber, E., 1961, The cytoarchitecture of the brain stem of the cat. I. Brain stem nuclei of the cat, *J. Comp. Neurol.* **116**:27–70.

Takakusaki, K., Ohta, Y., and Mori, S., 1988a, Single medullary reticulospinal neurons exert postsynaptic inhibitory effects via inhibitory interneurons upon alpha-motoneurons innervating cat hindlimb muscles, *Exp. Brain Res.* **201**:1–13.

Takakusaki, K., Sakamoto, T., and Mori, S., 1988b, Chemical modulation of medullary output neurons which control excitability of hindlimb alpha-motoneurons in cats, *Soc. Neurosci. Abstr.* **14**:180.

Takeuchi, Y., McLean, J. H., and Hopkins, D. A., 1982, Reciprocal connections between the amygdala and parabrachial nuclei: Ultrastructural demonstration by degeneration and axonal transport of horseradish peroxidase in the cat, *Brain Res.* **239**:583–588.

Tanji, J., and Evarts, E. V., 1976, Anticipatory activity of motor cortex neurons in relation to direction of an intended movement, *J. Neurophysiol.* **39**:1062–1068.

Tebecis, A. K., 1972, Cholinergic and non-cholinergic transmission in the medial geniculate nucleus of the cat, *J. Physiol. (Lond.)* **226**:153–172.

Thierry, A. M., Chevalier, G., Ferron, A., and Glowinski, J., 1983, Diencephalic efferents of the medial prefrontal cortex in the rat: Electrophysiological evidence for the existence of branched neurons, *Exp. Brain Res.* **50:**275–282.

Thompson, A. M., 1986, Comparison of responses to transmitter candidates at an N-methylaspartate receptor mediated synapse in slices of rat cerebral cortex, *Neuroscience* **17:**37–47.

Thompson, A. M., 1988a, Inhibitory postsynaptic potentials evoked in thalamic neurones by stimulation of the reticular nucleus evoke slow spikes, *Neuroscience* **25:**491–502.

Thompson, A. M., 1988b, Biphasic responses of thalamic neurones to gamma-aminobutyric acid in isolated rat brain slices, *Neuroscience* **25:**503–512.

Thompson, S. H., 1977, Three pharmacologically distinct potassium channels in molluscan neurones, *J. Physiol. (Lond.)* **265:**465–488.

Tigges, J., and Tigges, M., 1985, Subcortical sources of direct projections to visual cortex, in: *Cerebral Cortex*, Vol. 3 (A. Peters and E. G. Jones, eds.), Plenum Press, New York, pp. 351–378.

Tigges, J., Tigges, M., Cross, N. A., McBride, R. L., Letbetter, W. D., and Anschel, S., 1982, Subcortical structures projecting to visual cortical areas in squirrel monkey, *J. Comp. Neurol.* **209:**29–40.

Tigges, J., Walker, L. C., and Tigges, M., 1983, Subcortical projections to the occipital lobe and parietal lobes of the chimpanzee brain, *J. Comp. Neurol.* **220:**106–115.

Tohyama, M., Sakai, K., Salvert, D., Touret, M., and Jouvet, M., 1979a, Spinal projections from the lower brain stem in the cat as demonstrated by the horseradish peroxidase technique. I. Origins of the reticulospinal tracts and their funicular trajectories, *Brain Res.* **173:**383–403.

Tohyama, M., Sakai, K., Salvert, D., Touret, M., and Jouvet, M., 1979b, Spinal projections from the lower brain stem in the cat as demonstrated by the horseradish peroxidase technique. II. Projections from the dorsolateral pontine tegmentum and raphe nuclei, *Brain Res.* **176:**215–231.

Tork, I., Halliday, G., Scheibner, T., and Turner, S., 1984, The organization of the mesencephalic ventromedial tegmentum (VMT) in the cat, in: *Modulation of Sensorimotor Activity during Alterations in Behavioural States* (R. Bandler, ed.), Alan R. Liss, New York, pp. 39–73.

Tortella, F. C., Eschevaria, E., Pastel, R. H., Cox, B., and Blackburn, T. P., 1988, Differential effects of ICI 169,369 and ritanserin on 24 h EEG sleep patterns in rats, *Br. J. Pharmacol.* **93:**196P.

Trachsel, L., Tobler, I., and Borbely, A., 1988, Effect of ritanserin on sleep and sleep EEG in the rat, *Abstr. Eur. Sleep Res. Soc.* 253.

Trétiakoff, C., and Bremer, F., 1920, Encephalite letargique avec syndrome Parkinsonien et catatonie. Rechute tardive, *Rev. Neurol. (Paris)* **7:**772–775.

Trulson, M. F., and Jacobs, B. L., 1979, Raphe unit activity in freely moving cats: Correlation with level of behavioral arousal, *Brain Res.* **163:**135–150.

Trulson, M. E., Howell, G. A., Brandstetter, J. W., Fredrickson, M. H., and Fredrickson, C. J., 1982, *In vitro* recording of raphe unit activity: Evidence for endogenous rhythms in presumed serotonergic neurons, *Life Sci.* **31:**785–790.

Trussell, L. O., and Jackson, M. B., 1985, Adenosine-activated potassium conductance in cultured striatal neurons, *Proc. Natl. Acad. Sci. U.S.A.* **82:**4857–4861.

Trussell, L. O., and Jackson, M. B., 1987, Dependence of an adenosine-activated potassium current on a GTP-binding protein in mammalian central neurons, *J. Neurosci.* **7:**3306–3316.

Tsumoto, T., Masui, H., and Sato, H., 1986, Excitatory amino acid transmitters in neuronal circuits of the cat visual cortex, *J. Neurophysiol.* **55:**469–483.

Ursin, R., and Sterman, M. B., 1981, *A Manual for Standardized Scoring of Sleep and Waking States in the Adult Gat*, Brain Information Service/BRI UCLA, Los Angeles.

Valverde, F., 1961, Reticular formation of the pons and medulla oblongata. A Golgi study, *J. Comp. Neurol.* **116:**71–99.

Valverde, F., 1962, Reticular formation of the albino rat's brain stem: Cytoarchitecture and corticofugal connections, *J. Comp. Neurol.* **119:**25–53.

van den Hoofdakker, R. H., and Beersma, D. G. M., 1985, On the explanation of short REM latencies in depression, *Psychiatr. Res.* **16:**155–163.

Van der Kooy, D., Kuypers, H. G. J. M., and Catsman-Berrevoets, C. E., 1978, Single mammillary cell bodies with divergent axon collaterals. Demonstration by a simple, fluorescent retrograde double labeling technique in the rat, *Brain Res.* **158:**189–196.

van der Loos, H., and Glaser, E. M., 1972, Autapses in neocortex cerebri: Synapses between pyramidal cell's axon and its own dendrites, *Brain Res.* **48:**355–360.

VanderMaelen, C. P., and Aghajanian, G. K., 1980, Intracellular studies showing modulation of facial motoneurone excitability by serotonin, *Nature* **287:**346–347.

VanderMaelen, C. P., and Aghajanian, G. K., 1983, Electrophysiological and pharmacological characterization of serotonergic dorsal raphe neurons recorded extracellularly and intracellularly in rat brain slices, *Brain Res.* **289:**109–119.

Vanderwolf, C. H., and Robinson, T. E., 1981, Reticulo-cortical activity and behavior: A critique of the arousal theory and a new synthesis (with commentaries), *Behav. Brain Res.* **4:**459–514.

van Dongen, P. A. M., 1980, Locus ceruleus region: Effects on behavior of cholinergic, noradrenergic and opiate drugs injected intracerebrally into freely moving cats, *Exp. Neurol.* **67:**52–78.

van Gisbergen, J. A. M., Robinson, D. A., and Gielen, S., 1981, A quantitative analysis of generation of saccadic eye movements by burst neurons, *J. Neurophysiol.* **45:**417–442.

Vanni-Mercier, G., Sakai, K., and Jouvet, M., 1984, Neurones specifiques de l'eveil dans l'hypothalamus posterieur du chat, *C.R. Acad. Sci. (Paris)* **298:**195–200.

Velasco, M., Velasco, F., Cepeda, C., and Romo, R., 1979, Effect of a push–pull perfusion of carbachol on the pontine reticular formation multiple unit activity, in: *Pharmacology of the States of Alertness* (P. Passouant and I. Oswald, eds.), Pergamon Press, New York, pp. 231–233.

Velayos, J. L., Jimenez-Castellanos, J., and Reinoso-Suarez, F., 1989, Topographical organization of the projections from the reticular thalamic nucleus to the intralaminar and medial thalamic nuclei in the cat, *J. Comp. Neurol.* **279:**457–469.

Verrier, R., 1988, Behavioral state and myocardial excitability, in: *Clinical Physiology of Sleep* (R. Lydic and J. F. Biebuyck, eds.), American Physiological Society, Bethesda, pp. 31–51.

Vertes, R. P., 1977, Selective firing of rat pontine gigantocellular neurons during movement and REM sleep, *Brain Res.* **128:**146–152.

Vertes, R. P., 1982, Brain stem generation of the hippocampal EEG, *Prog. Neurobiol.* **19:**159–186.

Vertes, R. P., 1984, Brainstem control of the events of REM sleep, *Progr. Neurobiol.* **22:**241–288.

Vertes, R. P., and Martin, G. F., 1988, Autoradiographic analysis of ascending projections from the pontine and mesencephalic reticular formation and the median raphe nucleus in the rat, *J. Comp. Neurol.* **275:**511–541.

Vertes, R. P., Martin, G. F., and Waltzer, R., 1986, An autoradiographic analysis of ascending projections from the medullary reticular formation in the rat, *Neuroscience* **19:**873–898.

Vijayan, V. K., 1979, Distribution of cholinergic neurotransmitter enzymes in the hippocampus and the dentate gyrus of the adult and developing mouse, *Neuroscience* **4:**121–137.

Villablanca, J., 1965, The electrocorticogram in the chronic *cerveau isolé* cat, *Electroencephalogr. Clin. Neurophysiol.* **19:**576–586.

Villablanca, J., 1974, Role of the thalamus in sleep control: Sleep–wakefulness studies in chronic diencephalic and athalamic cats, in: *Basic Sleep Mechanisms* (O. Petre-Quadens and J. D. Schlag, eds.), Academic Press, New York, pp. 51–78.

Villis, T., Hepp, K., Schwarz, U., Henn, V., and Haas, H., 1986, Unilateral riMLF lesions impair saccade generation along specific vertical planes, *Soc. Neurosci. Abstr.* **12:**1187.

Vincent, S. R., and Reiner, P. B., 1987, The immunohistochemical localization of choline acetyltransferase in the cat brain, *Brain Res. Bull.* **18:**371–415.

Vincent, S. R., Satoh, K., Armstrong, D. M., and Fibiger, H. C., 1983, Substance P in the ascending cholinergic reticular system, *Nature (Lond.)* **306:**688–691.

Vincent, S. R., Satoh, K., Armstrong, D. M., Panula, P., Vale, W., and Fibiger, H. C., 1986, Neuropeptides and NADPH–diaphorase activity in the ascending cholinergic reticular system of the rat, *Neuroscience* **17:**167–182.

Vivaldi, E., McCarley, R. W., and Hobson, J. A., 1980, Evocation of desynchronized sleep signs by chemical microstimulation of the pontine brain stem, in: *The Reticular Formation Revisited* (J. A. Hobson and M. A. B. Brazier, eds.), Raven Press, New York, pp. 513–529.

Vogel, G., 1960, Studies in the psychophysiology of dreams. III. The dream of narcolepsy, *Arch. Gen. Psychiatry* **3:**421–425.

Vogel, G., 1989, Sleep variables and the treatment of depression, in: *Principles and Practices of Sleep Medicine* (M. H. Kryger, T. Roth, and W. C. Dement, eds.), Saunders, New York, pp. 419–420.

Vogel, G. W., Vogel, F., McAbee, R. S., and Thurmond, A. J., 1980, Improvement of depression by REM sleep deprivation. New findings and a theory, *Arch. Gen. Psychiatry* **37:**247–253.

Volterra, V., 1931, *Lecons sur la Théorie Mathémaatique de la Lutte pour la Vie,* Gauthier-Villars et Cie., Paris.

Voorn, P., Jorritsma-Byham, B., Van Dijk, C., and Buijs, R. M., 1986, The dopaminergic innervations of the ventral striatum in the rat: A light and electron microscopical study with antibodies against dopamine, *J. Comp. Neurol.* **251:**84–99.

Wada, J. A., and Terao, A., 1970, Effect of parachlorophenylalanine on basal forebrain stimulation, *Exp. Neurol.* **28**:501–506.

Walker, L. C., Kitt, C. A., DeLong, M. R., and Price, D. L., 1985, Noncollateral projections of basal forebrain neurons to frontal and parietal neocortex in primates, *Brain Res. Bull.* **15**:307–314.

Walter, W. G., Cooper, R., Aldridge, V. J., McCallum, W. C., and Winter, A. L., 1964, Contingent negative variation: An electric sign of sensorimotor association and expectancy in the human brain, *Nature* **203**:380–384.

Walton, K., and Fulton, B. P., 1986, Ionic mechanisms underlying the firing properties of rat neonatal motoneurons studied *in vitro, Neuroscience* **19**:669–683.

Walton, K., and Llinás, R., 1986, Calcium-dependent low threshold rebound potentials and oscillatory potentials in neonatal rat spinal motoneurons *in vitro, Soc. Neurosci. Abstr.* **12**:382.

Waltzer, R., and Martin, G. F., 1984, Collateralization of reticulospinal axons from the nucleus reticularis gigantocellularis to the cerebellum and diencephalon. A double-labeling study in the rat, *Brain Res.* **293**:153–158.

Wang, R. Y., and Aghajanian, G. K., 1977, Physiological evidence for habenula as major link between forebrain and midbrain raphe, *Science* **197**:89–91.

Watkins, J. C., and Evans, R. H., 1981, Excitatory amino acid transmitters, *Annu. Rev. Pharmacol. Toxicol.* **21**:165–204.

Watkins, J. C., and Olverman, H. J., 1987, Agonist and antagonists for excitatory amino acid receptors, *Trends Neurosci.* **10**:265–272.

Watson, R. T., Heilman, B. D., Miller, B. D., and King, F. A., 1974, Neglect after mesencephalic reticular formation lesions, *Neurology (Minneap.)* **24**:294–298.

Webster, H. H., and Jones, B. E., 1988, Neurotoxic lesions of the dorsolateral pontomesencephalic tegmentum cholinergic area in the cat. II. Effects upon sleep–waking states, *Brain Res.* **458**:285–302.

Wehr, T. A., Wirz-Justice, A., Goodwin, F. K., Duncan, W., and Gillin, J. C., 1979, Phase advance of the circadian sleep–wake cycle as an antidepressant, *Science* **206**:710–713.

Weitzmann, E., 1961, A note on the EEG and eye movements during behavioral sleep in monkeys, *Electroencephalogr. Clin. Neurophysiol.* **13**:790–794.

Westbrook, G. L., and Mayer, M. L., 1987, Micromolar concentrations of zinc antagonize NMDA and GABA responses of hippocampal neurons, *Nature* **328**:640–643.

Westman, J., and Bowsher, D., 1971, Ultrastructural observations on the degeneration of spinal afferents to the nucleus medullae oblongatae centralis (pars caudalis) of the cat, *Brain Res.* **26**:395–398.

Wikler, A., 1952, Pharmacologic dissociation on behavior and EEG sleep patterns in dogs: Morphine, N-allylnomorphine and atropine, *Proc. Soc. Exp. Biol.* **79**:261–265.

Wiklund, L., and Cuénod, M., 1984, Differential labeling of afferents to thalamic centromedian-parafascicular nuclei with ^{3}H-choline and D-^{3}H-aspartate: Further evidence for transmitter specific retrograde labelling, *Neurosci. Lett.* **46**:275–281.

Wiklund, L., Léger, L., and Persson, M., 1981, Monoamine cell distribution in the cat brain stem. A fluorescence histochemical study with quantification of indolaminergic and locus coeruleus cell group, *J. Comp. Neurol.* **203**:613–647.

Wilcox, K. S., Gutnick, M. J., and Cristoph, G. R., 1986, Voltage dependence of patterned output of lateral habenula neurons, *Soc. Neurosci. Abstr.* **12**:853.

Wilcox, K. S., Grant, S. J., and Christoph, G. R., 1987, Electrophysiological properties of lateral dorsal tegmental neurons *in vitro, Soc. Neurosci. Abstr.* **13**:57.

Wilder, M. B., Farley, G. R., and Starr, A., 1981, Endogenous late positive component of the evoked potential in cats corresponding to P300 in humans, *Science* **211**:605–607.

Williams, J. T., 1988, Amino acid synaptic neurotransmission in locus coeruleus: Effects of field stimulation *in vitro, Soc. Neurosci. Abstr.* **14**:151.

Williams, J. T., and Marshall, K. C., 1987, Membrane properties and adrenergic responses in locus coeruleus neurons of young rats, *J. Neurosci.* **7**:3687–3694.

Williams, J. T., and North, R. A., 1985, Catecholamine inhibition of calcium action potentials in rat locus coeruleus neurones, *Neuroscience* **14**:103–109.

Williams, J. T., and North, R. A., 1987, Membrane properties and adrenergic responses in locus coeruleus neurons of young rats, *J. Neurosci.* **7**:3687–3694.

Williams, J. T., North, R. A., Shefner, S. A., Nishi, S., and Egan, T. M., 1984, Membrane properties of rat locus coeruleus neurones, *Neuroscience* **13**:137–156.

Williams, J. T., Henderson, G., and North, R. A., 1985, Characterization of alpha$_2$-adrenoceptors which increase potassium conductance in rat locus coeruleus neurones, *Neuroscience* **14**:95–101.

Williams, J. T., North, R. A., and Tokimasa, T., 1988a, Inward rectification of resting and opiate-activated potassium currents in rat locus coeruleus neurons, *J. Neurosci.* **8**:4299–4306.

Williams, J. T., Colmers, W. F., and Pan, Z. Z., 1988b, Voltage- and ligand-activated inwardly rectifying currents in dorsal raphe neurons *in vitro, J. Neurosci.* **8**:3499–3506.

Willis, W. D., Kenshalo, D. R., and Leonard, R. B., 1979, The cells of origin of the primate spinothalamic tract, *J. Comp. Neurol.* **188**:543–574.

Wilson, P. M., 1985, A photographic perspective on the origin, form, course and relations of the acetylcholinesterase-containing fibers of the dorsal tegmental pathways in the rat brain, *Brain Res. Rev.* **10**:85–118.

Wise, S. P., Weinrich, M., and Mauritz, K. H., 1983, Motor aspects of cue-related neuronal activity in premotor cortex of the rhesus monkey, *Brain Res.* **260**:301–305.

Wohlberg, C. J., Davidoff, R. A., and Hackman, J. C., 1986, Analysis of the responses of frog motoneurons to epinephrine and norepinephrine, *Neurosci. Lett.* **69**:150–155.

Wolfe, B. B., Harden, T. K., Sporn, J. R., and Molinoff, P. B., 1978, Presynaptic modulation of beta adrenergic receptors in rat cerebral cortex after treatment with antidepressants, *J. Pharmacol. Exp. Ther.* **207**:446–457.

Woody, C. D., Swartz, B. E., and Gruen, E., 1978, Effects of acetylcholine and cyclic GMP on input resistance of cortical neurons in awake cats, *Brain Res.* **158**:373–395.

Woody, C. D., Bartfai, T., Gruen, E., and Nairn, A. C., 1986, Intracellular injection of cGMP-dependent protein kinase results in increased input resistance in neurons of the mammalian motor cortex, *Brain Res.* **386**:379–385.

Woolf, N. J., and Butcher, L. L., 1986, Cholinergic systems in the rat brain. III. Projections from the pontomesencephalic tegmentum to the thalamus, tectum, basal ganglia and basal forebrain, *Brain Res. Bull.* **16**:603–637.

Woolf, N. J., Hernit, M. C., and Butcher, L. L., 1986, Cholinergic and non-cholinergic projections from the rat basal forebrain revealed by combined choline acetyltransferase and *Phaseolus vulgaris* leucoagglutinin immunohistochemistry, *Neurosci. Lett.* **66**:281–286.

Wouterlood, F. G., and Groenewegen, H. J., 1984, Neuroanatomical tracing by use of *Phaseolus vulgaris*-leucoagglutinin (PHA-L): Electron microscopy of PHA-L-filled neuronal somata, dendrites, axons and axon terminals, *Brain Res.* **326**:188–191.

Wright, J. J., and Craggs, M. D., 1978, Changed cortical activation and lateral hypothalamic syndrome: A study in the split-brain cat, *Brain Res.* **151**:632–636.

Wurtz, R. H., and Mohler, C. W., 1976, Enhancement of visual response in monkey striate cortex and frontal eye fields, *J. Neurophysiol.* **39**:766–772.

Wurtz, R. H., Goldberg, M. E., and Robinson, D. L., 1980, Behavioral modulation of visual responses in the monkey: Stimulus selection for attention and movement, in: *Progress in Psychobiology and Physiological Psychology*, Vol. 9, (J. M. Sprague and A. N. Epstein, eds.), Academic Press, New York, pp. 43–83.

Wurtz, R. H., Richmond, B. J., and Newsome, W. T., 1984, Modulation of cortical visual processing by attention, perception and movements, in: *Dynamic Aspects of Neocortical Function* (G. M. Edelman, W. E. Gall, and W. M. Cowan, eds.), Wiley-Interscience, New York, pp. 195–217.

Wyzinski, P. W., McCarley, R. W., and Hobson, J. A., 1978, Discharge properties of pontine reticulospinal neurons during the sleep–waking cycle, *J. Neurophysiol.* **41**:821–834.

Yaari, Y., Hamon, B., and Lux, H. D., 1987, Development of two types of calcium channels in cultured mammalian hippocampal neurons, *Science* **235**:680–682.

Yakel, J. L., Trussell, L. O., and Jackson, M. B., 1988, Three serotonin responses in cultured mouse hippocampal and striatal neurons, *J. Neurosci.* **8**:1273–1285.

Yamamoto, C., 1974, Electrical activity recorded from thin sections of the lateral geniculate body, and the effects of 5-hydroxytryptamine, *Exp. Brain Res.* **19**:271–281.

Yamamoto, K., Mamelak, A., Quattrochi, J., and Hobson, J. A., 1988, Localization of a D sleep induction site with short latency by microinjection of carbachol in a head-restrained cat, *Soc. Neurosci. Abstr.* **14**:1307.

Yamamoto, T., Samejima, A., and Oka, H., 1985, An intracellular analysis of the entopeduncular inputs on the centre median–parafascicular complex in cats, *Brain Res.* **348**:343–347.

Yamashita, H., Inenaga, K., and Kannan, H., 1987, Depolarizing effect of noradrenaline on neurons of the rat supraoptic nucleus *in vitro, Brain Res.* **405**:348–352.

Yamaoka, S., 1978, Participation of limbic–hypothalamic structures in circadian rhythm of slow wave sleep and paradoxical sleep in the rat, *Brain Res.* **151**:255–268.

Yarom, Y., Sugimori, M., and Llinás, R., 1985, Ionic currents and firing patterns of mammalian vagal motoneurons *in vitro, Neuroscience* **16**:719–737.

Yen, C. T., and Jones, E. G., 1983, Intracellular staining of physiologically identified neurons and axons in the somatosensory thalamus of the cat, *Brain Res.* **280:**148–154.

Yingling, C. D., and Skinner, J. E., 1975, Regulation of unit activity in nucleus reticularis thalami by the mesencephalic reticular formation and the frontal cortex, *Electroencephalogr. Clin. Neurophysiol.* **39:**635–642.

Yingling, C. D., and Skinner, J. E., 1977, Gating of thalamic input to cerebral cortex by nucleus reticularis thalami, in: *Attention, Voluntary Contraction and Event-Related Potentials* (J. E. Desmedt, ed.), S. Karger, Basel, pp. 70–96.

Yoshida, K., McCrea, R., Berthoz, A., and Vidal, P. P., 1981, Properties of immediate premotor inhibitory burst neurons controlling horizontal rapid eye movements in the cat, in: *Progress in Oculomotor Research* (A. F. Fuchs and W. Becker, eds.), Elsevier/North-Holland, New York, pp. 71–80.

Yoshimura, M., and Higashi, H., 1985, 5-Hydroxytryptamine mediates inhibitory postsynaptic potentials in rat dorsal raphe neurons, *Neurosci. Lett.* **53:**69–74.

Yoshimura, M., Polosa, C., and Nishi, S., 1987, Slow IPSP and the noradrenaline-induced inhibition of the cat sympathetic preganglionic neuron *in vitro, Brain Res.* **419:**383–386.

Yoss, R. E., and Daly, D. D., 1957, Criteria for the diagnosis of the narcoleptic syndrome, *Proc. Staff Meet. Mayo Clin.* **32:**320–328.

Young, W. S. III, and Kuhar, M. J., 1980, Noradrenergic alpha 1 and alpha 2 receptors: Light microscopic autoradiographic localization, *Proc. Natl. Acad. Sci. U.S.A.* **77:**1696–1700.

Zaborsky, L., Heimer, L., Eckenstein, F., and Leranth, C., 1986, GABAergic input to cholinergic forebrain neurons: An ultrastructural study using retrograde tracing of HRP and double immunolabeling, *J. Comp. Neurol.* **250:**282–295.

Zarcone, V., 1989, Sleep abnormalities in schizophrenia, in: *Principles and Practices of Sleep Medicine* (M. H. Kryger, T. Roth, and W. C. Dement, eds.), Saunders, New York, pp. 422–423.

Zarcone, V. P., Benson, K. L., and Berger, P. A., 1987, Abnormal rapid eye movement latencies in schizophrenia, *Arch. Gen. Psychiatry* **44:**45–48.

Zemlan, F. B., Behbehani, M. M., and Beckstead, R. M., 1984, Ascending and descending projections from nucleus reticularis magnocellularis and nucleus reticularis gigantocellularis: An autoradiographic and horseradish peroxidase study in the rat, *Brain Res.* **292:**207–220.

Ziegelsgänsberger, W., and Reiter, C. H., 1974, A cholinergic mechanism in the spinal cord of cats, *Neuropharmacology* **13:**519–527.

Zulley, J., 1979, *Der Einfluss von Zeitgebern auf den Schlaf des Menschen,* Rita G. Fischer Verlag, Frankfurt.

Zulley, J., 1980, Distribution of REM sleep in entrained 24 hour and free-running sleep-wake cycles, *Sleep* **2:**377–389.

Zulley, J., Wever, R., and Aschoff, J., 1981, The dependence of onset and duration of sleep on the circadian rhythm of rectal temperature, *Pflugers Arch.* **391:**314–318.

Index

INDEX

Burst neurons
    anatomic connectivity of, 289–292
    physiolology of, 286–289
b(X), in limit-cycle model, 390

Calcium action potentials
    blockade in LC neurons, 146–148
    of mPRF neurons, 130, 131–132
    TTX effect on, 132, 135
Calcium conductance. *see* Calcium spike
Calcium ion (Ca), potassium conductances dependent on, 160–161
Calcium spike
    high-threshold, 134, 136–137
        thalamic neurons and, 157, 159–160
    LC neurons and, 145
    low-threshold, 131–132
        modulation of, 132–134, 136
        thalamic neurons and, 153–158
Canonical reticular formation neuron, camera lucida drawing of, 109
cAMP. *see* Cyclic adenosine 3′,5′-monophosphate (cAMP)
Carbachol
    PRF neuronal response to, 164–169
    REM-sleep muscle atonia and, 324
3-[(+)-2-Carboxypiperazin-4-γ-1]-propyl-1-phosphonic acid (CPP), 199, 200
Cardiovascular system, state-related changes in, 344–345
Cataplexy, 396–397
Cell burst. *see* Burst
Cell groups
    homogeneity in mammalian brain, 22–23
    immunohistochemical identification of, 35–38
Center(s)
    behavioral state, 21–23
    cerebral structures as, 22–23
    defined, 21–23
Central nervous system (CNS)
    and norepinephrine receptors, 185
    simple reflex model, 419–421
    and state definitions, 12–14
Central tegmental field (FTC)
    and FTP distinction, 74
    reticular cholinergic nuclei in, 69
    and RRF distinction, 74
    unidentified transmitters in, 73–75
Centrolateral–paracentral (CL–PC) nuclei, 81, 83–89
    rostral intralaminar, 221–222
Centromedian parafascicular nuclei, 81, 83–89
Cerebellum, afferents and, 44
Cerebral cortex; *see also* Hippocampus; Neocortex
    ACh action on, 180–184

Cerebral cortex (*cont.*)
    and brainstem–thalamic projections link, 91, 93, 94–95
    neuronal recordings in monkeys, 253–256
    projections, cholinergic nuclei and, 75–77
    stimulation, thalamocortical cell response to, 160
Cerebral tone, passive sleep theory and, 15–18
Cerveau isolé preparation, 1–7, 5–7, 16–18
Cesium, hyperpolarizing potassium currents and, 137
cGMP. *see* Cyclic guanosine 3′,5′-monophosphate (cGMP)
Channels, and calcium action potentials, 131–132
Characterological depression, REM-sleep latency, 415
ChAT. *see* Choline acetyltransferase (ChAT)
p-Chlorophenylalanine (PCPA), active sleep theory and, 19–21
Cholecystokinin, immunoreactivity for, 38
Choline acetyltransferase (ChAT)
    immunohistochemistry
        for cell group identification, 35–38, 38
        and TMB procedure combined, 37
    neuronal staining
        in basal forebrain nuclei, 68, 69–73
        in brainstem reticular nuclei, 68
Cholinergic mesopontine reticular formation, brainstem and spinal cord projections of, 95–108
Cholinergic/noncholinergic projections, 95–108
Cholinergic nuclei
    of basal forebrain, 68–69
    nomenclature for, 68
    of reticular formation, 69–73
    rostral projections, 75–95
Cholinergic projections
    to bulb and spinal cord, 100–103
    to pontine FTG, 95–100
Circadian rhythm
    in depression, 412–413
    and REM sleep modulation, 374
CL-PC. *see* Centrolateral-paracentral (CL-PC) nuclei
Clinical syndromes, constituent mechanisms in, 396
CM-PF. *see under* Intralaminar nuclei
CNA. *see under* Amygdala
CNS. *see* Central nervous system (CNS)
CNV. *see* Contingent negative variation (CNV)
Cobalt, calcium current blockade in LC neurons, 146–148
Cognition, components in SEPs, 252–253
Collaterals. *see* Axon collaterals
Conductance
    agonist-induced (G_{ag}), 187, 189, 191